STUDENT WORKBOOK

Pearson's Comprehensive Medical Assisting

THIRD EDITION

NINA BEAMAN
KRISTIANA D. ROUTH
LORRAINE M. PAPAZIAN-BOYCE
JANET R. SESSER
HELEN MILLS
RON MALY

PEARSON

Boston Columbus Indianapolis New York San Francisco Upper Saddle River
Amsterdam Cape Town Dubai London Madrid Milan Munich Paris Montréal Toronto
Delhi Mexico City São Paulo Sydney Hong Kong Seoul Singapore Taipei Tokyo

10 9 8 7 6 5 4 3

PEARSON

ISBN 10:   0-13-356398-7
ISBN 13: 978-0-13-356398-6

Contents

INTRODUCTION

This student workbook is designed as a study guide and practice tool to accompany the student text, *Pearson's Comprehensive Medical Assisting, Third Edition*. Use the study guide to reinforce what you have learned. Test your knowledge of medical terminology by completing the variety of activities in the Key Terminology Review section. Measure whether you have achieved the learning objectives in each chapter by completing the exercises in the Applied Practice and Learning Activities sections of the workbook. Apply your knowledge to real-life situations by answering the Critical Thinking Questions. Use outside and Internet resources to complete the research activity at the end of each chapter.

Each chapter of this student workbook includes the following:

Student Study Guide: This is material presented in the chapter. Fill in the blanks, or answer the questions by following PowerPoint presentations in class, or reading through your text.

Applied Practice: Use the knowledge you learned in the chapter to complete these activities.

Learning Activities: These questions/tasks allow you to measure whether or not you have achieved the learning objectives for the chapter.

Key Terminology Review: This section tests your knowledge of the medical terminology presented in the chapter.

Critical Thinking Questions: These challenging questions allow you to apply your knowledge to real-life situations.

Research Activity: Use outside sources to complete these activities and go beyond the classroom.

Procedure Skill Sheets: These boxed procedures, found in the back of the workbook, correspond to those in the student textbook and allow students to demonstrate the skills needed to become a medical assistant. A space is included for your instructor to document that you have successfully completed the skill. Each step is weighted to better indicate proficiency in the skill.

Note: Answer key located in Instructor's Manual.

Mastery of Competency Skills

Procedure Number	Procedure Title	Date Mastered	Instructor's Signature
5-1	Effective Listening Skills		
5-2	Assisting the Hearing-Impaired Patient		
6-1	Handling a Fire in the Medical Office		
6-2	Proper Use of an Eyewash Device		
6-3	Housekeeping Using OSHA Guidelines		
7-1	Answering the Telephone and Placing Calls on Hold		
7-2	Taking a Telephone Message		
7-3	Taking a Prescription Refill Message		
7-4	Placing a Conference Call		
8-1	Opening the Office		
8-2	Registering a New Patient		
8-3	Collecting Copayments		
8-4	Closing the Office		
9-1	Scheduling Established Patients		
9-2	Scheduling a New Patient Appointment		
9-3	Arranging a Referral Appointment		
9-4	Scheduling Inpatient Surgical Procedures		
9-5	Scheduling Outpatient Surgical Procedures		
10-1	Maintaining Equipment		
10-2	Performing an Office Inventory and Ordering Office Supplies		
11-1	Composing a Business Letter		
11-2	Proofreading Written Documents		
11-3	Opening and Sorting the Daily Mail		
12-1	Installing Computer Hardware		
12-2	Installing Computer Software		
12-3	Using the Internet to Access Health Information		

Procedure Number	Procedure Title	Date Mastered	Instructor's Signature
13-1	Adding or Changing Items on a Patient's Record		
13-2	Organizing a Patient's Medical Record		
13-3	Collating Records		
13-4	Filing a Record Alphabetically		
13-5	Filing a Record Numerically Using the Terminal-Digit Filing System		
13-6	Locating Missing Files		
14-1	Correcting an Entry in the Electronic Medical Record		
14-2	Recording Vital Signs		
14-3	Sending Automated Orders		
15-1	Calculating Patient Financial Responsibility		
15-2	Verifying Eligibility		
15-3	Obtaining Insurance Company Authorizations		
15-4	Obtaining Managed Care Referrals		
15-5	Completing a CMS-1500 Claim Form		
15-6	Electronic Insurance Claims		
16-1	Performing ICD-10-CM Diagnostic Coding		
17-1	Coding for a Procedure		
18-1	Using a Computerized Billing System		
18-2	Correcting Account Posting Errors		
18-3	Posting NSF Checks		
18-4	Posting Insurance Payments		
18-5	Responding to a Denied Insurance Claim		
18-6	Preparing Patient Statements		
18-7	Processing Credit Balances and Refunds		
18-8	Making Collection Calls		
18-9	Writing a Collection Letter		

Procedure Number	Procedure Title	Date Mastered	Instructor's Signature
18-10	Posting a Payment from a Collection Agency		
19-1	Preparing a Deposit Slip		
19-2	Preparing Manual Checks		
19-3	Paying Bills with Accounts Payable Software		
19-4	Reconciling a Bank Statement		
19-5	Working with an Outside Payroll Service		
20-1	Staff Meeting Procedures		
20-2	Developing a Patient Information Booklet		
34-1	Disposal of Infectious Wastes and Substances		
34-2	Performing Hand Washing		
34-3	Applying and Removing Nonsterile Gloves		
34-4	Performing Transmission-Based Precaution: Isolation Techniques		
34-5	Sanitizing Instruments		
34-6	Wrapping and Labeling Instruments for Autoclaving		
34-7	Sterilizing Instruments in an Autoclave		
34-8	Chemically Sterilizing Instruments		
35-1	Measuring Adult Weight and Height		
35-2	Measuring Oral Temperature Using an Electronic Thermometer		
35-3	Measuring Rectal Temperature Using an Electronic Thermometer		
35-4	Measuring Axillary Temperature		
35-5	Measuring Temperature Using a Tympanic Membrane (Aural) Thermometer		
35-6	Measuring Temperature Using a Heat-Sensitive Wearable Thermometer		
35-7	Measuring Temperature Using a Temporal Artery Thermometer		
35-8	Measuring Radial Pulse		

Procedure Number	Procedure Title	Date Mastered	Instructor's Signature
35-9	Measuring Apical–Radial Pulse (Two Persons)		
35-10	Measuring Respirations		
35-11	Measuring Blood Pressure		
35-12	Measuring Systolic Blood Pressure Using the Palpatory Method		
36-1	Cleaning the Examination Room		
36-2	Documenting a Chief Complaint During a Patient Interview		
36-3	Interviewing a New Patient to Obtain Medical History Information and Preparing for a Physical Examination		
36-4	Positioning the Patient in the Supine Position		
36-5	Positioning the Patient in the Dorsal Recumbent Position		
36-6	Positioning the Patient in the Lithotomy Position		
36-7	Positioning the Patient in the Fowler's Position		
36-8	Positioning the Patient in the Prone Position		
36-9	Positioning the Patient in the Sims' Position		
36-10	Positioning the Patient in the Knee-Chest Position		
36-11	Assisting with a Complete Physical Examination		
37-1	Performing a Scratch Test		
37-2	Taking a Wound Culture		
37-3	Assisting with a Sigmoidoscopy		
37-4	Administering a Disposable Enema		
37-5	Instructing the Patient in Collecting a Stool Specimen		
37-6	Testing for Occult Blood		
37-7	Performing a Pupil Check on a Patient		

Procedure Number	Procedure Title	Date Mastered	Instructor's Signature
37-8	Assisting with a Neurologic Examination		
38-1	Instructing a Patient on Breast Self-Examination		
38-2	Assisting with a Pelvic Examination and Pap Test		
38-3	Instructing a Male Patient How to Perform a Testicular Self-Examination		
39-1	Testing Visual Acuity Using a Snellen Eye Chart		
39-2	Screening for Near Vision Acuity		
39-3	Screening for Color Vision Acuity		
39-4	Irrigation of the Eye		
39-5	Instilling Eye Medication		
39-6	Irrigation of the Ear		
39-7	Instilling Ear Medication		
39-8	Assisting with Audiometry		
39-9	Instilling Nasal Medications		
40-1	Wrapping an Infant or Small Child		
40-2	Measuring Pediatric Vital Signs		
40-3	Measuring the Weight and Length of an Infant		
40-4	Measuring the Head Circumference of an Infant or Small Child		
40-5	Measuring the Chest Circumference of a Child		
40-6	Calculating Growth Percentiles		
40-7	Applying a Pediatric Urine Collection Device		
41-1	Communicating Effectively with the Elderly		
42-1	Surgical Hand Hygiene/Surgical Scrub		
42-2	Surgical Gloving		
42-3	Opening a Sterile Packet		
42-4	Dropping a Sterile Item onto a Sterile Field		

Procedure Number	Procedure Title	Date Mastered	Instructor's Signature
42-5	Transferring Sterile Objects Using Transfer Forceps		
42-6	Transferring Sterile Solutions onto a Sterile Field		
42-7	Assisting with Minor Surgery		
42-8	Preparing the Patient's Skin for Surgical Procedures		
42-9	Assisting with Suturing		
42-10	Removing Sutures		
42-11	Changing a Sterile Dressing		
42-12	Applying a Bandage Over a Sterile Dressing		
43-1	Perform Adult Rescue Breathing and One-Rescuer or Two-Rescuer CPR		
43-2	Perform Infant Rescue Breathing		
43-3	Use an Automated External Defibrillator		
43-4	Respond to an Adult with an Obstructed Airway		
43-5	Administering Oxygen		
43-6	Demonstrate the Application of a Pressure Bandage		
43-7	Demonstrate the Application of Triangular, Figure-Eight, and Tubular Bandages		
43-8	Respond to a Patient Who Has Fainted		
43-9	Document an Incident		
43-10	Demonstrate the Application of a Splint		
43-11	Create a Medical Emergency Plan		
43-12	Develop an Environmental Exposure Safety Plan		
44-1	Completing a Laboratory Requisition and Preparing a Specimen for Transport to an Outside Laboratory		
44-2	Monitoring and Following Up on Laboratory Test Results		

Procedure Number	Procedure Title	Date Mastered	Instructor's Signature
44-3	Evaluating a Contour TS Glucometer Using Control Solutions		
44-4	Using and Cleaning the Microscope		
45-1	Obtaining a Throat Culture		
45-2	Obtaining a Sputum Specimen for Culture		
45-3	Obtaining a Stool Specimen for Ova and Parasites		
45-4	Obtaining a Stool Specimen for Examination for Pinworms		
45-5	Preparing a Smear		
45-6	Prepare a Wet Mount Slide		
45-7	Perform a Gram Stain		
45-8	Perform Rapid Group A Strep Testing		
46-1	Collecting a 24-hour Urine Specimen		
46-2	Collecting a Clean-Catch Midstream Urine Specimen		
46-3	Assisting with Straight Catheter Insertion and Collecting a Sterile Urine Specimen		
46-4	Evaluating the Physical Characteristics of Urine		
46-5	Measuring the Specific Gravity of Urine with a Refractometer		
46-6	Testing the Chemical Characteristics of Urine with Reagent Strips		
46-7	Testing for Glucose in Urine Using the Tablet Method		
46-8	Preparing a Urine Specimen for Microscopic Examination (for Classroom Evaluation Only)		
46-9	Performing a Urine Pregnancy Test Using the Enzyme Immunoassay Method		
46-10	Performing a Chain of Custody Urine Collection for Drug Analysis		
47-1	Perform a Capillary Puncture (Manual)		

Procedure Number	Procedure Title	Date Mastered	Instructor's Signature
47-2	Obtaining Venous Blood with a Sterile Syringe and Needle		
47-3	Performing Venipuncture using the Vacutainer Method		
48-1	Determining Hemoglobin Using the Hemoglobinometer		
48-2	Performing a Microhematocrit		
48-3	Perform an Erythrocyte Sedimentation Rate Test Using the Wintrobe Tube Method		
48-4	Preparing Slides		
48-5	Perform a Glycosylated Hemoglobin A1C Test Using a Bayer DCA Vantage Analyzer		
48-6	Perform a PKU Test		
48-7	Perform a Mono Test		
49-1	General X-Ray Examination		
50-1	Recording a 12-Lead Electrocardiograph		
50-2	Applying a Holter Monitor		
51-1	Performing a Spirometry Test to Measure Forced Vital Capacity		
51-2	Instructing Patients According to Their Needs: Teaching Peak Flow Measurement		
51-3	Measuring Oxygen Saturation		
51-4	Administer a Nebulizer Treatment		
52-1	Assisting with Assessing Gait, Using a Gait Belt		
52-2	Assisting with Assessing Ability to Use Stairs		
52-3	Application of a Hot Compress		
52-4	Application of a Hot Soak		
52-5	Application of a Heating Pad		
52-6	Application of a Cold Compress		
52-7	Application of an Ice Bag		
52-8	Application of a Cold Chemical Pack		

Procedure Number	Procedure Title	Date Mastered	Instructor's Signature
52-9	Instructing a Patient to Use Crutches Correctly		
52-10	Instructing a Patient to Use a Cane		
52-11	Teaching a Patient to Correctly Use a Walker		
52-12	Wheelchair Transfer to a Chair or Examination Table		
55-1	Administering Oral Medications		
55-2	Administering Sublingual or Buccal Medication		
55-3	Administering a Rectal or Vaginal Suppository		
55-4	Withdrawing Medication from Single-Dose or Multiple-Dose Vials		
55-5	Withdrawing Medication from an Ampule		
55-6	Administering a Z-Track Injection		
55-7	Administering Parenteral, Subcutaneous, or Intramuscular Injections		
55-8	Administering an Intradermal Injection		
55-9	Preparing an Intravenous Tray		
55-10	Reconstituting a Powdered Medication for Administration		
56-1	Creating a Community Resource Brochure		
56-2	Creating a Public Relations Brochure		
56-3	Instructing Patients According to Their Needs for Health Maintenance and Promotion		
57-1	Calculating Adult Body Mass Index		
57-2	Instruct a Patient According to Dietary Needs		
58-1	Role-Playing a Situation in Which a Patient Is from Another Culture		
58-2	Role-Playing a Situation in Which a Patient Is Frightened, Angry, or Anxious		

Procedure Number	Procedure Title	Date Mastered	Instructor's Signature
58-3	Develop a Patient Teaching Handout About Stress		
60-1	Conducting a Job Search		
60-2	Preparing Your Résumé and References		
60-3	Preparing a Cover Letter		
60-4	Role-Playing an Interview		
60-5	Preparing a Follow-Up Thank-You Letter		

CHAPTER 1
Medical Assisting: The Profession

STUDENT STUDY GUIDE

Use the following guide to assist in your learning of the concepts from the chapter.

I. The History and Training of Medical Assistants

  1. Steps in the History of Trained Medical Assistants

    A. Originally MAs received their training

    _____.

    B. The increase in responsibility and _____ issues led to the need for medical assistants to be more formally trained.

    C. Prior to the formal training of medical assistants, _____ were in higher demand to assist physicians.

  2. The AAMA

    A. The AAMA is the acronym for the

    _____.

    B. The AAMA was founded by _____.

    C. In the year _____, the AAMA was organized.

  3. AAMA Definition of a Medical Assistant

    A. According to the AAMA's definition of medical assistants, MAs work primarily in _____ settings.

    B. Medical assistants perform both _____ and _____ procedures.

  4. Formal Training for the Medical Assistant and Accreditation of Medical Assisting Programs

    A. Certificate training varies from _____ weeks to a yearlong program and focuses typically on _____ skills.

    B. Diploma MA programs are similar to certificate programs but focus on both _____ and _____ skills.

    C. Medical assistant degree programs are approximately _____ years in length.

    D. Accreditation is a(n) _____ process.

    E. Accreditation ensures that a program in a school meets or exceeds _____.

  5. The Medical Assisting Externship

    A. The externship is a(n) _____ component of an MA program.

    B. Externships take place in _____, _____, or _____ settings.

II. Role and Responsibilities of the Medical Assistant

  1. Role of the Medical Assistant

    A. The role of the MA is to _____ the physician.

2. Places of Employment for MAs

    i. _____

    ii. _____

    iii. _____

    iv. _____

    v. _____

3. Duties of the Medical Assistant

    A. Duties typically _____ from office to office.

    B. _____ and _____ of setting determine the types of duties the medical assistant will perform.

    C. Duties vary because of _____ and _____ regulations and guidelines.

4. Administrative Duties

    A. _____ nonpatients and visitors is one example of the MA's administrative duties.

    B. During the physician's absence it is up to the medical assistant to _____ the office.

5. Clinical Responsibilities

    A. Clinical responsibilities of the MA include _____ patients in preparation for physical exams and procedures.

    B. Prior to a physical exam, the MA may need to obtain a patient's _____ history.

    C. Inventory control may involve the _____ and _____ of supplies.

6. General, Clinical, and Administrative Skills of the CMA (AAMA)

    A. Identify three major categories of competences of entry-level MAs

        i. _____

        ii. _____

        iii. _____

7. General Characteristics of a Good MA and the Professional Image

    A. Ability to perform _____ and _____ skills.

    B. _____ cares about others.

    C. Ability to _____ and get along with others.

    D. Develop a basic _____ of human behavior.

    E. Exhibit good daily personal _____ and _____ habits.

    F. Provide _____ care.

III. Certification and Career Opportunities for the MA

1. MA Certifying Organizations

    i. _____

    ii. _____

    iii. _____

    iv. _____

2. American Association of Medical Assistants

    A. Headquarters are located in _____.

    B. Key association in the field of _____.

    C. Offers _____ credential.

3. AAMA Certification Exam

    A. Offered to graduates of programs accredited by _____ or _____.

    B. Computerized exams are available _____ the year.

    C. _____ indicates that the candidate has met the standards of the AAMA for being an MA.

4. American Medical Technologists
    A. Provides a(n) _____ certification exam for MAs.
    B. _____ is awarded to candidates who pass the AMT certification exam.
    C. RMA certification exam focuses on three areas:
        i. _____
        ii. _____
        iii. _____

5. AMT Certification Requirements for Applicants
    A. Be of good _____ character.
    B. Graduate must have graduated from a(n) _____ program/organization.
    C. Applicant must have completed a minimum of _____ clock-hours or _____.

6. General Medical Assisting Knowledge
        i. _____
        ii. _____
        iii. _____
        iv. _____
        v. _____
        vi. _____

7. National Center for Competency Testing
    A. Issues the _____ credential.
    B. Candidate must be a _____ graduate and have completed a(n) _____ program or provide documentation of 2 years of _____ experience.
    C. Continuation of certification requires _____ hours per year of continuing education.

8. National Certified Medical Office Assistant
    A. Offered by the _____.
    B. To qualify, a candidate must have a(n) _____ diploma and must have completed a medical assisting program.
    C. Those who are not graduates of an MA program but are able to provide documentation of _____ years of experience working as an MA are eligible to sit for the NCMA exam.

9. National Health Career Association
    A. Founded in the year _____.
    B. Grants the following two credentials: _____, _____.
    C. Qualified applicants must pass a _____ examination.

KEY TERMINOLOGY REVIEW

Complete the following sentences using the correct key terms found at the beginning of the chapter.

1. The _____ was previously known as the Kansas Medical Assistant Society.

2. _____ is the process in which an institution voluntarily completes a process of determining whether or not the school meets or exceeds standards set forth by an accrediting body.

3. _____ provides oversight for the registration and testing of medical assistants, medical technologists, and phlebotomists.

4. _____ is awarded to candidates who pass the AMT certification examination.

5. The credential issued by the National Center for Competency Testing is the _____.

APPLIED PRACTICE

Give two examples of each positive quality that a medical assistant should possess.

Quality	Examples
Integrity	
Empathy	
Discretion	
Confidentiality	
Thoroughness	
Punctuality	
Congeniality	
Proactivity	
Competence	
Appearance	

LEARNING ACTIVITY: TRUE/FALSE

Indicate whether the following statements are true or false by placing a T or an F on the line that precedes each statement.

_____ 1. Historically, medical assistants were trained on the job by physicians.

_____ 2. An externship is typically a paid position for a period of 160 hours.

_____ 3. A medical assistant can only call him- or herself a nurse if certified by either an ABHES- or a CAAHEP-accredited medical assisting program.

_____ 4. Membership in the AAMA is not necessary to take the certification examination.

_____ 5. For the MA credential to remain current, it must be revalidated every 3 years.

_____ 6. The RMT is a nonprofit certifying body.

_____ 7. Entry-level medical assistants may find work as office managers, medical records managers, hospital unit secretaries, and instructors for medical assistant programs.

_____ 8. A rehabilitation center provides care to patients who need immediate medical treatment.

_____ 9. If you witness behaviors that are unsafe to workers, you must notify OSHA.

_____ 10. As a medical assistant, it is a crime to perform procedures that only nurses or physicians are licensed to do.

CRITICAL THINKING

Answer the following questions to the best of your ability. Use the textbook as a reference.

1. Sara Dunn is taking an administrative medical assisting class as part of her training toward earning a medical assisting certificate. She has been assigned the task of writing a paper that outlines the history of medical assisting. Part of the assignment is to include the milestones reached by this profession over the past 50 years. How should Sara outline this paper?

   _____

   _____

   _____

2. Diane Luder, CMA (AAMA), has been working as an administrative medical assistant in a busy pediatric office for 5 years. Diane's job has been in the billing and coding department. Helga, a colleague of Diane's in the billing and coding department, tells Diane about the benefits of joining a professional organization of coders. How might Diane benefit from joining such a group?

   _____

   _____

   _____

RESEARCH ACTIVITY

Use Internet search engines to research the following topic and write a brief description of what is found. It is important to use reputable websites.

1. Research your state and local chapters of the American Association of Medical Assistants. What information is available? When and where are meetings located? If a chapter does not exist in your area, what are the requirements for starting a chapter?

   _____

   _____

   _____

   _____

   _____

CHAPTER 2

Medical Science: History and Practice

STUDENT STUDY GUIDE

Use the following guide to assist in your learning of the concepts from the chapter.

I. The History of Medicine

   1. Code of Hammurabi

      A. Used by _____ physicians in 3000 B.C.
      B. Laws related to the _____.
      C. Hammurabi was _____.

   2. Early Contributions

      A. Personal hygiene, the sanitary preparation of food, and other matters of public health were pioneered by the practices of the _____ culture.
      B. Some records of early _____ practitioners depict them using nonpoisonous snakes to treat the wounds of patients.

   3. Early Medicinal Remedies Still Used Today

      A. _____ is used to treat heart patients.
      B. _____ from the foxglove plant is used to regulate and strengthen the heartbeat.
      C. _____ is used to treat urinary tract infections.

   4. Fifth Century to 16th Century

      A. During this time frame, _____ progress was made in medical practices.
      B. The _____ swept across Europe, Asia, and North Africa, killing _____ the population.

   5. Hippocrates

      A. Known as the _____.
      B. Shifted medicine from _____ to science.
      C. Stressed the body's _____ nature.
      D. The Hippocratic Oath serves as a widely used _____ guide for physicians.
      E. When taking the oath, physicians pledge to work for the _____ of patients, to _____ no deadly drugs, and to do no _____ to patients.

   6. Galen

      A. Stressed the value of _____.
      B. Founded _____.
      C. Known as the _____.

   7. Other Influential Individuals of Early Medicine

      A. _____ was the first individual to use a telescope to study the skies, leading to the invention of the microscope.
      B. John Hunter is known as the founder of _____.
      C. The first individual to perform the first vaccination using the smallpox vaccine was _____.

8. Advancements Made in Medicine During the 19th Century
    A. It was discovered that certain diseases and wound infections were caused by
       _____.
    B. _____ microscopes were developed and used.
    C. The discovery of the _____ is considered to be one of the most enlightening
       discoveries of this era.
9. Other Major Advancements During the 19th Century
    A. _____ discovered X-rays.
    B. _____ and _____ discovered radium.
    C. _____ worked in the field of psychiatry.
10. Influential Women in Medicine
    A. _____ is known as the founder of modern nursing.
    B. _____ established the American Red Cross.

II. Medical Practitioners
    1. Title of Doctor
       A. Designates a person who holds a(n) _____ degree.
       B. Practicing medicine requires a minimum of _____ years of education and training.
    2. Doctor of Osteopathy
       A. Learns the skill of _____ therapy.
       B. Places greater emphasis on the relationship between the _____ and the
          _____.
       C. Attends school of _____.

III. Medical Practice Acts
    1. Ways a Medical License May Be Granted
       i. _____
       ii. _____
       iii. _____
    2. Causes for Suspension or Revoking of a Medical License
       i. _____
       ii. _____
       iii. _____

IV. Health Care Costs and Payments
    1. The _____ protects consumers who have pre-existing conditions.
    2. In 1963, Medicare instituted the _____ hospital payment system.

V. Types of Medical Practices
    1. List the six types of medical practices.
       i. _____
       ii. _____
       iii. _____
       iv. _____
       v. _____
       vi. _____

VI. Medical and Surgical Specialties

    1. Dermatologists specialize in diseases and problems of the _____.

    2. Physicians who specialize in bariatrics treat patients who are _____.

    3. _____ surgery is the surgical treatment of the heart and blood vessels.

VII. Health Care Institutions

    1. Categories of Hospitals

        i. _____
        ii. _____
        iii. _____
        iv. _____

    2. Outpatient Surgical Centers

        A. _____ procedures are performed in these facilities.
        B. Outpatient surgical centers are also known as _____ surgical centers.
        C. Surgeries typically require _____ recovery time.

    3. Urgent Care Centers

        A. These facilities offer quick care for non-_____ situations.
        B. In some managed care systems, these centers may be designated as a(n) _____ facility.

    4. Types of Long-Term Care Institutions

        i. _____
        ii. _____
        iii. _____
        iv. _____

    5. Hospice

        A. Hospice care emphasizes improved quality of care for the _____.
        B. Most hospice care is provided at _____.

VIII. Allied Health Professions

    1. "Meaningful use" is defined in the_____ Act and impacts electronic health records (EHRs).

    2. A(n) _____ is often the first person at the scene of an emergency.

    3. A Med Lab technician falls under the_____ career cluster.

IX. National Health Care Skill Standards

    1. The _____ is the largest medical research funding agency in the world.

    2. Centers for Disease Control and Prevention (CDC)

        A. The CDC is a division of the _____.
        B. Its purpose is to safeguard public health by _____ and _____ disease.
        C. It acts as a resource for the _____.

KEY TERMINOLOGY REVIEW

◼

Complete the following sentences using the correct key terms found at the beginning of the chapter.

1. _____ shows that an individual has met the educational/experience standards in his or her profession.

2. A disease that affects many people in different countries at the same time is called a _____.

3. _____ provides proof that the individual has been authorized by a government agency to perform work in his or her profession.

4. To numb the pain, Dr. Antolik gave his patient local _____ prior to the removal of an ingrown toenail.

5. Rates of disease or illness are called _____.

APPLIED PRACTICE

◼

Match the early contributor of medicine with his or her accomplishment.

a. Hippocrates   f. Leeuwenhoek

b. Galen   g. Fleming

c. Laennec   h. Salk

d. Franklin   i. Semmelweiss

e. Koch   j. Blackwell

1. _____ Discovered that colds could be passed from one person to another.

2. _____ First to study bacteria and protozoa using a microscope.

3. _____ His experiments with hand washing led to the reduced death rate of women who gave birth in hospitals.

4. _____ He practiced and taught medicine on the island of Kos, Greece. He is known as the "Father of Medicine."

5. _____ Discovered penicillin.

6. _____ Invented the stethoscope.

7. _____ Discovered the cause of tuberculosis.

8. _____ Developed vaccines.

9. _____ Founded experimental physiology.

10. _____ First female physician in the United States.

LEARNING ACTIVITY: TRUE/FALSE

◼

Indicate whether the following statements are true or false by placing a T or an F on the line that precedes each statement.

_____ 1. The Hippocratic Oath is no longer used, but it was around for nearly 2,000 years.

_____ 2. During the early part of the 20th century, the main form of medical practice was solo practice.

_____ 3. In a partnership practice, each partner is responsible for the actions of all partners.

_____ 4. Many early and historic plant remedies are still used today for heart conditions, indigestion, bleeding, and urinary tract infections.

_____ 5. An associate practice consists of three or more physicians who share the same facility and practice medicine together.

_____ 6. A group practice is managed by a board of directors.

_____ 7. A technician typically has an associate's degree from a 2-year community college or vocational program.

_____ 8. Registered nurses have more training than nurse practitioners.

_____ 9. Physical therapists develop programs that help restore the patient's ability to manage the activities of daily living.

_____ 10. In nearly every state, a physician's assistant can prescribe medications.

CRITICAL THINKING

Answer the following questions to the best of your ability. Use the textbook as a reference.

1. Robert Bautista is taking an administrative medical assisting course as part of his training to earn a certificate in medical assisting. He has been asked to write a paragraph outlining the contributions the Greek physician Galen made to medicine. Robert has been told to include the reasons why Galen's findings were not completely accurate. What could Robert write on this topic?

   _____

   _____

   _____

2. Willie Harrison is creating a presentation for a history class he is enrolled in. Because he is in a medical assisting program, he wants his history paper to focus on a medical topic. Willie has chosen to write about the history of the use of anesthesia in medicine. How should he start his outline for this presentation?

   _____

   _____

   _____

3. Olivia Denton is a medical assisting instructor discussing the Affordable Care Act (ACA) with students. What are four benefits of the ACA to consumers?

   _____

   _____

   _____

4. Who is Joseph Lister, and what major discovery did he make?

   _____

   _____

   _____

5. Discuss early anesthesia. What is it, who discovered it, how was it used, and what compound was first used extensively?

   _____

   _____

   _____

RESEARCH ACTIVITY

Use Internet search engines to research the following topics and write a brief description of what is found. It is important to use reputable websites.

1. Choose and research one of the early contributors to medicine and write a summary regarding your findings.

   _____

   _____

   _____

   _____

   _____

CHAPTER 3
Medical Law and Ethics

STUDENT STUDY GUIDE

Use the following guide to assist in your learning of the concepts from the chapter.

I. Law and Liability

  1. Classification of Law

    A. _____ law is made to protect the public as a whole from the harmful acts of others.

    B. _____ law concerns relationships between individuals or between individuals and the government.

    C. _____ law is concerned with a breach or neglect of an understanding between two parties.

  2. Civil Law

    A. _____ law falls under civil law and covers acts that result in harm to another.

    B. _____ occurs when the patient is injured as a result of the health care professional not exercising the ordinary standard of care.

    C. When an individual is being threatened with imminent bodily harm, the person doing the act could be charged with _____.

    D. A violation of the personal liberty of another person through unlawful restraint is known as _____.

  3. The Four Ds of Negligence

    i. _____

    ii. _____

    iii. _____

    iv. _____

  4. Name 4 Intentional Torts.

    i. _____

    ii. _____

    iii. _____

    iv. _____

    v. _____

  5. Standard of Care

    A. Asserts that the physician must provide the same _____, _____, and _____ that a similarly trained physician would provide under the same circumstances in the same locality.

    B. If the physician violates the standard of care, he or she is liable for _____.

II. Patient–Physician Relationship

  1. Physician Rights

    A. Both the physician and the patient must agree to _____ if there is to be a contract for service and treatment. The patient must confide _____ to the physician in order to receive proper treatment.

    B. Physicians have the right to _____ payment for the treatment given.

2. Patient Rights

    i. _____

    ii. _____

    iii. _____

    iv. _____

3. Patient Obligations

    i. _____

    ii. _____

4. Common Exceptions to Informed Consent

    A. A physician does not have to inform a patient about risks that are _____ known.

    B. If the physician feels that the disclosure of risks may be _____ to the patient, then he or she is not responsible for disclosing them.

    C. If the patient requests that the physician _____ disclose the risks, then he or she is not responsible for disclosing them.

5. Categories of Minors Who Can Give Consent

    i. _____

    ii. _____

6. Legal Implications to Consider When Treating a Minor

    i. _____

    ii. _____

    iii. _____

7. Durable Power of Attorney (DPOA)

    A. A DPOA allows an agent or _____ to act on behalf of the patient.

    B. An agent may be a(n) _____, _____, _____, or a(n) _____.

    C. A DPOA is used when a patient becomes physically or _____.

8. Uniform Anatomical Gift Act

    A. This act allows a person _____ years or older and of sound mind to make a gift of any or all parts of his or her body for the purposes of organ transplantation or medical research.

    B. A physician who is not involved in the transplant will determine the _____.

    C. No _____ is allowed to change hands for organ donations.

III. Documentation and Regulations

1. When a Medical Record Is Subpoenaed for Court

    A. Copy only the parts of the record that are _____.

    B. Send a(n) _____ unless the original record is subpoenaed.

    C. Place a(n) _____ for the subpoenaed record in the patient's file.

2. Considerations for Testifying in Court

    i. _____

    ii. _____

    iii. _____

    iv. _____

    v. _____

    vi. _____

3. Childhood Vaccines and Toxoids Required by Law

    i. _____

    ii. _____

    iii. _____

      iv. _____
      v. _____
      vi. _____

4. Drug Regulation Agencies

   A. The _____ has jurisdiction over testing and approving drugs for public use.
   B. The _____ is a branch of the U.S. Department of Justice.
   C. The _____ regulates the sale and use of scheduled drugs.

5. Requirements for Controlled Substances

   A. Controlled drugs must be kept in a(n) _____ cabinet.
   B. Any theft must be immediately reported to both the regional _____ office and local police.
   C. Federal regulations require a(n) _____ inventory of drug supplies.

6. Role of the Medical Assistant as Related to Controlled Substances

   A. The MA does not _____ controlled substances.
   B. The MA must be knowledgeable about the _____ governing the documentation and control of drugs.
   C. The MA must always _____ any unusual patient behavior indicating addictive drug use.

7. MA's Role Related to Drug Administration

   A. The MA may administer medication only under the _____ supervision of a physician.
   B. When preparing medications for administration, check the medication _____ times, as follows:
      i. _____
      ii. _____
      iii. _____

IV. Medical Ethics

1. Ethics and Medical Ethics

   A. Ethics is a branch of philosophy related to _____ or _____ principles.
   B. Medical ethics refers to the _____ conduct of people in medical professions.
   C. The members of the medical profession set _____ and _____ for themselves.

2. Areas covered in the AAMA code of ethics.

      i. _____
      ii. _____
      iii. _____
      iv. _____
      v. _____

3. Pledge Made Under the AAMA Code of Ethics

   A. Render service with full _____ for the _____ of humanity.
   B. Uphold the honor and high _____ of the profession and accept its _____.
   C. Seek to continually improve the _____ and _____ of medical assistants for the benefit of patients and professional colleagues.

4. HIPAA is organized into three parts.

      i. _____
      ii. _____
      iii. _____

5. The Patient's Bill of Rights

   A. Is now called the _____.
   B. Describes the _____ relationship.

6. HIPAA
   A. Defined as the _____ .
   B. Regulates the _____ of patient health information.

KEY TERMINOLOGY REVIEW

Write a sentence using the selected key terms in the correct context.

1. **Bioethics:**
   _____
   _____

2. **Contributory negligence:**
   _____
   _____

3. **Informed consent:**
   _____
   _____

4. **Living will:**
   _____
   _____

5. **Reasonable person standard:**
   _____
   _____

APPLIED PRACTICE

Provide answers to the following questions.

1. Considering the Latin terms discussed throughout the text, identify which of the Latin terms pertain to the following situations and then translate each term:
   A. A physician is sued because he amputates the wrong leg during surgery.
   _____
   _____

   B. Dr. Lin is being sued because his medical assistant injured a patient while suturing a 3-mm incision on the patient's lower leg, a procedure that is clearly outside the MA's scope of practice.
   _____
   _____

   C. Due to possible negligence by a physician, a child has been injured. When the case goes to court, an individual is appointed to represent the child.
   _____
   _____

LEARNING ACTIVITY: TRUE/FALSE

Indicate whether the following statements are true or false by placing a T or an F on the line that precedes each statement.

_____ 1. Although less serious in nature, misdemeanors may carry a punishment of jail time.

_____ 2. Medical malpractice can include medical errors, but every mistake or error is not considered malpractice.

_____ 3. Physicians have a duty to issue a legal certificate of death for natural and unnatural deaths.

_____ 4. Physicians have a duty to report all injuries of children.

_____ 5. The requirements of reporting elderly abuse vary by state.

CRITICAL THINKING

Answer the following questions to the best of your ability. Use the textbook as a reference.

1. Beth Clark is taking an administrative medical assisting course as part of her medical assisting training. She has been given the assignment of writing a paper that outlines the current ethical standpoints of the AMA. What points should Beth include?

   _____

   _____

   _____

2. Create a medical malpractice scenario in which the statute of limitations defense would apply.

   _____

   _____

   _____

3. Create a scenario, different from the one listed in the textbook, in which a health care worker would utilize the Good Samaritan Act as a defense in a lawsuit.

   _____

   _____

   _____

RESEARCH ACTIVITY

Use Internet search engines to research the following topic and write a brief description of what is found. It is important to use reputable websites.

1. Search for a medical malpractice case. Describe the case you find and include whether the patient or the physician won the case. Did you feel the case was decided fairly? Why or why not?

   _____

   _____

   _____

   _____

   _____

CHAPTER 4
Medical Terminology

STUDENT STUDY GUIDE

Use the following guide to assist in your learning of the concepts from the chapter.

I. Word Parts and Combining Forms
   1. Words for Forming Medical Terms
      A. Medical terms will often contain prefixes and suffixes, both of which add further _____ to the given term. If a word root is used, to prepare the word root for combining with another part, a(n) _____ is sometimes added.
   2. Combining Vowels
      A. If the suffix begins with a vowel, _____ the combining vowel from the combining form and _____ the suffix. If the suffix begins with a consonant, *keep* the combining vowel and _____ the suffix to the combining vowel.
   3. Prefix
      A. A prefix is a word element that is placed _____, or is _____ to the beginning of the word root.
   4. Suffix
      A. In medical terminology usage, a suffix is a word element that is affixed to the _____ of the word.

II. Writing and Pronouncing Medical Terms
   1. Spelling
      A. *Hyper–* means _____, whereas *hypo–* means_____.
   2. Plurals
      A. The plural form of the word *iris* is _____.
   3. Pronunciation
      A. When speaking with patients, the medical assistant must correctly _____all medical terms.

III. Gross Anatomy
   1. Anatomical Position
      A. Anatomical position is used when describing the _____ and _____ of a structure in the human body.
      B. It describes the position of the body standing _____ with arms _____ of the body, palms facing _____, eyes looking _____ ahead.
      C. The legs are _____, with the feet and toes pointing _____.

2. Body Planes (indicate the position of each of the body planes)

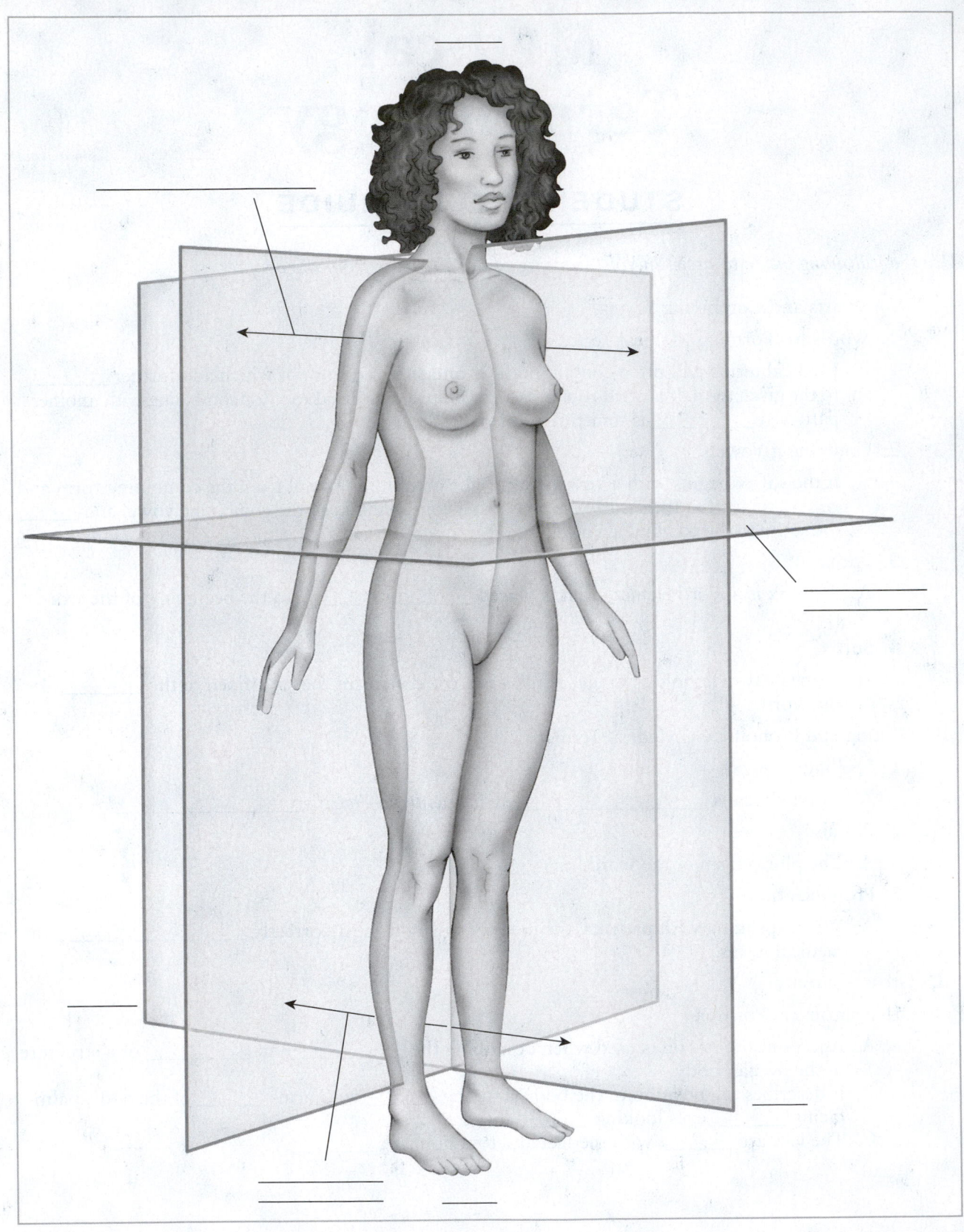

3. Directional Terms,
    A. Superior _____
    B. Anterior _____
    C. Posterior _____
    D. Cephalic _____
    E. Medial _____
    F. Lateral _____
    G. Proximal _____
    H. Distal _____

4. Body Cavities (explain each)

    A. The body's _____ are contained in cavities.
    B. The cranial cavity houses the _____.
    C. The chest, or _____, cavity holds the lungs and heart.
    D. Under the diaphragm, the _____ cavity holds other vital organs, including the intestines, stomach, and reproductive organs.

IV. Body Systems: Structure and Function

1. The Skeletal System

    A. The skeletal system consists of bones that are used to store _____, to give the body height and movement, and to _____ and _____ the body organs.
    B. The combining form for the word *bone* is _____.
    C. –*clast* is the combining form for _____.
    D. *cost/o* is the combining form for _____.

2. The Muscular System

    A. Muscles aid bones in _____.
    B. The combining forms used for muscles are _____ and _____.
    C. The word part –*trophy* means _____.

3. The Nervous System

    A. The nervous system helps the body to sense changes in the _____ and _____ environments.
    B. Pain is referred to with the suffixes _____ and _____.
    C. *cephal/o* means the _____, and *encephal/o* is _____.

4. Special Senses

    A. Special senses include _____, _____, taste, touch, and _____.
    B. The combining forms for the word *eye* are _____, _____, and _____.
    C. The combining forms for the word *ear* are _____ and _____.

5. The Circulatory System

    A. The circulatory system consists of the heart, the blood vessels, the blood, and the structures that make up the _____ system.

    B. The cardiovascular system is a subsystem of the _____ system and is comprised of the heart and its vessels.

    C. The combining form for the word *heart* is _____.

6. The Immune System

    A. The immune system protects the body from _____.

    B. The word part *bas/o* means _____.

    C. The combining form *–phage* means _____.

7. The Respiratory System

    A. The respiratory system exchanges oxygen (O_2) in the environment for _____ in the body.

    B. The main organs of respiration are the _____.

    C. _____ is a combining form that means "lung."

8. The Digestive System

    A. The digestive system either _____ or _____ food and drugs for the body.

    B. The _____ is another term for the mouth.

    C. A physician with specialized training in the digestive system is a(n) _____.

9. The Urinary System

    A. The urinary system rids the body of the toxic by-products of _____.

    B. The combining form for the word *kidney* is _____.

    C. A physician with specialized training related to the kidney is a(n) _____.

10. The Endocrine System

    A. The endocrine system is the ductless glandular system that controls other body systems by secreting _____ within the bloodstream.

    B. *Endo–* means _____ and *–crine* means _____.

    C. The word part *estr/o* means _____.

11. The Reproductive System

    A. The physician with specialized training in women's health is a(n) _____.

    B. The combining forms for the word *uterus* are _____ and _____.

    C. A common abbreviation related to the male reproductive system is _____.

V. Surgical and Diagnostic Terms

  1. Define each word part.

    A. *–graphy*: _____

    B. *–scopy*: _____

    C. *–tome*: _____

    D. *–stomy*: _____

    E. *–tomy*: _____

VI. Word Building

  1. What word parts make up each of the following terms?

    A. Melanoma _____

    B. Costectomy _____

    C. Arachnoid _____

    D. Phlebostasis _____

    E. Gastroenteritis _____

KEY TERMINOLOGY REVIEW

Write a sentence using each of the word parts listed. Note the word part by underlining it in your sentence.

1. *combining form:*
   _____
   _____

2. *combining vowel:*
   _____
   _____

3. *prefix:*
   _____
   _____

4. *suffix:*
   _____
   _____

5. *word root:*
   _____
   _____

APPLIED PRACTICE

For each of the following rules related to forming plurals, write a sentence without the use of the plural ending and then rewrite the sentence using the word with a plural ending.

1. Words ending in *on* will drop *on* and add *a*.
   _____
   _____

2. Words ending in *us* will drop *us* and add *l*.
   _____
   _____

3. Words ending in *um* will drop *um* and add *a*.
   _____
   _____

4. Words ending in *y* will drop *y* and add *ies*.
   _____
   _____

5. Words ending in *nx* will change the *x* to *g* and add *es*.
   _____
   _____

CRITICAL THINKING

Answer the following question to the best of your ability. Use the textbook as a reference.

1. Andrea Natal has been working as an MA for Dr. Smith for about a month. Andrea has just finished assisting with a patient examination. As Dr. Smith leaves the examination room, he hands Andrea the patient's chart and indicates that he has written down some instructions that need to be given to the patient. After the physician leaves the room, Andrea looks at the patient's chart and discovers that she is unable to decipher some of the information. What should Andrea say to the patient and do to ensure that the patient receives the correct information? What should Andrea *not* do?

_____

_____

_____

RESEARCH ACTIVITY

Use Internet search engines to research the following topic and write a brief description of what you find. It is important to use reputable websites.

1. Select one of the systems of the body described in your textbook. Using information obtained on the Internet, conduct research on the various conditions that can occur in that system. Prepare a short paper on what you learned about the system and the conditions that can occur within the system. Be sure to cite your sources at the end of your paper.

_____

_____

_____

_____

CHAPTER 7
Telephone Techniques

STUDENT STUDY GUIDE

Use the following guide to assist in your learning of the concepts from the chapter.

1. Guidelines for Answering the Office Telephone
    i. _____
    ii. _____
    iii. _____
    iv. _____
    v. _____

2. Elements of a Professional Greeting
    i. _____
    ii. _____
    iii. _____

3. Guidelines for Making Calls

    A. Access _____ line as required.
    B. Dial _____ code if necessary.
    C. Know the _____ of the office with regard to personal calls.

4. Guidelines for Taking a Message

    A. Many medical offices have _____ messages and notepads.
    B. All messages should include the _____ and _____ name of the caller.
    C. _____ the message with the caller.
    D. _____ the telephone number for a return call.
    E. Ensure that the telephone message is placed in the patient's chart as _____ of the call.
    F. Follow _____ rules with regard to patient information.

5. Pagers and Cell Phones

    A. You must know if any physician in your office carries a _____.
    B. Smart phones combine the features of _____ and _____.
    C. Follow hospital building policies on _____ of pagers and cell phones.

6. Prescription Refill Requests

    A. Due to a high volume of calls, _____ systems are often used.
    B. The MA is often responsible for _____ and _____ to messages.
    C. Messages should be checked at least _____ a day.
    D. A prescription refill request must be _____ on by a physician.
    E. A message may need to be attached to the _____ prior to obtaining a physician's approval.

7. Steps for Taking a Prescription Refill Message
    i. _____
    ii. _____
    iii. _____
    iv. _____
    v. _____
    vi. _____
    vii. _____
    viii. _____
    ix. _____
    x. _____
    xi. _____

8. Purposes for Using a Telephone Log
    A. Logs are typically used to keep track of _____ calls.
    B. A log helps to identify any _____ calls that are not _____ related.

9. Purposes for Using an Answering Service
    i. _____
    ii. _____
    iii. _____

10. Handling Emergency Calls
    A. Every office should have a(n) _____ protocol.
    B. Immediately get the caller's _____ and _____.
    C. If it is an emergency, alert the _____ and/or _____.
    D. Try to _____ the individual.

KEY TERMINOLOGY REVIEW

Complete the following sentences using the correct key terms found at the beginning of the chapter. Key terms may be more than one word in length.

1. Before seeing a specialist, Mrs. Smith has been told that she must get a(n) _____.

2. When the office is closed, the _____ will typically handle all emergency calls.

3. _____ refers to the quality or state of being understandable.

4. When calling a patient, it is important for the medical office to set up a system to block the office number from showing up on the patient's _____.

5. A medical assistant is on the phone with a patient; the process she uses to determine the order in which patients calls should be handled is called _____.

APPLIED PRACTICE

Using your textbook, complete the following activities and answer the following questions.

1. Using the box on the next page, create a message pad template that could be used in a medical office to take telephone messages. Consider the important information to be obtained from callers when they call the office.

2. Manuel Vargas is an administrative medical assistant. He receives a phone call from a patient requesting a refill for one of her prescription medications. How should Manuel handle this call? What information must Manuel obtain from the patient? What should he do with the message after the call has ended? Manuel needs to be sure that he is talking on a phone that cannot be overheard by other patients and visitors. In what law is this provision covered?

_____

_____

_____

_____

LEARNING ACTIVITY: MULTIPLE CHOICE

Circle the correct answer to each of the following questions.

1. Which of the following would be appropriate to play for callers who are on hold?
   a. A local radio station
   b. Pre-recorded music
   c. A message about seasonal allergies
   d. All of the above

2. Which of the following might be offensive or irritating for callers to listen to while they are on hold?
   a. Religious music
   b. Pre-recorded music
   c. A message about seasonal allergies
   d. A local radio station

3. How long is an acceptable period of time to leave a caller on hold?

    a. Less than 10 seconds
    b. 20–30 seconds
    c. 45–60 seconds
    d. 1–2 minutes

4. What items should a medical assistant have available before answering the office telephone?

    a. Pen or pencil
    b. Paper
    c. Telephone message pad
    d. All of the above

5. The medical office telephone should be answered within how many rings?

    a. On the first ring
    b. By the second ring
    c. By the third ring
    d. No more than five rings

6. What rule are you violating if a patient's private information is thrown into the trash?

    a. OSHA's privacy rule
    b. HIPAA's privacy rule
    c. AAMA's privacy rule
    d. AMA's privacy rule

7. Which of the following telephone calls should be taken care of first?

    a. A patient who says she needs to schedule her yearly mammogram
    b. An angry patient who is calling about her bill
    c. A patient who says he is having chest pains
    d. A patient who is calling to find out his laboratory results

8. What information would you expect to find in a telephone triage notebook?

    a. Driving directions to the medical office
    b. The hours the clinic is open
    c. The questions to ask a patient who complains of chest pains
    d. All of the above

9. In the event of a medical emergency in the office, what information should the medical assistant have available before calling for emergency services?

    a. The patient's name
    b. The patient's age
    c. The patient's gender
    d. All of the above

10. Which of the following emergency telephone numbers should the medical assistant have readily available at the front desk?

    a. Poison control
    b. The local police department
    c. The local fire department
    d. All of the above

CRITICAL THINKING

Answer the following questions to the best of your ability. Use the textbook and other resources such as the Internet in considering the following questions.

1. Rosie Sanchez, CMA (AAMA), has been working as an administrative medical assistant in an internal medicine clinic for the past year. A large part of her day is spent answering the office telephone and scheduling appointments. She would like the office to provide her with a hands-free headset for the telephone system. The clinic director has asked Rosie to create a list that outlines the benefits of having a hands-free headset over a conventional telephone headset. What should Rosie list?

   _____

   _____

   _____

2. Ron Douglas is a student in an administrative medical assisting class. He has been given an assignment to create an office policy that discusses how the speakerphone function of the front desk telephone system can be used without violating patient confidentiality. What should Ron write?

   _____

   _____

   _____

3. Martin Taylor, RMA, is working in an audiology clinic. The clinic is researching the possibility of purchasing a new telephone system that will include an automatic routing unit where callers can dial an extension to reach the desired party. Martin has been asked to create a list of pros and cons for this type of system. What should Martin include on his list?

   _____

   _____

   _____

RESEARCH ACTIVITY

Use Internet search engines to research the following topic and write a brief description of what you find. It is important to use reputable websites.

1. Search for on-call, after-hours answering services that are provided for medical offices. What types of services are offered by these companies? What is the general cost for on-call answering services?

   _____

   _____

   _____

   _____

   _____

CHAPTER 8
Patient Reception

STUDENT STUDY GUIDE

Use the following guide to assist in your learning of the concepts from the chapter.

I. Opening the Office and Receiving Patients

1. The Duties of a Receptionist

    A. _____ patients upon arrival.
    B. Assist new patients with _____ of proper forms.
    C. _____ copayments.
    D. Maintain a(n)_____ and _____ environment in the reception area.
    E. _____ any disturbances in the reception room.
    F. _____ return appointments.
    G. Make _____ calls for upcoming appointments.

2. The Reception Room

    A. Often, it is the MA's job to keep the reception room _____ and _____ of hazards.
    B. The reception room provides the _____ impression of the office.

3. The Image of the Medical Assistant

    A. Image is important because the MA is often the _____ person the patient meets.
    B. Attention should be paid to good _____ and _____ habits.
    C. Makeup, hairstyle, and jewelry should reflect _____.
    D. The MA's name _____ should always be visible.

4. Responsibilities in Opening the Office

    A. Arrive _____ minutes prior to office hours.
    B. Ensure that the day's charts have been _____ and _____.
    C. Ensure that _____ slips have been printed in advance for each patient.
    D. Print out _____ lists of patient appointments and distribute them.

5. The Task of Collating Records

    A. This is usually done the day _____ patients are seen.
    B. All necessary information should be received and in the record _____ to the patient's visit.
    C. In some offices, patient records are organized in the _____ in which patients will be seen.
    D. A(n) _____ appointment list is placed on top of the collated records.
    E. As patients arrive, the _____ should be verified on the schedule.

6. Collating records.

    A. Collating is filing all information and test results for a patient into that patient's _____ _____ , then sorting and organizing the charts in the order in which the _____ will be seen.
    B. An encounter form is also called a _____ _____.

40

© 2015 Pearson Education, Inc.

7. General Guidelines for Greeting Patients

    A. Patients should not be kept waiting more than a few _____.

    B. If possible, have emergency or _____ patients enter through a private entrance.

    C. Place _____ ahead of other visitors.

    D. Follow _____ guidelines.

8. Patient Sign-In

    A. The sheet is maintained at the _____ desk.

    B. The sheet provides a(n) _____ record of all patients who come to the office.

    C. _____ sign-in pads provide complete confidentiality.

    D. In order to be HIPAA compliant, all efforts should be made to protect _____.

9. Patient Registration Forms

    A. Forms are sometimes sent to patients _____ to their first appointment.

    B. Some offices request that patients arrive _____ minutes early to complete the forms.

    C. Forms contain _____ information.

    D. Forms should be _____ marked to indicate areas that patients need to complete.

    E. Patients should be provided _____ as needed to ensure the completeness of the forms.

    F. Many clinics have all patients (returning and new) sign a new HIPAA form for each visit. What does the term *HIPAA* mean? _____.

10. Registering New Patients

    A. Office billing and payment policies should be _____ explained to new patients.

    B. Obtain the patient's signature on a(n) _____ form.

    C. Ensure that forms are filled out _____ and _____, including signatures.

    D. Verify information with the patient's _____ card.

    E. Photocopy _____ of the insurance card.

    F. Determine if a(n) _____ is required.

11. Payment for Services

    A. Should be documented on the _____ slip.

    B. The charge slip contains a list of the most common _____ for procedures and diagnoses at that office.

    C. Payment or _____ should be made prior to the patient leaving the office.

12. Consideration for the Patient's Time

    A. Inform the patient when the wait for his or her appointment will be longer than _____ minutes.

    B. If the wait is going to be longer, then you should approach each patient and ask if the patient prefers to wait or wishes to _____.

II. Completing a Patient Visit

    1. Escorting the Patient to the Examination Room

        A. When calling the patient, verify the patient's _____ with the record and with the patient.

        B. Offer _____ to those who need it.

        C. Walk at a(n) _____ pace.

2. The Patient and the Examination Room
   A. Enter the room with the patient and _____ explain what clothing the patient should remove.
   B. _____ patients in disrobing if necessary.
   C. Make every effort to protect the patient's _____.
   D. Once the physician has completed the exam, return to the examination room and _____ before entering.
   E. _____ ask the patient if he or she has any additional questions.

3. Ensuring Effective Patient Education
   A. Ensure that patient education is adapted and provided at a(n) _____ that the patient understands.
   B. Assess the patient's level of understanding by asking the patient to _____ what he or she heard.
   C. If a misunderstanding is apparent, _____ the information to an appropriate level and ask the patient to repeat it again.
   D. Provide _____ information to which the patient can refer.
   E. Do not _____ to ask the physician or another individual in the office to help clarify information for the patient.

4. Assisting patients with intellectual disabilities.
   A. Intellectual disability, formerly called _____, is characterized by below-average intelligence and a lack of _____ necessary for daily life activities.
   B. A paitient with ID may have a condition that causes _____behavior.
   C. Treat them with courtesy and _____.

5. Guidelines for Dealing with Disturbances
   A. If possible, move angry or loud patients into a(n) _____ office area.
   B. Handle the situation as _____ and _____ as possible.
   C. Using a quiet, calm manner, _____ respond to the patient's complaint.
   D. Ask the patient to _____ the issue.
   E. Discuss _____ with the patient.
   F. Know office policy regarding when the _____ must be called.

6. Dealing with Children
   A. The children of adult patients are allowed in the examination room unless _____ is required.
   B. Rarely are children seen by physicians without the presence of a(n) _____.

7. Handling Medical Emergencies in the Reception Room (list the steps)
   A. The receptionist must be familiar with _____ _____ regarding regarding emergency treatment of patients.
   B. In certain emergency situations, the medical assistant may be required to start _____ _____ procedures.

8. Steps for Closing the Office
   A. Allow for _____ minutes at the end of the day to close the office.
   B. Check all _____ used during the day for any orders that may have been missed.
   C. _____, _____, and _____ all records for patients who will be seen the next day.
   D. Balance the _____ in the presence of another staff member.
   E. _____ or pull records for patients who will be seen the next day.
   F. Lock all _____ and _____, physician offices, and other individual offices within the medical practice.
   G. Some equipment, such as _____, fax machines, and computers, may require 24-hour operation.
   H. Turn off all _____ equipment and appliances.
   I. Know the name of the physician who is accepting _____ _____ or is on call until morning.
   J. _____ the reception room.
   K. _____ the security system.
   L. Double-check that the _____ is locked.

KEY TERMINOLOGY REVIEW

Choose the term that best represents each of the following statements.

   a. Copayments
   b. Demographic
   c. Medical emergency
   d. Overbooking
   e. No-show

1. _____ When more than one patient is scheduled for the same time slot.
2. _____ Designated amounts that some medical insurance plans require patients to pay for medical services.
3. _____ Information, such as age, gender, ethnic background, education, and Social Security number.
4. _____ Patient condition that requires the immediate attention of a physician.
5. _____ Patients who do not keep their appointment and do not call to cancel.

APPLIED PRACTICE

Using information from your textbook and other sources you may find on the topic, complete the following applied practice.

1. Aubrey Cody is a CMA (AAMA) who has been hired as a medical assistant for a new pediatric practice that is being built. The physicians within the practice have asked her to design and decorate the reception area. In the practice, there are three physicians who can see up to four patients each hour. How could Aubrey design the medical office reception area? What is the minimum amount of seating that should be in the reception area? What theme, toys, and reading materials would be appropriate for the reception area? Explain your answer after you have designed the reception area.

_____

_____

_____

LEARNING ACTIVITY: MULTIPLE CHOICE

Circle the correct answer to each of the following questions.

1. When mentioning another patient's name over the telephone or to another staff member within hearing distance of any patients in the reception room, the MA should

   a. use caution and speak in a low voice.
   b. be sure that the glass partition at the reception desk is closed so that others in the reception room are not able to hear the conversation.
   c. step into a private area where other patients are unable to hear the conversation.
   d. Any of the above

2. When an established patient checks in at the front desk, what information should the receptionist first confirm with the patient?

   a. That the patient's marital status has not changed since the last visit
   b. The type of medications that the patient is taking
   c. Current contact information
   d. All of the above

3. When using a sign-in sheet, HIPAA allows which of the following information to be requested?

   a. Patient's name
   b. Time of arrival
   c. Physician's name
   d. All of the above

4. In general, patients should not be made to wait longer than _____ minutes for their appointment.

    a. 10
    b. 15
    c. 20
    d. None of the above

5. How should the receptionist respond when confronted with an angry patient?

    a. Move the patient out of the front desk area.
    b. Ask the patient to sit down in the reception room until the patient has calmed down.
    c. Walk away from the front desk until the patient calms down.
    d. Any of the above

CRITICAL THINKING

Answer the following questions to the best of your ability. Use the textbook as a reference.

1. Marcus Winston, RMA, has been hired to work as an administrative medical assistant at the front desk in a small, one-physician medical office. Dr. Quan has been using a paper sign-in sheet for his patients for many years. Marcus has recently completed his medical assisting education and remembers learning that sign-in sheets must be HIPAA compliant. What can Marcus tell Dr. Quan about the paper sign-in system that he is currently using?

    _____

    _____

2. Sara Womack, CMA (AAMA), is the medical office manager in a women's clinic. She has two employees who share the job of front desk receptionist. Aaron Shelley, CMA (AAMA), doesn't like to work at the front desk. He is often short with the patients, some of whom have complained to the physician. Michael Sulley, RMA, is the other front desk receptionist. Michael has a sunny personality and thoroughly enjoys the fast pace at the front desk. Would Sara be better serving the patients at the women's clinic if she moved Aaron out of that position and had Michael work there full time? Why or why not? What sort of ramifications might occur if Sara leaves Aaron in the front desk position?

    _____

    _____

3. Marjorie Sorensen, CMA (AAMA), has just been hired to work as the office manager for Dr. Rodriguez. The doctor tells Marjorie that she has noticed that many tasks are being skipped by the front desk staff when opening the office in the morning. Dr. Rodriguez believes that the front desk staff is forgetting these tasks and has asked Marjorie to come up with a solution to this problem. What might Marjorie suggest?

    _____

    _____

4. Isaiah Chung is taking an administrative medical assisting course as part of his training to become a medical assistant. His instructor has assigned the task of creating an office policy for opening the medical office. What should Isaiah's policy include?

_____

_____

_____

RESEARCH ACTIVITY

Use Internet search engines to research the following topic and write a brief description of what you find. It is important to use reputable websites.

1. Using the information and décor theme of the reception area that you designed in the Applied Practice activity, search the Internet and obtain figures and estimates regarding the cost of decorating a reception area. Take into consideration paint, accessories, seating, tables, and so forth. Be sure to cite the websites that you use to find your information.

_____

_____

_____

_____

_____

CHAPTER 9
Appointment Scheduling

STUDENT STUDY GUIDE

Use the following guide to assist in your learning of the concepts from the chapter.

I. Scheduling Systems

  1. Factors to Be Considered in Selecting a Scheduling System

     i. _____

     ii. _____

     iii. _____

     iv. _____

     v. _____

     vi. _____

     vii. _____

  2. Purpose of a Scheduling System

    A. A scheduling system assists in the _____ of the office.

    B. It provides _____ management.

    C. It helps to prevent _____.

  3. Variations in Appointment Schedules

     i. _____

     ii. _____

     iii. _____

     iv. _____

     v. _____

     vi. _____

  4. Specified Times

    A. The length of appointment is determined by _____ needs.

    B. It is up to each staff member to reduce _____ time.

  5. Wave Scheduling

    A. All the patients are told to come in at the _____ of the hour in which they are to be seen.

    B. Its purpose is to _____ and _____ each hour on time.

    C. Each hour is divided into _____ amounts of time.

    D. Three _____ -minute or four _____ -minute appointments could be seen in an hour.

    E. Patients are seen in the _____ in which they arrive.

  6. Open Office Hours

    A. This is the _____ structured of all systems.

    B. Patients may arrive at _____ during business hours.

    C. This method is _____ by some because it avoids the disruption caused by missed appointments.

7. Advantages of Computerized Scheduling Systems

   A. It has the ability to access and view _____ with a click or touch of a button.
   B. Computerized appointment systems help to maximize workflow and ensure that _____ are followed.
   C. The computer searches for available _____ and provides a list of available _____.
   D. It provides the ability to track _____ in the medical practice.

8. Manual Scheduling Systems

   A. A manual scheduling system consists of a(n) _____ schedule book.
   B. The book is selected based on practice _____ and _____.

9. Requirements for Both Computerized and Manual Systems

   A. The appointment book is a legal document that can be _____ by the court.
   B. Appointment books should be _____ for future reference and kept for several years in the event of a court case.
   C. If there are any changes in the scheduled patients in the appointment book, these should be noted both in the _____ and in the _____.

II. Patient Scheduling Process

   1. The Appointment Matrix

      A. A matrix is a grid that shows the availability of each _____, as well as periods of time that are not _____ for appointments.
      B. A matrix is formed in advance for a period of _____ to _____ months.
      C. Cross out the _____ _____ _____ when the physician is unavailable and write the reason across the blocked-out space.

   2. Steps for Manually Scheduling Established Patients

      A. Use a(n) _____ so that appointments can be erased to make changes as needed.
      B. Set up a(n) _____ by blocking out all time periods when the physician is not available for appointments.
      C. Print the patient's _____ first and last names next to the appropriate time on the schedule.
      D. Add _____ for *junior* and _____ for *senior* if there are two patients with the same name in a family.
      E. Ask the patient for _____ work and home telephone numbers, including the area codes.
      F. Write these numbers next to the _____.
      G. Record the _____ for the visit on the schedule.

   3. Additional Steps Related to Scheduling Patients Electronically

      A. Log in to the scheduling system with your _____ and _____ that have been previously established..
      B. Search for the _____ patient.
      C. _____ that the telephone numbers in the system are correct.

   4. Steps for Scheduling New Patients

      A. _____ the necessary appointment scheduling equipment.
      B. Obtain the patient's full _____ name.
      C. Record the patient's chief _____ and _____.
      D. Request the name of the patient's insurance _____ and policy _____.
      E. Attempt to _____ the new patient's request for his or her preferred appointment time.
      F. Provide the new patient with _____ to the office.
      G. Welcome and thank the new patient by _____ for selecting your medical office.
      H. _____ new patient information in a new medical record.

5. Addressing Missed Appointments and No-Shows
   A. Charge the patient according to office _____.
   B. _____ the patient and reschedule.
   C. _____ the missed appointment and rescheduled date.
   D. _____l, legible documentation of missed appointments is necessary.

6. Advance Bookings and Follow-Up
   A. Advance bookings are done for _____ scheduled appointments.
   B. Ensure that the patient receives a(n) _____ card.
   C. Using an appointment reminder system is known as a _____ file.

7. Issues Related to Arranging a Referral Appointment
   A. Information required for an outgoing or incoming referral includes:
      i. _____
      ii. _____
      iii. _____
      iv. _____
      v. _____
      vi. _____
      vii. _____
   B. Depending on the type of insurance, _____ may be necessary before scheduling the appointment.

8. Steps for Arranging a Referral Appointment
   A. Before providing the patient's name and other information, _____ that the practice accepts the patient's medical insurance.
   B. Record the referral appointment information in the _____, as well as on an appointment _____ for the patient.
   C. Record the name of the individual with whom you spoke in the _____, as well as on the _____.
   D. Notify the patient of the _____ and _____ of the appointment.

9. Patient Information Supplied When Scheduling Hospital Admissions
   A. Ask patient to state _____ address.
   B. Verify the _____ of the patient's first and last names.
   C. Verify _____ _____ in patient record.
   D. Ask the patient for _____ phone number and area code.
   E. Give the physician's statement from the _____ as the reason for the admission.
   F. Fax copy of _____ card.

10. Steps for Scheduling an Inpatient Surgical Procedure
      i. _____
      ii. _____
      iii. _____
      iv. _____
      v. _____
      vi. _____
      vii. _____
      viii. _____
      ix. _____
      x. _____

11. Steps for Scheduling an Outpatient Procedure
      i. _____
      ii. _____

iii. _____

iv. _____

v. _____

vi. _____

vii. _____

viii. _____

ix. _____

x. _____

xi. _____

xii. _____

12. Considerations for Handling Nonscheduled Patients

A. Determine the _____ of the patient's condition.

B. Ask the patient for his or her telephone number and where he or she is calling from, and determine whether the patient is _____.

C. Follow office _____ and _____ regarding handling emergency situations.

D. Inform the _____ immediately regarding a potential emergency.

KEY TERMINOLOGY REVIEW

Match the following medical terms with the correct definitions.

a. catch-up

b. cycle time

c. double-booking

d. matrix

e. triage

1. _____ Also known as assigning priority.

2. _____ A time when appointments are not scheduled.

3. _____ Process of blocking out times in the appointment schedule when the provider is unavailable or out of the office.

4. _____ The length of time the average patient spends in the medical office.

5. _____ Scheduling more than one patient for the same appointment time.

APPLIED PRACTICE

Follow the directions as instructed for each of the following questions.

1. Using the following information and the manual schedule on the following pages, create a matrix for the medical office. *(Remember to use a pencil.)*

   a. The medical offices open at 8:30 A.M. every day.

   b. The last appointment for the day is scheduled no later than 3:30 P.M.

   c. The office is closed for appointments for lunch starting at 12:00 P.M.; it reopens at 1:15 P.M.

   d. Dr. Cho has hospital rounds every Wednesday from 7:30 A.M.–10:00 A.M.

   e. Dr. Jackson has hospital rounds every Thursday from 7:45 A.M.–10:15 A.M.

   f. On February 3, Dr. Cho has a meeting at Alliance Assisted Living that starts at 3:30 P.M.

   g. On February 2, Dr. Jackson has a meeting with a pharmaceutical representative that is scheduled for 12:45–1:30 P.M.

2. Schedule the following patients on the appointment schedule.

   a. LaToya Atwater is a new patient to see Dr. Cho. Wednesdays work best for LaToya.
   b. Sujin Dalywhal wants to see Dr. Jackson on Thursday afternoon for an abdominal suture removal.
   c. Jose Alvarez calls on Wednesday morning because he has had a terrible headache for the past 2 days.
   d. Anna Maria DeCamillo is a diabetic patient who wants to see Dr. Jackson for her 3-month diabetic checkup on Wednesday afternoon.
   e. Mark Tomlinson wants to see Dr. Cho for his annual checkup on Thursday.
   f. Aiden Taylor needs to be seen on Thursday morning for his 3-year well-child visit with Dr. Jackson.
   g. Dr. Cho requests that an appointment be made on Wednesday morning with her patient, Lydia Pazmino, regarding her blood test results.

Pearson Family Clinic

Wednesday, February 2, 20xx

	Dr. S. Cho	Dr. A. Jackson
7:30		
7:45		
8:00		
8:15		
8:30		
8:45		
9:00		
9:15		
9:30		
9:45		
10:00		
10:15		
10:30		
10:45		
11:00		
11:15		
11:30		
11:45		
12:00		
12:15		
12:30		
12:45		

Wednesday, February 2, 20xx

	Dr. S. Cho	Dr. A. Jackson
1:00		
1:15		
1:30		
1:45		
2:00		
2:15		
2:30		
2:45		
3:00		
3:15		
3:30		
3:45		
4:00		

Thursday, February 3, 20xx

	Dr. S. Cho	Dr. A. Jackson
7:30		
7:45		
8:00		
8:15		
8:30		
8:45		
9:00		
9:15		
9:30		
9:45		
10:00		
10:15		
10:30		
10:45		
11:00		
11:15		
11:30		

Thursday, February 3, 20xx

	Dr. S. Cho	Dr. A. Jackson
11:45		
12:00		
12:15		
12:30		
12:45		
1:00		
1:15		
1:30		
1:45		
2:00		
2:15		
2:30		
2:45		
3:00		
3:15		
3:30		
3:45		
4:00		

LEARNING ACTIVITY: MULTIPLE CHOICE

Circle the correct answer to each of the following questions.

1. How many minutes do most patients consider to be an acceptable wait time prior to seeing the doctor?

    a. 10
    b. 15
    c. 20
    d. None of the above

2. Which of the following is an acceptable way to note a missed appointment in a hard-copy appointment book?

    a. Use white correction fluid to cover the patient's name.
    b. Use a black marker to obliterate the patient's name.
    c. Use an eraser to remove the patient's name.
    d. Write no-show (NS) both on the appointment schedule and in the patient's chart.

3. What is one way to remind patients of their upcoming appointment in the medical office?

   a. Send out a reminder card to the patient just prior to the appointment.
   b. Call the patient to remind him or her of the appointment.
   c. Send an e-mail to the patient to remind him or her of the appointment.
   d. All of the above

4. The _____ method of scheduling is where two or three patients are scheduled at the beginning of each hour, followed by single patient appointments every 10 to 20 minutes for the rest of that hour.

   a. wave
   b. modified wave
   c. open hours
   d. fixed appointment

5. The _____ method of scheduling is where patients are scheduled only for the first half of each hour. The first patient to arrive is seen first.

   a. wave
   b. modified wave
   c. open hours
   d. fixed appointment

6. The _____ method of scheduling is most commonly used in walk-in clinics, laboratories, and X-ray facilities where patients are typically seen on a first-come, first-served basis.

   a. wave
   b. modified wave
   c. open hours
   d. fixed appointment

7. To eliminate the need to "squeeze in" an emergency or unscheduled appointment, the medical assistant should integrate _____ into the office schedule, if office policy allows.

   a. more time
   b. time patterns
   c. wave scheduling
   d. None of the above

8. Examples of emergency conditions that require patients to be seen immediately include

   a. skin rash.
   b. pain or burning on urination.
   c. chest pain.
   d. All of the above

9. When confirming an appointment with a patient on the telephone, the patient should be asked to repeat which of the following information?

   a. Location of the appointment
   b. Date of the appointment
   c. Time of the appointment
   d. All of the above

10. Triage

    a. becomes necessary when more than one seriously ill patient is waiting to see the physician.
    b. takes place each time a patient visits the office.
    c. is only done in a hospital setting.
    d. is a skill performed only by the physician.

CRITICAL THINKING

Answer the following questions to the best of your ability. Use the textbook as a reference.

1. Dylan Reilly, CMA (AAMA), is working in a busy family practice office. The physicians and staff all agree that the appointment scheduling system is not working and patients are frequently waiting long periods of time for appointments. How should Dylan go about creating a new scheduling procedure for this office?

   _____

   _____

2. Armando Alonso is taking an administrative medical assisting course as part of his medical assisting training. He has been given an assignment to create a list of the information the patient should be given when scheduling the patient in order to help prepare the patient for medical procedures. What sort of information should Armando list?

   _____

   _____

3. Anna Simonenko, CMA (AAMA), is working at the front desk in a family practice clinic. Anna has been asked to schedule Roger Edetsberger for a procedure to be performed in the hospital. Anna tells Roger that she will need to call his insurance company before she can schedule the procedure. Roger asks, "Why do you need to do that? Can't you just schedule the procedure now and call the insurance company some other time?" What can Anna say to Roger?

   _____

   _____

   _____

RESEARCH ACTIVITY

Use Internet search engines to research the following topic and write a brief description of what you find. It is important to use reputable websites.

1. Research various appointment scheduling software programs for medical offices.

   What products are available?
   What must be considered prior to purchasing medical office software?
   What type of technical support is available?

   _____

   _____

   _____

   _____

   _____

CHAPTER 10
Office Facilities, Equipment, and Supplies

STUDENT STUDY GUIDE

Use the following guide to assist in your learning of the concepts from the chapter.

I. Medical Office Facility and Equipment

  1. Desirable Characteristics of a Medical Facility

    A. It should adhere to federal, state, and local _____ and _____ regulations.

    B. Things to be considered in setting up and _____ a medical office include the office layout and design.

    C. It makes a good _____ impression.

    D. It generates positive employee _____.

  2. Americans with Disabilities Act (ADA)

    A. The ADA protects the rights of the disabled regarding access to _____, _____, _____, _____, _____, and _____.

  3. Lighting and Colors

    A. _____ colors are typically used.

    B. _____ art should hang on the walls.

    C. Fish tanks are _____ for children and adults.

  4. Reception Room Safety

    A. Frayed cords, _____ _____, and extension cords are examples of of situations that pose safety risks.

    B. Ensure that staff members understand their _____ during a fire.

    C. Post _____ plans in a central location within the office.

  5. Equipment Typically Found in Administrative Areas

    i. _____

    ii. _____

    iii. _____

    iv. _____

    v. _____

    vi. _____

    vii. _____

    viii. _____

    ix. _____

  6. Factors Promoted by an Effective Office Flow

    i. _____

    ii. _____

    iii. _____

    iv. _____

    v. _____

7. Considerations for the Patient Entrance

   A. The _____ should include handrails, elevators, ramps, wheelchair-accessible door frames, patient lifts if necessary, and well-lit walkways.
   B. High steps should be _____.
   C. Push and pull indicators should be placed on _____.

8. Considerations for the Reception Area

   A. The desk area should provide _____ and protect the confidentiality of information.
   B. The desk area should allow for ease of _____ to patient records but at the same time protect patient privacy.
   C. The waiting area should contain seats that can be _____ and that provide good _____.
   D. Toys in the waiting area should be _____ and _____.

9. Considerations for Office Bathrooms

   i. _____
   ii. _____
   iii. _____
   iv. _____
   v. _____
   vi. _____
   vii. _____

10. Electronic Postage

   A. Electronic postage requires the user to apply for and receive approval from the _____ prior to use.
   B. The user is required to determine the _____ of postage required for letters and packages and then a computer interfaces with the postal system to print the appropriate postage.
   C. This method may be used in offices with a lot of _____ mail.

II. Supplies and Inventory

   1. Factors Affecting the Selection of Vendors

      i. _____
      ii. _____
      iii. _____
      iv. _____
      v. _____

   2. Considerations for Supply Inventory Control

      A. Mark the _____ sheet whenever an item is removed from the supply cabinet.
      B. Expendable supplies are also called _____ supplies.
      C. The _____ _____ is the lowest amount of a supply item the office should have before reordering.
      D. The office should also establish specific _____ when orders will be placed, so that orders for multiple items can be processed at the same time.

   3. Establishing an Ordering System

      A. It is important to determine when _____ of the supply will have been used and how long an order takes to arrive.
      B. Use of _____ reminders or _____ reminder cards may be useful.
      C. _____ scanning systems can be purchased as an ordering system.

4. Drug Samples
   A. These are small packages of drug samples for physicians to distribute to _____.
   B. They are provided by _____ representatives.
   C. The discarding of samples must be done according to _____ and _____ regulations.

KEY TERMINOLOGY REVIEW

Complete the following sentences using the correct key terms found at the beginning of the chapter.

1. The _____ is the legislation that protects the rights of the disabled regarding access to employment, public buildings, transportation, housing, schools, and health care facilities.

2. Supplies that are used up quickly and have a relatively inexpensive unit cost are called _____ supplies.

3. _____ equipment refers to items that require a large dollar amount to purchase (generally more than $500) and have a relatively long life.

4. The medical facility generally has a flow that lends itself easily to teamwork, time management, organized and efficient office equipment usage, and patient flow. This is known as _____.

5. _____ refers to the positive or negative state of mind of employees with regard to their work or work environment.

APPLIED PRACTICE

Read the scenario and answer the questions that follow.

> ### Scenario
> Javier Gomez, CMA (AAMA), is working in the front office of a busy family practice. His manager, Chris, has asked him to create a detailed inventory list of all of the supplies needed for his station at the patient check-out desk. Here is the list that Javier has started:

Name	Company	Amount on Hand
Pens	Office Supplies R Us	14
Message pad	Office Supplies R Us	2 tablets
Ink pad	Office Supplies R Us	2 pads

1. Based on the inventory list, what additional important information should Javier include before submitting his list to Chris?

   _____

   _____

   _____

2. Considering that Javier is working at a patient check-out desk, where patients pay copayments and schedule follow-up appointments as needed, what additional items would Javier be likely to add to his inventory list? Name at least five additional items.

_____

_____

_____

LEARNING ACTIVITY: MULTIPLE CHOICE

Circle the correct answer to each of the following questions.

1. ADA regulations ensure that every public facility
   a. is made easily accessible to the handicapped.
   b. provides unrestricted hallways.
   c. has elevators or ramps available.
   d. All of the above

2. When addressing safety issues in the medical office, concerns noted may include
   a. the use of throw rugs.
   b. the culture of the office.
   c. the tone of the office.
   d. All of the above

3. Issues to be considered when setting up a medical office include the
   a. employees who work in the office.
   b. office design and layout.
   c. other offices in the building.
   d. None of the above

4. The first element of office flow is the
   a. restrooms.
   b. patient entrance.
   c. placement of examination rooms.
   d. staff offices.

5. Which of the following is considered to be capital equipment?
   a. Copy machine
   b. EKG paper
   c. Medications
   d. All of the above

6. Uses and advantages of using a postal meter include which of the following?
   a. Metered mail does not have to be stamped when it arrives at the post office.
   b. A postal meter will calculate the exact postage required and either print it directly onto the letter or print out a strip to be affixed to the package.
   c. A postal meter allows for postage to be printed directly onto an envelope or onto an adhesive-backed strip that is placed directly on an envelope or package.
   d. All of the above

7. Examples of expendable supplies include

    a. scanners.
    b. the telephone system.
    c. clinical supplies such as catheters.
    d. All of the above

8. An inventory list of all sample drugs must be maintained to adhere to _____ regulations.

    a. Drug Enforcement Administration (DEA)
    b. Americans with Disabilities Act (ADA)
    c. Food and Drug Administration (FDA)
    d. None of the above

9. Which of the following guidelines should be followed with regard to drug samples?

    a. They must be placed in a secure location.
    b. They should be kept all together by category.
    c. All samples should be rotated like other supplies, with newer samples placed in the back behind samples of the same medication and strength with earlier expiration dates.
    d. All of the above

10. A warranty

    a. is a manufacturer's guarantee in writing that its product will perform correctly under normal conditions.
    b. can be purchased to cover a period of time after the original warranty has expired.
    c. will state in detail what is actually covered by the contract.
    d. provides for replacement of defective parts but for an additional charge.

CRITICAL THINKING

Answer the following questions to the best of your ability. Use the textbook as a reference.

1. Corey Steinberg, CMA (AAMA), has recently been hired to work as an administrative medical assistant in a busy cardiology practice. Corey has been given the task of creating a manual that outlines the warranty information as well as the maintenance schedule for each piece of medical office equipment. How should Corey go about beginning this task?

    _____

    _____

    _____

2. Monte Beaton, RMA, is the office manager in a gastroenterology practice. Monte has recently hired three new medical assistants and wants to ensure that they are properly trained to use each piece of equipment in the medical office. How can Monte ensure that the training is done properly?

    _____

    _____

    _____

3. Krystle Shawger is taking an administrative class as part of her medical assisting training. She has been given an assignment to write an essay describing how an equipment maintenance log would be useful in the medical office. What might Krystle include in her paper?

_____

_____

4. Marian Harrison, RMA, is the administrative office manager in a family practice clinic. She is writing an office policy for the inventory of administrative office equipment. What might her policy include?

_____

_____

_____

5. Joanne Felmer, CMA (AAMA), works in a walk-in clinic. At the weekly office staff meeting, the office manager mentioned the need for purchasing a new EKG machine. The office manager has asked Joanne to research the various options available. How should Joanne handle this task?

_____

_____

_____

RESEARCH ACTIVITY

Use Internet search engines to research the following topic and write a brief description of what you find. It is important to use reputable websites.

1. Conduct an Internet search for office and medical supply companies in your area and outside your area. Compare prices. Which companies supply products at competitive prices? What are the shipping charges? Which company seems to have the best variety of products? How could this information be useful for medical offices?

_____

_____

_____

_____

CHAPTER 11

Written Communication

STUDENT STUDY GUIDE

Use the following guide to assist in your learning of the concepts from the chapter.

I. Written Communication in the Medical Office

1. How Professionalism Is Reflected in Written Communication

    A. Professionalism is reflected in the physical _____ of the letter.
    B. Professionalism is reflected in the _____ of the message being sent.
    C. Professionalism is reflected in the use of grammar and _____.

2. Elements to Be Included in a Professional Letter

    A. The message should be _____ and to the point.
    B. The expected outcome should be _____.
    C. Threats or derogatory comments should _____ be made.
    D. Negative _____ should be avoided.

3. Ways to Improve Sentences and Paragraphs

    A. Ensure that the sentence length never exceeds _____ words.
    B. Eliminate all words that are _____.
    C. Cover _____ point in each paragraph.
    D. Avoid use of the _____ pronoun.
    E. Avoid redundancy and _____.
    F. Eliminate inflated _____.

4. Active vs. Passive Voice

    A. When using the active voice, the subject of the sentence does the _____.
    B. The use of the active voice is considered to be more effective because it is _____ and more _____ than the use of the passive voice.
    C. When using the passive voice, the _____ receives the action.

5. Rules for Writing Numbers

    A. Numbers _____ through _____ are spelled out.
    B. Only Arabic _____ are used in tables, statistical data, dates, measurements, money, percentages, and time.
    C. When placing numbers in columns, align them as follows: Arabic integers are aligned on the _____. Decimal numbers are aligned on the _____ point. Roman numerals are aligned on the _____.
    D. Do not use _____ when writing on-the-hour time.

6. Eight Parts of Speech

    i. _____
    ii. _____
    iii. _____
    iv. _____
    v. _____

vi. _____

vii. _____

viii. _____

7. Standard Components of a Business Letter

i. _____

ii. _____

iii. _____

iv. _____

v. _____

vi. _____

vii. _____

8. Address of the Recipient

A. The address is typed along the _____ margin and is _____-spaced.

B. The company name is typed exactly as shown on the company's own _____.

C. The name of the city is followed by a _____.

D. The two-letter state abbreviation is followed by _____ spaces and then the ZIP code.

9. Guidelines for Using Courtesy Titles

A. _____ is always an appropriate title for men.

B. If there is a professional title, such as MD or PhD, this is used instead of the _____ title.

C. _____ is used when the marital status of a woman is unknown.

D. _____ is appropriate for unmarried women who prefer that title and is also used for young girls.

10. Body of the Letter

A. The body contains the _____ of the letter.

B. It begins _____ lines below the salutation.

C. The body is _____-spaced, with _____-spacing between each paragraph.

D. Paragraphs are either _____ or indented on the first line.

E. Most letters bearing a single message are usually _____ or _____ paragraphs in length and are confined to a(n) _____ page.

11. Signature Line

A. The signature line is typed _____ lines below the complimentary close.

B. If the name and title are on the same line, they are separated by a _____.

C. The _____ must be written directly over the typed signature line before the letter is sent.

12. Steps for Composing a Business Letter

i. _____

ii. _____

iii. _____

iv. _____

v. _____

vi. _____

vii. _____

viii. _____

ix. _____

13. Developing a Two-Page Letter

A. _____ stationery is used only for the top sheet.

B. A _____-inch margin is used at the bottom of the page.

C. All pages following the first page must begin with the _____ and the _____ _____ of the letter.

14. Letter Styles
    i. _____
    ii. _____
    iii. _____
    iv. _____

15. Editing
    A. When editing medical reports, do not change the _____ of the report or _____ the meaning in any way.
    B. If the meaning seems to be unclear, check with the writer of the report before any _____ changes are made.
    C. When editing material that you have composed, changes can be made to increase _____.

16. Medical Abbreviations
    A. _____ medical abbreviations can be used in medical reports and when filing insurance documents.
    B. The _____ has released a list of abbreviations that should never be used.

17. Reference Tools for Writing
    i. _____
    ii. _____
    iii. _____
    iv. _____
    v. _____

II. Handing Mail in the Medical Office

1. Tasks Related to the Handling of Incoming Mail
    i. _____
    ii. _____
    iii. _____

2. Sizes of Letterhead Stationery
    A. _____ letterhead is used for most office correspondence.
    B. _____ or _____ style is used by some physicians for their social correspondence.
    C. _____ letterhead is a half-sheet used for brief letters and memoranda.

3. Folding and Inserting Letters into a No. 10 Envelope
    A. Fold the bottom _____ of the letter upward and crease the fold.
    B. Fold the top of the letter downward to _____ inch from the previous crease and crease this fold.
    C. Place this edge into the envelope _____.

4. Folding and Inserting Letters into a No. 63/4 Envelope
    A. Bring the bottom edge up to _____ inch from the top edge.
    B. Fold the right edge _____ the width of the paper and crease this fold.
    C. Fold the left edge to _____ inch from the previous crease and insert this edge into the envelope first.

5. Guidelines for Optimal Efficiency of OCR Scanning
    A. The address must be typed on the envelope using _____-spacing and capital letters with no _____.
    B. The last line in the address must include the city, the two-digit state code, and the ZIP code. The line must not exceed _____ characters.

6. Considerations When Typing an Envelope
   A. The bottom margin of the No. 10 envelope should be _____ inch with _____-inch margins on the left and right sides.
   B. No. 6¾ envelopes should have a _____-inch margin on the left side, with the address _____ lines from the top of the envelope.
   C. The return address for the sender should always be placed in the upper-_____ corner of the envelope.

7. ZIP Codes
   A. ZIP stands for _____ _____ _____.
   B. The first _____ numbers identify the city and all five digits combine to identify the individual post office and _____ within the city.
   C. _____ additional digits have been added to the ZIP code by the USPS. These represent the addressee's _____ location.

8. Common Types of Mail
   i.   _____
   ii. _____
   iii. _____
   iv. _____
   v.   _____
   vi. _____

9. Size Requirements for Mail
   A. Domestic mail must be at least _____ inch thick.
   B. Mail that is _____ inch or less in thickness must be _____ inches in height and at least _____ inches long. All mail not meeting this requirement is considered to be _____.
   C. Items that are bulky and lightweight are charged a _____.

10. Guidelines for Preparing Mail That Is to Be Metered
    A. Separate all _____ mail from the _____ mail.
    B. Separate all mail destined to either _____ or _____ from the rest of the international mail.
    C. When mailing letter-size envelopes, flaps must be _____, _____, or _____.
    D. Envelopes larger than a(n) _____ size envelope must be sealed before being sent.

11. Issues Related to Electronic Mail
    A. Electronic mail cannot be used if the original _____ on the document must be sent.
    B. The _____ of the message should remain as professional as if you were typing a letter to be sent through the USPS.
    C. E-mail is not efficient for use in _____.
    D. It is imperative to adhere strictly to all _____ confidentiality laws when using e-mail.

12. Issues Related to Instant Messaging
    A. Instant messaging is a way to communicate with another person in _____.
    B. Instant messages are not _____ documents and cannot be attached to a person's _____ records or be used in a court of law.
    C. Abbreviating words when instant messaging is not acceptable for electronic messages sent from within the _____.

13. Steps in Opening and Sorting Mail
    i. _____
    ii. _____
    iii. _____
    iv. _____
    v. _____
    vi. _____
    vii. _____
    viii. _____
    ix. _____
    x. _____
    xi. _____

14. Guidelines for Sending a Fax

    A. The _____ document is inserted into the fax machine.
    B. The _____ sheet should be sent first.
    C. All fax cover sheets must be _____ compliant.

15. Contents of a Fax Cover Sheet

    i. _____
    ii. _____
    iii. _____
    iv. _____
    v. _____

KEY TERMINOLOGY REVIEW

Without using your textbook, write a sentence using each selected key term in the correct context.

1. *active voice*

  _____
  _____

2. *electronic mail*

  _____
  _____

3. *homophones*

  _____
  _____

4. *letterhead*

  _____
  _____

5. *reference initials*

  _____
  _____

APPLIED PRACTICE

Follow the directions for each assignment.

1. Using proofreader's marks, make the necessary corrections to the body of the business letter. (Refer to Figure 11-5 in your textbook.)

> Mr. SUSAN Rowe (8-12-1877 was seen in my office today. She presents with complaints of
>
> upper right quadrant pain times too weeks. Mrs. Rowe states that along with the pain, she is
>
> experiencing nausea and vomiting. Upon palpation the abdomen appears bloated and is
>
> sensitive to the touch

2. Using word processing software, create an interoffice memo. Andrew Edwards, CMA (AAMA), is the sender of the memo and all clinical staff members are intended to be the recipients. The purpose of the memo is to inform the clinical staff that a pharmaceutical sales representative will be presenting information on a new cardiac drug that Dr. Sheila Tyrone is considering using for patient therapy. The presentation will occur on Friday during the lunch hour.

LEARNING ACTIVITY: MULTIPLE CHOICE

Circle the correct answer to each of the following questions.

1. Which of the following is the size of a standard business envelope?
   a. 3½" × 8½"
   b. 4⅛" × 9½"
   c. 4¼" × 9¼"
   d. None of the above

2. How much postage is required to mail an interoffice memo?
   a. $0.31
   b. $0.23
   c. $0.20
   d. None of the above

3. In order to catch all of the errors in a written document, how many times should the medical assistant read a letter before sending it out?
   a. Once
   b. Twice
   c. Three times
   d. Four times

4. The _____ of a professional letter typically appears two lines down from the ending portion of the body.
   a. closing
   b. subject line
   c. salutation
   d. letterhead

5. Which of the following pieces of information is typically included in the office letterhead?

   a. Office name
   b. Office address
   c. Office e-mail address
   d. All of the above

6. Which of the following statements is written correctly?

   a. The patient is taking five milligrams of the medication every hour.
   b. The patient is taking 5 milligrams of the medication every hour.
   c. The patient is taking five (5) milligrams of the medication every hour.
   d. All of the above are correct.

7. Which of the following words is misspelled?

   a. foreign
   b. occurrence
   c. liaison
   d. None of above is misspelled.

8. The closing appears _____ spaces below the end of the body of the letter.

   a. one
   b. two
   c. three
   d. four

9. Which of the following parts of speech modifies a noun or a pronoun?

   a. Verb
   b. Adverb
   c. Adjective
   d. Preposition

10. Which of the following styles of letters is spaced with all lines flush with the left margin except for the first line of each paragraph?

   a. Modified block
   b. Simplified letter block
   c. Semi-simplified letter block
   d. None of the above

CRITICAL THINKING

Answer the following questions to the best of your ability. Use the textbook as a reference.

1. Missy Hurst, RMA, is working as an administrative medical assistant with a gastroenterology practice. Dr. Brown has asked Missy to annotate the laboratory reports that come back from the lab. What is he asking Missy to do?

   _____

   _____

   _____

2. Henry Connelly, CMA (AAMA), has just been hired to work at the front desk in a family practice clinic. Part of his job is to open and sort the mail. No written office policy about this task is currently on file in the office, so Henry decides to create one. How should Henry proceed and what might his policy look like?

_____

_____

_____

3. Willie Pachinko, RMA, has been working with Dr. Stuart for several years. Dr. Stuart asks Willie to contact Mr. Brocheer regarding his lab results from earlier this week. Willie looks into Mr. Brocheer's chart and sees that the patient has listed his work e-mail address. Willie isn't able to reach Mr. Brocheer by telephone and instead of leaving a voice mail message asking the patient to return his call, Willie decides to e-mail the patient with his lab results. Later that day, Mr. Brocheer calls the office very upset. He tells Willie that his boss intercepted the e-mail and now knows that his employee was screened for a possible sexually transmitted disease. What did Willie do wrong?

_____

_____

_____

4. Mallory Valdez is taking an administrative medical assisting class. She has been given the assignment of writing a short paper that outlines the various mailing services offered by the U.S. Postal Service. What should Mallory include in her paper?

_____

_____

_____

RESEARCH ACTIVITY

Use Internet search engines to research the following topic and write a brief description of what you find. It is important to use reputable websites.

1. Visit www.usps.com and research information regarding certified mail, rates, and extra services available. When could some of the "extra services" be useful when dealing with written correspondence between the medical office and patients?

_____

_____

_____

_____

CHAPTER 12
Computers in the Medical Office

STUDENT STUDY GUIDE

Use the following guide to assist in your learning of the concepts from the chapter.

I. Computers in the Medical Office

1. Administrative Functions of Computers in the Medical Office (List six general functions.)

   i. _____
   ii. _____
   iii. _____
   iv. _____
   v. _____
   vi. _____

2. Central Processing Unit (CPU)

   A. The CPU acts as a traffic controller, directing the computer's _____ and sending electronic signals to the right place at the right time.
   B. The transmission speed of these electronic signals is measured in _____.
   C. One _____ equals one _____ cycles per second.
   D. The higher the _____, the faster the _____.

3. Random Access Memory (RAM)

   A. RAM is available only as long as the computer is _____.
   B. Once the computer is turned off, or powered down, all information stored in RAM is _____.

4. Read-Only Memory (ROM)

   A. ROM is _____, _____ storage.
   B. ROM is used to make the computer _____.
   C. Users cannot _____ or _____ the data in ROM.

5. The Computer Monitor

   A. Allows the user to _____ information on the computer.
   B. Monitors are available in a variety of _____ and _____.
   C. The screen size is measured _____, in inches.
   D. A _____ monitor displays anywhere from 16 to more than 1 million different colors.

6. Storage

   A. A hard-disk drive is located inside the computer with _____ access to the user.
   B. CD-ROM stands for _____.
   C. DVD stands for _____ or _____.

7. Computer Office Security Considerations

   A. Position the computer _____ so that it cannot be easily seen by patients.

   B. Use a(n) _____ screen around the computer workstation.

   C. Use a screen _____.

   D. Use computer _____.

8. Describe the following kinds of HIPAA security rules.

   i. Administrative: _____

   ii. Physical: _____

   iii. Technical: _____

9. Chair Ergonomics When Working on the Computer

   A. Push your hips as _____ back in the chair as possible.

   B. Adjust the seat height so that your feet are _____ on the floor and your knees are _____, or _____ than, your hips.

   C. Adjust the back of the chair to a(n) _____ to _____ reclined angle.

   D. Make sure that your upper and lower back are _____.

10. Ergonomics When Working on the Keyboard

   A. If possible, adjust the keyboard height so that your shoulders are _____, your elbows are in a slightly _____ position, and your wrists and hands are _____.

   B. Wrist rests can help maintain a(n) _____ posture and pad hard surfaces.

   C. Wrist rests should only be used to rest the _____ of the hands between keystrokes.

11. The Monitor and Ergonomics

   A. Adjust the monitor and source documents so that your _____ is in a neutral, relaxed position.

   B. Position the top of the monitor approximately _____ to _____ inches above your seated eye level.

   C. To reduce glare, place the screen at a(n) _____ angle to windows and adjust curtains or blinds.

12. Body Ergonomics When Working on the Computer

   A. Take short _____ or _____-minute stretch breaks every _____ to _____ minutes.

   B. After each hour of work, take a break or change tasks for at least _____ to _____ minutes.

   C. Avoid eye fatigue by resting and _____ your eyes periodically.

   D. Rest your eyes by covering them with your palms for _____ to _____ seconds.

KEY TERMINOLOGY REVIEW

Match each of the following terms with the correct definition.

   a. central processing unit (CPU)

   b. Internet service provider (ISP)

   c. output devices

   d. universal serial bus (USB)

   e. World Wide Web (WWW)

1. _____ Provides access to the Internet.

2. _____ Allow the user to see what the computer has accomplished.

3. _____ Acts as a traffic controller, directing the computer's activities and sending electronic signals to the right place at the right time.

4. _____ Feeds data and instructions into a computer.

5. _____ A small portable storage device that can hold up to 64 GB or more of data.

APPLIED PRACTICE

Read the scenario and answer the questions that follow.

> **Scenario**
>
> Shane Eiler, RMA, is an office manager for Inner Harbor Sports Medicine. His office computer has had a recent attack from a malware program. This attack has left his computer unusable.

1. Shane has been asked to research the cost of purchasing a new computer for the medical office. Create a list of the steps he should take to determine the type of system that is best for the office.

   _____

   _____

2. The physicians have also asked Shane to create a list of suggestions for securing the office computers from unauthorized access. What suggestions should Shane make?

   _____

   _____

LEARNING ACTIVITY: MULTIPLE CHOICE

Circle the correct answer to each of the following questions.

1. _____ are devices that allow documents to be copied and transferred to the computer.
   a. Thumb drives
   b. Personal digital assistants
   c. Printers
   d. Scanners

2. The _____ is the computer equipment.
   a. hardware
   b. software
   c. peripheral
   d. USB

3. The computer's CPU is considered to be the computer's
   a. brain.
   b. memory.
   c. keyboard.
   d. mouse.

4. _____ makes it possible for a computer to temporarily store data and programs.
   a. A mass storage device
   b. Memory
   c. Software
   d. The CPU

5. The hard-disk drive, a magnetic storage media inside the computer, is usually called the _____ drive.
   a. A
   b. B
   c. C
   d. D

CRITICAL THINKING

Answer the following questions to the best of your ability. Use the textbook and other resources such as the Internet in considering the following questions.

1. Marcia Dukat is taking a computer applications class in the medical assisting program. She has been given an assignment to create a list of steps that medical office staff can take in order to protect the office computers from viruses. What should Marcia's list include?

   _____

   _____

2. Rolf Von Trapp, RMA, is discussing the need for a new computer system with the physician. Dr. Nyrse has asked Rolf to describe the difference between the hardware, the software, and the peripherals that go with the various computer systems. How might Rolf define these three components?

   _____

   _____

3. George El Fashir, CMA (AAMA), has been asked to describe the various computer drives that might be used to store information from the computer systems in his office. What information should George prepare?

   _____

   _____

4. Riley Gaddum is taking a computer class as part of his medical assistant training. He has been given an assignment to describe the difference between ROM and RAM. What might Riley write for this assignment?

   _____

   _____

   _____

RESEARCH ACTIVITY

Use Internet search engines to research the following topic and write a brief description of what you find. It is important to use reputable websites.

1. Use the Internet to research medical office software programs. What software program do you like the most? What features does it have? Why would you recommend its use?

   _____

   _____

   _____

   _____

CHAPTER 13

Managing Paper Medical Records

STUDENT STUDY GUIDE

Use the following guide to assist in your learning of the concepts from the chapter.

I. Managing Paper Medical Records

   1. Standard records and reports found in a medical record include:

      i. _____

      ii. _____

      iii. _____

      iv. _____

      v. _____

      vi. _____

      vii. _____

      viii. _____

      ix. _____

      x. _____

      xi. _____

      xii. _____

      xiii. _____

      xiv. _____

      xv. _____

      xvi. _____

   2. The Chronological Medical Record

     A. The chronological medical record follows the patient _____.

     B. Each visit consists of a new entry by _____ rather than by _____ or _____.

     C. This record can sometimes make it more difficult to "catch" _____.

   3. The Problem-Oriented Medical Record

     A. The problem-oriented medical record is used to identify patient problems and chart by those _____.

     B. The functional aspect of this type of charting is that the patient _____ list is found at the _____ of the chart.

     C. As new problems and diagnoses are identified, they are noted on the _____ list.

     D. This type of charting helps health care providers who do not already know a specific patient to obtain a(n) _____ regarding previous visits and problems at a glance.

   4. Sections of the Problems-Oriented Medical Record

      i. _____

      ii. _____

      iii. _____

      iv. _____

5. SOAP Charting
    A. "S" identifies the _____ information gathered from the patient.
    B. "O" stands for _____, the data gathered during the visit.
    C. "A" is for _____, the physician's _____ diagnosis.
    D. "P" indicates the _____ of the chart where _____ for the care of this patient are discussed.

6. The Source-Oriented Medical Record
    A. Patient information is placed in the medical record in _____ order and is organized in different sections.
    B. Each office determines which _____ to be used and in what order they are to appear in the medical chart.

7. Components of Medical Records
    i. _____
    ii. _____
    iii. _____
    iv. _____
    v. _____
    vi. _____
    vii. _____
    viii. _____
    ix. _____
    x. _____

II. Filing
    1. Categories of Medical Records
        i. _____
        ii. _____
        iii. _____

    2. The Vertical File Cabinet
        A. This type is set up _____ to _____ stacked pull-out drawers holding up to _____ files per drawer.
        B. A drawback of this method is that the files are _____ and consume _____.

    3. The Lateral File Cabinet
        A. This type is set up with _____ allowing for easy access to files by pulling them off the _____.
        B. This type uses a(n) _____ method for visual recognition of files.

    4. The Movable File Cabinet
        A. This type is set up with _____ powered or _____ controlled file units that move on tracks in the floor.
        B. This method is a type of _____ filing system.
        C. This method is _____ saving because the file units can be moved close together when they are not in use.
        D. This method is useful for _____ and _____ because the floor can be reinforced when the track is installed.

5. File Folders

    A. The patient's file typically has tabs on the _____ or _____ edge.

    B. These tabs are marked with _____ labels.

    C. It is easier to read the labels in the file drawer if the files have _____ tab cuts.

    D. File folders may be _____ to indicate the primary care physician.

6. Outguide

    A. The outguide is inserted where a file has been _____ to indicate the place to which the file should be _____.

    B. It can be used to indicate who has _____ the file and when it was _____.

    C. The outguide is especially helpful in a large office when trying to _____ charts.

    D. Usually a distinctive color, such as _____, is used to indicate that a file is missing.

7. The Purposes of Labels on File Folders

    A. The main purpose is to _____ what is in the file.

    B. The label can include a(n) _____ stripe that can be used for other purposes, such as identifying the _____ physician.

    C. Offices use special labels on charts to bring attention to patient _____, required _____, and the year of the last visit.

    D. Special labels help the staff find _____ information at a glance.

8. Rules for an Alphabetical Filing System

    A. A name with only a(n) _____ in place of the first name is filed before a(n) _____ name.

    B. Hyphenated names are treated as _____ unit.

    C. Apostrophes are _____.

    D. Titles and initials are _____, but placed in _____ after the name.

    E. Married women are to be indexed using their _____ name.

    F. Seniority units are filed _____.

9. Numerical Filing or Patient Identification System

    A. This type of system is used in _____ and many larger clinics.

    B. A number is assigned to each patient's _____.

    C. The number is generally a(n) _____-digit number divided into _____ sections of _____ digits each.

10. Straight Numerical Filing

    A. This is the _____ numerical method.

    B. Each record is filed _____ based on its assigned number.

    C. Numbers used in this system begin at _____ and continue upward.

11. Terminal-Digit Filing

    A. This method is based on the last digits of the _____ number.

    B. It evenly distributes the files within the entire filing system, eliminating the need for frequent _____ of files.

    C. It requires dividing the files into _____ primary sections, starting with _____ and ending with _____.

    D. Three sections of numbers assigned to each file are designated as _____, _____, and _____ sections, respectively.

12. Unit-Number Filing

    A. This method assigns a number to patients the _____ time that they are seen or admitted to a hospital.

    B. All other hospitalizations or hospital visits use the _____ number.

    C. This method requires that all of the records be kept at the _____ location.

13. Serial-Number Filing

    A. With this system, the patient receives a different medical record number for each _____ visit.

    B. The patient acquires _____ records that are stored at _____ locations.

    C. The assigned numbers are kept in a(n) _____ record in which numbers in sequential order have a(n) _____ placed next to them as each new _____ is entered.

14. Subject-Matter Filing

    A. This method is used for _____ files.

    B. This method is adequate as long as the files are relatively _____.

15. Color-Coding Systems

    A. These systems assign a(n) _____ for each number from _____.

    B. _____ bars on files correspond to the medical record number.

    C. The system allows for misfiles to be _____ seen.

16. The Alpha-Z System

    A. The system is based on _____ colors using _____ letters on a(n) _____ background for the first half of the alphabet, with the addition of a white stripe on the _____ background for the second half of the alphabet.

    B. The system uses _____ to denote the patient's name and a colored label with the letter of the alphabet to indicate the _____ unit.

    C. In large practices with several physicians, each physician may have a(n) _____ assigned to him or her.

17. Cross-Referencing Files

    A. Cross-referencing refers to alerting a health worker that a file may be found under a(n) _____.

18. Tips for Locating Missing Files

    i. _____

    ii. _____

    iii. _____

    iv. _____

    v. _____

    vi. _____

19. Tickler Files

    A. A tickler file is used to _____ the medical assistant of future events or actions.

    B. It should be reviewed _____.

    C. Contents may include _____, _____, _____, and _____.

III. Releasing, Retaining, and Storing Medical Records

  1. Authorizing the Release of Records

    A. The _____ owns the information on the medical record.

    B. The patient has the _____ right to access the record.

    C. A(n) _____ must be signed to authorize the release of a patient's record.

  2. Guidelines for Retaining Medical Records

    A. To be absolutely safe, medical records should be retained _____.

    B. The standard set by most states is to keep records _____ to _____ years after the last treatment or _____ years after the patient reaches the age of _____.

    C. The AMA recommends keeping the records for _____ years.

KEY TERMINOLOGY REVIEW

Match each of the following medical terms with the correct definition.

a. active records
b. inactive records
c. medical record
d. POMR
e. SOAP

1. _____ Source of all documentation related to the patient.

2. _____ Used to identify patient problems and chart by those problems.

3. _____ Patients who have been seen within the past 3 years and are currently being treated.

4. _____ A charting method that is distinct because of the four parts of the approach.

5. _____ Patients who have not been seen within the past 3 years or another period determined by office policy.

APPLIED PRACTICE

Follow the instructions for each question.

1. Indicate whether the following patients would be considered active, inactive, or closed patient files.

   a. Lori Hughes, a patient who has moved out of the state
      Patient file status: _____

   b. Quin Tao, a patient who has not been seen in the office for 5 years
      Patient file status: _____

   c. Gloria Sanchez, a patient who was in the office for care last week
      Patient file status: _____

   d. Sara Womack, a patient who died last year
      Patient file status: _____

2. Accurately place the statements below into SOAP format on the accompanying Progress Note form. Mario Reynolds, born August 12, 1990, presents to the office with the following:

   - T: 100.3°
   - Positive Rapid Strep Test
   - "My throat is sore."
   - Pharyngitis and Strep Throat
   - Throat appears red and white spots present on tonsils.
   - Penicillin V 250mg BID × 10 days
   - BP: 118/86
   - Wt: 192#
   - Patient has been sick with a fever for 3 days.

PROGRESS NOTE

Patient: _____ **DOB:** _____

	S	O	A	P	

LEARNING ACTIVITY: MULTIPLE CHOICE

Circle the correct answer to each of the following questions.

1. Under which of the following circumstances can the patient's medical record be copied and released?
   a. When the patient's spouse comes to the office to request a copy
   b. When the patient's employer calls the office to request a copy
   c. When the patient has signed a release form
   d. When the patient's brother sends a letter asking for a copy

2. The American Medical Association recommends keeping medical records
   a. for 2 years.
   b. for 5 years.
   c. for 10 years.
   d. indefinitely.

3. _____ patient files are the files of patients who have not been seen within the past 3 years or another period determined by office policy.
   a. Open
   b. Closed
   c. Inactive
   d. None of the above

4. The simplest numerical method of filing is
   a. straight numerical filing.
   b. terminal-digit filing.
   c. middle-digit filing.
   d. unit-number filing.

5. _____ is a type of medical charting that tracks a patient's problems throughout medical care by assigning a number to each of the patient's medical problems.
   a. Narrative notes
   b. SOAP notes
   c. POMR notes
   d. None of the above

CRITICAL THINKING

Answer the following questions to the best of your ability. Use the textbook and other resources such as the Internet in considering the following questions.

1. Chris Nichols, CMA (AAMA), has been given the task of deciding which patient files to purge from the clinic in order to create more storage space. How should Chris proceed with this project?

   _____

   _____

   _____

2. Michael Manson, RMA, has just been hired to work in a family practice clinic. On his first day in the office, he notices that many patients' records have words such as "problem" and "talker" listed on them. He asks the MA who is training him about these words and is told that it is the office's way of noting those patients who are difficult to work with or who talk excessively during their visit. What kinds of problems might this facility encounter when using these notations?

   _____

   _____

   _____

3. Susan Haufe, RMA, is working with a small, one-doctor internal medicine clinic. The physician, Dr. Chentow, is unable to retain his patient records indefinitely. What considerations must Susan give to the method of destruction?

   _____

   _____

   _____

RESEARCH ACTIVITY

Use Internet search engines to research the following topic and write a brief description of what you find. It is important to use reputable websites.

1. Research the types of filing systems that may be found in a medical setting. Describe the advantages and disadvantages of each system.

   _____

   _____

   _____

   _____

   _____

CHAPTER 14

Electronic Health Records

STUDENT STUDY GUIDE

Use the following guide to assist in your learning of the concepts from the chapter.

I. Electronic Health Records

  1. Electronic Health Records (EHRs)

    A. EHRs are sometimes called _____.

    B. The EHR is a means of _____, _____, and _____ information about the patient and the care received in the medical setting.

  2. Functions of the EHR

    i. _____

    ii. _____

    iii. _____

    iv. _____

    v. _____

    vi. _____

    vii. _____

    viii. _____

    ix. _____

    x. _____

    xi. _____

    xii. _____

    xiii. _____

  3. Converting from Paper to Electronic Health Records

    A. Some clinics are able to use a(n) _____ to _____ the patient's paper medical record for use in the EHR system.

    B. Other clinics may need to enter information from the paper medical record to the EHR _____.

  4. Data Backup System

    A. A backup system is mandated by _____.

    B. It must be used on a(n) _____ basis.

  5. Cost Savings of Using an EHR

    i. _____

    ii. _____

    iii. _____

    iv. _____

    v. _____

    vi. _____

    vii. _____

    viii. _____

6. Electronic Signatures
   A. Most electronic health records provide an electronic signature component that is based on the individual's _____ via his or her user name and _____.
   B. Once the entry is made into the patient's chart, the staff member or physician clicks _____ and the entry is electronically _____.

7. Avoiding Medical Errors
   A. EHR software typically has a(n) _____ mechanism built in that alerts the prescribing physician to any _____ medications that a particular patient may be taking.
   B. Studies have found that many medical errors are caused by _____ or _____ handwriting, a problem that would be eliminated if providers made their entries electronically.

8. Availability of Medical Records Online
   A. Some clinics allow patients to look up portions of their EHR via the _____.
   B. Using a _____-_____ system, patients can access a company's network or intranet for their laboratory results, dates of immunization, or history of medications prescribed.

KEY TERMINOLOGY REVIEW

Without using your textbook, write a sentence using each of the selected key terms in the correct context.

1. *Electronic health record*

   _____

   _____

2. *Electronic signature*

   _____

   _____

3. *Health Insurance Portability and Accountability Act (HIPAA)*

   _____

   _____

4. *Meaningful use*

   _____

   _____

   _____

APPLIED PRACTICE

Read the scenario and then answer the questions that follow.

Scenario

Jeffery Cody, RMA, is the office manager for Foothills Family Medicine. The office has slowly been transferring from paper medical records to electronic health records.

1. In the final stages of this process, how will the medical office include written reports and consultations from other facilities?

_____

_____

2. Jeffery is writing a memo to the office staff regarding making corrections to medical records. What information should he include in his memo?

_____

_____

LEARNING ACTIVITY: TRUE/FALSE

Indicate whether the following statements are true or false by placing a T or an F on the line that precedes each statement.

_____ 1. Electronic health records offer enhanced ease, efficiency, and accessibility.

_____ 2. Using electronic health records, a medical office can send reminder postcards to patients more easily than performing this task using paper medical records.

_____ 3. Using electronic health records, a medical office is able to perform many tests in the office and have the results shown immediately in the EHR.

_____ 4. Most EHR programs have drop-down menus that allow the user to choose information from a list.

_____ 5. EHR systems may alert health care providers to possible medication errors.

CRITICAL THINKING

Answer the following questions to the best of your ability. Use the textbook as a reference.

1. Rosa Valdez, CMA (AAMA), is working in the billing office of a urology practice. The office uses electronic health records for patient charting. Rosa frequently finds that she needs to alert other staff members of her need to speak with a patient about the patient's account. How might Rosa devise a way to alert her coworkers of her need to see a patient when that patient comes into the office?

_____

_____

2. Chris Hernandez, RMA, is the office manager of a busy family practice clinic. Chris has been asked by the physicians to come up with some ideas for using EHR software to create a marketing program. What kinds of ideas could Chris suggest for this project?

_____

_____

_____

3. Mickey Cape is taking a course on electronic health records. Mickey has been given an assignment to write a policy on how to dispose of paper medical records once the records have been converted to electronic form. What might Mickey come up with?

_____

_____

_____

4. Barret Risenhour, RMA, is the office manager in a women's clinic. The physicians in the clinic are considering moving to electronic health records from the paper records that they have been using for years. Barret has been asked to create a list of the pros and cons of using electronic health records versus paper records. What might Barret's list contain?

_____

_____

_____

5. Dr. Shawn Hagen has been using paper medical records in his practice for more than 20 years. He is reluctant to change to electronic health records because he feels that his computer skills are poor. What sort of information can his office manager give him about the ease of converting from paper to electronic health records?

_____

_____

_____

RESEARCH ACTIVITY

Use Internet search engines to research the following topic and write a brief description of what you find. It is important to use reputable websites.

1. Locate three companies that sell EHR software. Create a list of the advantages and disadvantages of each system.

_____

_____

_____

_____

_____

CHAPTER 15
Medical Insurance

STUDENT STUDY GUIDE

Use the following guide to assist in your learning of the concepts from the chapter.

I. Health Insurance and Managed Care

    1. A medical office must operate as a(n) _____.

    2. The Basics of Insurance

        A. Insurance provides protection from _____ and _____ loss.
        B. Money is paid to the _____.
        C. Premiums are paid for by the _____.

    3. Medical Insurance

        A. The person who owns the policy is the _____, the _____, the _____, or the _____.
        B. Family members covered by the policy are called _____.
        C. Premiums are usually paid _____.
        D. In _____ coverage, the employer often pays the _____ of the premium.

    4. Health Maintenance Organization (HMO)

        A. An HMO is a type of _____ plan.
        B. The original intent was to _____ health care costs.
        C. Membership is limited to certain _____.
        D. Services are provided for a(n) _____ fee.
        E. Patients must see the plan's _____ physicians.
        F. Emphasizes the _____ of health.

    5. Preferred Provider Organization (PPO)

        A. The purpose is to _____ costs.
        B. Patients must use _____ providers.
        C. Members are not restricted to designated _____ or _____.

    6. Point-of-Service Plan (POS)

        A. A POS is a type of _____ plan.
        B. It offers more _____ than some HMOs and PPOs.
        C. An out-of-network or _____ provider may be seen.

II. Group-Sponsored or Individual (Commercial) and Government Plans

    1. Commercial Insurance Carriers

        A. These are typically _____ organizations.
        B. They often offer both traditional _____ service plans and _____ plans.
        C. They require subscribers to pay a(n) _____ for membership.

    2. Contents of a Health Insurance Card

        i. _____
        ii. _____

iii. _____

iv. _____

v. _____

vi. _____

vii. _____

3. Blue Cross/Blue Shield

   A. Patients may have Blue Cross (BC) and Blue Shield (BS) plans through _____ health coverage or individual insurance.

   B. Historically, BC plans provided _____ service benefits and BS plans provided _____ service benefits.

4. Medicare

   A. Medicare is health coverage provided by the _____.

   B. It is available to persons who are age _____ and older and those who are _____.

   C. It is operated by the _____.

   D. Medicare is the single _____ payer of health care services in the United States.

5. Medicare Parts A and B

   A. Part A provides coverage for _____ expenses.

   B. No _____ is paid for Part A.

   C. A(n) _____ deductible must be met for Part B.

6. Medicare Coverage

   A. Medicare pays all expenses for the first _____ days of hospitalization.

   B. Medicare Part _____ does cover Skilled nursing facility (SNF) care (facility for long-term care where patients must be monitored by nursing staff regularly).

   C. One very important aspect to billing Medicare is a form called the _____ (ABN)

7. Medicare Part D

   A. Part D is offered by _____ insurance companies.

   B. IPart D covers _____ and _____ drugs at participating pharmacies.

   C. It covers a(n) _____ list of prescription drugs at participating pharmacies.

   D. Part D has an a _____ _____, _____ or coinsurance, and a _____ benefit level.

8. Medigap Plans

   A. Medigap (MG) is a _____ _____ policy that supplements Medicare coverage.

   B. Medigap is billed _____ Medicare has determined its portion of the payment.

9. Medicaid

   A. Medicaid is health coverage for _____ patients.

   B. It is paid for by _____ and _____ governments.

   C. Low-income elderly or disabled patients often have both _____ and _____ coverage.

   D. The rules of eligibility and payment _____ by state.

   E. Typically, individuals must qualify on a(n) _____ basis.

10. Workers' Compensation

   A. Occupational injuries are those that occur during the course of _____.

   B. A workers' compensation claim is initiated by filing the _____ _____ of Illness or Injury.

   C. There are three types of claims: _____, _____, and _____.

11. Claims

   A. The physician fee schedule is determined by _____ fees.

   B. Resource-based fee schedules are also known as _____, or ROVs.

12. Preauthorization
    A. Preauthorization is also called _____, _____.
    B. It must be acquired prior to the patient's appointment, unless it is a(n) _____.
    C. Failure to obtain preauthorization may _____ treatment.
    D. If service is provided without preauthorization, the insurance carrier may _____ to pay.

13. Calling the Insurance Carrier for Precertification
    A. Preauthorizations may be valid for a _____ period of time.
    B. Gather all pertinent _____ information prior to calling the insurance carrier.

14. Verification of Benefits
    i. _____
    ii. _____
    iii. _____
    iv. _____
    v. _____

15. Steps for Obtaining Approval
    i. _____
    ii. _____
    iii. _____
    iv. _____
    v. _____

16. Steps to Take When Preauthorization Is Denied
    i. _____
    ii. _____
    iii. _____

17. Referrals
    A. A referral requires paperwork to be sent to the _____ physician.
    B. The referral recommendation must be made _____.
    C. Documentation must be placed in the _____.

18. Steps in Obtaining a Managed Care Referral
    i. _____
    ii. _____
    iii. _____
    iv. _____
    v. _____
    vi. _____
    vii. _____

KEY TERMINOLOGY REVIEW

Match each of the following selected key terms with the correct definition.

a. claim
b. deductible
c. formulary

d. premium
e. referral

1. _____ The portion the patient must pay before the insurance company will pay any benefits.
2. _____ An approved list of medications specific to each insurance carrier.
3. _____ Used to send a patient for treatment to another facility or physician.
4. _____ A fixed monthly fee or semimonthly fee.
5. _____ A written and documented request for reimbursement.

APPLIED PRACTICE

Complete the activity and answer the questions that follow. Select and complete Activity 1 if you currently have health insurance. Select and complete Activity 2 if you currently do not have health insurance.

1. If you have health insurance, do you know everything about your plan? Conduct research either through the Internet or by calling your insurance company to find out the following information:

   a. What conditions does the insurance plan not cover?

   _____

   _____

   b. For conditions not covered, is it possible to receive coverage for an additional fee?

   _____

   _____

   c. When is preauthorization required, who typically should perform this activity?

   _____

   _____

2. If you do not have health insurance, begin to research the types of health insurance plans that may be affordable for you in your area.

   a. Does your school offer health insurance for students? If so, what is the cost and what type of coverage is offered?

   _____

   _____

   b. List two other types of insurance plans you found in your area that may be affordable for you. If your school offers health insurance, what is the difference between these two other plans and the plan offered by the school?

   _____

   _____

   c. When is preauthorization required for the plans you researched, and who typically should perform this activity?

   _____

   _____

3. Complete the CMS-1500 form (Figure 15-8) using the patient registration form, the encounter form, and the fee schedule that is provided.

AUDIOLOGY SERVICES		
Screening audio air only	92551	$ 38.00
Pure tone air	92552	$ 37.00
Pure tone air and bone	92553	$ 50.00
Comprehensive audio	92557	$101.00
Loudness balance test	92562	$ 38.00
Tone decay	92563	$ 41.00
Tympanography	92567	$ 40.00
Acoustic reflex	92568	$ 42.00
Reflex decay	92569	$ 43.00
Visual reinforced audio	92579	$ 78.00
Brain stem audiogram	92585	$327.00

CRITICAL THINKING

Answer the following questions to the best of your ability. Use the textbook and other resources such as the Internet in considering the following questions.

1. Monica Swinger is taking an administrative medical assisting course. She has been given the assignment of writing an essay describing how health insurance began in the United States. What information should Monica include?

   _____

   _____

2. Erica Owsley, CMA (AAMA), is working with Charles Wong, a patient in the clinic where Erica works. Charles tells Erica he has the option of buying into the group insurance plan that his employer offers or he can buy an individual policy on his own. He isn't sure which option to choose and asks Erica if she can tell him the differences between individual and group insurance plans. What should Erica tell Charles?

   _____

   _____

RESEARCH ACTIVITY

Use Internet search engines to research the following topic and write a brief description of what you find. It is important to use reputable websites.

1. Using the Internet as a research source, find your state's Medicaid website and research the criteria for being covered under Medicaid in your state. Write an essay describing the persons who may be covered under Medicaid in your state.

   _____

   _____

   _____

   _____

   _____

CHAPTER 16
Diagnosis Coding

STUDENT STUDY GUIDE

Use the following guide to assist in your learning of the concepts from the chapter.

I. ICD-10-CM Coding

1. The Role of Medical Assistants (MAs) in Coding

   A. MAs assist in communication between the _____ and the _____ when questions arise.
   B. MAs provide _____ when an insurance preauthorization is needed for a procedure.
   C. MAs facilitate communication with _____ who may need information when representing a patient.
   D. MAs answer _____ questions about the meanings of the codes on their insurance paperwork.
   E. MAs review _____ documentation.

2. The History of Coding

   A. Historically, diagnosis coding was used to track the study of _____ and the _____ of _____.
   B. WHO is the _____.

3. ICD-10-CM

   A. There are _____ codes in ICD-10-CM.
   B. The codes are _____ to _____ characters long.
   C. The seventh character is used for _____.
   D. The _____ character is always alphabetic.
   E. The _____ character is always numeric.
   F. The _____ is mandatory after the third character.
   G. The character "X" is known as a(n) _____.

4. Compliance Programs Characteristics

   i. _____
   ii. _____
   iii. _____
   iv. _____
   v. _____
   vi. _____
   vii. _____

5. Organization of the ICD-10-CM Manual

   A. Introductory material includes _____-_____; _____; _____; and _____.
   B. The Index includes _____; _____; _____; _____ and _____.
   C. The Tabular List includes _____.

6. Conventions

    A. Conventions are specialized rules, _____, _____, and symbols.

    B. _____ notes appear immediately under a code in the tabular text.

    C. Excludes2 means that the condition _____ part of the condition represented by the code.

7. Index to Diseases and Injuries

    A. The index is organized _____ by main term and subterm.

    B. A table of _____ and chemicals is also found in the index.

8. Tabular List

    A. The Tabular List is an alphanumerically sequenced list based on _____.

    B. Chapter 9 of the Tabular List covers _____.

    C. The code range for Chapter 15 of the Tabular List is _____.

9. How to Code

    A. Three basic steps of diagnosis coding are _____, _____, and _____.

    B. Medical assistants _____ information from the medical record to identify the information necessary to code for answers.

    C. After determining the diagnoses in the patient's medical record, use the _____ to assign an actual code number.

    D. Preliminary codes found in the index must be verified in the _____.

    E. Reporting incorrect codes on an insurance claim can create problems such as _____, _____, _____, and _____.

KEY TERMINOLOGY REVIEW

Match each of the following selected key terms with the correct definition.

    a. ICD-10-CM   d. OGCR

    b. compliance   e. PPACA

    c. fraud

1. _____ Contains numeric and alphanumeric diagnostic codes.

2. _____ Patient Protection and Affordable Care Act.

3. _____ Following the rules.

4. _____ Knowingly billing for services that were never given.

5. _____ Official Guidelines for Coding and Reporting.

APPLIED PRACTICE

ICD-10-CM Coding Exercises

For each of the following, underline the main term. Look up each condition in the ICD-10-CM Index to Diseases, and then verify the code in the Tabular list. Write the code on the line provided.

1. _____ Pain in the right shoulder

2. _____ Plantar wart

3. _____ Cluster headache syndrome, not intractable

4. _____ Encounter for routine child health examination, without abnormal findings

5. _____ Atypical atrial flutter

6. _____ Kidney stones (calculi)

7. _____ Addison anemia

8. _____ Open bite, right thigh, initial encounter

9. _____ Malignant neoplasm of the large intestine

10. _____ Paralytic lagophthalmos, left lower eyelid

11. _____ Diaper rash

12. _____ Celiac disease

13. _____ Congenital glaucoma

14. _____ Type 2 diabetes with diabetic nephropathy

15. _____ Chronic fatigue

16. _____ Acute bronchitis due to *Streptococcus*

17. _____ Incomplete spontaneous abortion, without complication

18. _____ Cannabis abuse with intoxication delirium

19. _____ First degree burn, left shoulder, subsequent encounter

20. _____ Cholesteatoma of the tympanum, right ear

CRITICAL THINKING

Answer the following questions to the best of your ability. Use the textbook as a reference.

1. Teresa Clymer is taking a course in medical insurance billing as part of her medical assistant training. She has been asked to write a paper describing how proper diagnostic coding is linked to proper reimbursement from insurance carriers. What information should Teresa include in her paper?

   _____

   _____

2. Mavis Raschenko, RMA, has been asked by her office manager to explain the difference between ICD-9 and ICD-10. Cite the differences and the benefits of the revisions.

   _____

   _____

RESEARCH ACTIVITY

Use Internet search engines to research the following topic and write a brief description of what you find. It is important to use reputable websites.

1. Go to your state's website for the Department of Health. Research the laws that apply to billing for medical services in your state. Create a list of the laws that are relevant to the issue of fraudulent practices in billing and coding.

   _____

   _____

   _____

   _____

   _____

CHAPTER 17
Procedural Coding

STUDENT STUDY GUIDE

Use the following guide to assist in your learning of the concepts from the chapter.

I. Procedural Coding

1. Procedure Coding

   A. Procedure coding is the act of _____ to procedures and services that physicians provide to patients.
   B. Procedure codes have been standardized since _____.
   C. CPT means _____.
   D. Medical assistants are often involved with assigning procedure codes to _____ procedures and services.
   E. If medical assistants have questions about assigning a code, they should reach out to a(n) _____.

2. Fraud and Abuse

   A. Fraud is _____ for services _____ provided.
   B. Abuse is _____ behavior and _____ that result in improper financial gain but are not fraudulent.
   C. Coding for a higher level of service than originally provided is _____.
   D. List four examples of Medicare abuse.
      i. _____
      ii. _____
      iii. _____
      iv. _____

3. The CPT Manual

   A. Covers all procedures approved by the _____ and _____ administration.
   B. It lists over _____ codes.
   C. The CPT manual is updated _____.
   D. The CPT manual consists of a(n) _____, a(n) _____, and several _____.
   E. Inside the front cover or the first several pages of the manual is a list of commonly used _____, _____, and _____.
   F. Appendix J contains codes for _____.
   G. _____ codes describe widely used services and procedures.
   H. Category II codes are _____ codes used to collect and track data for performance assessment.
   I. Category III codes are _____ codes.
   J. The CPT appendices provide _____ information.

4. Procedure Coding
   A. Step One: _____ procedures from the medical file.
   B. Step Two: Look up the procedure(s) in the _____.
   C. Step Three: Verify the code in the _____.
   D. This section contains an index of injuries resulting from _____ causes.

5. Evaluation and Management
   A. These codes describe patient _____ for the evaluation and management of a health problem.
   B. They are the most _____ used codes in the medical office.
   C. Step One: _____ the type of service.
   D. Step Two: Determine the _____ and _____ factors.
   E. Step Three: Verify the _____ with the documentation.
   F. Step Four: Identify _____ and _____ services.
   G. Step Five: Append _____.
   H. In addition to coding for office visits, MAs may need to code for _____, radiology, and _____.

6. Health Care Common Procedure Coding System (HCPCS)
   A. The HCPCS is usually referred to as _____ in the industry.
   B. The level II HCPCS code range for chemotherapy drugs is _____ to _____.
   C. The HCPCS modifier for the lower right eyelid is _____.

KEY TERMINOLOGY REVIEW

Match each of the following selected key terms with the correct definition.

a. modifier
b. principal diagnosis
c. procedural coding

d. symbols
e. upcoding

1. _____ Used in circumstances in which the procedure code does not accurately describe the procedure.

2. _____ Used in the CPT Manual to distinguish changes or give instructions to be used when coding.

3. _____ The process of translating a narrative description of procedures into numbers.

4. _____ The reason that the patient sought care on a particular date.

5. _____ Contains increased specificity and includes recently discovered or diagnosed diseases.

APPLIED PRACTICE

CPT Coding Exercises

For each of the following, underline the main term. Look up each procedure in the CPT Index, and then select and verify the code in the Tabular List. Write the code on the line provided.

1. _____ Surgical laparoscopy with partial nephrectomy
2. _____ Allergy patch application test, 5 tests
3. _____ Repair of blood vessel, direct, right hand

4. _____ Evaluation and management of a new patient, for an office visit that includes an expanded problem-focused history, an expanded problem-focused examination, and straightforward medical decision making

5. _____ Urinalysis, non-automated, without microscopy

6. _____ Gill operation

7. _____ Needle biopsy of cervical lymph node

8. _____ Anesthesia for an open total hip arthroplasty

9. _____ Diagnostic thyroid uptake scan, nuclear medicine

10. _____ Partial laryngectomy, laterovertical

11. _____ Nephrostomy with drainage

12. _____ X-ray of the cervical spine, 4 views

13. _____ Flexible colonoscopy, proximal to splenic flexure, diagnostic

14. _____ Excision of a malignant lesion from the skin of the right arm, excised diameter 1.1 to 2.0 cm

15. _____ Routine obstetric care including antepartum care, vaginal delivery, and postpartum care

16. _____ Myringotomy including aspiration

17. _____ Nissen fundoplasty via laparotomy

18. _____ Routine ECG, 12 leads, with interpretation and report

19. _____ Incision and drainage of a bursa on the left foot

20. _____ Lipid panel laboratory test

LEARNING ACTIVITY: MULTIPLE CHOICE

Circle the correct answer for each of the following questions.

1. The CPT Manual has _____ major sections.
   a. three
   b. four
   c. five
   d. six

2. All CPT codes are _____ digits long.
   a. four
   b. five
   c. six
   d. All of the above

3. Within the CPT Manual, _____ indicate(s) that this is a new code.
   a. a black circle
   b. a triangle
   c. two triangles
   d. a circle with an inner dot

4. Within the CPT Manual, _____ indicate(s) that this is a revised code.
   a. a black circle
   b. a triangle
   c. two triangles
   d. a circle with an inner dot

5. Within the CPT Manual, _____ indicate(s) a new or revised description.
   a. a black circle
   b. a triangle
   c. two triangles
   d. a circle with an inner dot

CRITICAL THINKING

Answer the following questions to the best of your ability. Use the textbook as a reference.

1. Kira Stansfield, CMA (AAMA), is working with Dr. Ramey in an internal medicine clinic. Dr. Ramey is unsure of which evaluation and management code to choose for certain patients whom she has seen. How can Kira advise Dr. Ramey in choosing the appropriate code?

   _____
   _____
   _____

2. Gloria Heritage, RMA, is working in the billing office of a pediatric practice. One of the physicians in the practice frequently chooses a high-level E/M code when billing for his patients. When Gloria consults the patients' charts, she finds that there is not sufficient information to use the higher billing codes and determines that lower codes would be more appropriate. What can Gloria do in this situation?

   _____
   _____
   _____

RESEARCH ACTIVITY

Use Internet search engines to research the following topic and write a brief description of what you find. It is important to use reputable websites.

1. Go to the appropriate website and list five of the changes to the CPT that have occurred this year.

   _____
   _____
   _____
   _____
   _____

CHAPTER 18
Patient Billing and Collection

STUDENT STUDY GUIDE

Use the following guide to assist in your learning of the concepts from the chapter.

I. Patient Accounting

1. List the seven steps in the accounts receivable cycle.

   i. _____
   ii. _____
   iii. _____
   iv. _____
   v. _____
   vi. _____
   vii. _____

2. Accounts Receivable Transactions

   A. A(n) _____ is the monetary cost for services or supplies.
   B. A payment is the receipt of money that decreases the account balance, sometimes referred to as a(n)_____.
   C. An adjustment is a(n) _____ or negative change to a patient's account balance.
   D. _____ is a running total of all patient account transactions each day and is an important _____ tool.
   E. At the end of each day, the day sheet should be reconciled with individual encounter forms, total charges from encounter forms, and the _____.
   F. The patient ledger or ledger card is a(n) _____ record of charges, adjustments, payments, and current balances for a specific patient.

3. Accounts Receivable Systems

   A. Patient accounting software is also referred to as a(n) _____.
   B. A typical PMS includes the following components:

   i. _____
   ii. _____
   iii. _____
   iv. _____
   v. _____
   vi. _____
   vii. _____
   viii. _____
   ix. _____

   C. The pegboard system is also known as the _____ method.

4. Fees and Copayments

   A. Medical offices should post a(n) "_____" sign prominently.
   B. A copayment is a(n) _____ that patients' insurance policies may require them to pay for certain types of visits.

C. When a copayment is required by the _____, the health care provider must collect it.

D. Always create a(n) _____ receipt when taking a co-payment.

5. Insurance Payments

A. After an insurance carrier has processed a claim, a check is sent to the health care provider with a(n) _____ or a(n) _____.

B. A(n) _____ EOB lists multiple claims for multiple patients.

C. The allowed amount is sometimes called the _____.

6. What are the 15 steps for posting insurance payments? (Check your procedures!)

i. _____

ii. _____

iii. _____

iv. _____

v. _____

vi. _____

vii. _____

viii. _____

ix. _____

x. _____

xi. _____

xii. _____

xiii. _____

xiv. _____

xv. _____

7. List seven reasons for the denial of an insurance claim.

i. _____

ii. _____

iii. _____

iv. _____

v. _____

vi. _____

vii. _____

8. Patient Billing

A. The faster you bill the patient, the faster you will receive the _____.

B. In monthly billing, statements for all patients are generated _____ a month on the same day of each month.

C. In cycle billing, about _____ of patient accounts are billed each week.

II. Patient Collections

1. Collection Techniques

i. _____

ii. _____

iii. _____

iv. _____

v. _____

2. Guidelines for Making Collection Calls

A. Avoid placing calls earlier than _____ A.M. or later than _____ P.M. and on Sundays and holidays.

B. Do not call the patient's _____.

C. _____ the person prior to discussing the account.

D. Be _____ regarding who you are and the intent of the call.

E. Do not _____ or intimidate the patient.

F. Ask the patient when payment should be expected and _____ this information in the patient's record.

G. Politely _____ the patient for his or her time and repeat back to the patient the terms agreed upon.

3. Guidelines for Sending a Personalized Letter

   A. Insert the letter with the _____ statement.

   B. The letter should inquire _____ the bill has not been paid.

   C. In the letter, an offer should be made to assist the patient with making payment _____.

   D. The letter must convey the message that _____ will be taken to resolve the payment obligation.

4. Basic Guidelines for Drafting a Collection Letter

   i. _____

   ii. _____

   iii. _____

   iv. _____

   v. _____

   vi. _____

   vii. _____

   viii. _____

   ix. _____

   x. _____

5. "Skips"

   A. Steps for Finding Skips

      i. Check the _____ form to confirm the information.

      ii. Call the telephone numbers and _____ to try to locate the individual.

      iii. Ensure that _____ has been indicated on the billing envelope.

6. Collection Agencies

   A. Posting a Payment from a Collection Agency

      i. Log in to the PMS using your previously established _____ and password.

      ii. Access the patient's account or the _____ _____ account.

      iii. Enter the date the _____ was received.

      iv. Enter the _____ _____ of the check.

      v. Post an _____ for the amount of the collection agency fee.

      vi. Post an adjustment to write off the remaining _____ as bad debt.

      vii. Verify that all entries are _____.

KEY TERMINOLOGY REVIEW

Match each of the following selected key terms with the correct definition.

a. bad debt

b. copayment

c. professional courtesy (PC)

d. statute of limitations

e. Truth in Lending Form

1. _____ Physician opts not to charge other physicians, staff, family members, or clergy.

2. _____ An amount owed and not collected.

3. _____ Refers to the amount of time a legal collection suit may be brought against a debtor.

4. _____ If credit is extended and it is determined that the patient will make set payments to the physician over four or more installments, the patient must sign this document.

5. _____ A predetermined amount of money that the patient must pay for medical services at every visit, as determined by the insurance company.

APPLIED PRACTICE

Complete the activities and answer the questions that follow.

1. Call a local medical office in your area and ask to speak to someone in the billing office. Interview this person about his or her job function. Ask the person the following questions:

   a. What type of system does the person's office use for billing (manual or computerized)?

   _____

   _____

   b. If the office uses a computer system for billing, what is the name of the software used?

   _____

   _____

   c. What functions does the computer system have that helps the billing office staff better perform their jobs?

   _____

   _____

2. Read the following scenario and answer the accompanying questions.

> ### Scenario
> Kaley McManus, RMA, works for Havensburg Audiology. The payment policy for the audiology practice states that all copayments are expected at the time of service. The patient, Arturo Alamos, is responsible for paying 20% of all services and his insurance company, Healthy Care, will reimburse the physician the remaining 80%.
>
> Mr. Alamos was seen today by Dr. Lynst. Two procedures were performed: a comprehensive audio examination and a tympanography. Following is the fee schedule for the office.

New Patient Examinations		
Office Visit, Level 1	99201	$ 55.00
Office Visit, Level 2	99202	$110.00
Office Visit, Level 3	99203	$154.00
Office Visit, Level 4	99204	$226.00
Office Visit, Level 5	99205	$299.00
Established Patient Examinations		
Office Visit, Level 1	99211	$ 45.00
Office Visit, Level 2	99212	$ 60.00
Office Visit, Level 3	99213	$ 80.00
Office Visit, Level 4	99214	$123.00
Office Visit, Level 5	99215	$199.00

a. How much will Kaley collect from Mr. Alamos today?

_____

_____

b. How much will Healthy Care be billed for the services provided to Mr. Alamos?

_____

_____

c. As Mr. Alamos gets ready to pay for his office visit, he realizes that he has only a $20 bill. What should Kaley do?

_____

_____

LEARNING ACTIVITY: MULTIPLE CHOICE

Circle the correct answer for each of the following questions.

1. _____ are documents that detail the money owed to the medical practice and how long the account has been outstanding.
   a. Accounts payable
   b. Aging reports
   c. Superbills
   d. None of the above

2. The fee is determined by the physician or the practice's partners as a result of taking which of the following into consideration?
   a. Services involved
   b. Economic level of the community
   c. Prevailing fees in the community
   d. All of the above

3. The customary fee refers to

   a. what a physician usually charges for a procedure or service.
   b. the fee charged for the same procedure by the majority of physicians with the same or similar training.
   c. what a physician charges for a modified procedure or service that is more difficult and requires more time and effort than a standard procedure.
   d. None of the above

4. Cycle billing requires

   a. statements leave the office in time to reach the patient no later than the last day of the month.
   b. certain portions of the accounts receivable (AR), or money owed to the practice, are billed at given times during the month.
   c. offices have a software medical billing program.
   d. All of the above

5. The accounting term "debit" indicates _____.

   a. that a payment has been received on an account.
   b. that a charge has been entered into the account record.
   c. the difference between the money owed and the credit.
   d. that a charge has been entered and added to the account balance.

CRITICAL THINKING

Answer the following question to the best of your ability. Use the textbook and other resources such as the Internet in considering the following questions.

1. Dr. Roger Dominguez operates a single-physician practice. Dr. Dominguez employs one medical assistant, Garrick Sinclair, CMA (AAMA). The clinic has been using a manual accounting system for many years, and Dr. Dominguez has asked Garrick to research the pros and cons of moving to a computerized system versus keeping the manual system. What might Garrick list as pros and cons for using a computerized system versus a manual system?

   _____

   _____

   _____

RESEARCH ACTIVITY

Use Internet search engines to research the following topic and write a brief description of what you find. It is important to use reputable websites.

1. Look up three collection agencies that offer their services for medical accounts in your area. List the advantages and disadvantages for using each of these three companies.

   _____

   _____

   _____

   _____

   _____

CHAPTER 19

Banking and Practice Finances

STUDENT STUDY GUIDE

Use the following guide to assist in your learning of the concepts from the chapter.

I. Online Banking and Writing Checks

1. Basic Banking Functions (list six general functions)

   i. _____

   ii. _____

   iii. _____

   iv. _____

   v. _____

2. Types of Bank Accounts

   i. _____

   ii. _____

   iii. _____

3. Checking Account

   A. A checking account allows the owner of the account to _____ money from the account.

   B. It is not usually a(n) _____ account.

   C. Some accounts earn interest only if there is a(n) _____ balance in the account.

4. Savings Account

   A. This is a(n) _____ account where funds that are not needed for daily expenses are placed.

   B. Interest is earned _____ or _____.

   C. Cash can be withdrawn or transferred in to a(n) _____ account.

5. Money Market Account

   A. A money market account is used more as a(n) _____ tool; it usually pays a(n) _____ rate.

   B. It typically requires a minimum balance of _____ to _____.

6. Online Banking

   A. The functions that customers can perform include _____ the account, comparing the account with the bank's records, paying bills, and _____ data from the bank.

   B. This is a(n) _____ system that requires notations to be entered into the _____ records.

7. Computerized Accounting Systems

   A. List the three abilities of computerized accounting systems.

   i. _____

   ii. _____

   iii. _____

   B. Each user of a computerized accounting system should have a(n) _____.

8. Online Banking

    A. Online banking provides the customer access to his or her bank account _____ a day, _____ week.

    B. Online banking is a(n) _____ system.

9. Preventing Financial Fraud

    A. _____ is a set of internal controls that reduce the risk of fraud and embezzlement by dividing financial responsibilities into distinct tasks and assigning each task to a different individual.

    B. A(n) _____ bond discourages employee dishonesty.

10. Checks

    A. A check is a document that orders a bank to _____ or _____ money.

    B. It is _____ on demand.

    C. It is a(n) _____ instrument.

11. Preprinted Information on Checks

    i. _____

    ii. _____

    iii. _____

    iv. _____

    v. _____

    vi. _____

    vii. _____

    viii. _____

    ix. _____

    x. _____

    xi. _____

12. Magnetic Ink Character Recognition

    A. MICR increases the speed and accuracy of processing _____ and check sorting.

    B. The first series of numbers identifies the _____ and its _____.

    C. The second series of numbers identifies the _____.

13. Cashier's Check

    A. A cashier's check is written using the bank's own check or form; it is issued by the _____.

    B. Funds to pay the check are _____ against the payer's account when the check is issued to the bank.

    C. It can be requested from a bank by _____ holders who do not have a checking account.

14. Bank Draft and Limited Check

    A. A bank draft is a check that is drawn up by a bank against funds that are _____ into its account in another bank.

    B. A limited check is issued on a(n) _____ form that indicates a preprinted _____ dollar amount for which the check can be written.

    C. A(n) _____ limit may exist for a limited check.

    D. Limited checks are used for _____ checks and _____ payments.

15. Money Order

    A. Money orders are purchased for the _____ value embossed on the check.

    B. They can be purchased from _____, the _____, and other authorized agents.

    C. Money orders are frequently used by individuals who do not have _____ accounts and who do not want to send cash by mail.

    D. They are considered safe to accept as payment because they are _____ at the value embossed on the check.

16. Traveler's Check

    A. Traveler's checks are _____ and _____ in certain dollar amounts.

    B. They are considered a safe means for carrying money when _____.

    C. The check contains _____ spaces for the signature of the _____, one space that is signed upon purchase of the check, the other for when the check is presented in payment.

17. The Write-It-Once System

    A. This system allows a record to be kept of the _____, _____, _____, and net amount of the check.

    B. The _____ system, the check _____ sheet, and the checks with a(n) _____ writing strip on the back are used for this method.

    C. A check _____ sheet is placed over the pegs of the _____.

    D. Checks must be _____ when using this method.

    E. The check register has space for _____ checks to be recorded on one page.

18. Steps for Preparing a Check

    i. _____

    ii. _____

    iii. _____

    iv. _____

    v. _____

    vi. _____

    vii. _____

    viii. _____

    ix. _____

    x. _____

    xi. _____

    xii. _____

    xiii. _____

    xiv. _____

19. Errors in Writing Checks

    A. Banks are very suspicious of _____ on a check.

    B. For checks with major errors, _____ a(n) _____ through the check and write _____ in ink across the check.

    C. Keep the _____ _____ so that it is not considered missing.

20. Risky Checks

    i. _____

    ii. _____

    iii. _____

    iv. _____

21. Third-Party Check

    A. A third-party check is a check written by a party _____ to you.

    B. The patient is considered the _____ party.

    C. The first party is the medical office staff who is _____ the money.

22. "Paid-in-Full" Checks

    A. Checks written with the statement _____ added are to be avoided.

    B. If the check is deposited, you are _____ that this is correct, making it difficult to collect any further payments.

23. Considerations for Endorsing a Check

    A. Place the endorsement on the _____ of the check within the top _____ inches on the left-hand side of the check as it is turned over.

    B. An endorsement can either be a payee's written signature or a(n) _____.

    C. To prevent theft, checks should be endorsed for _____ as soon as they are received.

    D. Endorsements are regulated by the _____.

24. Types of Check Endorsements (list and explain each)

    i. _____

    ii. _____

    iii. _____

25. Reasons for Returned Checks

    i. _____

    ii. _____

    iii. _____

26. Guidelines for Handling Deposits

    i. _____

    ii. _____

    iii. _____

    iv. _____

    v. _____

    vi. _____

27. Steps for Completing a Deposit Slip

    i. _____

    ii. _____

    iii. _____

    iv. _____

    v. _____

    vi. _____

    vii. _____

    viii. _____

    ix. _____

    x. _____

II. Bank Statements and Payroll

  1. Bank Statement

    A. A bank statement provides _____ of the funds in an account.

    B. It assists in _____ errors made by the office or bank bookkeeping system.

    C. It includes all _____ and _____ processed.

  2. Information Included on a Bank Statement

    i. _____

    ii. _____

    iii. _____

    iv. _____

    v. _____

    vi. _____

    vii. _____

    viii. _____

    ix. _____

    x. _____

3. Instructions for Reconciling a Bank Statement
   A. Compare the _____ balance of the current statement with the _____ balance of the previous statement.
   B. Write the current _____ balance in the appropriate space on the reverse side of the bank statement.
   C. Compare the _____ noted on the statement against your records or _____ by making a check mark next to each correct number.
   D. List _____ all outstanding deposits.
   E. Add these together, and place the total on the _____ side of the statement in the space provided.
   F. Add the _____ balance to the total of the deposits not already included, and write this amount on the _____ line.
   G. Compare the value of the checks listed on the statement with the value listed in the _____ or check stubs, and place a check mark next to each correct number.
   H. Note all numbers missing from the _____ list of check numbers.
   I. List all _____ checks.
   J. Add the total for the _____ checks and place that figure on the line indicated on the back of the statement.
   K. Subtract the total for the checks outstanding from the _____ total on the _____ of the statement to determine the current balance.
   L. The current balance should _____ with the amount in your checkbook or stub balance.

4. Documents Used to Verify Banking Procedures
   i. _____
   ii. _____
   iii. _____
   iv. _____
   v. _____

5. Petty Cash
   A. Petty cash must be _____ and recorded in a(n) _____ financial log.
   B. A(n) _____ is used to replenish petty cash.
   C. It is typically handled by _____ individual in the office.
   D. It is kept under _____ and _____ for security purposes.

6. Payroll Periods
   i. _____
   ii. _____
   iii. _____
   iv. _____

7. Payroll Information That Employers Must Maintain
   i. _____
   ii. _____
   iii. _____
   iv. _____
   v. _____
   vi. _____

8. Working with an Outside Payroll Service
   i. _____
   ii. _____
   iii. _____
   iv. _____
   v. _____
   vi. _____
   vii. _____

9. Information to Be Included on the W-4 Form
   A. Employee's name and _____.
   B. Employee's _____ number.
   C. Employee's _____ status.
   D. The number of _____ that the employee is claiming.

KEY TERMINOLOGY REVIEW

Match each of the following selected key terms to the correct definition.

   a. accounts payable (AP)
   b. audit
   c. cash disbursement

   d. debits
   e. embezzlement

1. _____ Refers to an official inspection of an individual's or organization's accounts, typically by an independent body.

2. _____ The unauthorized taking of funds; involves a breach of trust.

3. _____ Charges against an account.

4. _____ Actualizes or permits the transfer of cash money to another person.

5. _____ Money that is owed to vendors, suppliers, utility companies, and others for services rendered.

APPLIED PRACTICE

Read the scenario and answer the questions that follow.

Scenario
Daniel Evans, CMA (AAMA), works as the administrative medical assistant for Happy Valley Medical Center. Handling payroll, accounts payable, and banking procedures is part of his work responsibilities. It is Thursday and he must perform these duties.

1. Daniel must calculate the gross earnings for the two clinical medical assistants who work in the back office. The office pays its employees every week, for the previous week's work. For every hour over 40 hours worked, employees get paid time and a half. Last week, Shelby Coleman worked 43.5 hours. She earns $13.00 per hour. Chantal Jefferson worked 45 hours last week. Chantal earns $13.75 per hour.

   a. What are Shelby's gross earnings?
   _____

   b. What are Chantal's gross earnings?
   _____

2. Daniel Smith has received an invoice from a vendor that supplied the physician with new business cards. The invoice reads as follows:

SELECT STATIONERY UNLIMITED

Bill to: Happy Valley Medical Center
1129 Felicity Road
Springfield, PA 00010
Account #: 288901HVMC

Remit Payment to: Select Stationery Unlimited
PO Box 588
New York, NY 11110

Item Number	Description	Price	Total
0123	250 Business Cards	32.99	32.99
		Tax (5%)	1.65
		Shipping and Handling	4.95
		Total	$ 39.59

---

   a. Complete the check according to how Daniel should pay this bill.

Happy Valley Medical Clinic   **13003**
1129 Felicity Road   Date _____ 20_____
Springfield, PA 00010

Pay to the order of: _____

_____

_____dollars

MEMO: _____   _____

LEARNING ACTIVITY: MULTIPLE CHOICE

Circle the correct answer to each of the following questions.

1. Which of the following would be considered a deduction for the purposes of employee payroll?

   a. Federal tax withholding
   b. Vacation pay
   c. Overtime pay
   d. All of the above

2. Petty cash is available for incidentals such as

   a. small purchases.
   b. reimbursements.
   c. miscellaneous expenses.
   d. All of the above

3. In order to have a negotiable instrument, the check must

   a. be written and signed by an authorized payer of the check.
   b. state a sum of money to be paid.
   c. be payable on demand or at a fixed date in the future.
   d. be payable to the holder (the payee) of the check.
   e. All of the above

4. Types of checks include

   a. bank drafts.
   b. money orders.
   c. All of the above

5. The American Bankers Association (ABA) number is always located

   a. in the phone book.
   b. in the upper-right-hand corner of a printed check.
   c. in the lower-left-hand corner of a printed check.
   d. None of the above

6. What are check stubs used for?

   a. As a permanent record of the date, amount, payee, and purpose of the check
   b. As a bookmark
   c. As an example of the correct way to write a check
   d. The quarterly form

7. How much is typically paid to employees as overtime wages?

   a. Twice the employee's normal rate of pay
   b. One and a half times the employee's normal rate of pay
   c. Three times the employee's normal rate of pay
   d. None of the above

8. The _____ IRS form is used to calculate the correct amount of federal withholding tax for an employee.

   a. quarterly report
   b. W-2
   c. Circular E
   d. None of the above

9. A money market account
   a. is an interest-bearing account.
   b. is used more as an investment tool.
   c. typically requires a minimum balance of $500.
   d. All of the above

10. Banking is one of the critical office procedures because
    a. it requires careful handling of money and records.
    b. many offices do not have a bookkeeper or medical assistant assigned to perform this duty.
    c. it requires specialized training.
    d. All of the above

CRITICAL THINKING

Answer the following questions to the best of your ability. Use the textbook and other resources such as the Internet in considering the following questions.

1. Francie Crook, RMA, has been newly hired to work in a busy family practice clinic. When Francie looks at her first paycheck, she notices that a tax has been taken out for something called FICA. She asks her office manager to explain what this tax is. How might the office manager explain this tax to Francie?

   _____

   _____

   _____

2. Linnea Wagner is responsible for training new employees in the correct way to write checks. In order to do this, she must also explain the parts of the check. What might Linnea include in her instructional sessions?

   _____

   _____

   _____

RESEARCH ACTIVITY

Use Internet search engines to research the following topic and write a brief description of what you find. It is important to use reputable websites.

1. Look up three different software programs that can perform the payroll function. Create a list of the advantages and disadvantages of these three programs, as well as manual versus computerized payroll systems.

   _____

   _____

   _____

   _____

   _____

CHAPTER 20
Medical Office Management

STUDENT STUDY GUIDE

Use the following guide to assist in your learning of the concepts from the chapter.

I. Managing the Medical Office

   1. General Skills for Office Management

      i. _____

      ii. _____

      iii. _____

   2. General Duties of the Office Manager list any three

      i. _____

      ii. _____

      iii. _____

   3. Critical Resources Used in Managing a Medical Office

      i. _____

      ii. _____

      iii. _____

   4. Personnel Management Responsibilities

      A. Personnel management responsibilities include hiring new employees and establishing _____ training.

      B. Responsibilities also include performing _____ reviews.

      C. Disciplinary measures should occur as soon as they are warranted and not be held over until a(n) _____.

   5. Employee Records

      A. Federal law requires records to be maintained for _____ employee.

      B. Payroll records must include the following:

         i. _____

         ii. _____

         iii. _____

         iv. _____

   6. Elements of Financial Management

      i. _____

      ii. _____

      iii. _____

      iv. _____

7. Effective Scheduling
    A. Effective scheduling can contribute to the _____ level of the practice.
    B. If the office staff is continuously scheduled inappropriately, it affects _____ and may cause _____ among the physicians and patients.
    C. _____ must be built into the staff schedule to allow for _____ occurrences such as sick days and business appointments.

8. Elements of Facility and Equipment Management
    i. _____
    ii. _____
    iii. _____
    iv. _____
    v. _____
    vi. _____

9. Communications
    A. To be effective, one must be able to communicate at _____.
    B. Effective communication contributes significantly to the _____ of the staff.
    C. Communication includes _____ and _____ materials.

10. The Basic Duties of the Office Manager
    A. The office manager acts as a liaison between the _____ and the _____.
    B. The office manager conducts _____ and _____ reviews.
    C. The office manager _____ responsibilities to staff.
    D. The office manager maintains the office procedures _____.
    E. The office manager oversees HIPAA _____.
    F. The office manager plans and _____ staff meetings.
    G. The office manager prepares _____ educational materials.
    H. The office manager supervises employees on a(n) _____ basis.
    I. The office manager supervises the purchase and _____ of equipment and supplies.

11. Qualities of a Good Manager
    i. _____
    ii. _____
    iii. _____
    iv. _____
    v. _____
    vi. _____
    vii. _____
    viii. _____
    ix. _____
    x. _____
    xi. _____
    xii. _____

12. Managing the Monthly Planning Calendar
    A. Develop a system in which the schedule for the _____ is laid out on a calendar.
    B. List _____ vacations on a calendar because it helps to prevent overlapping of vacations, which can leave an office _____.
    C. Note all physicians' _____, _____, _____, accountant meetings, and vendor visits.
    D. Ensure that all vacations have been _____.
    E. Compare the office's calendar with the _____ calendar on a periodic basis and update the office's _____ calendar as necessary.

13. Staff Meetings

    A. Staff meetings facilitate communications between _____ and the _____.

    B. The meeting time, date, and agenda are created by the _____ with input from the _____.

    C. Ensure that staff meetings are _____ to help minimize wasted time.

    D. The minutes and the _____ of attendees should be recorded.

14. Equipment Needed for a Staff Meeting

    i. _____

    ii. _____

    iii. _____

    iv. _____

15. Preparing for the Staff Meeting

    A. _____ week before the meeting, request agenda items from the _____.

    B. Before the meeting, create a meeting _____ that includes all topics that need to be discussed.

    C. On the agenda, include the following:

        i. _____

        ii. _____

        iii. _____

16. Ensuring the Success of Staff Meetings

    A. Start the meeting _____.

    B. Begin by _____ reviewing the last meeting.

    C. Address each topic within its _____ amount of _____.

    D. Allow for time at the end of the meeting to have _____ of any new business.

    E. After the meeting, the _____ of the meeting should be distributed to _____.

17. The Staff's Expectations of Management

    i. _____

    ii. _____

    iii. _____

    iv. _____

    v. _____

    vi. _____

    vii. _____

    viii. _____

    ix. _____

    x. _____

    xi. _____

    xii. _____

18. Ways to Show Respect

    A. Greet employees in a(n) _____ manner.

    B. Always _____ employees' hard work.

    C. Never _____ employees in front of their peers.

    D. Be _____ and listen to employees when they need to talk.

    E. Take employees' suggestions into _____.

    F. Work toward having _____ employees.

    G. When possible, provide _____ space for each employee.

    H. Create a sense of _____ with the medical office.

    I. Ensure that employees feel that they have been _____ for the amount of work that they accomplish.

J. Provide employees with _____ beyond pay.

K. Maintain a cohesive work environment by ensuring that communication is _____ and _____.

II. Leadership and Team Accountability

1. Attributes of Good Leaders

    i. _____

    ii. _____

    iii. _____

    iv. _____

    v. _____

2. Attributes of Authoritarian Leaders

    A. Authoritarian leaders make most decisions on their own without the _____ of others.

    B. Authoritarian leaders are not as likely to be team _____ as are solid _____.

    C. Authoritarian leaders want _____ and _____ from their staff.

    D. Authoritarian leaders use _____ to achieve obedience from their staff.

    E. Authoritarian leaders are motivated by _____ and _____ authority.

    F. Authoritarian leaders work best under great _____ and in _____.

3. Attributes of Democratic Leaders

    A. Democratic leaders concentrate more on the relationships among _____ and emphasize _____ in the office.

    B. Democratic leaders are motivated from _____ to provide a comfortable work environment for all employees.

    C. A democratic leadership style often results in a(n) _____ staff.

4. Attributes of Permissive Leaders

    A. Permissive leaders are not strict with regard to _____ and _____.

    B. A permissive leadership style may result in _____ and even _____ conditions in the work environment.

    C. Permissive leaders are self- _____.

5. Attributes of Bureaucratic Leaders

    A. Bureaucratic leaders very strongly _____ rules.

    B. Bureaucratic leaders are motivated by _____ factors.

    C. Bureaucratic leaders rely on _____ management methods for office matters.

    D. Bureaucratic leaders are _____ because they do not trust themselves when making decisions that affect the office.

    E. Bureaucratic leaders are very _____ and formal.

6. Types of Power (*List and briefly describe each type*)

    i. _____

    ii. _____

    iii. _____

    iv. _____

    v. _____

    vi. _____

7. Methods for Providing the Job Application

    A. Send the job application to the applicant by _____ and have him or her bring the application to the interview.

    B. Provide a(n) _____ to the online version.

    C. Have the applicant fill out the form at the time of the _____.

8. The Benefits of Having the Application Completed at the Interview

    A. You will see how the applicant handles filling out forms under _____.
    B. You will obtain a visual of the applicant's _____.
    C. You will learn how _____ the applicant is at completing a required task.

9. Areas for Consideration During the Interview

    i. _____
    ii. _____
    iii. _____

10. The Contents of Questions Prohibited by the Equal Employment Opportunity Act

    i. _____
    ii. _____
    iii. _____
    iv. _____
    v. _____

11. Information to Be Obtained About an Applicant

    A. Obtain information about past office _____.
    B. Obtain information about the types of _____ with whom the applicant has worked.
    C. Obtain information about the applicant's ability to _____ on his or her feet.

12. Possible Office Requirements for an Applicant

    i. _____
    ii. _____
    iii. _____
    iv. _____
    v. _____

13. The Purpose of the Probationary Period

    A. A probationary period allows the supervisor to _____ the new employee at work and to _____ if he or she is suited to the position.
    B. During the probationary period, an employee can be _____ without cause.
    C. After _____ days, the employer must show just cause, or reason, to dismiss an employee.

14. The Contents of an Orientation Checklist

    i. _____
    ii. _____
    iii. _____
    iv. _____
    v. _____
    vi. _____
    vii. _____
    viii. _____
    ix. _____
    x. _____
    xi. _____
    xii. _____
    xiii. _____

15. Types of Reviews (*Explain each type*)

    A. Orientation or training: _____
    B. Routine performance review: _____
    C. Poor performance review: _____
    D. Salary review: _____

16. Steps for Creating a Time Management System
    A. Define the office _____ in consultation with the _____.
    B. Create a(n) _____ list of _____.
    C. Incorporate the _____ list into a(n) _____ list.

17. Information Found in an Employee Handbook
    i. _____
    ii. _____
    iii. _____
    iv. _____
    v. _____

18. The Office Procedures Manual
    A. The procedures manual contains detailed descriptions of _____ and how to perform both _____ and _____ tasks.
    B. The terms "policy" and "procedure" are used _____ in many offices.

19. The Primary Functions of a Procedures Manual
    i. _____
    ii. _____
    iii. _____

20. The Benefits of an Effective Patient Information Booklet
    A. It reduces the number of _____ by telephone from _____.
    B. It enhances the office's _____.
    C. It reduces the number of patients who _____ to remember instructions.
    D. It is useful either for _____ with _____ or for teaching methods of _____ prevention.

KEY TERMINOLOGY REVIEW

Without using information from the textbook, write a sentence using each selected key term in the correct context.

1. *Colleagues*

   _____
   _____

2. *Discriminatory*

   _____
   _____

3. *Grievance*

   _____
   _____

4. *Itinerary*

   _____
   _____

5. *Probationary period*

   _____
   _____

APPLIED PRACTICE

Complete the following activity.

1. Develop a patient information booklet, as described in Procedure 20-2 in Chapter 20 of your textbook. Your booklet will be graded on accuracy, completeness, and appearance. In addition to other items that may be considered, the following items should be part of the booklet:

   a. Regular office hours
   b. Special services offered by the practice or clinic, such as patient education classes or blood pressure screening
   c. Written procedures for handling prescription refills
   d. Written procedures for how medical insurance forms are processed
   e. General statement about the payment of fees, especially if payment is expected at the time of the delivery of services
   f. Information about the physician and the staff
   g. Written procedures on how emergencies are handled

LEARNING ACTIVITY: TRUE/FALSE

Indicate whether the following statements are true or false by placing a T or an F on the line that precedes each statement.

_____ 1. Personnel management usually requires a performance review every 6 months for each employee.

_____ 2. The clinical aspects of office management are separate from the administrative aspects.

_____ 3. The office manager's time is generally spent on employee and administrative issues.

_____ 4. A good office manager strives to become the boss.

_____ 5. Many office managers are promoted based on seniority.

CRITICAL THINKING

Answer the following questions to the best of your ability. Use the textbook as a reference.

1. Teresa Clymer, CMA (AAMA), has just been promoted to office manager. In order to create a team atmosphere, what factors should Teresa consider to ensure the building of a successful team?

   _____

   _____

   _____

2. Mavis Raschenko, RMA, must fill an open medical assistant position. What methods might Mavis choose, and why?

   _____

   _____

   _____

3. When hiring individuals, what cultural aspects need to be considered?

_____

_____

_____

RESEARCH ACTIVITY

Use Internet search engines to research the following topic and write a brief description of what you find. It is important to use reputable websites.

1. Determine the importance of conducting performance evaluations and explore the tools used to perform this task. Write an essay explaining what you have learned through your research. Cite your sources at the end of your essay.

_____

_____

_____

_____

_____

CHAPTER 21

Body Structure and Function

STUDENT STUDY GUIDE

Use the following guide to assist in your learning of the concepts from the chapter.

I. Organization of the Human Body

   1. Organization of the Human Body (Diagram the organization of the body. Refer to Figure 21-1 in your textbook.)

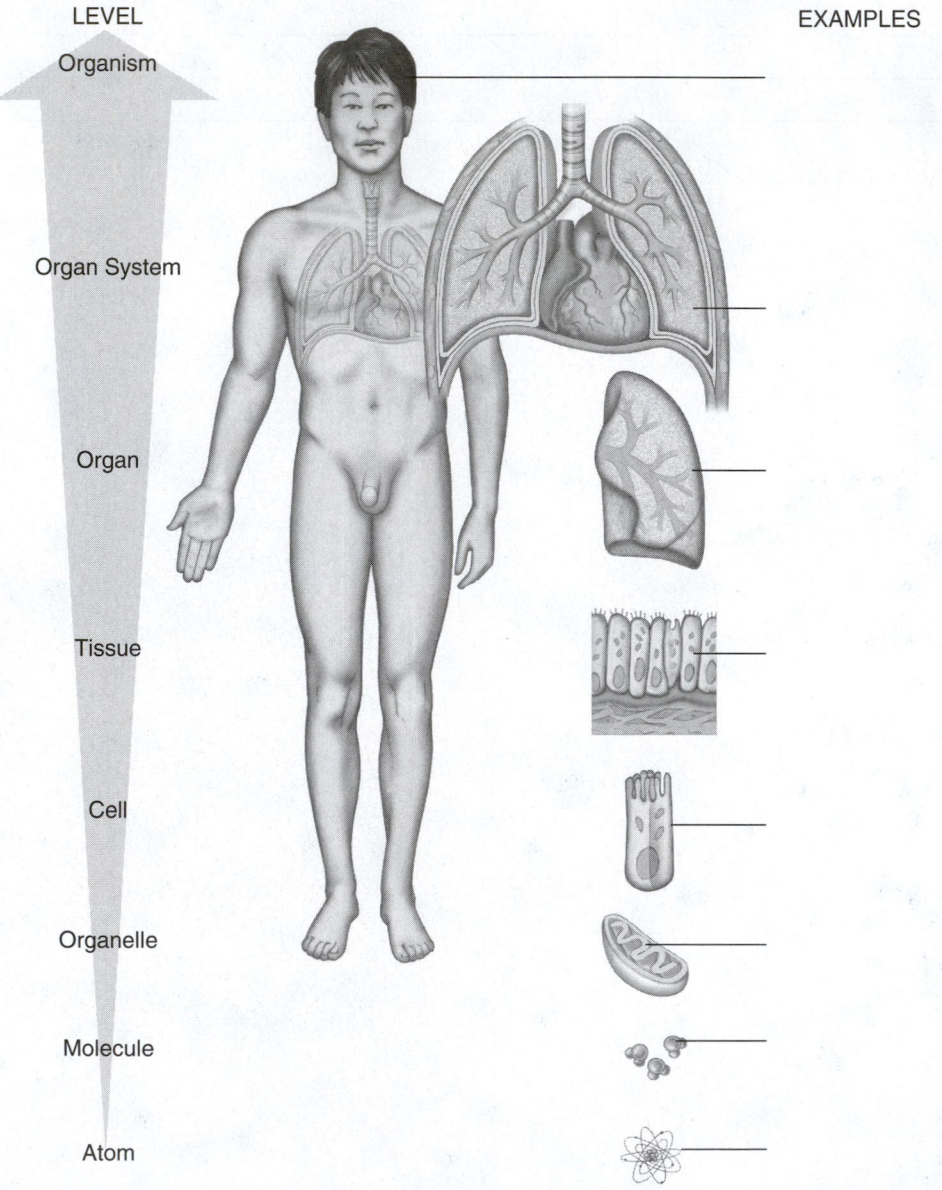

LEVEL

Organism

Organ System

Organ

Tissue

Cell

Organelle

Molecule

Atom

EXAMPLES

2. Atom
   A. _____ and _____ constitute the majority of the anatomic mass and reside within the nucleus.
   B. _____, _____, and _____ combine to create elements.

3. Elements Found in the Human Body
   i. _____
   ii. _____
   iii. _____
   iv. _____
   v. _____
   vi. _____
   vii. _____
   viii. _____
   ix. _____
   x. _____
   xi. _____
   xii. _____
   xiii. _____
   xiv. _____
   xv. _____
   xvi. _____
   xvii. _____
   xviii. _____
   xix. _____

4. Molecules
   A. Molecules can take the form of _____, _____, or _____.
   B. Water contains _____ of molecules.

5. Components of a Cell
   i. _____
   ii. _____
   iii. _____

6. Cell Membrane
   A. The cell membrane helps maintain the _____ shape.
   B. It allows some substances to pass into and out of the cell while _____ the passage of other substances.

7. Cilia
   A. Cilia _____ the overall surface area of a cell.
   B. It propels substances along a cell's surface, which increases the cell's ability to absorb _____ and _____.

8. Cytoplasm
   A. Cytoplasm is _____ percent water; it is generally _____ in color, resembling a _____.
   B. It provides _____ and work areas for the cell.

9. Organelles
   A. Each organelle has a specific function and purpose in maintaining the vitality of the _____.
   B. Organelles include _____, _____, _____, _____, _____, and _____.

10. Nucleus

    A. The nucleus is the _____ of the cell.

    B. Within the nucleus are the cell's _____.

11. Nucleic Functions

    i. _____

    ii. _____

    iii. _____

    iv. _____

    v. _____

12. Organs

    A. Composed of several types of _____.

    B. Perform _____ functions.

13. Passive and Active Transport

    A. Passive transport involves a number of processes, including _____, _____, and _____.

    B. Through active transport, _____ are able to obtain what they need through _____ fluid.

14. Electrolytes

    A. An electrolyte is an electrically charged _____ that moves to either a(n) _____ or a(n) _____ electrode.

    B. Electrolytes are used to carry _____ impulses to other cells.

    C. Electrolytes must be _____ to keep their concentrations in the body fluids constant.

15. Electrolytes in the Human Body

    i. _____

    ii. _____

    iii. _____

    iv. _____

    v. _____

    vi. _____

    vii. _____

    viii. _____

II. Genetics and Heredity

  1. Genetic Engineering

    A. Genetics is the study of the _____ makeup of animals or plants.

    B. Genetic engineering is generally considered to be the use of technology by scientists intentionally to make _____ to the genetic makeup.

  2. Heredity

    A. Heredity is the transmission of genes from _____ to _____.

    B. Individuals carry _____ genes for each _____.

  3. Genetic Disorders

    A. Mutations are changes in the _____ sequence of a(n) _____.

    B. Genetic mutations can occur at any time during _____.

4. Albinism

  A. Albinism is a common _____ disorder.
  B. It is a congenital but _____ disorder.
  C. A mutation in a recessive gene causes a hereditary lack of pigment in the _____, _____, and eyes.
  D. The patient may complain of _____ and is prone to _____ because protective melanin is not present.

5. ADHD

  A. ADHD stands for _____.
  B. It is characterized by a person having difficulty _____ and completing a task.
  C. It may be caused by _____ factors. It is _____ times more prevalent in _____ than in _____.

6. Cleft Palate

  A. Cleft palate is a(n) _____ defect in the roof of the mouth that occurs when the _____ bones of the skull do not close properly.
  B. The cleft causes a(n) _____ between the mouth and the nasal cavities.
  C. This defect also may be accompanied by a cleft _____.
  D. It affects _____ more often than _____.

7. Color Deficiency

  A. This disorder was previously called _____.
  B. It often entails difficulty in distinguishing between _____ and _____.
  C. This condition is a(n) _____, sex-linked disorder, usually passed from mother to _____.
  D. With total color deficiency, a person is unable to perceive any color at all because of a defect in or absence of _____ in the _____.

8. Cystic Fibrosis

  A. Cystic fibrosis is a chronic and _____ disease, usually diagnosed in _____.
  B. This disease causes mucus to become _____, _____, and sticky.
  C. Mucus builds up and clogs passages, primarily in the lungs and the _____.

9. Down Syndrome

  A. Down syndrome occurs when a person has a(n) _____ copy of _____ 21.
  B. A mother who gives birth after age _____ has a higher risk of delivering an infant with Down syndrome.
  C. _____ is generally used as a tool for diagnosing this disorder.

10. Fragile X Syndrome

  A. Fragile X syndrome also is known as _____ syndrome, _____ syndrome, and _____ syndrome.
  B. This condition is the most common form of inherited _____.
  C. Generally, _____ are affected with moderate mental retardation and _____ with mild mental retardation.

11. Hemochromatosis

  A. Hemochromatosis is an inherited disorder in which the body accumulates an excessive amount of _____.
  B. It is common among the _____ population, affecting approximately _____ in _____ individuals of _____ ancestry.
  C. _____ deposits in the skin will eventually cause _____ of the skin.

12. Hemophilia

A. Hemophilia is a(n) _____, _____ disorder in which the time it takes for blood to coagulate is greatly increased.
B. It is caused by a(n) _____ gene mutation in the _____ chromosome.
C. Females carry the _____ gene and transmit the disorder to their _____ offspring.

13. Klinefelter's Syndrome

A. Klinefelter's syndrome is a congenital _____ disorder.
B. Primary _____ failure occurs, which usually is not evident until puberty.
C. This disorder also can lead to _____ intelligence.

14. Muscular Dystrophy

A. Muscular dystrophy is a genetic disease that is characterized by a gradual _____ and _____ of the muscles.
B. It occurs most frequently in _____.
C. The most common type is _____ muscular dystrophy, which accounts for _____ of all cases.
D. Death often occurs within _____ to _____ years after the onset of symptoms.

15. PKU

A. PKU stands for _____.
B. It is caused by a recessive gene _____.
C. If the condition is not treated early, _____ occurs because of brain damage.

16. Spina Bifida

A. Spina bifida is a congenital _____ tube defect.
B. The posterior vertebral arch has a(n) _____ anomaly.
C. Most often the abnormality occurs in the _____ region.

17. Tay-Sachs Disease

A. Tay-Sachs disease is an inherited disorder that tends to affect people of _____ and _____ European Jewish or French-Canadian ancestry.
B. It is caused by a faulty gene that targets the _____.
C. Symptoms first appear at around _____ months of age in an otherwise healthy baby.

18. Turner's Syndrome

A. Turner's syndrome is a congenital disorder caused by the failure of the _____ to respond to the stimulation of _____ hormones.
B. _____ may be impaired.
C. The patient is usually _____ in stature.

1. Label the various cells found in this image.

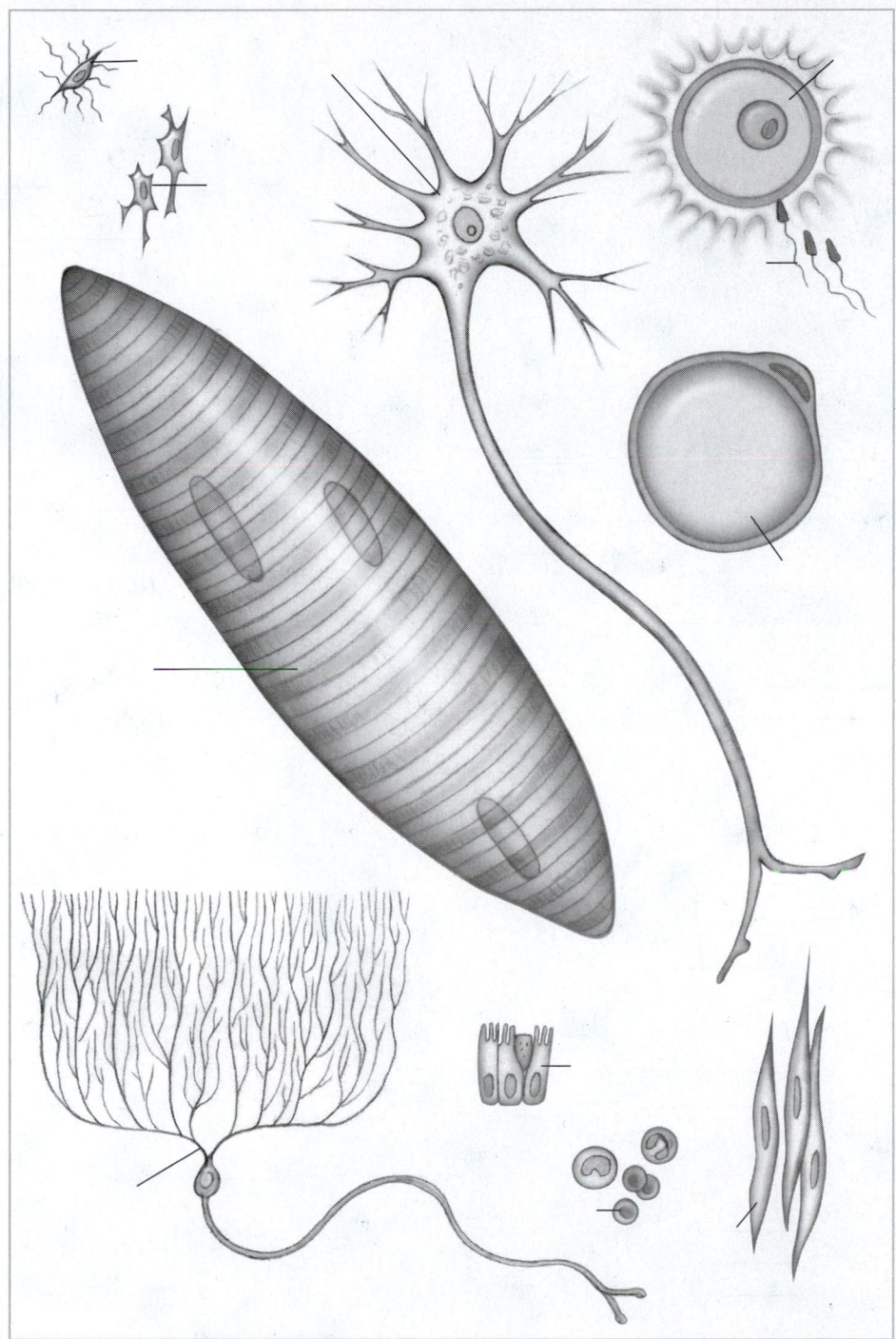

Body Structure and Function **125**

2. Label the types of tissue found in this image.

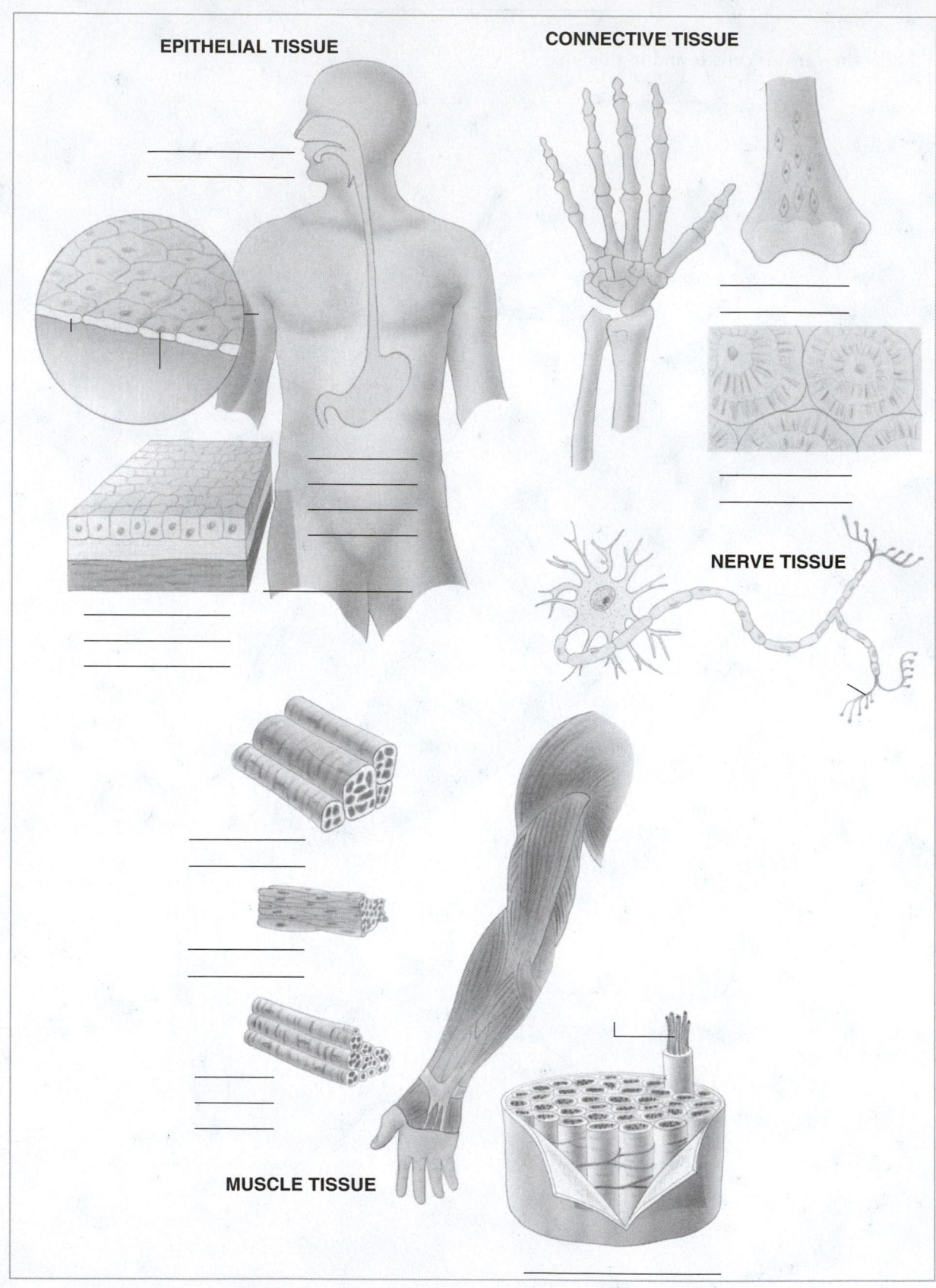

LEARNING ACTIVITY: TRUE/FALSE

Indicate whether the following statements are true or false by placing a T or an F on the line that precedes each statement.

_____ 1. Atoms are found at the most basic level of organization.

_____ 2. Molecules cannot move and thus take the form of solids, liquids, or gases.

_____ 3. DNA is shaped in a single helix.

_____ 4. The golgi apparatus is the location for the production of protein that is essential to the vitality of the cell.

_____ 5. Epithelial tissue is found on the outer layer of skin.

_____ 6. Involuntary or smooth muscle tissues are controlled by the autonomic nervous system.

_____ 7. In the phagocytosis method, the cell "drinks" the fluid required.

_____ 8. The muscular system transmits impulses, responds to change, is responsible for communication, and exercises control over all parts of the body.

_____ 9. Cells utilize electrolytes to maintain voltage or electrical force across their cell membranes.

_____ 10. Genetic disorders are considered medical conditions.

CRITICAL THINKING

Answer the following questions to the best of your ability. Use the textbook as a reference.

1. Why is it important for a medical assistant to understand the structures and functions of the human body?

    _____

    _____

    _____

    _____

2. When documenting a patient's treatment, why should documentation always take place after the procedure has been performed?

    _____

    _____

    _____

    _____

RESEARCH ACTIVITY

Use Internet search engines to research the following topic and write a brief description of what you find. It is important to use reputable websites.

1. Conduct further research on genetic engineering. Discover more about this fascinating topic and write a brief essay to explain what you learned through your research. Be sure to cite your sources.

   _____

   _____

   _____

   _____

   _____

CHAPTER 22
The Integumentary System

STUDENT STUDY GUIDE

Use the following guide to assist in your learning of the concepts from the chapter.

I. The Integumentary System

  1. The Skin and the Accessory Organs, Known as the Integumentary System

    A. The skin weighs more than _____ (in adults).

    B. It covers _____ of the body.

    C. The integumentary System is made up of the following organs:

      i. _____

      ii. _____

      iii. _____

      iv. _____

      v. _____

  2. The Functions of the Integumentary System

      i. _____

      ii. _____

      iii. _____

      iv. _____

      v. _____

  3. Temperature Regulation

    A. The integumentary system aids in the _____ of body temperature.

    B. To _____ heat, superficial blood vessels in the skin _____, bringing more blood to the surface of the skin.

    C. To _____ heat, superficial blood vessels _____, keeping warm blood away from the surface.

    D. A continuous layer of _____ fat acts as insulation.

  4. Sensory Receptors

    A. Sensory receptors detect temperature, pain, _____, and _____.

    B. They are located in the _____.

    C. Nerve endings in the _____ layer of skin convey _____ to the brain and spinal cord.

  5. The Three Layers of Skin

    A. The epidermis is divided into _____ layers.

    B. The dermis ("true skin") is the _____, _____ connective tissue layer.

    C. The subcutaneous tissue is the _____ layer.

6. The Layers of the Epidermis: Stratum Corneum
   A. The stratum corneum is the _____ layer of skin that consists of dead cells filled with a protein called _____.
   B. It forms a protective _____ for the body.
   C. The _____ of the layer depends on the part of the body.

7. The Layers of the Epidermis: Stratum Lucidum
   A. The stratum lucidum is the _____ layer lying directly beneath the _____.
   B. In thinner skin, it is often _____.
   C. Cells in this layer are either _____ or _____.

8. The Layers of the Epidermis: Stratum Granulosum
   A. The stratum granulosum consists of several layers of _____ cells that become part of the _____ lucidum and stratum _____.
   B. Cells actively become _____, or hardened, after they lose their _____.

9. The Layers of the Epidermis: Stratum Germinativum
   A. The stratum germinativum is made of several layers of living cells that are still capable of _____, or cell division.
   B. It is most responsible for the _____ of the epidermis.

10. The Dermis
    A. The dermis is the _____ layer of the skin.
    B. It is composed of _____ tissue containing nerves and nerve endings, blood vessels, sebaceous and _____ glands, hair follicles, and _____ vessels.
    C. It is further divided into two layers: the _____ layer and the _____ layer.

11. The Subcutaneous Layer
    A. The subcutaneous layer is composed of _____ tissue.
    B. This tissue helps support, nourish, insulate, and _____ the skin.

12. Accessory Organs: Hair
    A. The visible portion of hair is the _____.
    B. The _____ + _____ is found at the base of each hair follicle.
    C. With the exception of the _____ of the hands and the _____ of the feet, the entire body is covered by a very thin layer of hair.

13. Accessory Organs: Nails
    A. Fingernails and toenails are composed of _____.
    B. The nail bed is also called the _____.
    C. Nail _____ may be adversely affected by disease.
    D. Average nail growth is about _____ per week.
    E. The light-colored, half-moon area at the base is the _____.

14. Accessory Organs: Fluid-Producing Glands
    A. Sweat glands assist the body in maintaining its _____ temperature.
    B. Sweat glands create a(n) _____ effect when _____ evaporates.
    C. Sebaceous glands are _____ glands.

15. Summary of the Integument

    A. Label the structures of the integument.

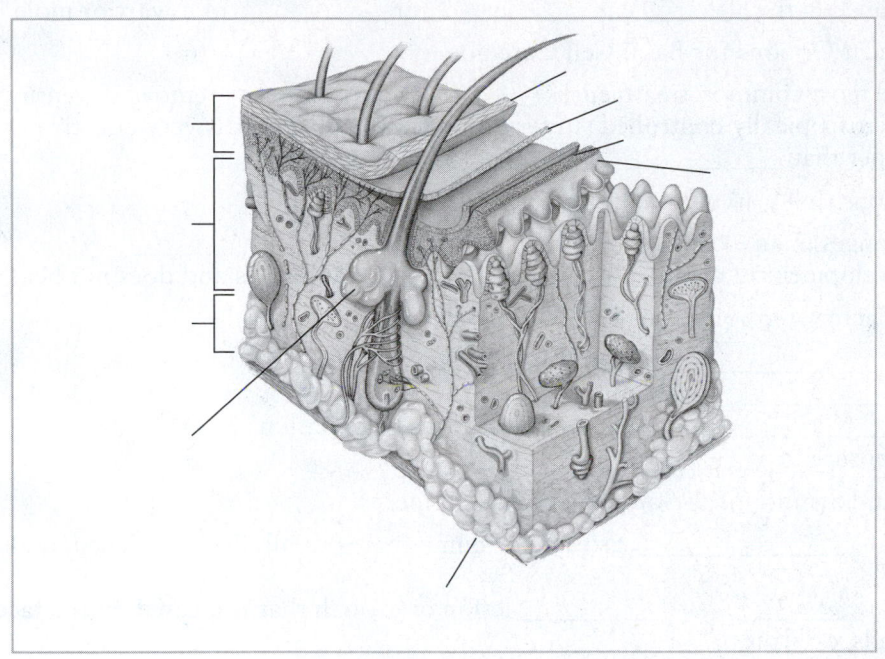

II. Pathology of the Integumentary System

  1. Facts About Skin Cancer

    A. Skin cancer is the most _____ of all cancers.
    B. It affects more than _____ people each year in the United States.

  2. How Skin Cancer Occurs

    A. Skin cancer occurs when normal skin cells undergo a change during which they _____ and _____ without the normal controls.
    B. As the cells multiply, they form a mass called a(n) _____.
    C. Tumors of the skin are often referred to as _____.
    D. Malignant tumors encroach on neighboring tissues, especially _____, because of their uncontrolled growth.

  3. Basal Cell Carcinoma

    A. Basal cell carcinoma is the most _____ form of skin cancer.
    B. It is most often caused by _____ to the sun.
    C. It often appears as a change in the skin, such as a(n) _____, a(n) irritation or _____ that does not heal, or a change in a(n) _____ or mole.
    D. Although the _____ is the most common site, it may affect the head, neck, back, chest, or shoulders.
    E. Exposure to _____ is the most common cause of this type of cancer.

  4. Signs and Symptoms of Basal Cell Carcinoma

    A. Firm, _____, including tiny blood vessels with a spiderlike appearance (telangiectasias)
    B. Red, tender, _____ that bleeds easily
    C. Small, fleshy bump with a smooth, pearly appearance, often with a(n) _____ center
    D. Smooth, shiny bump that may look like a(n) _____ or _____

E. _____ patch of skin, especially on the face, that is firm to the touch
F. Bump that itches, bleeds, _____, and then repeats the cycle, and has not healed in _____
G. Change in the _____, _____, or _____ of a wart or mole

5. Treatment Options for Basal Cell Carcinoma

   A. The most common treatment is _____ to destroy or remove the entire skin growth.
   B. Microscopically controlled surgery to remove skin cancer is very effective, with cure rates of higher than _____.

6. Squamous Cell Carcinoma: Indicators

   A. Changes in an existing wart, mole, or other _____
   B. Development of a(n) _____ that ulcerates and does not heal well

7. Risks Factors for Squamous Cell Carcinoma

   A. _____ predisposition
   B. _____ pollution
   C. _____ to X-rays or other forms of radiation
   D. Exposure to _____

8. Signs and Symptoms of Squamous Cell Carcinoma

   A. A(n) _____, growth, or bump that is small, firm, reddened, nodular, coned, or flat
   B. A(n) _____ or _____ lesion or growth that is located on the face, ears, neck, hands, or arms
   C. Occasionally, the growth may occur on the _____, _____, _____, or _____.

9. Treatment Options for Squamous Cell Carcinoma

   A. Treatment options include surgical removal of the tumor, which may include _____ of the _____ around the tumor.
   B. _____ (Mohs' micrographic surgery) may remove small tumors.
   C. _____ may be needed if broad areas of skin are removed.
   D. Another option is _____ treatment.

10. Malignant Melanoma

    A. A malignant melanoma originates in the _____ of the skin.
    B. It develops when the cells do not respond to the normal control mechanisms of _____ growth.
    C. The primary tumor begins in the _____.

11. Signs and Symptoms of Malignant Melanoma (list the signs and symptoms)

    i. _____
    ii. _____
    iii. _____
    iv. _____
    v. _____
    vi. _____
    vii. _____

12. Acne Vulgaris

    A. Acne vulgaris occurs when oil and _____ cells clog the skin's pores.
    B. It most often affects _____, with more than 85% of them developing at least a mild form of this condition.
    C. Whereas mild acne is merely annoying, severe acne can lead to _____ and _____ scars.
    D. Most people outgrow acne by the time they are in their _____ and _____.

13. Signs and Symptoms of Acne Vulgaris

   A. Skin blemishes are often _____ and _____.
   B. With a mild case of acne, only _____ and _____ may be present.
   C. Severe acne can mean hundreds of _____ or _____ that can cover the face, neck, chest, and back.
   D. _____ are pimples that are large and deep. These lesions are often painful and can leave scars on the skin.

14. Treatment Options for Acne Vulgaris

   A. The _____ of the acne will determine the most useful and beneficial treatment.
   B. Sometimes treatments will be combined to get the best results and to avoid the development of _____ bacteria.

15. Alopecia

   A. Alopecia is the condition of _____ or _____ of hair.
   B. The most common form is _____, also known as androgenic alopecia.

16. Alopecia Areata

   A. Alopecia areata affects about _____ in _____ people, mostly teenagers and young adults.
   B. It causes patches of baldness that are about the size of a(n) _____, usually appearing on the _____, but can occur anywhere on the body, including the beard, eyebrows, and eyelashes.

17. Male-Pattern Baldness

   A. Male-pattern baldness tends to follow a(n) _____.
   B. The first stage is usually the _____ of the _____.
   C. The second stage is thinning of the hair on the _____ and _____.
   D. When these two areas meet in the middle, the hair around the back and sides of the head resembles a(n) _____.
   E. Eventually the person may become _____.

18. Treatments for Addressing Baldness

   A. There are drugs that treat both _____ and _____ baldness.
   B. _____ can be rubbed on the scalp.
   C. Shampoos and formulas are available for _____ to the scalp.

19. Contact Dermatitis

   A. Contact dermatitis is a(n) _____ of the skin caused by irritating substances.
   B. Causes include exposure to _____ _____, _____ _____, _____ (especially on jewelry or jeans snaps), lotions, detergents, or other chemicals.

20. Signs and Symptoms of Contact Dermatitis

   A. Signs and symptoms include _____ and _____ skin.
   B. Vesicles (_____) and a rash may appear.
   C. _____ and _____ may be present.
   D. Serious allergic reactions may result in _____.

21. Treatment Options for Contact Dermatitis

   A. _____ (anti-allergy medicines)
   B. _____ creams to reduce inflammation
   C. _____ (oral medications)

22. Calluses and Corns

   A. Calluses and corns are caused by excessive growth of the _____ layer of the epidermis and often occur on the hands and feet.
   B. They can be caused by _____ or by other factors such as ill-fitting shoes and unprotected hands during manual labor.

23. Signs and Symptoms of a Callus
    A. Signs and symptoms of a callus include an area of _____ _____ that does not have an identifiable border.
    B. The area may appear _____, _____, or even _____ while being painless, or may feel tender, throb, or burn.

24. Signs and Symptoms of a Corn
    A. A corn has a(n) _____ _____ with various textures; it appears most often on the feet.
    B. Corns may be hard or soft; they are _____ _____.

25. Decubitus Ulcer
    A. A decubitus ulcer is also called a(n) _____ _____ or a(n) _____.
    B. It refers to an area of skin and tissue that _____.
    C. It typically occurs when _____ _____ is maintained on a specific area of the skin.
    D. The constant pressure on the area _____ the blood supply, causing the _____ of the affected tissue.
    E. Common locations include the _____, _____, _____, _____, _____, and the back of the head.

26. The Four Stages of the Decubitus Ulcer
    A. Stage I: _____ area on the skin that does not blanch (turn white) when pressed.
    B. Stage II: The skin has a(n) _____ or a(n) _____ _____. The area around the site may be red and irritated.
    C. Stage III: The skin looks like a(n) _____ with damage to the tissue below the skin.
    D. Stage IV: The wound becomes so deep that there is damage to the tissue beneath the _____ _____, including damage to _____ and muscle.

27. Eczema
    A. Eczema is also called _____ _____.
    B. It is a chronic skin condition caused by a(n) _____ _____ on the skin.
    C. _____ tends to play a role.
    D. it is most common in infants; about half of the cases disappear by _____.
    E. Signs and symptoms include _____, _____, and _____.
    F. Lesions may appear dry or scaly, as well as have a(n) _____ appearance.

28. Treatment Options for Eczema
    A. Weeping lesions are treated with _____ _____ and dressings.
    B. Severe cases and dry, scaly lesions may be treated with mild, _____ _____ or low-potency topical _____.
    C. Very severe cases may require _____ and _____ _____ (TIMs).
    D. Sometimes, short exposures in a(n) _____ _____ are useful to dry up the lesions.

29. Folliculitis
    A. Folliculitis is an infection or inflammation of the _____ _____.
    B. It can occur anywhere that there is _____ _____.
    C. It most often appears in areas that become irritated by shaving, the rubbing of clothes, or where follicles and pores are blocked by _____ and _____.
    D. Common sites include the _____, the _____, _____, and on the legs.

30. Signs and Symptoms of Folliculitis
    A. A(n) _____ _____
    B. Raised, red, often _____ lesions around hair follicles
    C. _____ that occur in areas with a high concentration of hair follicles, such as the face, under the arms, on the scalp, and in the groin area, and eventually crust over
    D. _____ at the site of the rash and pimples

31. Treatment Options for Folliculitis

    A. Treatment generally involves taking steps to _____ _____ to the hair follicles by avoiding clothes that rub against the skin.

    B. Shave with a(n) _____ _____ instead of a razor blade.

    C. Keep the skin clean using soap and water and _____ _____.

    D. Apply _____ _____.

32. Treatment Options for Shingles

    A. Early treatment can help shorten a shingles _____ and reduce the risk of complications.

    B. Oral antiviral medications are generally prescribed within _____ to _____ hours after the first sign of the rash.

    C. _____ are sometimes prescribed in order to reduce swelling and pain.

    D. When pain is severe, _____ _____ or a skin patch that contains a pain-relieving medication may be required.

33. Keloids

    A. Keloids are often referred to as _____ _____.

    B. They typically appear following _____ or a(n) _____.

    C. _____ and _____ have been known to cause keloids.

34. Pediculosis

    A. Pediculosis is a(n) _____ by eggs, larvae, or adult lice.

    B. Forms of pediculosis include *Pediculus humanus capitis* (_____ _____), *Pediculus humanus corporis* (_____ _____), and *Pthirus pubis* (_____ _____).

35. Signs and Symptoms of Pediculosis

    A. The most common symptom among all types of lice is _____.

    B. Head lice tend to cause itching on the back of the _____ or around the _____.

    C. Itching around the _____ is an indication of pubic lice.

    D. Body lice tend to travel to the body to feed on _____ and then return to _____.

36. Psoriasis

    A. Psoriasis affects an estimated _____ Americans.

    B. It most commonly affects persons between ages _____ and _____.

    C. The condition has _____ and _____ characteristics.

    D. It is thought to be caused by a buildup of _____.

37. Signs and Symptoms of Psoriasis

    A. Signs and symptoms include episodes of redness, itching, and _____, _____ on the skin.

    B. _____ can be gradual or abrupt.

    C. _____ have been attributed to infection, obesity, and lack of sunlight, as well as sunburn, stress, poor health, and cold climate.

    D. When the case is severe and widespread, large quantities of _____ can be lost, causing _____ and severe secondary infections that can be serious.

38. Treatment Options for Psoriasis

    A. Treatment options include analgesics, sedation, _____ _____, retinoids, and antibiotics.

    B. Mild cases are treated at home with topical medications such as prescription or nonprescription _____ _____, _____, or other corticosteroids, and antifungal medications.

    C. Severe lesions may require _____ for proper treatment.

39. Rosacea

    A. Rosacea is a disorder primarily of the _____.

    B. It is often characterized by _____ and _____.

    C. It affects an estimated _____ Americans.

40. Signs and Symptoms of Rosacea

    A. _____ on the cheeks, nose, chin, or forehead

    B. Small visible _____ _____ on the face, _____ on the face, and watery or irritated eyes

    C. Over time, the _____ becomes ruddier and more persistent.

41. Scabies

    A. Scabies is a(n) _____ _____ disorder of the skin.

    B. It is caused by the scabies mite or human _____ _____.

    C. It is spread by _____ _____, such as shaking hands; sleeping together; or close contact with infected articles such as clothing, bedding, or towels.

    D. Common among schoolchildren, roommates, and sexual partners, scabies is usually found where people are _____ _____.

    E. The sides of the _____, the backs of the _____, wrists, heels, elbows, armpits, inner thighs, and the waistline are common locations for scabies.

42. Signs and Symptoms of Scabies

    A. A very small _____ blister

    B. Intense _____ and a red _____ that occurs around the area

43. Treatment Options for Scabies

    A. Treatment includes application of a lotion or cream with a 6–10% concentration of _____.

    B. _____ and _____ are often used to relieve itching.

44. Seborrheic Dermatitis

    A. Seborrheic dermatitis is a(n) _____ condition of the sebaceous or oil glands caused by an increase in sebum.

    B. It is most common in infants and children; frequently known as _____.

45. Signs and Symptoms of Seborrheic Dermatitis

    A. Yellow or white scales that attach to the _____ _____

    B. Thick or patchy crusts on the _____

    C. Itching or soreness, as well as _____

46. Treatment Options for Seborrheic Dermatitis

    A. Application of low-strength _____

    B. Shampooing the scalp daily with _____

47. *Tinea Corporis*

    A. *Tinea corporis* is sometimes called _____.

    B. It is not actually a worm, but instead an integumentary disorder caused by a(n) _____.

    C. It can appear _____ on the body.

    D. If the fungus is on the head, it is called _____ _____.

    E. On the feet, it is known as _____ _____, or athlete's foot.

    F. When found in the genital area, it is referred to as _____ _____.

    G. *Tinea cruris* is more commonly known as _____ _____.

    H. Elsewhere on the body, the fungus is called _____ _____.

48. Urticaria

  A. Urticaria is better known as _____.
  B. It causes severe _____ because of an acute hypersensitivity to medications or environmental stimuli.
  C. A major concern is that it can obstruct the _____ _____.
  D. Because of the possibility of _____ _____, it is important to observe all patients after an injection or allergy test.

49. Signs and Symptoms of Urticaria

  A. Signs and symptoms include _____ areas of pink, itchy, swollen patches of skin.
  B. _____ or _____ sensations are common.
  C. Hives may vary in size from the diameter of a(n) _____ _____ to the diameter of a cereal bowl.
  D. Many times, the hives may _____, forming an even larger area of irritation and swelling.

50. Treatment Options for Urticaria

  A. Removal of _____ _____
  B. Treatment with _____ and _____

51. Vitiligo

  A. Vitiligo is also known as _____.
  B. This disorder causes white patches and large areas of decreased _____ to form on the skin.
  C. Patches form because of the destruction of _____, which are the cells that produce _____.
  D. It is often linked to immune system disorders such as _____ _____ or pernicious anemia.
  E. It affects persons with _____ disorders.

52. Treatment Options for Vitiligo

  A. Treatment is often aimed at _____ skin tone and color.
  B. This is accomplished through _____, _____, or _____ means.
  C. Avoiding tanning and using sunscreen will help make the _____ less noticeable.
  D. _____ and _____ lotions may also be used to even out the skin tone.
  E. Medical treatments may include the use of _____, as well as topical ultraviolet therapy.
  F. _____ _____, as well as a form of tattooing called _____, may also be successful.

53. Warts (Verruca)

  A. Warts are an infection caused by viruses in the _____ _____ (HPV) family.
  B. At least _____ types of HPV viruses cause warts.
  C. Warts can grow on all parts of the body, including the _____, the inside of the mouth, the genitals, and the _____ _____.
  D. A common wart is the _____ wart, which occurs on the soles of the feet.

54. Signs and Symptoms of Warts

  A. The _____ and _____ of a wart will vary with its location.
  B. Warts may appear _____ or _____, and may vary in color from flesh-toned to red, pink, or white.
  C. Warts may also appear as raised or _____ _____ _____.

55. Treatment Options for Warts

    A. Over-the-counter topical medications that contain _____ _____

    B. _____, which freezes the wart

    C. Various _____ _____

    D. In severe cases, _____ _____ may be an option.

III. Skin Care Treatments

1. Botox

    A. Botox injection is a popular procedure that is indicated for reducing _____ _____.

    B. A very small, diluted amount of the toxin _____ _____ is injected into the wrinkle lines.

    C. The procedure is usually repeated every _____ to _____ months.

    D. Temporary side effects include headaches, bruising, and _____ _____.

2. Light Chemical Peel

    A. The purpose of this treatment is to reduce the size of _____, make the skin appear _____, and produce more _____ in the skin.

    B. During a light chemical peel, only the _____ layer of the skin is stripped.

    C. The procedure is completed in about an hour and it leaves the skin _____, which disappears over time.

3. Medium Chemical Peel

    A. The purpose of this treatment is to _____ _____, resulting in a much smoother skin than that achieved with the light chemical peel.

    B. This treatment will strip the _____ _____ and some underlying cells, causing collagen and elastin to be stimulated.

    C. Recovery from a medium chemical peel can take up to _____ days because of the peeling, swelling, and redness that occur after treatment.

4. Deep Chemical Peel

    A. An aggressive treatment that can affect the layers of skin down to the _____ layer.

    B. Results are aimed at reducing all _____ in the face, with the exception of certain areas.

    C. This level of treatment can improve conditions such as _____ _____ and remove precancerous lesions.

    D. The healing process includes _____ _____, often felt up to 12 hours after surgery.

    E. _____ medications are required.

    F. It may take _____ for additional peeling, swelling, and redness to subside.

5. Laser Resurfacing

    A. In laser resurfacing, short, pulsated _____ _____ are used to vaporize damaged or troublesome areas of the skin.

    B. Full-face laser resurfacing takes approximately _____ hours.

    C. Partial-face resurfacing takes _____ minutes.

    D. Resurfacing results in the stimulation and production of new _____ and skin cells.

    E. Immediately following the procedure, _____ _____ and sterile _____ are applied to reduce the incidence of infection.

6. Microdermabrasion

    A. Microdermabrasion involves removing the top layer of _____ _____ _____.

    B. _____ are used with abrasion and suction devices to produce healthier-looking skin.

    C. This non- _____ and non- _____ approach is appealing to many patients who do not wish to pursue more aggressive skin-freshening treatments.

APPLIED PRACTICE

1. Using information found in the textbook, fill out the following table regarding infectious skin disorders.

Disorder	Symptoms	Diagnosis	Treatment
Furuncles/Carbuncles			
Herpes Simplex			
Herpes Zoster (Shingles)			

(continue)

Disorder	Symptoms	Diagnosis	Treatment
Impetigo			

2. Label the structures of the nail bed.

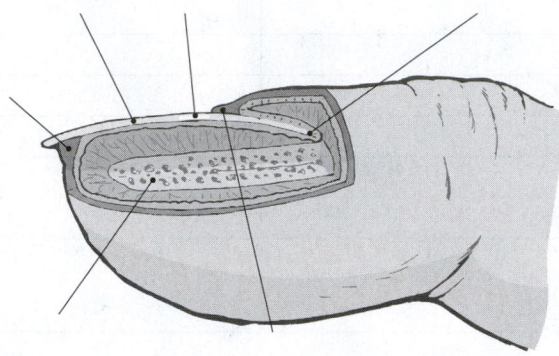

LEARNING ACTIVITY: FILL IN THE BLANK

Using words from the list below, fill in the blanks to complete the following statements.

ABCD rule

appearance

blood and lymphatic

common

connective tissue

curable

cushions

dehydration

dermis

diagnosed early

fat cells

generalized illness

hair growth

heat and cold

inflammation and infection

insulation

irritations or lesions

microorganisms

nails

nerve

polycystic

Staphylococcus

subcutaneous

subcutaneous tissue

support

sweat and sebaceous

toxins

temperature

tumors

vitamin D

1. Skin cancers are initially diagnosed according to their _____. Malignant melanoma is identified by the _____.

2. The integumentary system includes the _____, hair, and _____ glands.

3. Skin cancers are the most _____ type of cancer, as well as the most _____ when _____.

4. The skin serves as a barrier to prevent _____ and other foreign bodies from entering; regulates _____; protects against _____; acts as an environmental sensor for pain, temperature, and touch; synthesizes _____ from sunlight; and excretes _____ in perspiration.

5. The dermis contains _____ vessels, _____ cell endings, and skin _____ organs.

6. Hirsutism is a condition of excessive _____, which may be caused by _____ ovaries or _____ of the adrenal glands and ovaries.

7. A break in the defense system of the skin may result in _____, as well as localized _____.

8. Cellulitis is a disease of the skin and subcutaneous tissue that presents as _____. It is commonly caused by _____.

9. Sweat glands are located in the _____ and the _____.

10. The innermost layer of skin, the _____ tissue, is made up of _____ and _____. This layer acts as _____ for the body, provides protection against extreme _____ and against heat loss, and _____ and protects underlying structures.

CRITICAL THINKING

Answer the following questions to the best of your ability. Use the textbook as a reference.

1. As you are assisting a geriatric patient to get into a gown for an examination, you notice that she has a dime-sized mole with an irregular border on her back. You realize that the patient likely cannot see it and may be unaware of it. Would you mention it to the patient or only to the physician? State the reason for your answer.

_____
_____
_____

2. Utilize Internet search engines to locate a reputable site that provides pictures of various skin conditions, including lice. Draw a picture of head lice and state how this condition is treated.

_____
_____
_____

3. What possible advice could you give to a patient who has had a skin cancer removed today and works daily as a lifeguard in the sun?

_____
_____
_____

RESEARCH ACTIVITY

Use Internet search engines to research the following topic and write a brief description of what you find. It is important to use reputable websites.

1. Visit the Skin Cancer Foundation at www.skincancer.org. After reviewing the website, answer the following questions:

   a. What "Prevention" information do you find most interesting. Why?
   b. After reading "Skin Cancer Facts," which facts do you find most surprising?
   c. What can you do to further reduce your risk of developing skin cancer?

   _____
   _____
   _____
   _____
   _____

CHAPTER 23
The Skeletal System

STUDENT STUDY GUIDE

Use the following guide to assist in your learning of the concepts from the chapter.

I. The Skeletal System

1. Bone Classification

    i. _____
    ii. _____
    iii. _____
    iv. _____
    v. _____
    vi. _____

2. The Six Main Functions of Bones

    A. Bones provide _____, _____, and the framework of the body.
    B. They provide _____ for the body's internal organs.
    C. They serve as a storage place for _____, _____, and _____.
    D. They play an important role in the formation of blood cells as _____ takes place in the _____.
    E. They provide an area for the attachment of _____ muscle.
    F. They help to make movement possible through _____.

3. Bone Markings

    i. _____
    ii. _____
    iii. _____
    iv. _____
    v. _____
    vi. _____
    vii. _____
    viii. _____

4. Joints

    A. The positioning of the bones at the joint determines the _____ that the joint performs.
    B. Joints are always classified according to the _____ that they provide.

5. The Rib Cage

    A. The ribs form a protective cage that houses the _____, _____, and other vital components of the human body.
    B. The rib cage consists of _____ pairs of ribs.

II. The Pathology of the Skeletal System

1. Scoliosis

   A. Scoliosis is often diagnosed early in _____, _____ and _____.
   B. Persons who have scoliosis may often appear as if either their _____ or _____ are uneven.

2. Lordosis

   A. Lordosis is a(n) _____ curvature of the _____ spine.
   B. When diagnosed in adults, may be commonly found in persons who are _____ and in _____ women.
   C. When diagnosed in children, the most common symptom is a prominently protruding _____ and _____.

3. Kyphosis

   A. Kyphosis is an exaggeration of the _____ curvature.
   B. The normal _____ curvature may become exaggerated because of a _____ defect.

4. Arthritis

   A. Causes include _____ injury, _____ disorders, and normal to _____ wear and tear on the joints.
   B. Arthritis can occur at any age; however, it most commonly develops in _____ adults.

5. Treatment for Arthritis

   A. Treatment depends on the _____, _____, and _____ of the patient.
   B. Modification of daily activities and low-impact _____ exercise are helpful.

6. Osteoarthritis

   A. Osteoarthritis most frequently occurs in the _____, _____, and finger joints of _____ patients.
   B. Obesity, a history of _____, and various genetic and _____ diseases increase the risk of osteoarthritis.

7. Carpal Tunnel Syndrome

   A. Carpal tunnel syndrome is caused when pressure is placed on the _____.
   B. Certain conditions increase the risk of carpal tunnel syndrome, including _____, _____, and _____ arthritis.
   C. Treatment of carpal tunnel syndrome includes the use of proper _____ when engaging in computer use and other activities.

8. Treatment for Fractures

   A. Fractures are generally casted by a(n) _____.
   B. At times, with severe fractures, _____ intervention must be performed.
   C. Pain and _____ medications are often prescribed for patient comfort.

9. Treatment for Dislocations

   A. Dislocations are treated in a(n) _____ department.
   B. Reduction is used to _____ and _____ the joint.
   C. Administer pain relievers and _____ medications.

10. Osteoporosis

    A. Osteoporosis affects more than _____ Americans, mostly women ages _____ to _____ years old.

    B. Persons with osteoporosis are subject to increased _____ potential, especially in the _____, _____, and _____.

11. Individuals at Higher Risk for Osteoporosis

    i. _____

    ii. _____

    iii. _____

    iv. _____

    v. _____

    vi. _____

12. Signs, Symptoms, and Treatment for Osteoporosis

    A. The most common sign is decreased _____ and a(n) _____ posture.

    B. Additional signs and symptoms include _____ pain and frequent _____.

    C. Treatment includes _____ and _____ supplements.

13. Signs, Symptoms, and Treatment for Gout

    A. A _____ joint is often very warm and very sore to the touch.

    B. After joints have been persistently affected by gout, they may become _____.

    C. Treatment includes a diet rich in colorful _____ and _____.

14. Hallux Valgus

    A. Hallux valgus is the enlargement of the inner portion of the _____ joint at the base of the _____ toe.

    B. Signs and symptoms include _____ skin around the inflamed joint of the _____ toe.

    C. The joint may be filled with _____ and feel _____ to the touch.

15. Treatment for Hallux Valgus

    A. Properly _____ should be worn.

    B. Proper _____ and _____ of the joint should be considered.

    C. _____ surgery and pain medications may be required for severe cases.

16. Hammer Toe

    A. Signs and symptoms include _____ and visible joint _____.

    B. Treatment includes wearing specially designed _____.

17. Rickets

    A. Rickets results in bone _____, especially _____ legs.

    B. Signs and symptoms include _____ and _____ of the bones.

    C. Treatment includes increasing _____ and _____ intake.

18. Osteomalacia

    A. Osteomalacia is caused by deficiencies in _____ and _____.

    B. Symptoms include _____ pain, _____ legs, and _____ fractures.

    C. Treatment is similar to the treatment for _____.

APPLIED PRACTICE

1. Label the bones found on the images of the anterior and posterior views of the skeletal system.

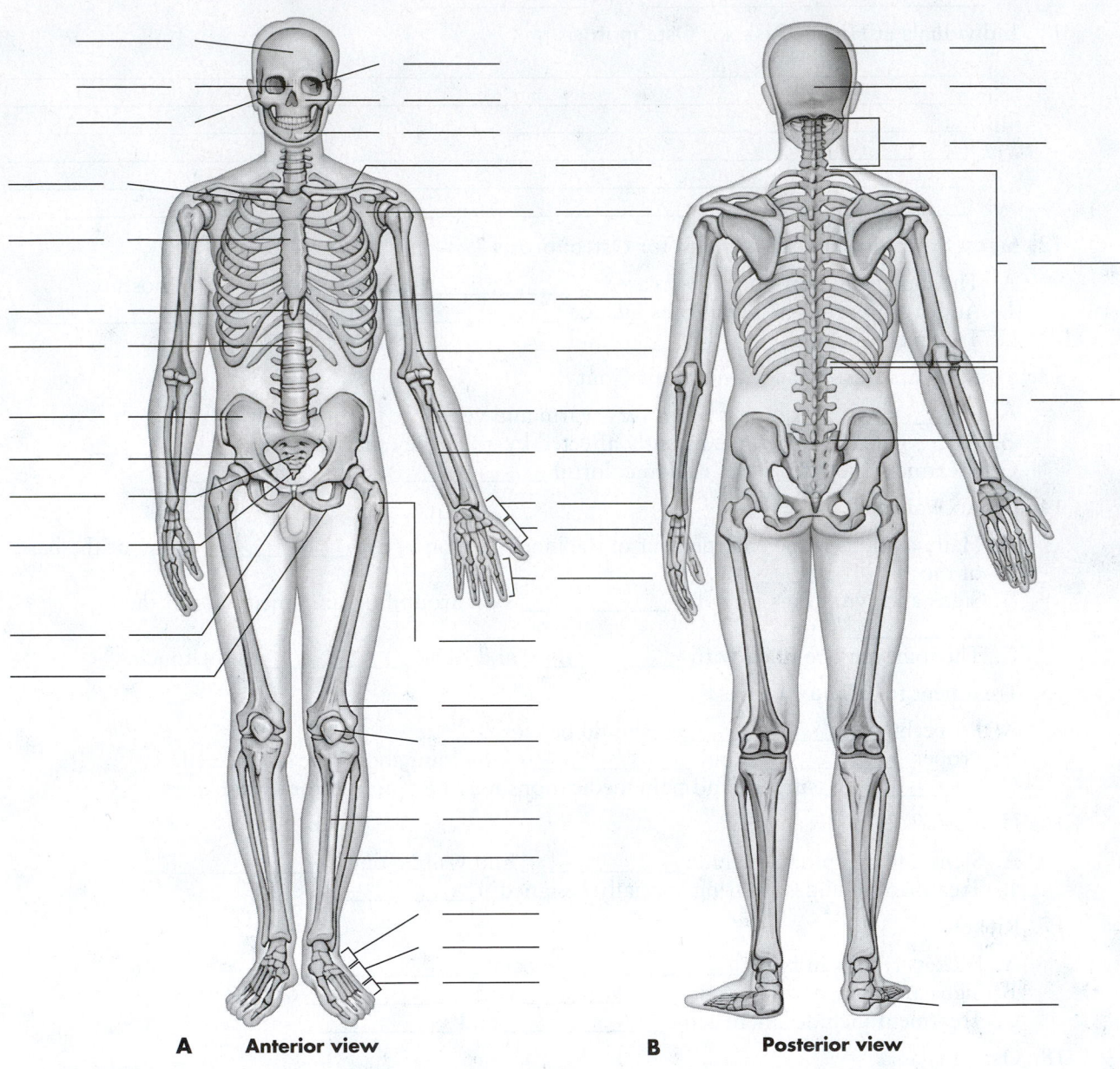

A   Anterior view   B   Posterior view

2. Label the types of fractures found in this image.

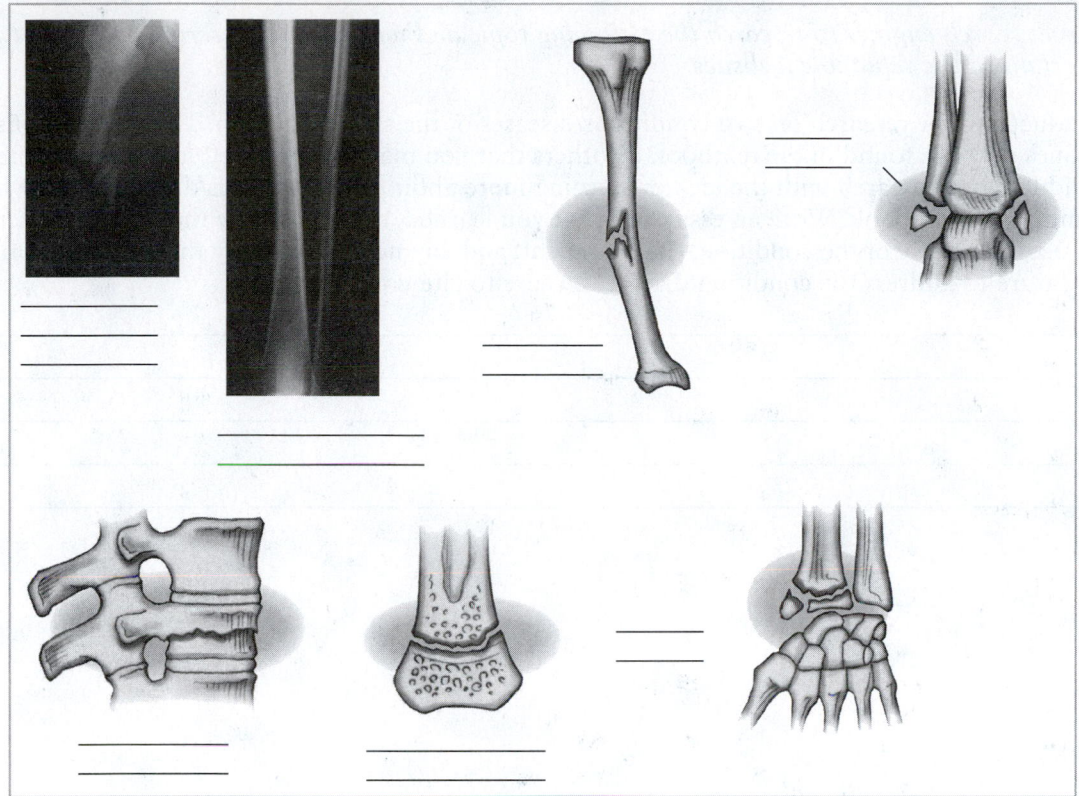

CRITICAL THINKING

Answer the following questions to the best of your ability. Use the textbook as a reference.

1. If a patient has an injury to the skeletal system, how might the medical assistant be able to assist the patient?

_____

_____

_____

2. How can the medical assistant stay current with new information that may be occurring in medicine? Why is staying current in one's field so critical?

_____

_____

_____

3. When obtaining a medical history from a patient, why is it important to check the patient's past medical history?

_____

_____

_____

RESEARCH ACTIVITY

Use Internet search engines to research the following topic and write a brief description of what you find. It is important to use reputable websites.

1. Conduct further research on two conditions/diseases of the skeletal system. These conditions can be ones that are found in the textbook or others that you may be interested in learning more about. Conduct your research with the idea of learning more about the conditions/diseases than what is found in the textbook. Write an essay on what you learned, including how the disease presents itself, the possible cause of the condition, the treatment, and any new technology that may be available in the future to address the condition/disease. Be sure to cite your sources.

_____

_____

_____

_____

_____

CHAPTER 24

The Muscular System

STUDENT STUDY GUIDE

Use the following guide to assist in your learning of the concepts from the chapter.

I. The Muscular System

   1. Muscle Characteristics

      A. Each muscle is made of specialized cells called muscle _____.

      B. The muscle fibers are held together by _____ tissue.

      C. Connective tissue is held together by a fibrous sheath called _____.

      D. Muscles make up more than _____ of body weight.

   2. The Functions of the Muscular System

      i. _____

      ii. _____

      iii. _____

      iv. _____

      v. _____

   3. Skeletal Muscles

      A. Skeletal muscles are attached to _____ bones.

      B. They are wrapped in layers of _____ tissue.

      C. They are stimulated by _____ neurons.

   4. Smooth Muscles

      A. Smooth muscles are found in tissue in the walls of _____ organs.

      B. They are responsible for the movement of _____ organs.

   5. Adenosine Triphosphate (ATP)

      A. ATP is the type of chemical energy needed for _____ or repeated muscular _____.

      B. It can be produced by either _____ or _____ means.

   6. The Effects of Oxygen Debt

      A. Oxygen debt occurs when skeletal muscles are used for more than _____ or _____ minutes.

      B. Lack of oxygen intake reduces the body's ability to produce energy _____, causing _____ production.

      C. The body can only utilize this energy for about _____ seconds, depending on the individual, before severe fatigue sets in, making it very difficult to recover.

      D. Oxygen "owed" to body is the debt and can only be recovered by _____ respiration, which allows more oxygen into the _____ to reach the _____.

II. The Pathology of the Muscular System

   1. Atrophy

      A. Lipoatrophy is atrophy of the _____ _____.

      B. The signs and symptoms of atrophy include the apparent _____ of a muscle group and extreme _____ and _____ associated with atrophic muscle groups.

      C. Treatment includes _____ exercises of the immobilized muscle.

2. Fibromyalgia

    A. Fibromyalgia is more common in _____ than _____.

    B. The signs and symptoms include mild to severe _____ pain and _____.

    C. _____ _____ syndrome is a common symptom.

3. Criteria for Determining Fibromyalgia

    A. The American College of _____ identified specific criteria.

    B. The patient must show _____ to _____ trigger or tender points to be considered for this diagnosis, as well as a history of widespread pain lasting at least _____ months.

4. Treatment for Fibromyalgia

    A. Treatment is geared toward improving the quality of _____ and reducing _____.

    B. Common medications used in treatment include the following:

        i. _____

        ii. _____

        iii. _____

        iv. _____

        v. _____

5. Ganglion Cyst

    A. Ganglion cysts are more common in _____ than _____.

    B. The signs and symptoms include masses occurring typically on the _____, _____, and _____.

    C. _____ swelling can occur.

6. Treatment for a Ganglion Cyst

        i. _____

        ii. _____

        iii. _____

7. Lyme Disease

    A. Lyme disease is carried by _____ and transmitted through the bite of an infected _____.

    B. The signs and symptoms include the following:

        i. _____

        ii. _____

        iii. _____

        iv. _____

8. The Prevention of and Treatment for Lyme Disease

    A. Prevention includes the following:

        i. _____

        ii. _____

        iii. _____

    B. Treatment includes the use of _____, _____, or _____.

9. Muscular Dystrophy

    A. There are _____ major forms of muscular dystrophy.

    B. The signs and symptoms include _____, _____, and _____.

10. Treatment for Muscular Dystrophy

    A. _____ _____ to prevent contraction

    B. _____ for support

    C. Corrective _____ surgery

    D. The Emery-Dreifuss and myotonic forms may necessitate a(n) _____ because of the cardiac problems associated with these forms

11. Rotator Cuff Tears

    A. Rotator cuff tears are common in _____ muscles/tendons.
    B. They are caused by many years of _____ of these muscles/tendons.
    C. They also may be caused by one single _____ injury.

12. Treatment for Rotator Cuff Tears

    i. _____
    ii. _____
    iii. _____
    iv. _____
    v. _____
    vi. _____

13. Shin Splints

    A. Shin splints are usually caused by _____ or _____ conditioning of the leg muscles.
    B. They are often found in persons with _____ feet or _____ arches.
    C. The signs and symptoms include the following:
        i. _____
        ii. _____
        iii. _____

14. Treatment for Shin Splints

    i. _____
    ii. _____
    iii. _____
    iv. _____

15. Sprains

    A. Sprains are very common in _____.
    B. A sprain often occurs in the _____ of major joints.
    C. The signs and symptoms include the following:
        i. _____
        ii. _____
        iii. _____
        iv. _____

16. Strains

    A. A chronic strain occurs from _____ and _____ movement.
    B. An acute strain can occur from _____ lifting of a heavy object.
    C. The signs and symptoms include the following:
        i. _____
        ii. _____
        iii. _____
        iv. _____
        v. _____
        vi. _____
        vii. _____

17. The Signs, Symptoms, and Treatment for Tendonitis

    A. The signs and symptoms include pain and _____ in the affected area.
    B. Treatment involves physical therapy, including _____ to increase range of motion.

18. Tetanus

   A. Tetanus is an often fatal, _____ disease.

   B. It is caused by _____ bacterium.

   C. The signs and symptoms include the following:

   i. _____

   ii. _____

   iii. _____

   iv. _____

   v. _____

APPLIED PRACTICE

1. Label the muscles found on the images of the anterior and posterior views of the muscular system.

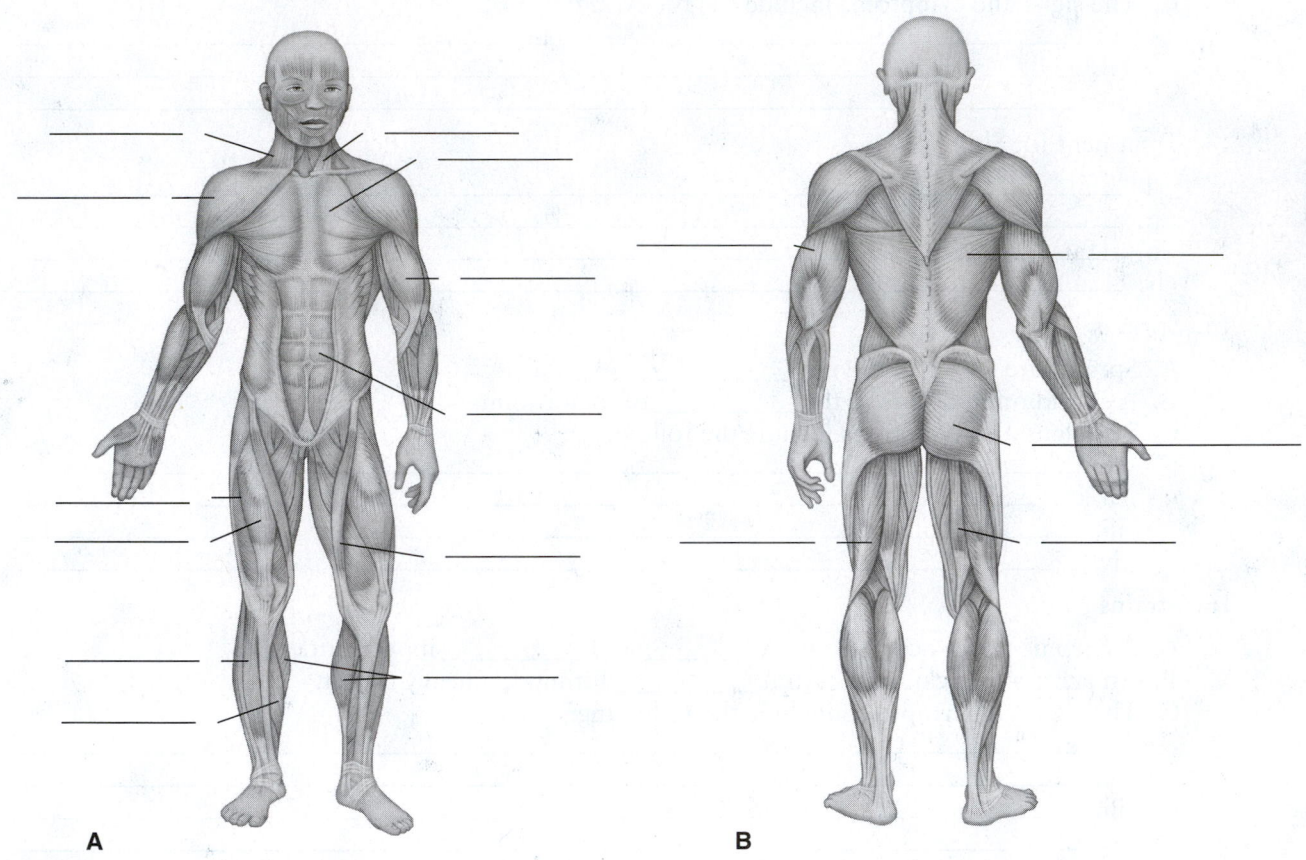

A

B

2. Label the muscles of the head, neck, and face found in this image.

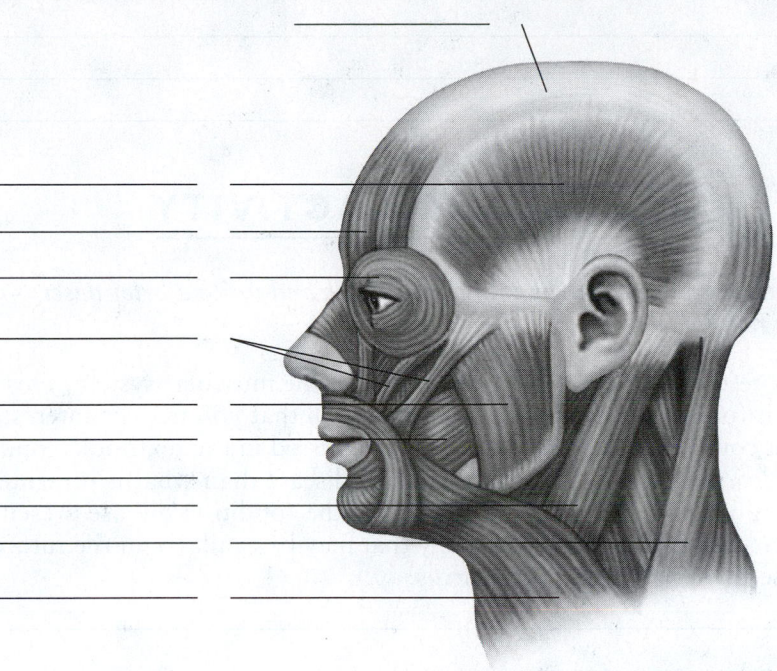

CRITICAL THINKING

Answer the following questions to the best of your ability. Use the textbook as a reference.

1. When giving children injections, why are injections usually given in the vastus lateralis muscle? When should the gluteus maximus muscle be used when giving an injection to an adult?

_____

_____

_____

2. As a medical assistant, what should you do if a patient is upset or concerned about his or her health?

_____

_____

_____

3. How does regular exercise help older adults stay healthy?

_____

_____

_____

4. What is aspiration? For what conditions would aspiration be necessary?

_____

_____

_____

5. Discuss tetanus and its symptoms. How can it be prevented?

_____

_____

_____

RESEARCH ACTIVITY

Use Internet search engines to research the following topic and write a brief description of what you find. It is important to use reputable websites.

1. Conduct further research on one condition/disease of the muscular system. This condition/disease can be one that is found in the textbook or a condition that you may be interested in learning more about that is not covered in the textbook. If it is discussed in the textbook, conduct your research with the idea of learning more about the condition/disease than what is presented in the textbook. Write an essay on what you learned, including how the condition/disease presents itself, the possible cause, the treatment, and any new technology that may be available in the future to address the condition/disease. Be sure to cite your sources.

_____

_____

_____

_____

_____

CHAPTER 25
The Nervous System

STUDENT STUDY GUIDE

Use the following guide to assist in your learning of the concepts from the chapter.

I. An Overview of the Central Nervous System

   1. The Nervous System

      A. The nervous system acts to correlate both _____ and _____ factors that affect our bodies by gathering, storing, and deciphering both external and internal information.

      B. It decides how to _____ and _____ in an appropriate manner in order to satisfy certain needs.

      C. Of these needs, the most important is _____.

   2. Types of Neurons: Motor Neurons

      A. Motor neurons usually have several _____ and only one _____.

      B. Axons may be several feet long and reach from the _____, _____ to the area that is to be activated.

      C. Dendrites resemble _____ and are unsheathed.

   3. Motor Neurons: On the following image, indicate the location of the axon, dendrite, and myelin sheath.

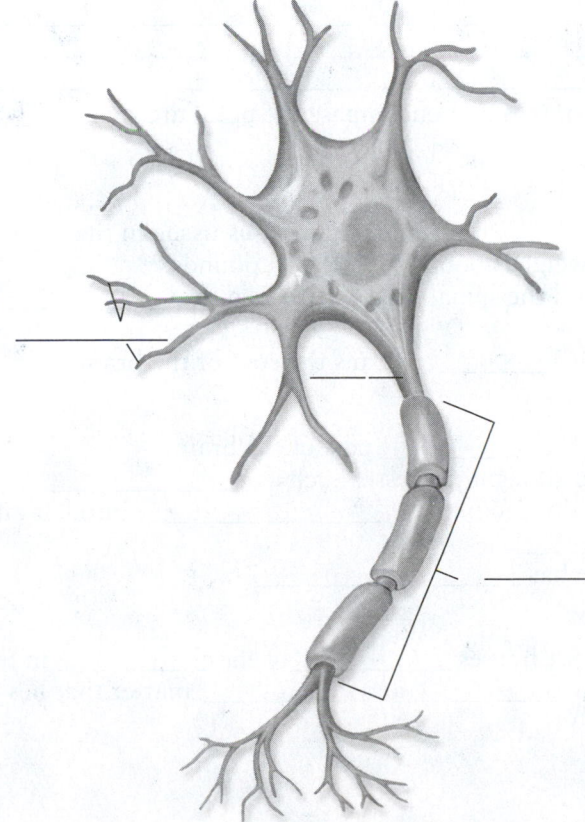

4. Sensory Neurons

   A. Sensory neurons lack true _____, are sheathed, and more closely resemble _____.

   B. They transmit impulses directly to the _____ _____ _____.

5. Nerve Fibers

   A. A nerve fiber is a single, elongated process, usually an axon or _____ process, from a _____ neuron.

   B. Nerve fibers in the peripheral nervous system (PNS) are wrapped in _____.

   C. Nerve fibers in the central nervous system (CNS) do not contain _____, and thus damage to the CNS is permanent, whereas damage to a(n) _____ nerve can be reversed.

6. Myelinated Sheaths

   A. Myelin is a thick _____ substance.

   B. Myelin sheaths have both an inner sheath of _____ and an outer sheath, or _____, composed of Schwann cells.

   C. _____ _____ are needed for the process of regenerating a damaged nerve fiber.

7. Tracts

   A. All nerve fibers that are housed within the nerve tract must have the same _____, _____, and _____.

   B. The spinal cord contains _____ tracts that are _____, which ascend to the brain, and _____ tracts that descend from the brain.

8. Nerve Impulses and Synapses

   A. Each receptor has its own _____ at which it will react to a stimulus, and each will only respond when its _____ has been reached.

   B. The impulse is then transmitted via a(n) _____, which is a knoblike branch ending.

   C. The process is similar to the _____.

9. An Overview of the Brain

   i. _____

   ii. _____

   iii. _____

   iv. The three membranes that encompass the brain are the _____, the _____, and the _____.

10. The Brain

   A. The brain is the _____ mass of nervous tissue in the body.

   B. The male brain weighs about _____ pounds.

   C. Both the brain and the spinal cord are divided into _____ matter and _____ matter.

   D. The _____ _____ forms the core of the brain.

11. The Cerebrum

   A. The cerebrum is the _____ part of the brain.

   B. It controls higher thought processes such as _____, reasoning, and judgment.

   C. The cerebrum is divided by the _____ into left and right halves called _____.

   D. Each hemisphere has _____.

12. The Cerebral Cortex

   A. The cerebral cortex houses _____ of the _____ in the entire nervous system.

   B. It is composed of _____ and _____ matter that lies directly below it.

    C. It is responsible for interpreting sensory information and initiating _____.

    D. It stores _____ and creates _____.

13. The Diencephalon

    A. "Diencephalon" literally means the _____ portion of the brain.

    B. It is made up of the _____ and the _____.

14. The Thalamus

    A. The thalamus is two large masses of _____ cell bodies connected by a third mass.

    B. It serves as a relay center for all sensory impulses, with the exception of _____.

15. The Hypothalamus

    A. The hypothalamus lies beneath the _____.

    B. It primarily regulates the _____ nervous activity associated with behavior and emotional expression.

    C. It is responsible for a variety of _____ functions that occur throughout the body.

16. The Brainstem

    A. The brainstem resembles a(n) _____.

    B. It contains the _____, the _____, and the _____.

    C. These structures relay important information to the cerebrum, including _____, _____, and other sensory data.

17. The Midbrain

    A. The midbrain is located just below the _____ and above the _____.

    B. It is associated with _____ _____ and the tracking movements of the eyes.

    C. The lower two segments are associated with the sense of _____.

18. The Pons

    A. The pons is a broad band of white matter anterior to the _____ that is between the midbrain and the _____ _____.

    B. It contains _____ _____ linking the cerebellum and medulla oblongata to higher cortical areas.

    C. It plays a vital role in _____ and _____ motor control.

19. The Medulla Oblongata

    A. The medulla oblongata connects the _____ and the rest of the brain to the spinal cord.

    B. The nerve centers in this area are vital to the body's _____ because they exert control of the circulation of blood by regulating both the _____ and arterial blood pressure.

    C. Different areas of the medulla oblongata are also responsible for involuntary bodily functions, including _____, _____, _____, _____, and _____.

20. The Cerebellum

    A. The cerebellum is located in the back of the skull below the cerebrum and behind the pons and the _____.

    B. The cerebellum is the _____ largest portion of the brain.

    C. The surface has a large _____ of gray cell bodies and white matter on its interior.

    D. It coordinates voluntary and involuntary _____ of movement.

    E. It adjusts muscles to automatically maintain _____.

21. A Review of the Brain: Label the parts of the brain as found on the image.

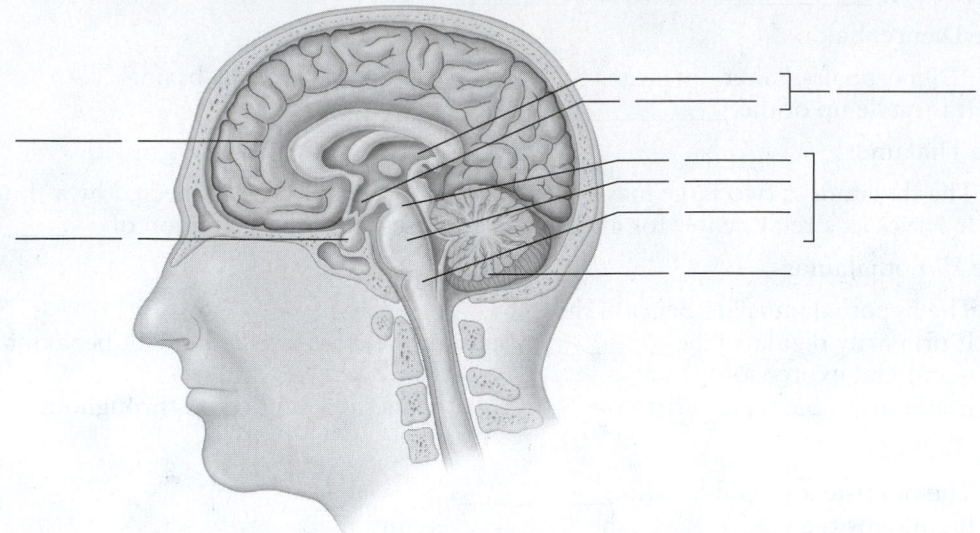

22. The Spinal Cord

   A. The spinal cord connects the brain with the _____ nerves.
   B. It consists of gray matter (cell bodies) in the _____ _____.
   C. It consists of white matter (_____ _____ _____) in the outer layer.
   D. Like the brain, it is surrounded by _____ fluid.
   E. Impulses are transmitted through the spinal cord along _____.
   F. The spinal cord is encased in the _____.
   G. The four divisions of the spinal cord are _____, _____, _____, and _____.

   H. The levels of the spinal column are numbered (e.g., cervical level 5 is noted as _____).
   I. Spinal nerves exit through _____ (openings) in the vertebrae.

23. Cerebrospinal Fluid

   A. Cerebrospinal fluid circulates around the brain and spinal cord in the _____ space.
   B. It provides _____ and _____ for the brain and spinal cord.
   C. It provides nourishment and _____.
   D. It is produced in the _____ of the ventricles of the brain.

24. Cranial Nerves and Their Functions: Name the nerves that provide each function listed.

   A. _____: Provides the sense of smell.
   B. _____: Provides vision.
   C. _____: Conducts motor impulses to four of the six external muscles of the eye and to the muscle that raises the eyelid.
   D. _____: Conducts motor impulses to control the superior oblique muscle of the eyeball.
   E. _____: Provides sensory input from the face, nose, mouth, forehead, and top of the head; motor fibers to the muscles of the jaw (chewing).
   F. _____: Conducts motor impulses to the lateral rectus muscle of the eyeball.
   G. _____: Controls the muscles of the face and scalp, the lachrymal glands of the eye and the submandibular and sublingual salivary glands, and input from the tongue for the sense of taste.
   H. _____: Provides input for hearing and equilibrium.
   I. _____: Provides a general sense of taste, regulates swallowing, and controls the secretion of saliva.

J. _____: Controls the muscles of the pharynx, larynx, thoracic, and abdominal organs; swallowing; voice production; the slowing of the heartbeat; and the acceleration of peristalsis.

K. _____: Controls the trapezius and sternocleidomastoid muscles, permitting movement of the head and shoulders.

L. _____: Controls tongue movement.

25. Spinal Nerves: Indicate the number of each.

A. _____ pair(s) of cervical spinal nerves
B. _____ pair(s) of thoracic spinal nerves
C. _____ pair(s) of lumbar spinal nerves
D. _____ pair(s) of sacral spinal nerves
E. _____ pair(s) of coccygeal spinal nerves

26. The Autonomic Nervous System

A. The final division of the nervous system occurs in the _____ _____.

B. The autonomic nervous system is further divided into the _____ and _____ nervous systems.

27. The Sympathetic Division

A. The sympathetic division branches from the _____ thoracic and the first three _____ spinal nerves form the first part of the sympathetic division of the ANS.

B. The cell bodies of these nerve fibers are located in the _____ _____ of the spinal cord.

C. The axons of the nerve cells leave the spinal nerves and enter almost immediately into masses of nerve cell bodies, which are called _____ _____.

D. Spinal nerves that synapse with the _____ _____ tend to produce widespread _____ when activated.

E. This occurrence is thought to prepare the body for _____ or _____.

F. During fight or flight, a person experiences increased alertness in conjunction with an increase in _____ _____ and other bodily functions.

G. At this point, the somatic nervous system stimulates the _____ _____ to release _____, the hormone that causes the familiar adrenaline rush.

28. The Parasympathetic Division

A. Long fibers that branch from _____ _____ III, VII, IX, and X in conjunction with the long fibers of _____ _____ II, III, and IV form the first stage of the parasympathetic division.

B. Cranial nerve fibers extend via the _____ nerve to ganglia serving the thoracic, abdominal, and pelvic viscera.

C. The fibers of the sacral spinal nerves form the _____ nerve, which branches to synapse with small ganglia near or within the organs to be innervated.

D. The cell bodies of these ganglia serve the _____ _____, _____, _____, and _____ _____.

E. The parasympathetic division works to conserve energy and innervate the digestive system; thus, its function earned the nickname "_____."

F. Instead of the adrenaline rush that is felt with the somatic nervous system, a(n) _____ in metabolism and bodily function occurs.

II. The Pathology of the Nervous System

1. Alzheimer's Disease

A. _____ history often plays a role in the development of this disease, along with _____ and _____.

B. Onset is most frequent in the later stages of life, generally ages _____ to _____.

2. Signs and Symptoms of Alzheimer's Disease

   A. Mild _____ of recent events is the first symptom.
   B. The ability to think and rationalize _____.
   C. Thought processes are _____.
   D. _____ may become difficult to understand.
   E. _____ and _____ skills dissipate.
   F. _____ patterns change during the later stages.
   G. Patients (may) become _____, _____, aggressive, or _____.
   H. Eventually, patients are unable to _____, _____, or _____ for themselves.

3. Treatment for Alzheimer's Disease

   A. Medications may _____ the progression of the disease in the _____ stages.
   B. Patients must continue to take medication throughout their lives to avoid _____.

4. Amyotrophic Lateral Sclerosis (ALS)

   A. ALS breaks down the _____ that are responsible for _____.
   B. The disease is also known as motor _____ disease.

5. Signs and Symptoms of Amyotrophic Lateral Sclerosis

   A. Signs and symptoms include loss of control of _____ muscle movement, including that of the arms, legs, and trunk.
   B. _____ muscle movement, such as that associated with the _____ of the heart and the smooth muscle of the internal organs, is not generally affected.
   C. Depending on the form of ALS, the loss of _____ (dementia) or sensory symptoms may occur.

6. Bell's Palsy

   A. Bell's palsy is generally not a serious condition, but does affect the _____ of the face.
   B. It is caused by damage to a(n) _____; a facial nerve runs beneath each ear to the muscles on that side of the face.
   C. It is also known as _____ palsy.
   D. It was named after Dr. Charles Bell, who first documented the disorder in _____.

7. Signs, Symptoms, and Treatment of Bell's Palsy
Signs and symptoms include the following:

   A. _____ of the face
   B. Facial _____ and lack of expression on the afflicted side. Treatment includes the following:
   A. _____ at the onset ensures good recovery.
   B. Without treatment, it may resolve on its own in a few _____ or _____.

8. Disk Disorders

   A. Disk disorders include painful deterioration of the disks that support the _____.
   B. Signs and symptoms include the following:
      i. _____
      ii. _____
      iii. _____
      iv. _____

9. Treatment for Disk Disorders

      i. _____
      ii. _____
      iii. _____
      iv. _____
      v. _____

10. Encephalitis

    A. Encephalitis is often caused by a(n) _____.

    B. It primarily affects _____ and the_____.

11. Epilepsy and Seizures

    A. The cause of epilepsy is _____.

    B. Epilepsy is often the result of another condition, such as a(n) _____ _____, _____, _____, or _____.

    C. Seizures affect about _____ of the population.

12. Types of Headaches

    i. _____

    ii. _____

    iii. _____

    iv. _____

13. Huntington's Chorea

    A. Huntington's chorea is a hereditary degenerative disorder of the cerebral and _____ _____.

    B. It is also referred to as _____ _____.

    C. Generally, onset begins during the mid- to late _____; it sometimes occurs in juveniles.

14. Signs and Symptoms of Huntington's Chorea

    i. _____

    ii. _____

    iii. _____

    iv. _____

    v. _____

    vi. _____

15. Treatment for Huntington's Chorea

    A. _____ and _____ are used to regulate pain, spasms, and seizures.

    B. Death occurs within _____ years of diagnosis.

16. Hydrocephalus

    A. Hydrocephalus commonly occurs in _____.

    B. It is characterized by an excessive amount of cerebrospinal fluid _____ in the brain, causing the brain to _____ against the skull.

    C. Without proper treatment, this condition can result in _____.

17. Signs and Symptoms of Hydrocephalus

    i. _____

    ii. _____

    iii. _____

    iv. _____

18. Signs and Symptoms of Meningitis

    i. _____

    ii. _____

    iii. _____

    iv. _____

    v. _____

19. Treatment for Meningitis

    i. _____

    ii. _____

    iii. _____

    iv. _____

    v. _____

    vi. _____

20. Multiple Sclerosis (MS)

    A. MS is a chronic, debilitating autoimmune disease that affects the _____ and the _____ _____.

    B. There is no known _____.

    C. The body directs the _____ and white blood cells to attack the _____ _____ surrounding the nerves in the brain and the spinal cord.

    D. _____ and injury to the sheath and nerves result; _____ is possible.

    E. Transmission of nerve impulses is impeded, making _____, _____, or _____ difficult.

21. Signs and Symptoms of Multiple Sclerosis

    i. _____

    ii. _____

    iii. _____

    iv. _____

    v. _____

    vi. _____

    vii. _____

    viii. _____

    ix. _____

    x. _____

22. Neuralgia

    A. Neuralgia is a general term for _____ _____.

    B. The signs and symptoms of neuralgia include the following:

        i. _____

        ii. _____

23. Treatment for Neuralgia

    A. Rest, stretching, and _____

    B. Aspirin, _____, or ibuprofen

    C. Narcotic pain killers, _____, and anesthetic agents administered via _____ injection

    D. Surgical procedures to decrease _____

24. Parkinson's Disease

    A. Parkinson's disease is a(n) _____ disorder.

    B. It is caused by the _____ of nerve cells in the parts of the brain that control _____.

    C. Because of degeneration, there is a shortage of the neurotransmitter _____, causing the _____ impairment that characterizes the disease.

    D. Parkinson's disease causes _____, _____ changes, _____, _____ disturbances, _____ impairment, and _____ difficulties.

    E. _____ over time.

25. Signs and Symptoms of Parkinson's Disease

    i. _____

    ii. _____

    iii. _____

    iv. _____

    v. _____

    vi. _____

26. Treatment for Parkinson's Disease

    A. _____ is administered.

    B. _____ must eventually be discontinued because of _____ _____.

    C. _____ intervention helps minimize involuntary movement.

27. Signs and Symptoms of Sciatica

    A. Signs and symptoms of sciatica include sharp pain from the _____, down the back of the _____.

    B. Pain may be worse during periods of _____, as well as at _____.

    C. Pain is increased when the _____ changes.

28. Treatment for Sciatica

    i. _____

    ii. _____

    iii. _____

    iv. _____

    v. _____

    vi. _____

29. Spina Bifida

    A. Spina bifida is the most frequently _____, permanently _____, and devastating of all birth defects.

    B. It affects approximately 1 out of every _____ newborns in the United States.

    C. More children have spina bifida than _____, _____, and _____ _____ combined.

    D. The spine fails to _____ properly during the first month of pregnancy.

    E. All nerve damage is _____.

30. Forms of Spina Bifida

    i. _____

    ii. _____

    iii. _____

    iv. _____

31. Signs and Symptoms of Spina Bifida: Closed Neural Tube

    A. Defects are _____.

    B. Some individuals show no _____.

    C. Others have _____, causing _____ and _____ dysfunction.

32. Signs and Symptoms of Spina Bifida: Meningocele

    A. The _____ protrude from the spinal opening.

    B. There may be no _____.

    C. Symptoms are similar to those of _____ neural tube defects.

33. Signs and Symptoms of Spina Bifida: Myelomeningocele

    A. Myelomeningocele is the most _____ form.

    B. The entire spinal cord is _____.

    C. _____ may be partial or complete below the area of the _____.

34. Treatment for Spina Bifida

    A. Some children may need _____ intervention as they grow and develop.

    B. _____ forms may not require any _____.

    C. Surgery _____ has been tried; however, complications can be great for both the mother and the fetus.

35. Treatment for the Complications of Paralysis

    A. Treatment is aimed at reducing _____.

    B. _____ therapy may be helpful in hemiplegic patients with complications due to stroke.

36. Complications Associated with Paralysis

    i. _____

    ii. _____

    iii. _____

    iv. _____

37. Strokes

    A. Strokes are the _____ leading cause of death in the United States.

    B. The _____ dies when the blood supply to the brain is decreased by _____ or _____.

    C. Brain cells can die when the _____ supply is interrupted for more than a few minutes.

    D. _____ is important in the diagnosis and treatment of strokes.

38. Signs and Symptoms of a Stroke

    i. _____

    ii. _____

    iii. _____

    iv. _____

    v. _____

    vi. _____

39. Treatment for a Stroke

    A. _____ intervention is vital.

    B. Stabilizing the patient's condition by either _____ blood clots or stopping the _____.

    C. _____ may be necessary.

    D. Administer medications to control _____ of the brain and _____.

    E. Medications and treatments are given after the incident to _____ the chance of _____.

40. Transient Ischemic Attacks (TIAs)

    A. TIAs are frequently precursors of _____.

    B. _____ can last anywhere from a few seconds to hours.

41. Signs and Symptoms of Transient Ischemic Attacks

    i. _____

    ii. _____

    iii. _____

42. Treatment for Transient Ischemic Attacks

    i. _____

    ii. _____

43. Methods for Reducing the Risk of Future Transient Ischemic Attacks

    i. _____

    ii. _____

    iii. _____

    iv. _____

    v. _____

44. Types of Trauma to the Brain

    A. A subdural _____ cause pressure in the brain that must be relieved by _____.

    B. A(n) _____ is an injury caused by abrupt jarring of, or a blow to, the head.

    C. A(n) _____ is bruising of the brain.

    D. Skull fractures known as _____ can cause brain injury.

45. Signs and Symptoms of Brain Trauma

    i. _____

    ii. _____

    iii. _____

    iv. _____

    v. _____

    vi. _____

    vii. _____

APPLIED PRACTICE

Read the following scenarios and answer the questions that follow.

Scenario 1

A 20-year-old female patient presents to your office with the following symptoms: Headache ×3 days, temperature of 103.2°F, dizziness, and blurred vision. She said that since she woke up this morning she has not been able to move her head. In her medical chart, you make a note that "the patient states 'My neck is so stiff, I can't bend it.'" Her head appears bent forward toward her chest.

1. What would you suspect the diagnosis might be based on her symptoms? *(Medical assistants never make a diagnosis; this is a question about your knowledge of the signs and symptoms of various conditions.)*

    _____

Scenario 2

A 59-year-old male patient presents to your office with observable right-side facial drooping, specifically near the mouth. The patient states that he "woke up this way" and he "can't feel anything on the entire right side of my face."

1. What would you suspect the diagnosis might be on the basis of his symptoms? *(Medical assistants never make a diagnosis; this is a question about your knowledge of the signs and symptoms of various conditions.)*

    _____

2. What is the treatment for this condition?

    _____

LEARNING ACTIVITY: MULTIPLE CHOICE

Circle the correct answer to each of the following questions.

1. Which of the following applies to a cerebrovascular accident?

   a. It is the third leading cause of death in the United States.
   b. It is caused by a virus.
   c. Brain tissue dies when the blood supply to a part of the brain is decreased.
   d. All of the above

2. Which of the following are signs and symptoms of encephalitis?

   a. Headache
   b. Stiff neck and back
   c. Drowsiness
   d. All of the above

3. Sciatica

   a. usually causes very intense pain.
   b. is caused by inflammation due to a pinched root.
   c. usually occurs on one side of the body.
   d. All of the above

4. Which of the following diseases has a cause that is unknown?

   a. ALS
   b. TIA
   c. Trigeminal neuralgia
   d. Multiple sclerosis

5. The corpus callosum

   a. controls most of the body's functions.
   b. joins the right and left hemispheres of the brain.
   c. is divided into gray and white matter.
   d. All of the above

6. Which of the following makes up the central nervous system?

   a. Nerves
   b. Cells
   c. Brain and spinal cord
   d. All of the above

7. Which of the following applies to epidural and subdural hematomas?

    a. They develop when the head receives a blow.
    b. They are typically seen in the elderly.
    c. They are a bruising of the brain.
    d. None of the above

8. Which of the following are associated with epilepsy?

    a. It often occurs after a head or neck injury has healed.
    b. The cause is unknown.
    c. It is a weakness or paralysis of the muscles that control expression on one side of the face.
    d. It is an inflammation of the brain caused by a virus.

9. Which of the following is not associated with meningitis?

    a. It is similar to encephalitis.
    b. It may be caused by a virus or bacteria.
    c. It has a high death rate if untreated.
    d. It is an autoimmune disease.

10. Motor neurons are

    a. greatly affected in ALS.
    b. considered afferent nerves.
    c. housed within the nerve tract.
    d. structurally like a stem.

CRITICAL THINKING

Answer the following questions to the best of your ability. Use the textbook as a reference.

1. A patient, a 57-year-old female named Katie Gilpatrick, has come into the office and is exhibiting signs of high stress. How can the medical assistant help relieve the patient's stress?

2. A fellow health care worker comes to work and states that she cannot do very much because she has "a migraine." She was out late last night at a party and states that the headache is not because she had some drinks. She hopes that you will help her through the day by taking care of some of her patients. She is incorrect in diagnosing herself with a migraine because it is a specific type of headache, and she has not been diagnosed with migraines by a physician. Explain why it is unlikely that someone with a true migraine would be able to come to work and function even at a slow pace.

3. Why is it important to be aware of the laws in your state regarding driving and neurological disorders?

4. What is a cerebrovascular accident?

_____

_____

_____

5. A patient comes to your clinic and complains of headache, stiff neck and back, drowsiness, and a fever. Could these be signs of encephalitis? Meningitis? Why or why not? What would you note in the patient's file?

_____

_____

_____

RESEARCH ACTIVITY

Use Internet search engines to research the following topic and write a brief description of what you find. It is important to use reputable websites.

1. Visit the Parkinson's Disease Foundation at www.pdf.org. Click on the "News and Events" tab on the top of the page, and then select "Science News." Choose an article of interest and provide a summary of the information discussed within the article. Discuss what interested you most about the article that you selected.

_____

_____

_____

_____

_____

CHAPTER 26
The Special Senses

STUDENT STUDY GUIDE

Use the following guide to assist in your learning of the concepts from the chapter.

I. The Eye and the Sense of Vision

    1. An Overview of the Eye and the Sense of Vision

        A. The eye is a(n) _____, _____ organ composed of specialized structures that work together to facilitate vision.

        B. Light rays pass through the _____, _____, _____, and vitreous humour to the retina where they stimulate sensory receptors.

        C. Nerves in the eye control the amount of _____ entering the eye through the _____, the focusing of the light by the lens on the _____, and the transmission of the resulting images to the _____.

        D. The eye is made up of the eyeball and its internal structures, which perform the complex process of translating _____ into _____, and external structures that support and protect the eyeballs.

        E. The eye contains three layers: the _____, the _____ and the _____.

    2. The Iris

        A. The iris is part of the _____ layer.

        B. It contains the _____, or eye color.

        C. It has a(n) _____ in the center, called the _____, that controls the amount of light entering the eye.

    3. The Innermost Layer of the Eye

        A. The innermost layer of the eye contains the _____ cells in the retina called _____ and _____ that translate light rays into nerve impulses that are transmitted to the brain.

        B. The fovea centralis retinae contains only _____.

        C. The optic nerve enters at the _____ disk and carries this information from the eye to the brain.

        D. A reflexive process called _____ adjusts the eye's optical powers to maintain a clear image at various distances.

    4. Eyelids, or Palpebrae

        A. Eyelids close over the eyeballs, protecting them from _____ _____, _____ _____, and _____.

        B. They also keep the eyes moist by preventing _____ from evaporating.

        C. _____ in the margins protect the eye from foreign matter.

        D. The superior and inferior _____ meet at the _____ at each corner of the eye.

5. The Lacrimal Apparatus

   A. The lacrimal gland secretes _____ through ducts on the surface of the _____ of the _____ lid.
   B. _____ cleanse the eyes and keep them moist.
   C. At the inner corner of each eye are two ducts, the _____ _____, which collect and drain the tears in the lacrimal _____.

6. Extrinsic Eye Muscles

   A. Six short extrinsic eye muscles connect the eyeball to the _____ _____.
   B. Muscles provide the eyeball with support and _____ movement.

7. The Characteristics of Refractive Disorders of the Eye

   A. Refractive disorders are the most _____ disorders of the eye.
   B. They are characterized by the _____ of the eye to _____ correctly.
   C. They are caused by factors such as _____ and changes in the _____ of the eyeball and the various eye muscles.

8. Astigmatism

   A. Astigmatism is caused by irregularities in the _____ of the _____ and _____ that cause light to focus on the retina but spread out over an area.
   B. Signs and symptoms include _____ near or distance vision.
   C. Treatment involves the use of _____ lenses or surgery to reshape the _____.

9. Myopia

   A. Myopia is also known as _____.
   B. The lens focuses the light in front of the _____.

10. Hyperopia

    A. Hyperopia is also known as _____.
    B. The lens focuses light behind the _____.
    C. _____ objects are seen more clearly than objects that are _____.

11. Presbyopia

    A. Presbyopia is characterized by a loss of _____ in the lens, usually as a result of _____.
    B. Signs and symptoms include difficulty in focusing on _____ objects.

12. Strabismus

    A. Strabismus is also called _____ eyes or _____ eyes.
    B. Signs and symptoms include poor _____ _____ and diplopia, or _____ vision.
    C. Treatment for Strabismus
        i. _____
        ii. _____
        iii. _____
        iv. _____

13. Blepharoptosis

    A. Blepharoptosis is usually a(n) _____ condition that occurs when the muscles of the eyelid are not strong enough to _____ it.
    B. Signs and symptoms include abnormal _____ of one or both _____.
    C. _____ is the only treatment option.

14. Exophthalmos

    A. Exophthalmos is usually caused by _____ or _____ disease.
    B. Unilateral exophthalmos may be caused by a(n) _____ _____.
    C. Signs and symptoms include _____ _____ of one or both eyeballs.

15. Blepharitis
    A. Blepharitis is an inflammation of the _____ of the _____.
    B. Signs and symptoms include redness, _____, and swelling of the eyelids.
    C. Treatment includes warm _____ and _____ antibiotic therapy.

16. Conjunctivitis
    A. Conjunctivitis is a(n) _____ of the conjunctiva.
    B. It is commonly known as _____.
    C. Causes of Conjunctivitis
        i. _____
        ii. _____
        iii. _____
        iv. _____
        v. _____

17. Hordeolums
    A. Hordeolums are caused by _____, generally *Staphylococcus*.
    B. They may accompany blocked or infected eyelid _____ or _____ eyelids.
    C. Contaminated _____ that touch the eye area may cause the infection.
    D. Painful hordeolums can occur _____ the eyelids.
    E. Signs and Symptoms of Hordeolums
        i. _____
        ii. _____
        iii. _____
        iv. _____
    F. Treatment includes a warm, wet _____ applied to the area that may help to relieve the pain.

18. Cataracts
    A. Cataracts are a clouding or _____ of the _____ that prevents light from entering.
    B. The cause is unclear, but there may be a correlation between the formation of cataracts and _____, _____, and excessive exposure to _____.
    C. Signs and Symptoms of Cataracts
        i. _____
        ii. _____
        iii. _____
    D. Treatment for Cataracts
        i. _____
        ii. _____

19. Dry Macular Degeneration
    A. Dry macular degeneration is the deterioration of the macula, the _____ portion of the _____.
    B. Small yellow deposits called _____ form under the macula, causing it to thin and dry out, leading to a loss of _____ vision.
    C. This form has a(n) _____ progression than does the wet type; however, it sometimes turns into the wet type.

20. Wet Macular Degeneration
    A. _____ new blood vessels grow under the _____ and the macula.
    B. These blood vessels may then _____ and leak fluid, which causes the macula to _____ or lift up, impairing or destroying the central vision.
    C. Vision loss may be _____ and _____.

21. Treatment of Macular Degeneration
    A. There is _____ _____ _____or cure for dry macular degeneration.
    B. _____ _____ y is currently the best treatment for wet macular degeneration.

22. Amblyopia
    A. Amblyopia is also called _____.
    B. This disorder, seen in _____, occurs when the muscles are weaker in one eye than in the other.
    C. Patients with more severe amblyopia may suffer from various vision-related disorders, such as _____ _____ _____.
    D. For treatment, a(n) _____ may be worn over the stronger eye to strengthen the muscles of the weaker eye.

23. Corneal Abrasion
    A. A corneal abrasion results from _____, _____, or both.
    B. It can be very _____.
    C. The patient will be very sensitive to _____ and will have difficulty opening the affected eye.
    D. Treatment may include mild _____ and resting the eye.

24. Retinal Detachment
    A. Retinal detachment occurs when a retina has separated from the underlying _____ layer.
    B. Damage may start out as _____ _____ or _____.
    C. _____ are particles that float slowly within the viewer's eyes.

25. Glaucoma
    A. Glaucoma is characterized by _____ pressure in the eye brought on by an excessive amount of _____ humor.
    B. If left untreated, the _____ can lead to damage of the _____ and, eventually, blindness.
    C. Types of glaucoma include _____ and _____.
    D. Glaucoma has no symptoms, so it must be diagnosed by _____ in a doctor's office.
    E. Treatment includes eye drops to lower _____ _____, as well as possible _____ or conventional surgery.

26. Nystagmus or Nystaxis
    A. Nystagmus or nystaxis is characterized by _____, _____, _____ eye movements.
    B. It may be _____ or acquired.
    C. It usually results in some _____ of vision.
    D. Signs and symptoms include _____ eye movements that may be _____, _____, or even _____.

27. Retinopathy
    A. Patients with _____ are prone to diabetic retinopathy.
    B. This nerve damage is a result of _____ _____ and can lead to permanent blindness.

II. The Senses of Hearing, Taste, and Smell

1. The Three Main Divisions of the Ear
    i. _____
    ii. _____
    iii. _____

2. The Structure and Function of the External Ear
    A. The pinna, or auricle, funnels sound waves through the _____ _____ to the _____ membrane.
    B. The auditory canal, or auditory meatus, is S-shaped and secretes _____, or _____.
    C. The tympanic membrane, or eardrum, separates the _____ ear from the _____ ear.

3. The Structure and Function of the Middle Ear
    A. The middle ear is a tiny cavity in the _____ bone of the skull.
    B. It contains three small bones: the _____ (hammer), the _____ (anvil), and the _____ (stirrup).
    C. The function of the middle ear
        i. The inner ear transmits _____ _____.
        ii. It _____ air pressure on both sides of the tympanic membrane.
        iii. It protects the ear from _____ _____.
        iv. Sound vibrations are transmitted by _____ from the tympanic membrane to the _____ _____ and into the inner ear.

4. The Structure and Function of the Inner Ear
    A. The inner ear is a bony labyrinth in the temporal bone that is made up of the _____, the _____, and _____ semicircular canals.
    B. The bony and membranous labyrinths are separated by _____.
    C. Tiny _____ cells function as receptors for hearing and balance.
    D. The cochlea resembles a(n) _____ _____.
    E. The cochlear duct runs between the _____ and _____ chambers.

5. The Two Most Common Types of Hearing Disorders
    A. Conductive
        i. This is a temporary form of hearing loss; sound is not conducted efficiently through the _____ _____ to the _____ and _____ _____.
        ii. _____ _____ can be corrected.
    B. Sensorineural
        i. This is a permanent type of hearing loss caused by damaged _____ or _____ _____ from the inner ear to the brain.
        ii. _____ _____ cannot be corrected.

6. Impacted Cerumen
    A. Cerumen is produced by the _____ _____ as lubrication.
    B. Impacted cerumen obstructs the _____ _____.
    C. Impacted cerumen affects _____ adults.
    D. The condition is exacerbated by the use of a(n) _____ swab.
    E. Signs and symptoms include blocked or _____ hearing, a(n) _____ feeling in the ear, and _____.

F. Treatment includes softening the _____, then flushing with a(n) _____.

G. If left untreated, impacted cerumen leads to _____.

7. Ruptured Tympanic Membrane

   A. A ruptured tympanic membrane is caused by _____ or _____ air pressure on both sides of the membrane.

   B. Signs and Symptoms of a Ruptured Tympanic Membrane

      i. _____

      ii. _____

   C. Treatment for a Ruptured Tympanic Membrane

      i. _____

      ii. _____

      iii. _____

8. Otitis Media

   A. _____ _____(swimmer's ear) is an inflammation of the outer ear.

   B. _____ _____ is an inflammation of the middle ear.

   C. Signs and Symptoms of Otitis Media

      i. _____

      ii. _____

      iii. _____

      iv. _____

      v. _____

   D. Treatment for Otitis Media

      i. Eliminating the cause of the _____

      ii. Oral _____ and decongestants

      iii. _____ _____ every 1 to 2 days

9. Otosclerosis

   A. Otosclerosis is a(n) _____ condition.

   B. The tissue surrounding the stapes grows _____.

   C. It prevents _____ from transmitting sound vibrations.

   D. Signs and symptoms include hearing loss in one or both ears, _____, and _____.

   E. Treatment includes the use of a(n) _____ or surgery.

10. Tinnitus

   A. Causes of Tinnitus

      i. _____

      ii. _____

      iii. _____

      iv. _____

      v. _____

   B. Signs and symptoms include _____ or _____ in one or both ears.

   C. Some relief is provided by the use of _____, _____, _____, and therapies including relaxation techniques.

11. Ménière's Disease

    A. Ménière's disease is caused by changes in _____ volume in the _____ ear.

    B. Signs and Symptoms of Ménière's Disease

        i. _____

        ii. _____

        iii. _____

        iv. _____

        v. _____

        vi. _____

        vii. _____

        viii. _____

        ix. _____

    C. Treatment for Ménière's Disease

        i. _____

        ii. _____

        iii. _____

        iv. _____

        v. _____

12. Presbycusis

    A. Presbycusis is caused by loud noises, _____, _____, or the side effects of medications.

    B. It occurs in both ears and affects _____ and _____ tones.

    C. Treatment typically involves the use of a(n) _____ _____.

13. How the Senses of Taste and Smell Function Together

    A. _____ cells respond to the changes in the chemical concentrations that activate the smell _____.

    B. Receptors send information to the brain via _____ _____.

    C. _____ move from the nose to the mouth region, stimulating the _____ _____.

14. The Four Types of Taste Cells

        i. _____

        ii. _____

        iii. _____

        iv. _____

15. The Sense of Touch

    A. The sense of touch is the oldest, most _____ sense.

    B. It is the first sense that humans experience in the _____ and the last one lost before _____.

    C. It is found over the _____ body.

    D. It originates in the _____.

    E. Nerve endings in the _____, called receptors, transmit _____ to the brain via the spinal cord.

    F. More nerve endings equal more _____.

APPLIED PRACTICE

1. On the image provided, label the parts of the eyeball and its anatomical structures.

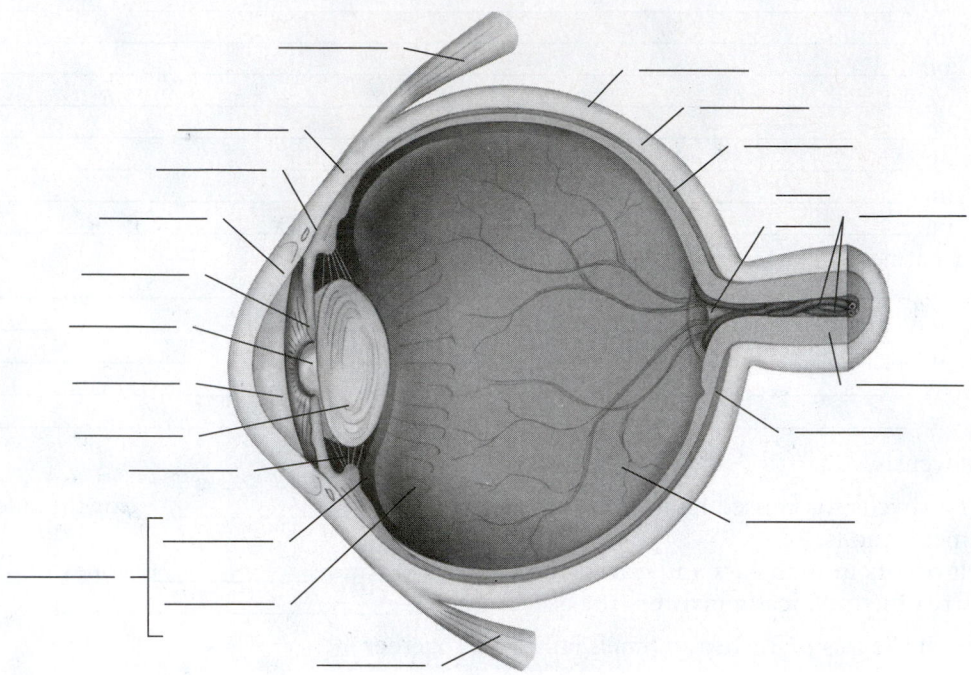

2. On the image provided, label the parts of the ear and its anatomical structures.

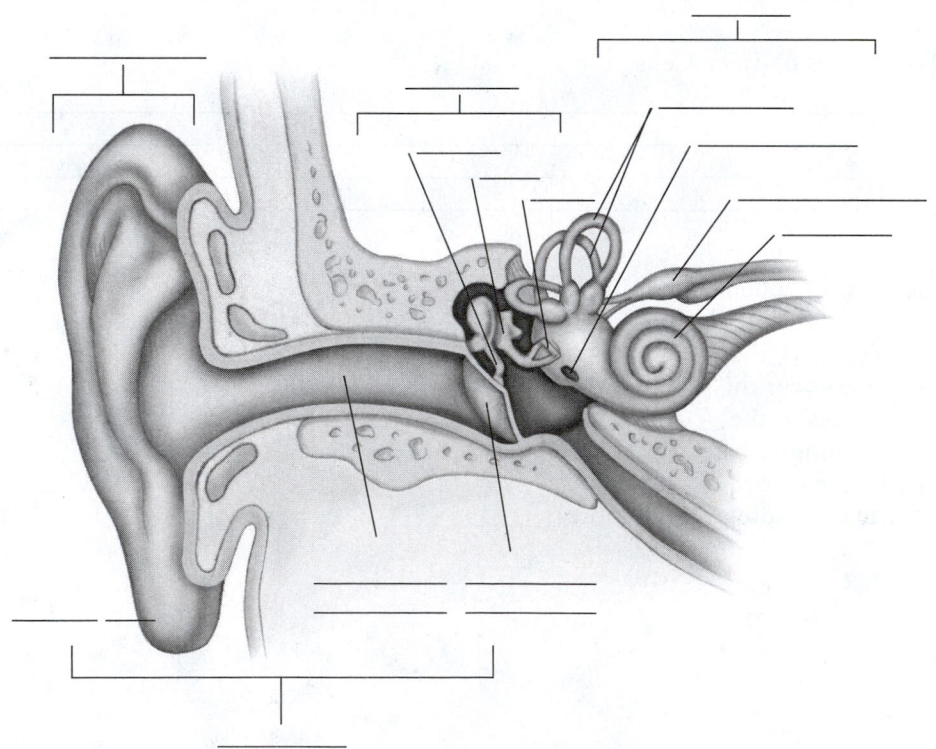

LEARNING ACTIVITY: MULTIPLE CHOICE

Circle the correct answer for each of the following questions.

1. Which of the following may develop due to maternal infections during the first 5 or 6 weeks of pregnancy?
   a. Strabismus
   b. Sensorineural deafness
   c. Congenital ear problems
   d. All of the above

2. How can intraocular pressure be reduced?
   a. Eyedrops
   b. Oral medications
   c. Surgery
   d. All of the above

3. Labyrinthitis is also known as
   a. otosclerosis.
   b. otitis media.
   c. nyctalopia.
   d. presbycusis.

4. The developing infant
   a. has poor visual acuity.
   b. is often farsighted.
   c. lacks color vision and depth perception at birth.
   d. All of the above

5. Refraction problems
   a. involve the inability to focus correctly and occur because light rays change direction when they pass through the eye.
   b. are typically seen more in children than in the elderly.
   c. include conditions such as blepharoptosis.
   d. All of the above

6. The use of an eye patch is recommended for which of the following conditions?
   a. Glaucoma
   b. Nystagmus
   c. Corneal abrasion
   d. Diplopia

7. Hypertensive retinopathy is caused by
   a. a variety of factors.
   b. hypertension.
   c. hypotension.
   d. diabetes.

8. Recurrent ear infections may be treated with
   a. myringotomy.
   b. keratotomy.
   c. osteotomy.
   d. None of the above

9. Tastes and smells are most acute
   a. at birth.
   b. by the toddler stage.
   c. in young adults.
   d. None of the above

10. The eyes continue to grow and mature
    a. throughout one's life.
    b. until adulthood.
    c. until the eighth or ninth year of life.
    d. None of the above

CRITICAL THINKING

Answer the following questions to the best of your ability. Use the textbook as a reference.

1. When dealing with patients who have visual difficulties, why should you understand the rules for driving in your state?

   _____

   _____

   _____

2. If the physician is running behind schedule and patients must wait, what should you do?

   _____

   _____

   _____

RESEARCH ACTIVITY

Use Internet search engines to research the following topic and write a brief description of what you find. It is important to use reputable websites.

1. Visit different websites that deal with speech and hearing loss. What information can you find to help families with speech and hearing deficiencies? What websites did you find most useful? Could these websites be beneficial to staff members of an eye, ear, nose, and throat (EENT) practice? If so, why?

   _____

   _____

   _____

   _____

CHAPTER 27
The Cardiovascular System

STUDENT STUDY GUIDE

Use the following guide to assist in your learning of the concepts from the chapter.

I. An Overview of the Cardiovascular System

  1. The Heart

    A. The heart is responsible for _____ the blood thorough the blood _____ throughout the body.
    B. It provides _____ blood to and removes _____ from the cells of the body.
    C. Is made up of three layers: _____, _____, and _____.
    D. It beats about _____ times a minute.
    E. It is about the size of a _____ and weighs approximately _____ ounces.
    F. It is _____ _____, with the apex at the most inferior (lowest) point.
    G. The tip of the heart at the lower edge is called the _____.
    H. The _____ is located directly in front of the heart.

  2. Blood flow through the Heart

    A. The mechanical, or pumping, action of the heart occurs with the _____ of the cardiac muscle.
    B. During this muscular contraction, an intricate _____ process occurs.

  3. The Blood

    A. The blood carries the _____ and waste products through the _____.
    B. ack of blood flow to the heart is known as myocardial _____.

  4. Vascular System of the Heart

    A. The _____ supply oxygenated blood to the heart.
    B. It is also a part of the _____ system.

  5. The Chambers of the Heart

    A. The heart is divided into _____ chambers.
    B. The _____ are the receiving chambers of the heart.
    C. The _____ are the pumping chambers.

  6. Heart Valves

    A. Healthy valves function as _____, never allowing the blood to flow backward.
    B. The valve that connects the right atrium to the right ventricle is the _____ valve.
    C. The blood leaves the left atrium through the _____ valve which is also called the _____ valve.

  7. The Tricuspid Valve

    A. The tricuspid valve is a(n) _____ valve.
    B. The prefix *tri*–, meaning _____, indicates that this valve has _____ leaflets or _____.

8. The Pulmonary Valve

    A. The pulmonary valve is also called the _____ valve.

    B. It is located between the right _____ and the pulmonary artery.

9. The Mitral Valve

    A. The mitral valve is also called the _____ valve.

    B. It has _____ cusps.

    C. Blood flows through the _____ valve to the left ventricle.

10. The Valves of the Heart (label the location of each valve of the heart)

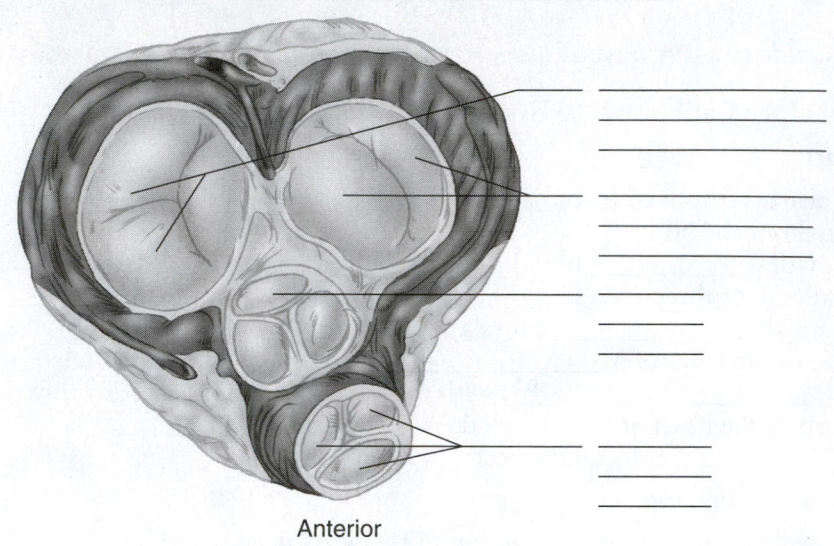

Anterior

11. The Great Vessels of the Heart (explain what each vessel does)

    A. The aorta _____.

    B. The pulmonary arteries _____.

    C. The pulmonary veins _____.

    D. The inferior and superior vena cava _____.

12. The Normal Flow of Blood Through the Heart

    A. _____ blood returns from the upper and lower body to fill the right atrium of the heart creating a pressure against the tricuspid valve.

    B. This pressure of the returning blood forces the tricuspid valve open and begins filling the _____.

    C. The final filling of the ventricle is achieved by the contracting of the right _____.

    D. Pressure closes the tricuspid valve and forces open the _____ semilunar valve.

    E. Oxygenated blood returns from the _____ via the pulmonary vein.

    F. The final filling of the left ventricle is achieved by the _____ of the left atrium.

    G. The left ventricle contracts, increasing internal pressure. This pressure closes the bicuspid valve and forces open the _____ _____.

13. The Conduction System of the Heart
    A. The _____ _____ system controls the heart rate.
    B. Special tissue conducts _____ impulses that _____ different chambers to _____ in the correct order.

14. The Phases of the Cardiac Cycle
    A. Phase 1: _____
    B. Phase 2: _____
    C. Phase 3: _____
    D. Phase 4: _____

15. Blood Pressure
    A. Blood pressure is a measurement of the force exerted by blood against the walls of a(n) _____.
    B. During ventricular contraction, blood pressure is at its highest in the arteries. The measurement obtained at this point is called the _____ blood pressure.
    C. Diastolic blood pressure is the measurement obtained when the ventricles relax and blood pressure is at its _____.

16. The Three Types of Blood Vessels (list and explain each type)
    i. _____
    ii. _____
    iii. _____

17. Veins
    A. Veins transport blood from _____ tissues to the heart.
    B. They have thin walls that contain _____.
    C. _____ force blood to flow toward the heart, preventing blood from _____ in the lower _____.
    D. Veins are more _____ than arteries.

18. Heart Sounds
    A. A heartbeat produces sounds commonly known as the _____.
    B. Listening for the flow of blood with a stethoscope is known as _____.

19. The normal blood pressure of a healthy young adult is _____.
    A. Newborn: _____
    B. 6–9 years: _____
    C. 10–15 years: _____
    D. 16 years to adulthood: _____

20. Physiological Factors Affecting Blood Pressure
    i. _____
    ii. _____
    iii. _____
    iv. _____

21. Pulmonary Circulation

    A. Pulmonary circulation is the route that blood takes from the _____ to the _____ and then back to the _____.

    B. The function of pulmonary circulation is to _____ the blood.

II. The Composition and Function of Blood

  1. The Blood

    A. The average adult has about _____ liters of blood.

    B. It circulates through the body in the vessels of the _____ system.

  2. The Functions of Blood

    i. _____

    ii. _____

    iii. _____

  3. Erythrocytes

    A. Erythrocytes are _____ blood cells.

    B. There are _____ erythrocytes per cubic millimeter of _____.

  4. Leukocytes

    A. Leukocytes are _____ blood cells.

    B. They provide protection against _____.

    C. There are _____ leukocytes per cubic millimeter of _____.

  5. Neutrophils

    A. Neutrophils are the most common _____.

    B. They are categorized as _____.

    C. They develop in the _____ marrow.

  6. Eosinophils

    A. Eosinophils are one of the least common _____.

    B. They are categorized as _____.

  7. Basophils

    A. Basophils are categorized as _____.

    B. Basophils are further classified as _____.

  8. Lymphocytes

    A. Lymphocytes are categorized as _____ because the granules in their cytoplasm are nearly invisible.

    B. They begin their development in the _____ marrow.

    C. Lymphocytes secrete _____ into the blood.

9. Monocytes
    A. Monocytes are _____ that engulf and destroy all types of invading microorganisms, cancerous cells, dead leukocytes, and cellular debris.
    B. This process is called _____.

10. Thrombocytes (Platelets)

    A. Platelets are different from other blood cells because they are only _____

    _____.
    B. They are active in the _____ process.
    C. They begin their development in the red marrow as stem cells, which then become _____.
    D. Thrombocytes are the smallest of all the elements of the _____.
    E. They are not _____ cells.
    F. They are critical in _____, or hemostasis.
    G. Thrombocytes lead to the formation of _____, which converts fibrinogen to fibrin.

11. Blood Types (list the four blood types)
    i. _____
    ii. _____
    iii. _____
    iv. _____

12. Universal Donor

    A. Because type _____ blood has neither marker _____ nor _____, it will not react with _____ or _____ antibodies.
    B. In an emergency, type _____ blood may be given to a person with any of the other blood types.
    C. A person with type _____ blood has no _____ against the other blood types and, therefore, in an emergency, can receive any type of blood.

13. The Rh Factor

    A. A person who is Rh-negative does not have the _____.
    B. Because this person has the Rh factor, he or she will not make _____ antibodies.
    C. A person without the Rh factor is Rh _____.

III. The Pathology of the Circulatory System

    1. Anemia

        A. Anemia is a condition characterized by abnormally _____ numbers of healthy _____ blood cells circulating in the body.
        B. It is often considered to be the most common dysfunction of the _____ blood cells.
        C. It affects about _____ Americans.

2. Common Signs and Symptoms of Anemia

    i. _____

    ii. _____

    iii. _____

    iv. _____

    v. _____

    vi. _____

    vii. _____

    viii. _____

    ix. _____

    x. _____

3. Causes of Anemia

    A. _____ production of healthy red cells by the bone marrow

    B. _____ erythrocyte destruction

    C. _____ and _____ deficiencies in the diet that can also slow down the production of _____

4. Iron Deficiency Anemia

    A. Iron deficiency anemia occurs when there is not enough _____ in the body.

    B. It is the most _____ type of anemia.

    C. _____ or pregnant women may require iron supplements.

5. Vitamin Deficiency Anemia

    A. Vitamin B_{12} is essential for normal _____ production. Some people have difficulty absorbing B_{12}, resulting in a vitamin B_{12} deficiency, a condition known as _____ anemia.

6. Hemolytic Anemia

    A. Hemolytic anemia occurs when there are not enough _____ blood cells in the blood.

    B. It is caused by a(n) _____ destruction of red blood cells with which the bone marrow cannot keep up.

7. Sickle Cell Anemia

    A. The abnormal _____ shape and sharp edges of this sickled _____ are very different from the smooth, rounded contours of a normal erythrocyte.

    B. Repeated sickling causes these fragile _____ to have a shortened life span, resulting in _____.

8. Aplastic Anemia

    A. Aplastic anemia occurs when the body stops producing enough _____ blood cells.

    B. Aplastic anemia is a rare and _____ condition.

    C. Treatment includes _____, _____, and a(n) _____.

9. Aneurysm

   A. An aneurysm is an abnormal _____ or _____ of a portion of a(n) _____, related to a weakness in the vessel wall.

   B. It can be congenital or _____.

   C. High blood pressure and _____ disease may contribute to the formation of certain types of aneurysms.

10. Treatment for Aneurysms

   A. Surgical intervention may be required to repair the _____ and prevent _____.

   B. Some patients may also be candidates for _____ placement within the affected vessel.

11. Arrhythmias

   A. An arrhythmia is a(n)_____ heartbeat caused by a disturbance of the normal _____ activity of the heart.

   B. Arrhythmias can be _____, especially when they significantly impact the pumping function of the blood.

12. Causes of Arrhythmias

   i. _____

   ii. _____

   iii. _____

   iv. _____

13. Signs and Symptoms of Arrhythmias

   i. _____

   ii. _____

   iii. _____

   iv. _____

   v. _____

   vi. _____

   vii. _____

14. Treatment for Arrhythmias

   i. _____

   ii. _____

   iii. _____

15. Arteriosclerosis

   A. Arteriosclerosis is often referred to as _____.

   B. Arteriosclerosis is the thickening and loss of _____ of the _____.

   C. Causative factors include the following:

      i. _____

      ii. _____

      iii. _____

      iv. _____

16. Symptoms of and Treatment for Arteriosclerosis

   A. Symptoms include:

      i. _____

      ii. _____

      iii. _____

   B. Treatment includes relieving the _____ and _____.

17. Atherosclerosis

   A. Atherosclerosis is the narrowing and _____ of the vessel _____ of the _____.

   B. It is caused by a buildup of _____ material and _____ within the vessel.

18. Cardiogenic Shock

   A. Cardiogenic shock is the collapse of the _____ system.

   B. It is characterized by _____ and fluid shifting away from the heart.

19. Symptoms of and Treatment for Cardiogenic Shock

   A. Symptoms of Cardiogenic Shock

      i. _____

      ii. _____

      iii. _____

      iv. _____

   B. Treatment for Cardiogenic Shock

      i. _____

      ii. _____

      iii. _____

      iv. _____

20. Cardiomyopathy

   A. Cardiomyopathy is a disease of the _____, or heart muscle, resulting in _____ dysfunction.

   B. It is thought to be _____ and idiopathic.

21. Fibrillation

   A. Fibrillation is _____ quivering or contractions of heart fibers.

   B. When this occurs within the fibers of the _____, arrest and death can occur.

      i. _____

      ii. _____

      iii. _____

22. Endocarditis

   A. Endocarditis is an inflammation of the _____ of the heart, including the heart _____.

   B. It is most commonly caused by a _____ infection.

   C. It frequently affects patients with existing abnormal conditions of the heart _____.

23. Symptoms of and Treatment for Endocarditis

   A. Symptoms of Endocarditis

      i. _____

      ii. _____

      iii. _____

      iv. _____

      v. _____

   B. Treatment generally consists of _____.

24. Myocarditis

    A. Myocarditis is an inflammation of the _____ layer of the heart.

    B. The most common cause is a(n) _____ infection.

25. Symptoms of and Treatment for Myocarditis

    A. Symptoms of Myocarditis

        i. _____

        ii. _____

        iii. _____

        iv. _____

        v. _____

        vi. _____

    B. The best treatment is the _____ of the inflammation, bed rest, and a _____ diet.

26. Pericarditis

    A. Pericarditis is an inflammation of the _____.

    B. It is most commonly seen as a complication of a(n) _____ or _____ infection.

27. Symptoms of and Treatment for Pericarditis

    A. Symptoms of Pericarditis

        i. _____

        ii. _____

        iii. _____

        iv. _____

    B. Treatment for Pericarditis

        i. _____

        ii. _____

        iii. _____

28. Cerebrovascular Accident

    A. A cerebrovascular accident occurs when the blood flow to the brain stops, allowing brain cells to _____.

    B. The two types of stroke are _____ and _____.

29. Symptoms of a Cerebrovascular Accident

        i. _____

        ii. _____

        iii. _____

        iv. _____

        v. _____

30. Causes of Congestive Heart Failure

        i. _____

        ii. _____

        iii. _____

        iv. _____

        v. _____

        vi. _____

31. Signs and Symptoms of Congestive Heart Failure

        i. _____

        ii. _____

        iii. _____

32. Treatment for Congestive Heart Failure
    i. _____
    ii. _____
    iii. _____
    iv. _____

33. Cor Pulmonale
    A. Cor pulmonale is also known as _____ heart disease.
    B. It causes the _____ ventricle to _____.
    C. A symptom of corn pulmonale is _____, or an _____ heart.

34. Coronary Heart Disease
    A. Coronary heart disease is also called _____ disease.
    B. It is a(n) _____ of the blood vessels that supply blood and oxygen to the heart muscle.

35. Factors that Increase the Risk of Coronary Heart Disease
    i. _____
    ii. _____
    iii. _____
    iv. _____
    v. _____
    vi. _____
    vii. _____
    viii. _____

36. Symptoms of and Treatment for Coronary Heart Disease
    A. Symptoms of Coronary heart Disease
        i. _____
        ii. _____
        iii. _____
    B. Treatment includes _____ and _____.

37. Myocardial Infarction
    A. Myocardial infarction affects more than _____ people each year.
    B. A heart attack may or may not lead directly to _____ _____.

38. Treatment for Myocardial Infarction
    i. _____
    ii. _____
    iii. _____
    iv. _____

39. Leukemia
    A. Leukemia is a malignant cancer of the _____ and _____.
    B. It involves the uncontrolled growth of _____ cells.
    C. It can be acute or _____.

40. Symptoms of Leukemia

    i. _____

    ii. _____

    iii. _____

    iv. _____

    v. _____

    vi. _____

    vii. _____

    viii. _____

    ix. _____

    x. _____

    xi. _____

41. Treatment for Leukemia

    A. _____ is used to kill leukemia cells with strong anticancer drugs.

    B. _____ therapy is used to kill cancer cells by exposure to high-energy _____.

    C. A(n) _____ transplant may be indicated.

42. Mitral Stenosis

    A. Mitral stenosis is caused by insufficient closing of the _____.

    B. It leads to _____, or a(n) _____ backward.

    C. It may cause a(n) _____.

    D. Treatment includes _____ to strengthen heart function.

43. Varicose Veins

    A. Varicose veins are enlarged walls that are _____ and _____ above the surface of the skin.

    B. They occur when the _____ in the veins _____.

    C. They affect _____ out of _____ people in the United States.

44. Signs of Varicose veins

    i. _____

    ii. _____

    iii. _____

45. Symptom Relief of Varicose Veins

    i. _____

    ii. _____

    iii. _____

    iv. _____

    v. _____

1. List the primary pulse points of the body.

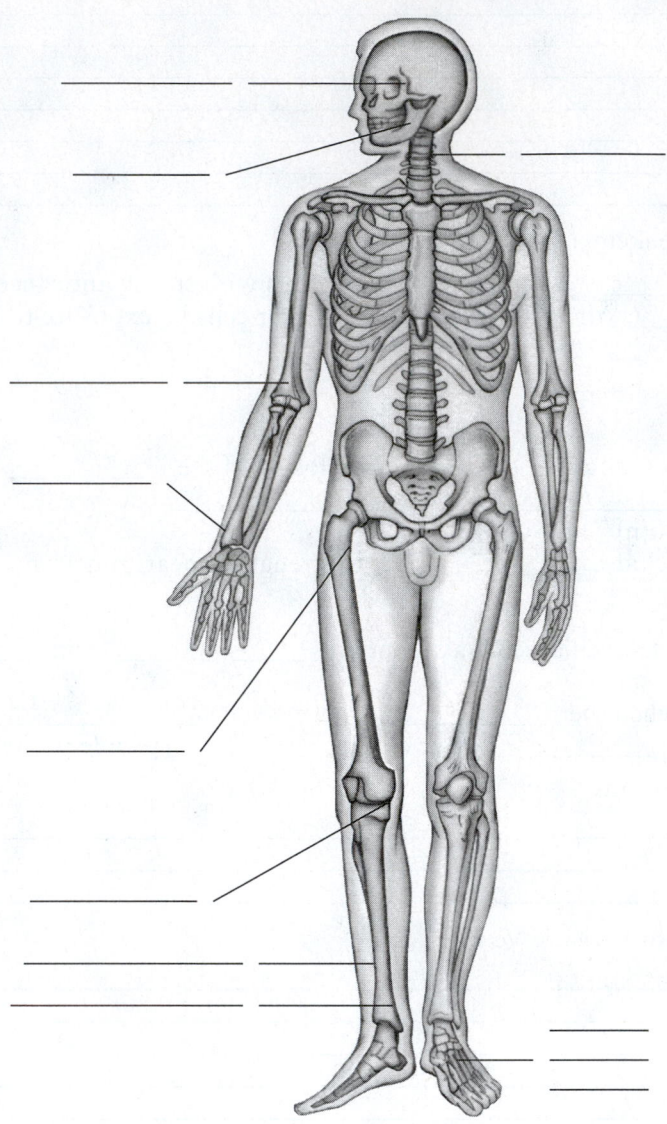

2. Provide the names of the ducts and nodes of the lymphatic system.

3. Provide the name of each formed element of blood.

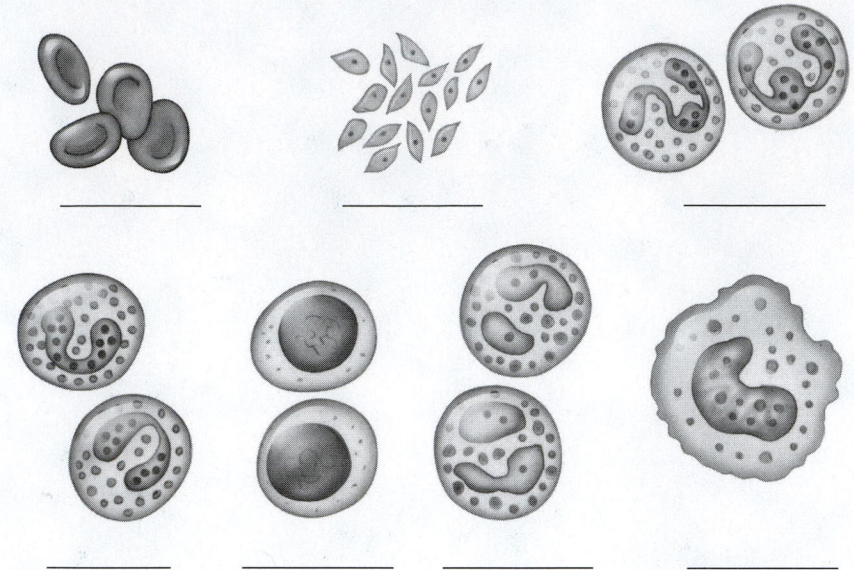

LEARNING ACTIVITY: FILL IN THE BLANK

Using words from the list below, fill in the blanks to complete the following statements.

agglutination	flutter	pulmonary artery
aneurysm	hypertension	pulmonary vein
buffers	hypotension	septum
cardiac arrest	myocardial infarction	tachycardia
cardiac tamponade	myocardium	tricuspid valve
congestive heart failure	pericardium	venipuncture
fibrillation	prehypertension	

1. A systolic pressure of greater than 120 is considered borderline _____.

2. The middle layer, or heart muscle, is called the _____.

3. _____ is the process of removing blood from the veins for examination.

4. _____ is defined as congestion of the heart muscle and the restriction of heart movement.

5. _____ is a condition in which the heart is unable to pump sufficient blood to the other organs.

6. Symptoms of a(n) _____ include a squeezing pain or heavy pressure in the middle of the chest.

7. When the electrical system has problems, _____ can occur.

8. The AV bundle extends from the AV node into the intraventricular _____.

9. The _____ is the outer lining of the heart.

10. _____ occurs when an antigen on the surface of red blood cells binds to antibodies in the plasma.

11. On its return from the lungs, oxygenated blood enters the left atrium via the _____.

12. When an occlusion leads to the heart stopping, it is known as _____.

13. Blood pressure ranging from 120/80 to 139/89 is a symptom of _____.

14. The blood contains _____, which are mechanisms within the blood that balance the pH level.

15. _____ is an abnormally fast heartbeat of more than 100 beats per minute.

16. _____ is an abnormal condition in which a person's blood pressure is much lower than usual.

17. After going through the _____, the blood enters the right ventricle.

18. Common locations for a(n) _____ include the aorta, brain, leg, and intestine.

19. Blood leaves the right ventricle through the pulmonary valve to go to the lungs, via the _____.

20. If the heart trembles, it is known as _____.

CRITICAL THINKING

Answer the following questions to the best of your ability. Use the textbook as a reference.

1. You are working at the front desk and looking out at the patients who have been waiting for their appointments. One man appears to be holding his left hand in front of his chest, he seems to be SOB, and his face looks sweaty or clammy. What is your first thought about this patient? Describe what the danger signs are to you even though the patient has not come up to the desk to voice a complaint about how he is feeling. What might you ask the patient, and how would you handle this situation?

   _____

   _____

   _____

2. You are performing an EKG. As it is printing, you notice that there is a normal waveform and complex, but the number of beats per minute is more than 100. What do you think the problem could be? Speculate on what the doctor might diagnose.

   _____

   _____

3. When providing care to a patient, how can you help to ensure that the patient's privacy is protected?

   _____

   _____

   _____

RESEARCH ACTIVITY

Use Internet search engines to research the following topic and write a brief description of what you find. It is important to use reputable websites.

1. Visit www.americanheart.org and navigate through the website. Pay particular attention to the link entitled "For Healthcare Professionals." Explain what information you think is most useful in this section and why.

   _____

   _____

   _____

   _____

   _____

CHAPTER 28
The Immune System

STUDENT STUDY GUIDE

Use the following guide to assist in your learning of the concepts from the chapter.

I. The Immune System

  1. The Composition of the lymphatic System

      i. _____

      ii. _____

      iii. _____

      iv. _____

      v. _____

  2. The Structures Central to the Immune System

    A. Central lymphoid tissue is composed of _____ _____.

    B. Peripheral lymphoid tissue consists of the _____ _____, _____, and _____ lymphoid tissue.

  3. The lymphatic system

    A. The lymphatic system is a network of _____, _____, and _____

    B. The structures are part of the _____ system, which is a subsystem of the _____ system.

    C. The primary function of the lymphatic system is to defend the body against invasion by pathogens such as _____, _____, and _____.

    D. Through the immune response, the _____, _____, and _____ work together to attack organisms and substances that invade body systems and cause disease.

    E. _____, or white blood cells (WBCs), combine to seek out and destroy harmful organisms.

    F. _____ medications and _____ can suppress the immune system.

  4. The Bone Marrow

    A. Bone marrow comprises the _____ _____ tissue.

    B. It contains _____ cells that create all of the cells that make up the tissues and structures of the immune system.

    C. It produces _____ _____ cells, _____ _____ cells, and platelets, along with _____ cells and natural killer cells.

  5. The Location and Purpose of the Thymus Gland

    A. The thymus is an _____ gland.

    B. It is located posterior to the _____, in the anterior _____.

    C. It manufactures infection-fighting _____ cells and helps distinguish normal _____ cells from those that attack the body's own tissues.

6. The Compartments of the Thymus Gland
    A. The thymus gland consists of an outer _____ and an internal _____.
    B. _____ lymphoid cells enter the cortex, reproduce, and mature; they then move to the medulla where they reenter the _____.

7. The Peripheral Lymphatic System
    A. The peripheral lymphoid tissue consists of the lymphatic pathways, lymph nodes, _____ and _____.
    B. Lymphatic _____, lymphatic _____, and lymphatic _____ are part of the peripheral lymphatic system.

8. Lymph Nodes
    A. Lymph nodes take many different _____ and _____.
    B. Most are _____ _____ and are about 1 inch long.
    C. They are covered with a _____, _____ capsule.
    D. The node is subdivided into different compartments by _____ _____.

9. B Lymphocytes
    A. The _____ _____ are the primary locations where B lymphocytes reproduce prolifically.
    B. B lymphocytes are responsible for the production of circulating _____.
    C. Each unique type of B cell produces only one type of _____.
    D. When a(n) _____ enters the body, these B lymphocytes rapidly undergo _____ and divide.

10. The Spleen
    A. The spleen is located in the _____ of the abdomen.
    B. It consists of lymphatic tissue that is highly _____ by blood vessels.
    C. The spleen's blood vessels are lined with _____, which swallow and digest debris in the blood such as worn-out red blood cells and _____.

11. Tonsils
    A. The tonsils are located in the depressions of the mucous membranes of the _____ and the _____.
    B. The function of the tonsils is to _____ _____ and aid in the _____ of white blood cells.

12. Phagocytes
    A. Phagocytes are a type of white blood cell that attacks the _____ _____.
    B. A number of different cells are considered to be phagocytes, but the most common are _____, which primarily fight bacteria.

13. Lymphocytes
    A. A lymphocyte is a type of white blood cell that allows the body to _____ and _____ previous invading organisms.
    B. It originates in the _____ _____ and either stays there and matures into B cells or moves to the _____ _____, where it matures into a T cell.

14. B and T Lymphocytes
    A. B lymphocytes and T lymphocytes have _____ _____ within the immune system.
    B. B lymphocytes seek out invading _____ and send _____ to attach onto them.
    C. T cells _____ the organisms that the B lymphocytes have _____.

15. Antibodies
    A. Immunoglobulins are _____ that function as antibodies.
    B. The terms *antibody* and _____ are often used interchangeably.
    C. Antibodies are found in _____, _____ _____, and many secretions.

16. The B Cells of the Immune System
    A. B cells are activated upon _____ to their specific antigen and _____ into plasma cells.
    B. Although antibodies can recognize an antigen and lock onto it, they are not capable of _____ it; that is the job of the _____ cells.

17. T Cells
    A. T cells are a part of the system that destroys antigens that have been tagged by antibodies or cells that have been infected or _____ _____.
    B. T cells assist other cells, such as _____.
    C. Antibodies can _____ toxins produced by different organisms.
    D. Antibodies can activate a group of proteins called _____, which are also part of the immune system.

18. Innate Immunity
    A. Everyone is born with innate, or _____, immunity.
    B. Innate immunity is provided, in part, by the external barriers of the body, including the _____ and _____ _____ that line the _____, _____, and _____ tract.
    C. If this outer defensive wall is broken, such as by a cut in the skin, _____ _____ _____ on the skin attack any invading microorganisms.

19. Active Immunity
    A. Active immunity is _____.
    B. The individual has lifelong _____ against the disease.

II. The Pathology of the Immune System

    1. Allergies
       A. A(n) _____ is any substance capable of causing an allergic reaction.
       B. Most allergic reactions are a result of an immune system that responds to a(n) _____ _____.
       C. When a harmless substance such as pollen is encountered by a person who is allergic to that substance, the immune system may react dramatically by producing _____ that attack the allergen.

    2. Anaphylaxis
       A. Anaphylaxis sometimes occurs after a(n) _____ or _____ is introduced into the patient.
       B. During anaphylaxis, _____ of the neck can cause breathing to be impeded, which can lead to _____ and death.

    3. Signs and Symptoms of Allergies
         i. _____
        ii. _____
       iii. _____
        iv. _____
         v. _____
        vi. _____
       vii. _____

4. Treatments for Allergies

    A. _____ or _____ can help combat allergy symptoms.

    B. Reactions to certain _____ _____ may be treated by the use of air filters and dehumidifiers.

    C. Alternative treatment includes _____ and _____ treatment.

    D. In severe cases, optimal treatment may be identified only through _____ _____ and desensitization.

    E. If anaphylaxis occurs, it is important for the physician to immediately order medications (such as _____) that will stop the process.

5. Cancer

    A. Cancer is a group of many related diseases that all pertain to _____.

    B. Cancer cells are unlike normal cells, which grow and, through _____, divide. Normal cells "know" when to stop growing.

6. Cancer Cells

    A. Cancer cells do not _____ or _____ like normal cells; they grow and spread very rapidly.

    B. Cancer cells continue to _____ and _____ erratically and do not die.

    C. They are not well _____, nor do they work on behalf of the body.

    D. They also make use of the body's resources at the expense of _____ cells.

    E. Usually, cancer cells clump together to form _____.

    F. A(n) _____ tumor can destroy the _____ cells around it, damaging the body's healthy tissue.

    G. Sometimes cancer cells break away from the _____ and travel to other areas of the body, where they keep growing, and form new tumors; this process is called _____.

7. Signs and Symptoms of Cancer

    i. _____
    ii. _____
    iii. _____
    iv. _____
    v. _____
    vi. _____

8. Treatment for Cancer

    A. _____, _____, _____, or a combination of all three

    B. The choice of treatment generally depends on the _____ of cancer and the _____ to which the cancer has spread within the body.

9. Surgery

    A. Cancer surgery is performed to remove cancerous _____.

    B. It is commonly used for _____ _____, and prostate cancer.

    C. During surgery, some _____ cells or tissue may also be removed to ensure that all of the cancer is removed.

10. Chemotherapy

    A. Chemotherapy refers to medicines that are sometimes taken in pill form but are more often given _____.

    B. Chemotherapy is usually given over a number of _____ or _____.

    C. Often, a permanent IV catheter, called a(n) _____, is placed under the skin into one of the larger blood vessels of the _____ _____.

11. Radiation Therapy

   A. Radiation therapy uses high-energy waves, such as _____, to damage and destroy cancer cells.
   B. It causes tumors to _____ and, in some cases, _____ completely.
   C. Radiation therapy is one of the most _____ treatments for cancer.

12. Immunotherapy

   A. Immunotherapy is the most _____ form of cancer therapy.
   B. It is a technique that involves creating _____ _____ _____ that are "programmed" to specifically target cancer cells.
   C. It empowers the body's own _____ _____ to target only cancer cells, rather than also destroying healthy cells.

13. Possible Causes of Chronic Fatigue Syndrome

   i. _____
   ii. _____
   iii. _____
   iv. _____
   v. _____

14. Signs and Symptoms of Chronic Fatigue Syndrome

   i. _____
   ii. _____
   iii. _____

15. Treatment for Chronic Fatigue Syndrome

   A. Treatment generally begins with a thorough evaluation of the patient's _____ _____ history.
   B. Both the _____ and _____ of sleep are important.
   C. Educating the patient, with emphasis on becoming a(n) _____ _____ in the treatment regimen, is extremely important in the treatment of chronic fatigue syndrome.

16. Infectious Mononucleosis

   A. Infectious mononucleosis is characterized by an increase in white blood cells that are _____, that is, containing a(n) _____ _____.
   B. It often develops in young adults between the ages of _____ and _____.
   C. It is commonly referred to as _____.
   D. The _____ period for mononucleosis is generally between 4 and 8 weeks.

17. Signs and Symptoms of Mononucleosis

   i. _____
   ii. _____
   iii. _____
   iv. _____

18. Treatment for Mononucleosis

   A. Getting plenty of _____
   B. Gargling with _____ or using _____ to soothe the throat
   C. Taking _____ and _____ medications to reduce fever and relieve sore throat and headache

19. Types of Lymphedema

   A. Primary lymphedema can be _____ and has several stages.
   B. Secondary lymphedema is generally caused by a(n) _____ of or _____ to the lymph system that interrupts the normal lymphatic flow.

20. Causes of Primary Lymphedema

    i. _____
    ii. _____
    iii. _____

21. Causes of Secondary Lymphedema

    i. _____
    ii. _____
    iii. _____

22. Treatment for Lymphedema

    A. Treatment includes _____ (CDT) and _____ (MDT).
    B. CDT is used primarily in the treatment of lymphedema and _____.
    C. Other treatments for lymphedema include:
       i. _____
       ii. _____
       iii. _____
       iv. _____
       v. _____

23. Rheumatoid Arthritis

    A. One out of every _____ persons suffers from chronic rheumatoid arthritis.
    B. Individuals with a family history of rheumatoid arthritis are _____ times more likely to develop the disease.
    C. Rheumatoid arthritis occurs when the body's immune defences attack tissue in the _____, leading to pain and degeneration of the _____.
    D. The disease and its treatment also increase _____; patients often have a shorter life expectancy than their healthy peers.

24. Signs and Symptoms of and Treatment for Rheumatoid Arthritis

    A. Signs and symptoms include pain and _____ in the joints.
    B. Treatment is based on medication regimens and educating the patient on how to _____.
    C. Drugs are used to _____ and _____ the symptoms, and help the patient to function at a more productive level.

25. Systemic Lupus Erythematosus (SLE)

    A. SLE is called a(n) _____ disorder because its effects may appear in many parts of the body.
    B. Ninety percent of patients with SLE are women, who are generally diagnosed before _____.
    C. There is a(n) _____ as well; the risk of developing SLE rises if a close family member has it.
    D. It is a chronic, lifelong condition with periods of _____ and _____.

26. Possible Signs and Symptoms of Systemic Lupus Erythematosus

    A. _____ and _____ in the joints
    B. General _____, _____, _____, and _____
    C. _____ (discoid) lesions that are raised and scaly
    D. _____, or inflamed blood vessels, characterized by red marks in any area of the body
    E. Sometimes, the appearance of _____, especially on the leg, where they may develop into _____
    F. In some people, the tips of the fingers and toes may develop _____.

27. Treatment of Systemic Lupus Erythematosus

    A. Treatment is usually aimed at reducing the immune response using drugs such as _____.

    B. The course of the disease for a given individual is difficult to predict, but with immediate treatment, most patients can expect to have a(n) _____ invade body systems and cause disease.

APPLIED PRACTICE

1. Label the components of the lymphatic system.

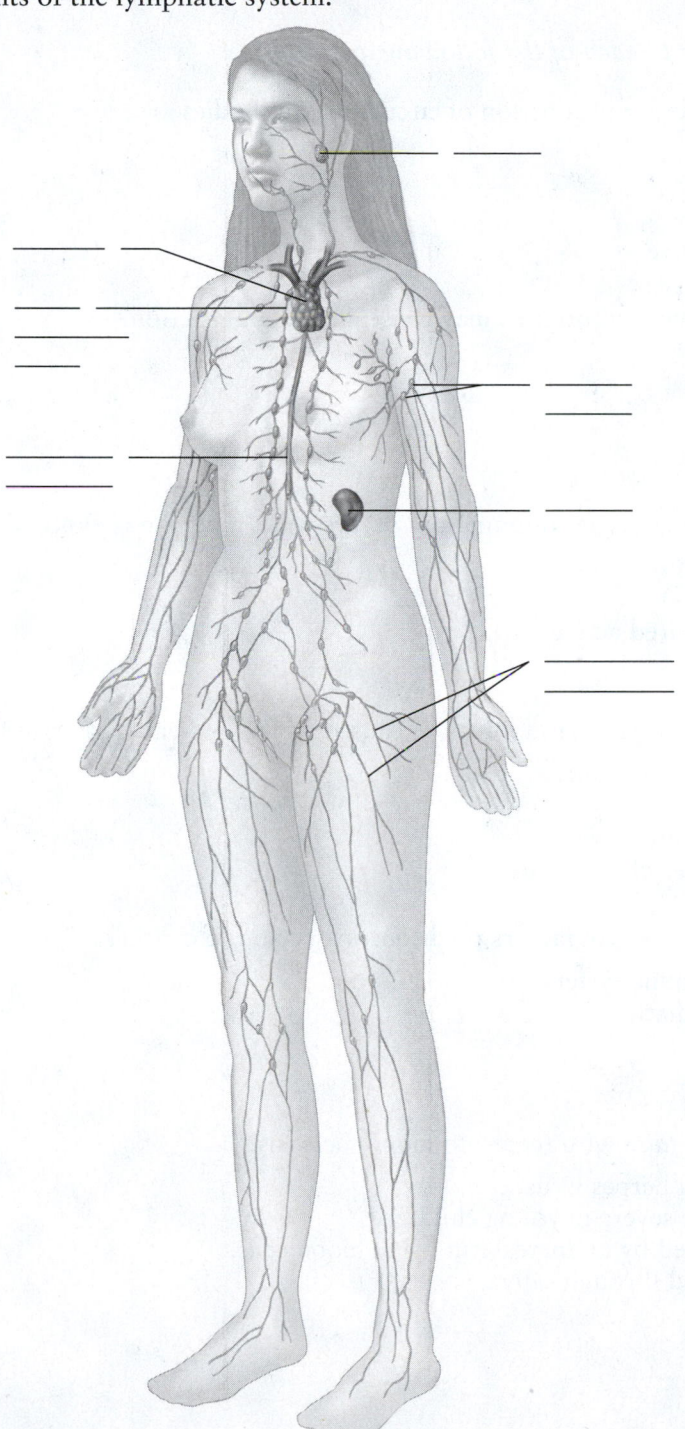

2. A patient has just been diagnosed with several allergies. It is her first visit and you are providing patient education and various instructions. How would you explain (in layperson's terms) antigens and allergens to the patient?

_____

_____

_____

LEARNING ACTIVITY: MULTIPLE CHOICE

Circle the correct answer to each of the following questions.

1. The cells responsible for production of circulating antibodies are

   a. T cells.
   b. B cells.
   c. A cells.
   d. None of the above

2. Which of the following substances may cause an allergic reaction?

   a. Dust
   b. Mold
   c. Pollen
   d. All of the above

3. Which of the following types of immunity occurs when a person is exposed to a live pathogen?

   a. Active
   b. Acquired active
   c. Artificially acquired active
   d. Natural

4. Which of the following is a viral infection caused by the Epstein-Barr virus?

   a. Chronic fatigue syndrome
   b. Lymphedema
   c. Infectious mononucleosis
   d. Systemic lupus erythematosus

5. Which of the following risk factors predisposes a person to cancer?

   a. Suppressed immune system
   b. Exposure to radiation
   c. Viruses
   d. All of the above

6. Which statement is *false* with regard to mononucleosis?

   a. It is caused by a herpes virus.
   b. It is much more severe in young children.
   c. It is characterized by an increase in white blood cells.
   d. It is often spread through saliva.

7. Which of the following allow the body to remember and recognize previous invading organisms?
    a. Lymphocytes
    b. Neutrophils
    c. Phagocytes
    d. Leukocytes

8. When an antigen is detected, several types of cells work together to recognize and respond to it. These cells trigger the lymphocytes to produce antibodies. This process is known as
    a. active immunity.
    b. acquired active immunity.
    c. humoral immunity.
    d. None of the above

9. The thymus gland enlarges during
    a. birth.
    b. childhood.
    c. puberty.
    d. None of the above

10. Which of the following contains stem cells that create all the cells that make up the tissues and structures of the immune system?
    a. Bone marrow
    b. Liver
    c. Thymus gland
    d. Lymph nodes

CRITICAL THINKING

Answer the following questions to the best of your ability. Use the textbook as a reference.

1. Why do the frequency and severity of infections and incidence of autoimmune disease generally increase in elderly persons?

_____

_____

_____

2. While at work, why should medical assistants not wear strong-smelling perfumes or aftershave lotions?

_____

_____

_____

RESEARCH ACTIVITY

Use Internet search engines to research the following topic and write a brief description of what you find. It is important to use reputable websites.

1. Research an autoimmune disease that is of interest to you. Identify the signs and symptoms of the disease, how a diagnosis is made, and treatment options. Also, research support groups, societies, or foundations for that disease. Write an essay on your findings and be sure to cite the websites where you found your information.

   _____

   _____

   _____

   _____

   _____

CHAPTER 29
The Respiratory System

STUDENT STUDY GUIDE

Use the following guide to assist in your learning of the concepts from the chapter.

I. The Respiratory System

1. The Process of Breathing

    A. When we breathe, we inhale _____ and exhale _____.
    B. Respiration is achieved through the _____, _____, _____, _____, and _____.
    C. Oxygen enters the respiratory system through the _____ and the _____.

2. The Path Taken by Oxygen During Breathing (list the path that oxygen takes during breathing)

    i.   Oxygen passes through the _____.
    ii.   It also passes through the _____, where speech sounds are produced.
    iii. It passes through the lungs and the bronchioles that connect to tiny sacs, the _____.
    iv.   After the gas exchange, it then diffuses through the _____ into the _____.
    v.   The waste-rich blood from the veins releases _____ _____ into the _____.
    vi.   The _____ helps pump air into and carbon dioxide out of the _____.
    vii. Upon _____, carbon dioxide follows the reverse of the path taken by oxygen flowing into the lungs.

3. The Functions of the Nose

    A. The nose_____ and moistens inhaled air.
    B. It warms the _____.
    C. It assists with _____.

4. The Internal Structure of the Nose

    A. The septum is a(n) _____ structure.
    B. The septum is lined with _____ membrane.
    C. The conchae connect the _____ tube, the _____, and the _____ duct.
    D. The palatine bone of the skull makes up the _____ palate and separates the nose from the _____.

5. The Pharynx

    A. The pharynx is a(n) _____ tube that is about _____ inches long.
    B. It contains the _____.
    C. It consists of three parts: the _____, the _____, and the _____.

6. The Larynx ("Voice Box")

    A. The epiglottic cartilage, also called the _____, closes over the _____ during swallowing to keep food out of the _____.
    B. The cricoid cartilage serves as a landmark for performing a(n) _____ when the airway is obstructed.

7. The Trachea
    A. The trachea is a cartilaginous tube about _____ inch wide and _____ inches long that extends between the _____ and the main _____.
    B. The interior of the trachea is lined with _____ _____ and _____ that trap foreign matter.
    C. The most important function of the trachea is to serve as a(n) _____ _____ through which air reaches the lungs.
    D. The epiglottis is a flap of _____ that covers the trachea when swallowing occurs to prevent food from entering the trachea.

8. The Main Branches of the Trachea
    A. The main branches of the trachea that extend into the lungs are called the _____.
    B. The right bronchus is the _____, _____ branch located along the _____ side of the heart.
    C. The left bronchus is _____ and more _____.
    D. After entering the lungs at the hilum, the _____ subdivide into the _____ tree, which continues to branch out into smaller and smaller branches called _____.

9. Alveoli
    A. The alveoli are small air _____ at the terminal end of the _____.
    B. They _____ and _____ with inhalation and exhalation.
    C. They are surrounded by a network of _____ for gas exchange.

10. The Structure of the Lungs
    A. The lungs contain _____, _____, and _____.
    B. The lungs are spongy, _____, and highly _____.

11. The Functions of the Lungs
    i. _____
    ii. _____
    iii. _____

12. The two processes of Ventilation
    i. _____
    ii. _____

13. The Action of the Diaphragm
    A. The diaphragm _____ and moves downward.
    B. This movement causes a(n) _____ in pressure, or _____ thoracic pressure, within the chest cavity.
    C. Air enters the lungs to _____ the pressure during _____.

14. Intercostal Muscles
    A. External intercostal muscles assist _____, raise the _____, and enlarge the _____ cavity.
    B. Internal intercostal muscles assist _____, reduce the size of the _____ cavity, and force air from the _____.

II. The Pathology of the Respiratory System

   1. Asthma

      A. Asthma is a chronic _____ disease of the _____.

      B. Causes of Asthma

         i. Irritations that cause _____ and, which

         ii. Affect the _____ and/or _____ _____,

         iii. Resulting in _____, which adds to the irritation.

      C. Treatment includes a(n) _____ for acute episodes and long-term _____ for
      the prevention of episodes.

   2. Chronic Obstructive Pulmonary Disease (COPD)

      A. COPD is a combination of related diseases—chronic _____ and _____.

      B. _____ is a major cause.

      C. Air and other _____ may increase risk.

      D. A diagnosis is made through _____ and _____.

      E. Signs and symptoms of chronic obstructive pulmonary disease include:

         i. _____

         ii. _____

         iii. _____

         iv. _____

      F. Treatment for chronic obstructive pulmonary disease includes:

         i. _____

         ii. _____

         iii. _____

         iv. _____

   3. Bronchitis

      A. Bronchitis is a respiratory disease in which the _____ _____ in the _____
      passages become _____.

      B. As the irritated _____ swells and grows thicker, it narrows or shuts off the tiny
      airways to the _____.

   4. Signs and Symptoms of Acute Bronchitis

         i. _____

         ii. _____

         iii. _____

         iv. _____

         v. _____

         vi. _____

5. Signs and Symptoms of Chronic Bronchitis

   A. A persistent cough that produces _____, white, or _____ phlegm
   B. Sometimes _____ and breathlessness
   C. The symptoms of chronic bronchitis are worsened by _____ _____.

6. Treatment for Acute Bronchitis

   A. Conventional treatment for acute bronchitis include:
      i. _____
      ii. _____
      iii. _____
      iv. _____

7. Emphysema

   A. Emphysema is a long-term, _____ lung disease in which the _____ that support the physical shape and function of the _____ are destroyed.
   B. Deterioration is _____ and may go unnoticed.
   C. _____ smoking is by far the most common cause.

8. Risk Factors for Emphysema

      i. _____
      ii. _____
      iii. _____
      iv. _____
      v. _____
      vi. _____

9. Signs and Symptoms of Emphysema

      i. _____
      ii. _____
      iii. _____

10. Treatment for Emphysema

      i. _____
      ii. _____
      iii. _____
      iv. _____
      v. _____

11. The Common Cold

   A. A common cold is an inflammation of the _____ respiratory tract.
   B. Many cold viruses are highly _____.
   C. The common cold can be spread by _____.

12. Signs and Symptoms of the Common Cold

      i. _____
      ii. _____
      iii. _____
      iv. _____
      v. _____
      vi. _____
      vii. _____
      viii. _____
      ix. _____
      x. _____
      xi. _____

13. Treatment for the Common Cold
   A. Antibiotics are _____ against cold viruses.
   B. Over-the-counter cold preparations do not cure a common cold or _____ its duration.
   C. For fever, sore throat, and headache, mild _____ _____ may be helpful.
   D. For a runny nose and nasal congestion, _____ or _____ may be useful.

14. Measures for Slowing the Spread of the Common Cold
   i. _____
   ii. _____
   iii. _____
   iv. _____

15. Hay Fever
   A. Hay fever is also called _____ _____ _____ or pollinosis.
   B. It is a seasonal allergy in which the _____ _____ of the nose and eyes become _____.
   C. About _____ million Americans experience hay fever symptoms each month.

16. Hay Fever
   A. Symptoms of Hay Fever
      i. _____
      ii. _____
      iii. _____
      iv. _____
      v. _____
      vi. _____
   B. Treatment for Hay Fever
      i. _____
      ii. _____
      iii. _____

17. Influenza
   A. Influenza is an illness caused by _____ that infect the respiratory tract.
   B. It is often more serious than the _____.
   C. Most people who get the flu recover completely in ____ to ____ weeks.

18. Signs and Symptoms of Influenza
   i. _____
   ii. _____
   iii. _____
   iv. _____
   v. _____

19. The Flu Vaccine
   A. The flu vaccine is the best defense against _____.
   B. The flu vaccine should be received by _____, the _____, those who are _____, and _____.

20. Lung Cancer
   A. Lung cancer is the leading cause of _____ deaths in both women and men in the United States and throughout the world.
   B. _____ percent of the cases occur in _____ and former _____.
   C. Other causes are _____, _____, and _____ exposure.

21. Treatment for Lung Cancer
    i. _____
    ii. _____
    iii. _____

22. Pleurisy

    A. Pleurisy is a(n) _____ of the _____ that surrounds and protects the lungs.
    B. Causes of Pleurisy
        i. _____
        ii. _____
        iii. _____
        iv. _____
    C. Symptoms of Pleurisy
        i. _____
        ii. _____
        iii. _____
        iv. _____
        v. _____
    D. Treatment includes _____ drugs and _____ medicine.

23. Pneumonia

    A. Pneumonia is an inflammation of the lung or lungs caused by _____, _____, _____, or _____.
    B. _____ *pneumoniae* is the most common bacteria.
    C. Symptoms of Pneumonia
        i. _____
        ii. _____
        iii. _____
    D. Treatment for Pneumonia
        i. _____
        ii. _____
        iii. _____

24. Legionnaire's Disease

    A. Legionnaire's disease is a type of _____.
    B. It usually affects _____ or _____ persons.
    C. It is caused by the _____ germ, which is spread throughout _____.

25. Pneumothorax

    A. A pneumothorax occurs when air enters the chest _____ of the lungs.
    B. It occurs most frequently when the lung has been _____ through trauma.
    C. Signs and symptoms are _____, _____, _____, and _____.
    D. Treatment must be given quickly to prevent _____ of the heart and lungs.

26. Pulmonary Edema

    A. Pulmonary edema is a condition in which _____ accumulates in the lungs.
    B. It can be a(n) _____ condition, or it can develop suddenly and quickly become life threatening.
    C. Most cases are caused by a failure of the heart's _____ chamber, the left _____, to pump adequately.

D. Symptoms include shortness of breath with _____, respiratory distress after _____, _____ breathing, and coughing.

E. Treatment must be _____ to reduce the amount of fluid.

27. Pulmonary Embolism

A. A pulmonary embolism is a(n) _____ clot that travels to the _____.

B. The result is a(n) _____ infarct.

C. Causes include extended periods of _____, surgery or _____, obesity, and _____ disease.

D. Symptoms of a Pulmonary Embolism
    i. _____
    ii. _____
    iii. _____
    iv. _____
    v. _____
    vi. _____

E. Treatment includes medications to eliminate the _____ or thin the blood and _____ the blood pressure.

28. Sinusitis

A. Sinusitis is an infection of the _____ of the sinuses.

B. Infection occurs because of lack of _____.

C. It is usually caused by a(n) _____ infection, a(n) _____, or a(n) _____ infection.

D. Symptoms include _____ and _____ in the facial area and green or _____ nasal discharge.

E. Treatment includes _____, moist heat for _____, and prevention of sinus ____.

29. Tuberculosis

A. Tuberculosis is caused by the _____ tuberculosis complex of bacteria.

B. Individuals become infected by inhaling _____ from an infected person.

C. Symptoms of Tuberculosis
    i. _____
    ii. _____
    iii. _____
    iv. _____
    v. _____
    vi. _____
    vii. _____

1. Label the sections of the nasal cavity and the pharynx.

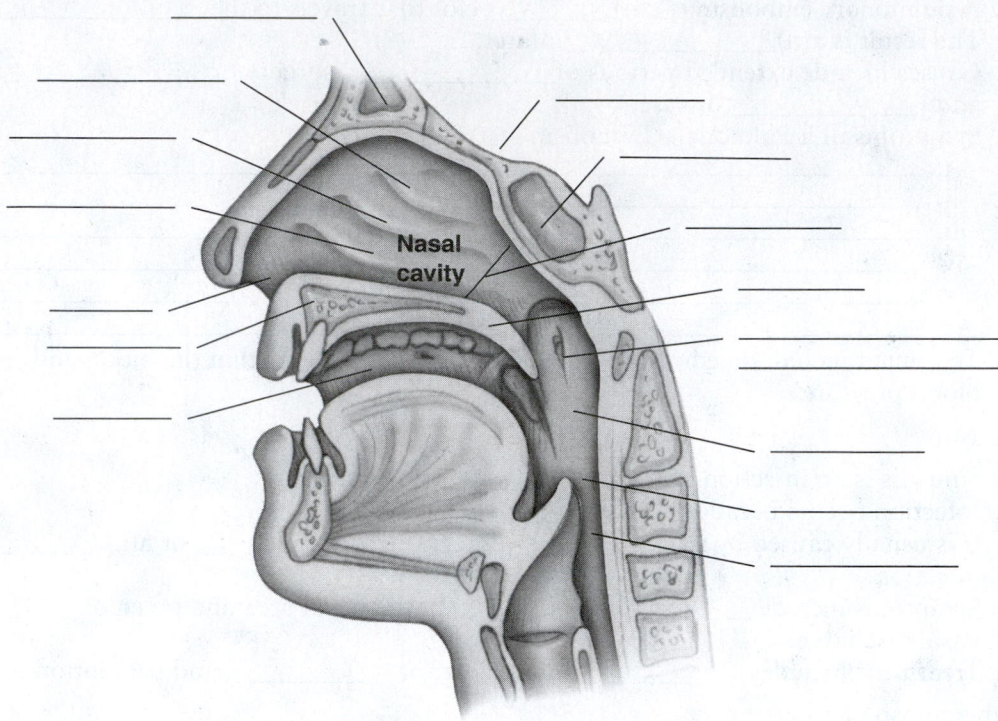

2. When working with children who have asthma, why should you be aware of the medication requirements of the school districts in your area?

LEARNING ACTIVITY: TRUE/FALSE

Indicate whether the following statements are true or false by placing a T or an F on the line that precedes each statement.

_____ 1. The upper respiratory tract includes the larynx, the trachea, the bronchioles, and the lungs.

_____ 2. The nose is part of the apparatus of respiration and voice.

_____ 3. The pharynx consists of two parts: the nasopharynx and the oropharynx.

_____ 4. The tonsils are part of the immune system and help with infection control.

_____ 5. The thyroid cartilage, or Adam's apple, is the smallest of the cartilage structures.

_____ 6. When the vocal cords are long and relaxed, high sounds are produced.

_____ 7. The respiratory rates in older adults may lower as the cumulative effects of pollution, smoking, and disease wear on the integrity of the tissues.

_____ 8. At birth, the lungs are pinkish in color, but as adulthood approaches they turn a dark slate-gray.

_____ 9. The right lung has three lobes, but the left lung only has two.

_____ 10. Asthma is related to the same process that causes allergic reactions.

CRITICAL THINKING

Answer the following questions to the best of your ability. Use the textbook as a reference.

1. You have a patient with obstructive lung disease who wants to know why he has a hard time breathing. This person has a form of COPD that does not allow him to exhale very much. Explain briefly here, as if explaining to the patient, why he feels so short of breath.

   _____

   _____

   _____

2. Severe acute respiratory syndrome (SARS) was spread from China to North America by infected persons traveling by airplane. How can we control the entry of microbes into a country? What should China have done to prevent the spread of the disease within and outside of China? Should the Chinese government have shared information about SARS with the world immediately in case it spread?

   _____

   _____

   _____

RESEARCH ACTIVITY

Use Internet search engines to research the following topic and write a brief description of what you find. It is important to use reputable websites.

1. Visit www.lungusa.org. What information do you think will be most useful with regard to patient education? Complete a search on "hidden" asthma. What is "hidden" asthma, and what age group does it commonly affect? How can this information be useful to patients?

   _____

   _____

   _____

   _____

CHAPTER 30

The Digestive System

STUDENT STUDY GUIDE

Use the following guide to assist in your learning of the concepts from the chapter.

I. The Digestive System

  1. The Digestive System

    A. The digestive system _____ food, _____ food, and _____ waste products.

    B. The three main functions are _____, _____, and _____.

    C. Name the four layers of the digestive system wall.

      i. _____

      ii. _____

      iii. _____

      iv. _____

  2. The Tongue

    A. The tongue is a(n) _____ muscle covered with a(n) _____ membrane.

    B. The three areas of the tongue are:

      i. _____

      ii. _____

      iii. _____

    C. Papillae and taste buds are located on the _____ of the tongue.

  3. The Teeth (list the types of teeth)

      i. _____

      ii. _____

      iii. _____

      iv. _____

  4. The Structure of the Tooth

    A. The _____ is the portion embedded in the top of the gum between the crown and the root.

    B. The _____ is the portion embedded in the gums.

    C. The _____ covers the exposed part of the crown.

  5. The Anatomy of the Tooth—From the Crown to the Root

    A. _____ is the calcified, mostly mineral tissue that forms the bulk of the tooth.

    B. _____ are the fibers that anchor teeth to bony sockets in the maxillary bone and the mandible.

    C. The _____ is the protective layer on the dentin that anchors the periodontal ligament.

  6. The Pharynx

    A. The pharynx is the beginning of the _____.

    B. It also opens to the _____.

7. The Esophagus

    A. The esophagus carries food to the _____.

    B. It is about _____ inches long.

    C. Wavelike muscular contractions, called _____, move food to the _____.

8. The Stomach

    A. The stomach can hold _____ to _____ liters.

    B. It secretes _____ that aid in digestion.

    C. It processes food into a(n) _____ state.

    D. It prepares food for further _____ and _____ in the small intestine.

9. The Sphincters of the Stomach

    A. The sphincters of the stomach are muscular _____.

    B. They allow the flow of food in a(n) _____ direction.

    C. The stomach has _____ sphincters.

    D. The lower esophageal sphincter is found between the _____ and the top of the stomach.

    E. The pyloric sphincter is located between the _____ and the _____.

10. The Stomach's Role in Digestion

    i. _____

    ii. _____

    iii. _____

    iv. _____

11. The Small Intestine

    A. The small intestine is a tube about _____ feet long, _____ inch in diameter.

    B. It attaches to the _____ at the _____ sphincter.

    C. It ends at the _____ orifice at the beginning of the large intestine.

12. The Sections of the Small Intestine (list the three sections)

    i. _____

    ii. _____

    iii. _____

13. The Large Intestine

    A. The large intestine begins at the _____ orifice.

    B. The large intestine is about _____ feet long.

    C. The functions of the large intestine include:

        i. _____

        ii. _____

        iii. _____

14. The Sections of the Large Intestine (list the four sections)

    i. _____

    ii. _____

    iii. _____

    iv. _____

15. The Salivary Glands (list the three pairs)

    i. _____

    ii. _____

    iii. _____

16. The Liver

    A. The liver stores _____ and several vitamins.
    B. The products of the liver include _____, _____, _____, _____, and _____.

17. The Pancreas

    A. The pancreas is about _____ to _____ inches long.
    B. It produces _____ enzymes.
    C. It serves the _____ function.
    D. It is part of two body systems: _____ and _____.
    E. Its function is to secret the hormone _____.

II. The Pathology of the Digestive System

    1. Appendicitis

        A. Appendicitis is a(n) _____ of the appendix.
        B. Symptoms include acute pain on the _____ point of the abdomen.
        C. Treatment is _____ of the appendix.

    2. Cirrhosis

        A. Cirrhosis is damage to the liver caused by _____.
        B. Chronic _____ of the liver prevents normal liver function.
        C. Symptoms of Cirrhosis
            i. _____
            ii. _____
            iii. _____
            iv. _____
            v. _____
            vi. _____
            vii. _____
            viii. _____
            ix. _____

    3. Treatment for Cirrhosis
        i. _____
        ii. _____
        iii. _____
        iv. _____
        v. _____

    4. Colitis

        A. Colitis is an inflammation of the _____ intestine.
        B. Symptoms of Colitis
            i. _____
            ii. _____
            iii. _____
            iv. _____
            v. _____

    5. Colorectal Cancer

        A. Colorectal cancer begins as _____ polyps.
        B. Treatment includes _____, _____, and _____.

6. Symptoms of Colorectal cancer

   A. Causes of Constipation

      i. _____

      ii. _____

      iii. _____

      iv. _____

      v. _____

      vi. _____

      vii. _____

      viii. _____

7. Crohn's Disease

   A. Crohn's disease is a chronic _____ of the _____.

   B. Common symptoms include _____, _____, and _____.

8. Diverticulosis

   A. Diverticulosis is outpouching in the _____ intestinal wall.

   B. There is a higher incidence in the _____.

   C. It can be prevented with a(n) _____ diet.

9. Diverticulitis

   A. Diverticulitis is an inflammation of the diverticulum in the walls of the _____.

   B. Symptoms of Diverticulitis

      i. _____

      ii. _____

      iii. _____

      iv. _____

      v. _____

      vi. _____

      vii. _____

10. Gastroesophageal Reflux Disease (GERD)

   A. GERD is a backflow of the _____ juices into the _____.

   B. The lower _____ sphincter does not close.

   C. Symptoms of Gastroesophageal Reflux Disease

      i. _____

      ii. _____

      iii. _____

      iv. _____

      v. _____

      vi. _____

   D. Complications of Gastroesophageal Reflux Disease

      i. _____

      ii. _____

      iii. _____

      iv. _____

      v. _____

      vi. _____

11. Hemorrhoids

   A. Hemorrhoids are dilated veins in the walls of the _____.

B. Symptoms include _____ with elimination.

C. Treatment involves _____ changes, topical medication, and _____ (if severe).

12. Hiatal Hernia

   A. In a hiatal hernia, the upper stomach protrudes into the chest through the _____ hiatus.

   B. Causes of a Hiatal Hernia

      i. _____

      ii. _____

      iii. _____

      iv. _____

      v. _____

      vi. _____

      vii. _____

      viii. _____

   C. Symptoms of a Hiatal Hernia

      i. _____

      ii. _____

      iii. _____

      iv. _____

      v. _____

      vi. _____

13. Inguinal Hernia

   A. In an inguinal hernia, the intestine pushes through the _____ wall in _____ area.

   B. Causes include _____ in the abdominal wall; heavy lifting; and _____ as a result of coughing, laughing, or bending.

   C. Symptoms include a bulge in the abdomen when _____, _____, or _____.

   D. The only treatment is _____.

14. Irritable Bowel Syndrome (IBS)

   A. IBS is a common _____ condition.

   B. Causes include _____.

   C. Treatment includes _____ modifications, medications, and _____.

   D. Symptoms of IBS

      i. _____

      ii. _____

      iii. _____

      iv. _____

      v. _____

      vi. _____

      vii. _____

15. Oral Cancer

   A. Risk factors for oral cancer include age, _____, smoking, the use of _____, _____ exposure, some _____ medications, and _____.

   B. Symptoms of Oral Cancer

      i. _____

      ii. _____

      iii. _____

      iv. _____

      v. _____

   C. Treatment for oral cancer includes _____, _____, and _____.

16. Pancreatic Cancer

    A. The most common type is _____ of the pancreas.

    B. Symptoms of Pancreatic Cancer

        i. _____

        ii. _____

        iii. _____

        iv. _____

        v. _____

        vi. _____

    C. Treatment includes _____, _____, and _____.

17. Peptic Ulcer Disease (PUD)

    A. PUD is characterized by a lesion in the lining of the _____, _____, or

       _____.

    B. _____ ulcers are common.

    C. PUD can be aggravated by _____ infection.

    D. Symptoms of PUD

        i. _____

        ii. _____

        iii. _____

        iv. _____

18. Treatment for Peptic Ulcer Disease

        i. _____

        ii. _____

        iii. _____

        iv. _____

        v. _____

19. Pyloric Stenosis

    A. Pyloric stenosis is a condition where the _____ sphincter _____ and thickens.

    B. Symptoms include _____, _____, and _____.

    C. Treatment for pyloric stenosis is _____.

APPLIED PRACTICE

1. Label each part of the digestive system.

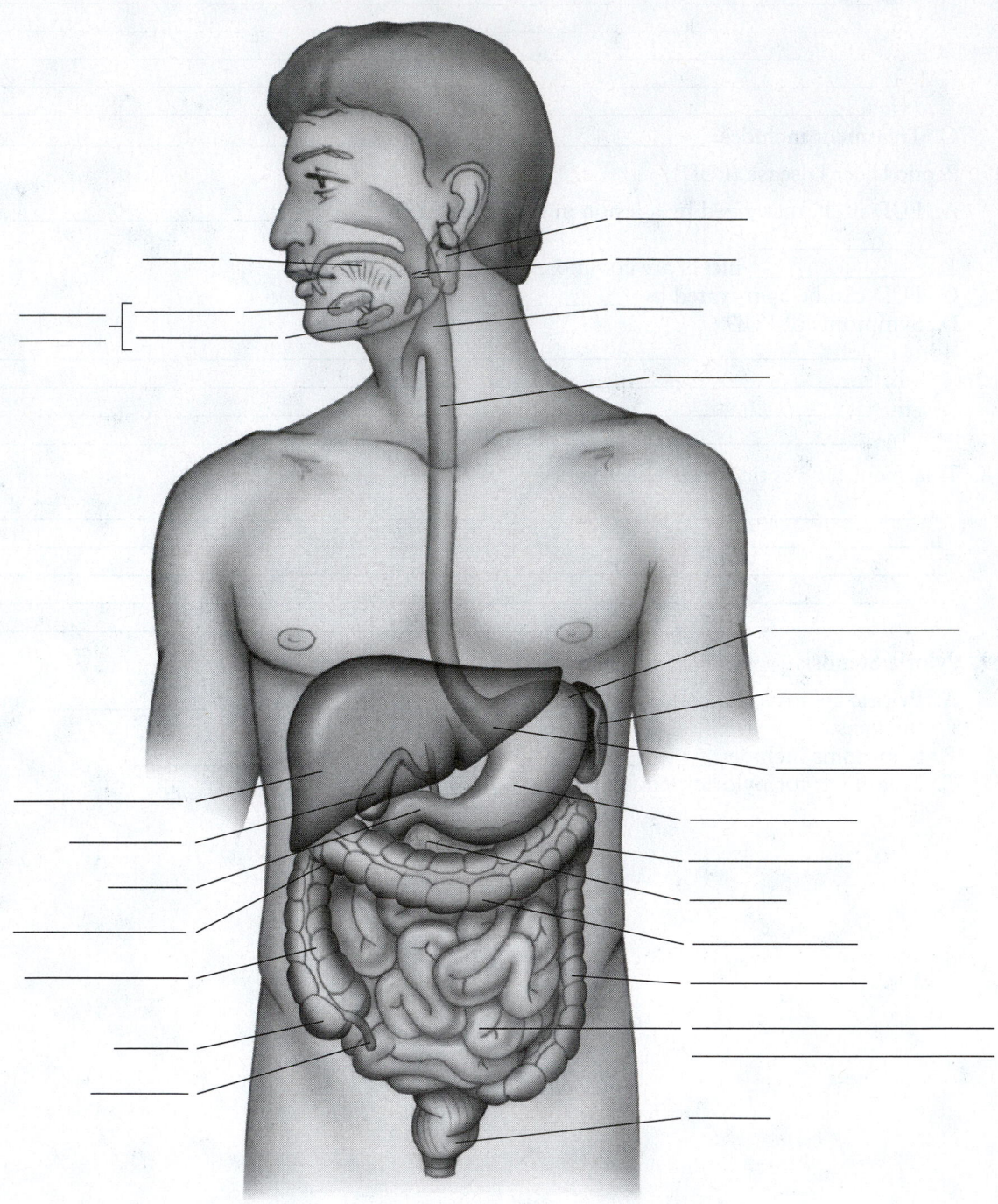

2. Label each part of the oral cavity.

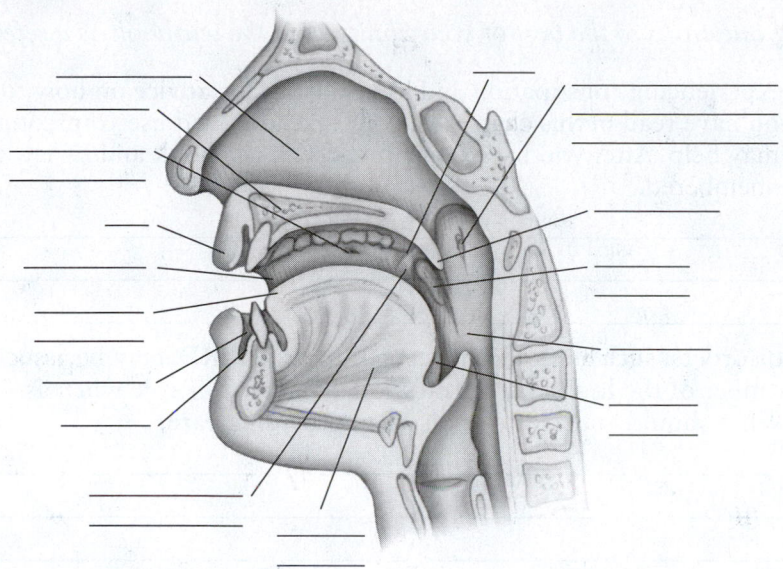

LEARNING ACTIVITY: TRUE/FALSE

Indicate whether the following statements are true or false by placing a T or an F on the line that precedes each statement.

_____ 1. There are three types of taste buds.

_____ 2. The main part of the digestive system is the digestive or gastrointestinal tract.

_____ 3. Humans have two sets of teeth: 25 deciduous teeth (the baby teeth) and 35 permanent teeth.

_____ 4. The incisor teeth are the largest teeth in the permanent set.

_____ 5. Enamel is the hardest and most compact part of the tooth.

_____ 6. Deciduous teeth erupt from the gums from the age of about 7 months to about 2 1/2 years.

_____ 7. The submandibular glands are located below the tongue.

_____ 8. Anyone can get appendicitis, but it occurs most often between the ages of 10 and 30.

_____ 9. Volvulus is the condition in which the bowel twists on itself and causes an obstruction that is painful and requires immediate surgery.

_____ 10. Crohn's disease is contagious.

_____ 11. A hiatal hernia is thought to contribute to the weakening of this sphincter muscle.

_____ 12. There is no cure for irritable bowel syndrome.

_____ 13. Age increases the risk of oral cancer.

_____ 14. About 50% of pancreatic cancers can be surgically removed at the time of diagnosis.

_____ 15. The accessory organs of digestion are the mouth, pharynx, esophagus, stomach, small intestine, large intestine, and rectum.

CRITICAL THINKING

Answer the following questions to the best of your ability. Use the textbook as a reference.

1. Mr. McNeill is experiencing constipation and has called in for advice on how to deal with this. Try to recall what you have read in this chapter of your textbook and use your common sense to list a few things that may help. After you have done that, check the book and review the items that you may not have remembered.

   _____

   _____

   _____

2. Some digestive disorders, such as stomach ulcers, IBS, and GERD, may be associated with a person's lifestyle. As a member of the health care profession, what is your role when assisting in the care of these patients? What should you avoid doing when providing care?

   _____

   _____

   _____

RESEARCH ACTIVITY

Use Internet search engines to research the following topic and write a brief description of what you find. It is important to use reputable websites.

1. As a medical assistant, it will be your responsibility to instruct patients on how to prepare for certain types of diagnostic tests, such as a colonoscopy, endoscopy, or sigmoidoscopy. Select a condition from your textoook, research the types of tests performed for diagnosis, select one of the tests, and research the instructions that would be provided to patients. Write a short essay explaining the condition, the procedure, and the preparatory instructions that patients should be given prior to the procedure. Cite your Internet sources.

   _____

   _____

   _____

   _____

   _____

CHAPTER 31

The Urinary System

STUDENT STUDY GUIDE

Use the following guide to assist in your learning of the concepts from the chapter.

I. The Urinary System

  1. Urine

    A. Urine is the waste product produced by the _____.

    B. It contains mostly water, as well as _____ and _____ compounds.

    C. It drains from the _____, through the _____, to the _____.

  2. The Structure of the Kidneys

    A. The kidney located at the back of the _____, against the muscles of the back, and on either side of the _____.

    B. The kidneys are encased in three capsules for protection: the _____, the _____, and the _____.

  3. The Nephron

    A. Each kidney contains more than 1 _____ nephrons.

    B. A nephron consists of a(n) _____ capsule and a renal _____.

  4. Ureters

    A. Ureters are composed of three layers:

      i. _____

      ii. _____

      iii. _____

    B. They are about _____ to _____ inches long.

  5. The Urinary Bladder

    A. The urinary bladder consists of four layers:

      i. _____

      ii. _____

      iii. _____

      iv. _____

    B. It stretches to hold _____.

  6. The Urethra

    A. In males, the urethra is approximately _____ cm long and transports urine and _____.

    B. The male urethra has three sections: the _____, the _____, and the _____.

    C. In females, the urethra is approximately _____ cm long and transports only urine.

    D. The external opening of the female urethra is situated between the _____ and the opening of the _____.

7. Facts About Urine

    A. Urine consists of about 95% _____ and 5% _____.

    B. An adult passes about _____ to _____ mL of urine daily.

    C. Characteristics of Normal Urine

        i. _____

        ii. _____

        iii. _____

        iv. _____

II. The Pathology of the Urinary System

  1. Cystitis

    A. Cystitis is caused by a(n) _____ infection of the _____ tract.

    B. It is most prevalent in _____ active women, ages _____ to _____, because of anatomical configuration.

    C. Symptoms include _____ and _____ urination.

    D. Treatment includes _____ and _____.

  2. Renal Failure

    A. Renal failure inhibits filtration of the _____.

    B. _____ occurs when there is a change in the filtering function of the kidneys.

    C. Acute kidney failure has no _____ signs.

    D. Dialysis uses a filter other than the kidneys to remove _____ and maintain _____ balance.

  3. Glomerulonephritis

    A. Glomerulonephritis can lead to _____ failure.

    B. Causes include _____, _____, _____, and _____.

    C. Symptoms of Glomerulonephritis

        i. _____

        ii. _____

        iii. _____

        iv. _____

        v. _____

        vi. _____

    D. Treatment includes _____, _____, _____, and _____.

  4. Incontinence

    A. Incontinence is commonly seen in women who have had _____.

    B. Types of incontinence include _____, _____, _____, and _____.

    C. Treatment includes _____, _____, _____, and _____.

  5. Kidney Stones, or Renal Calculi

    A. Kidney stones are harmless in the _____.

    B. They become problematic when passed into the _____.

    C. Symptoms include _____, _____, and _____.

    D. Treatment includes _____ and _____.

    E. Prevention includes controlling the _____ and _____.

6. Polycystic Kidney Disease (PKD)

   A. Symptoms of PKD

      i. _____

     ii. _____

    iii. _____

    iv. _____

     v. _____

    vi. _____

   B. _____ focuses on the symptoms and their complications.

7. Pyelonephritis

   A. Causes of Pyelonephritis

      i. _____

     ii. _____

    iii. _____

    iv. _____

   B. Symptoms of Pyelonephritis

      i. _____

     ii. _____

    iii. _____

    iv. _____

     v. _____

   C. Treatment is typically the use of _____.

   D. If left untreated, _____ and possible kidney _____ may occur.

8. Types of Dialysis (list and briefly explain the two types)

      i. _____

     ii. _____

APPLIED PRACTICE

Using the information found in the chapter, answer the questions following the scenario below.

Scenario

Mr. Bai Feng, born 8-13-66, presents to the office today with a fever of 99.7°F, noticeable beads of sweat on his brow, and complaints of right-sided pain in his lower back. He states, "I am in so much pain I can't stand up straight, and I feel like I always have to urinate." A urine specimen is obtained for urinalysis and shows positive for blood in the urine, as well as other abnormalities. His urine specimen is sent to the laboratory for further testing.

1. Based on his urinalysis and symptoms, what would be a likely diagnosis? (Keep in mind that a medical assistant never diagnoses a patient; this is your opinion based on information found in the textbook.)

   _____

   _____

2. Draw a picture of the urinary system (kidneys, ureters, urinary bladder, and urethra). Circle the area of the urinary system that is likely to be the causative factor for Mr. Feng's pain.

LEARNING ACTIVITY

Match each of the following vocabulary terms to the correct definition.

a. acute renal failure
b. cortex
c. frequency
d. glomerulonephritis
e. incontinence
f. interstitial cystitis
g. kidney stones
h. kidneys

i. medulla
j. polycystic kidney disease (PKD)
k. pyelonephritis
l. ureters
m. urethra
n. urinary bladder
o. void

1. _____ Caused by deposits of mineral salts in the kidney.
2. _____ The outer layer of a kidney.
3. _____ A muscular sac in the pelvic cavity that serves as a reservoir for urine.
4. _____ A kidney disease that hampers the kidneys' ability to remove waste and excess fluids.
5. _____ The involuntary and unpredictable flow of urine.
6. _____ The middle portion of the kidney.
7. _____ Two muscular tubes that carry the newly formed urine from each kidney down to the bladder.
8. _____ The need to void often.
9. _____ An infection of the kidney and renal pelvis.
10. _____ A musculomembranous tube extending from the bladder to the urinary meatus.

11. _____ Occurs when something causes a change in the filtering function of the kidneys.

12. _____ A pair of bean-shaped organs located at the back of the abdominal cavity.

13. _____ A painful inflammation of the bladder wall.

14. _____ To urinate.

15. _____ A disorder in which clusters of cysts develop primarily within the kidneys.

CRITICAL THINKING

Answer the following questions to the best of your ability. Use the textbook as a reference.

1. Why are the elderly more susceptible to becoming dehydrated?

   _____

   _____

   _____

2. When discussing urinary issues with patients, what cultural considerations are important?

   _____

   _____

   _____

RESEARCH ACTIVITY

Use Internet search engines to research the following topic and write a brief description of what you find. It is important to use reputable websites.

1. Visit www.kidney.org. As you navigate through the site, what information do you find that would be helpful for a patient who is in need of a kidney transplant? What information is available for health care technicians? How could this website be beneficial for a urology/nephrology office?

   _____

   _____

   _____

   _____

CHAPTER 32

The Endocrine System

STUDENT STUDY GUIDE

Use the following guide to assist in your learning of the concepts from the chapter.

I. The Endocrine System

   1. Types of Glands

      A. Exocrine glands secrete _____ to a(n) _____ surface, but do not circulate into the _____.

      B. Endocrine glands secrete _____ that _____ within the body.

   2. The Functions of the Endocrine System

      i. _____

   3. The Connection Between the Nervous and Endocrine Systems

      A. The nervous system works closely with the _____ system.

      B. The nervous system helps maintain _____.

      C. The _____, located in the brain, is the link between the two systems.

   4. The Pituitary Gland

      A. The pituitary gland regulates all of the other _____ in the _____ system.

      B. It is located near the _____ of the _____.

      C. It is attached to the _____ by the _____ stalk.

      D. The pituitary gland has two lobes: the _____ and the _____.

   5. Anterior Lobe Hormones (list each hormone)

      i. _____

      ii. _____

      iii. _____

      iv. _____

      v. _____

      vi. _____

      vii. _____

   6. The Hormones and the Functions of the Posterior Lobe of the Pituitary Gland (list the functions of each hormone)

      A. Antidiuretic Hormone (ADH)

B. Oxytocin

    i. _____

    ii. _____

7. The Pineal Gland

  A. The pineal gland is located at the _____ end of the _____.

  B. It secrets _____.

8. The Thyroid Gland

  A. The thyroid gland is located anterior to the _____, just below the _____ cartilage.

  B. Two _____ of the thyroid give the gland its butterfly-shaped appearance.

  C. The lobes are connected in the center by a band of tissue called the _____.

  D. It secretes _____ hormones.

9. The Parathyroid Glands

  A. The parathyroid glands are located around the _____ and lower aspect of the thyroid gland.

  B. Each gland is _____ mm in diameter.

  C. They do not share any function with the _____.

  D. Each gland secretes parathyroid _____.

10. Parathyroid Hormone (PTH)

  A. The Functions of PTH

    i. _____

    ii. _____

11. The Pancreas

  A. The pancreas contains small clusters of cells called the _____ that secrete hormones.

  B. _____ types of cells make up the islets of Langerhans.

12. Pancreatic Cells (list each cell and briefly explain its function)

    i. _____

    ii. _____

    iii. _____

13. The Adrenal Gland

  A. The adrenal gland is _____ in shape.

  B. The adrenal _____ is the outer portion of the gland.

  C. The adrenal _____ is the inner portion of the gland.

14. The Adrenal Cortex (list the three types of hormones manufactured by the adrenal cortex)

    i. _____

    ii. _____

    iii. _____

15. The Adrenal Medulla

  A. The adrenal medulla is the _____ portion of the _____ glands.

  B. It synthesizes, _____, and stores _____.

16. Primary Catecholamines (list the functions of each hormone)

  A. Dopamine

    i. _____

    ii. _____

    iii. _____

B. Epinephrine

    i. _____

    ii. _____

    iii. _____

C. Norepinephrine

    i. _____

    ii. _____

    iii. _____

II. The Pathology of the Endocrine System

1. Acromegaly

A. Acromegaly commonly affects _____ adults.

B. The most serious health consequences of acromegaly are the following:

    i. _____

    ii. _____

    iii. _____

    iv. _____

C. Acromegaly is commonly characterized by abnormal growth of the _____ and _____.

2. Signs and Symptoms of Acromegaly

    i. _____

    ii. _____

    iii. _____

    iv. _____

    v. _____

    vi. _____

    vii. _____

    viii. _____

    ix. _____

    x. _____

    xi. _____

    xii. _____

    xiii. _____

    xiv. _____

    xv. _____

    xvi. _____

3. Treatment for Acromegaly

A. Reduce _____ production to _____ levels.

B. Surgical removal of the _____

C. _____ therapy

D. _____ therapy of the pituitary gland

4. Addison's Disease

A. Addison's disease is a(n) _____ disease in which the body attacks itself.

B. It may be caused by _____ of the adrenal glands, cancer, or _____ into the glands.

C. It is a rare condition that occurs in _____ in _____ Americans.

D. It is diagnosed by _____ and _____ tests that measure _____ hormone levels.

5. Signs and Symptoms of Addison's Disease

    i. _____

    ii. _____

    iii. _____

    iv. _____

v. _____

vi. _____

vii. _____

viii. _____

ix. _____

x. _____

xi. _____

xii. _____

6. Treatment for Addison's Disease

   A. Replace the _____ hormones and prescribe sodium _____.
   B. Administer intramuscular _____ injections.

7. Cushing's Syndrome

   A. Cushing's syndrome is possibly caused by a(n) _____.
   B. Treatment includes _____ and _____.

8. Signs and Symptoms of Cushing's Disease

   i. _____

   ii. _____

   iii. _____

   iv. _____

   v. _____

   vi. _____

9. Diabetes Mellitus

   A. In diabetes mellitus, the body is unable to produce enough _____ to properly control _____ levels.
   B. The lack of insulin in the body can be caused by a lack of production by the _____.

10. Type 1 Diabetes

    A. Juvenile diabetes is typically diagnosed in _____ who cannot produce sufficient quantities, if any, of _____.
    B. Patients are dependent on _____ injections for the rest of their lives.

11. Type 2 Diabetes

    A. Type 2 diabetes is the most _____ form of the disease.
    B. It results from _____ resistance combined with a relative _____ deficiency.
    C. There is a very strong correlation between _____ and type 2 diabetes.

12. Signs and Symptoms of Diabetes

    A. _____ (frequent urination)
    B. _____ (excessive thirst)
    C. _____ (excessive hunger)

13. Treatment for Diabetes

    A. Type 1 diabetes can usually be treated only by _____ the _____.
    B. Type 2 diabetes is treated with _____, _____, and oral _____ medications.
    C. May be preventable with modest lifestyle changes, including a healthy _____, _____, and _____ management.

14. Achondroplasia

    A. Achondroplasia is the most common type of _____, occurring in 1 in 25,000 children.
    B. Abnormal _____ growth is usually diagnosed at birth.
    C. Development of motor skills may be _____, but intellectual development is normal.

15. Physical Characteristics of Achondroplasia

    i. _____
    ii. _____
    iii. _____
    iv. _____
    v. _____
    vi. _____
    vii. _____
    viii. _____

16. Treatment for Achondroplasia

    A. In addition to social and family support, treatment focuses on the _____ and _____ of medical complications.
    B. _____ may be performed to relieve pressure on the _____ system.
    C. Dental and _____ work may be necessary to correct _____ and preserve dental health.

17. Signs and Symptoms of and Treatment for Gigantism

    A. Signs and symptoms of Gigantism

       i. _____
       ii. _____
       iii. _____

    B. Treatment includes _____ therapy and _____ removal of the tumor.

18. Signs and Symptoms of Hyperthyroidism

    i. _____
    ii. _____
    iii. _____
    iv. _____
    v. _____
    vi. _____
    vii. _____
    viii. _____
    ix. _____
    x. _____
    xi. _____

19. Treatment for Hyperthyroidism

    A. _____ medications
    B. Radioactive _____ to destroy the thyroid
    C. _____

20. Hypothyroidism and Other Disorders of the Endocrine System

    A. Because it develops slowly, only about half of the _____ million cases in the United States are diagnosed early.
    B. Untreated, it can lead to other conditions. Constant stimulation causes the release of _____ hormones, which can cause the _____ gland to _____.
    C. Untreated hypothyroidism is associated with a higher risk of _____ disease because of the high levels of _____ (LDL).
    D. Other complications include _____, _____, and _____.

APPLIED PRACTICE

Follow the directions as instructed for each of the following questions.

1. Using the information from the following patient chart, correctly identify the possible endocrine gland disorder based on the patient's signs and symptoms.

Mikovich, Anya, 10-26-1982

4/02/20XX, 3:45 P.M.

Wt: 134 lbs T: 98.6°F P: 104 bpm, bounding

BP: 118/78

cc: Pt presents to office complaining of restlessness, heart palpitations, tremors, sweating. She states, "I am unable to relax and have been sweating a lot recently. I always feel hot." She is displaying exophthalmos and has lost 6 lbs since her last visit 3 months ago, although she claims she hasn't been trying to lose weight.

Adam Bello, RMA

---

2. Label the primary gland of the endocrine system on the image provided.

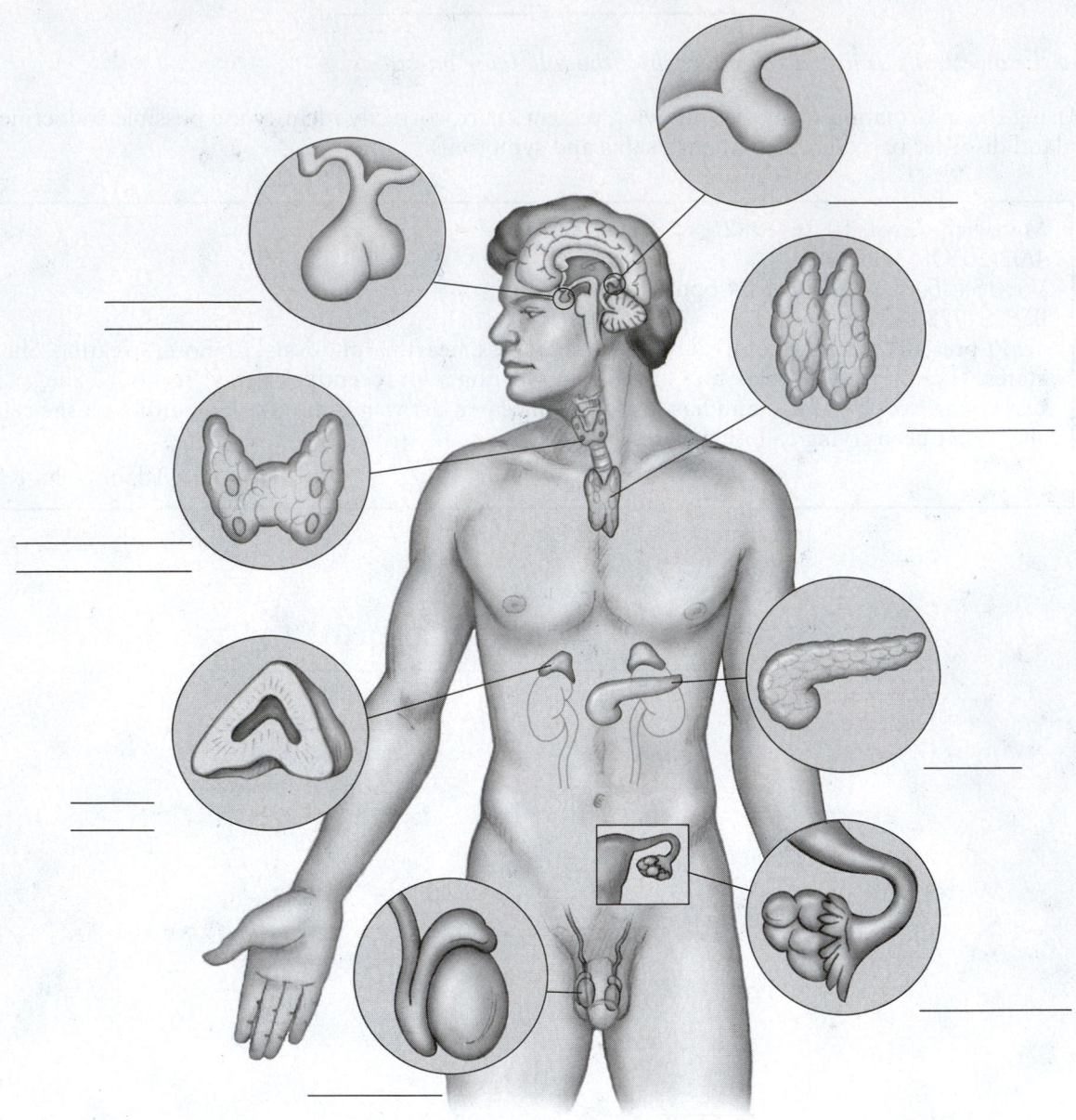

LEARNING ACTIVITY: TRUE/FALSE

Indicate whether the following statements are true or false by placing a T or an F on the line that precedes each statement.

_____ 1. The nerve cells in the hypothalamus control the pituitary gland by producing chemicals that either suppress or stimulate hormone secretion from the pituitary gland.

_____ 2. Depression is commonly associated with disorders related to the hormone serotonin.

_____ 3. Diabetes mellitus is very rare in children.

_____ 4. A myxedema coma can be triggered by sedatives, infection, or other stress.

_____ 5. Insulin and glucagon are secreted by the pancreas.

_____ 6. Hyposecretion of the adrenal cortex results in dwarfism.

_____ 7. Progesterone is a steroid hormone.

_____ 8. Copulation can occur without testosterone.

_____ 9. The thymus is part of the endocrine gland.

_____ 10. Von Rechlinghausen's disease results in degeneration of the bones due to excessive production of parathyroid hormone.

CRITICAL THINKING

Answer the following questions to the best of your ability. Use the textbook as a resource.

1. A pregnant patient who is overdue for going into labor may need a hormone to help stimulate the process of uterine contractions. What hormone may be given? What endocrine gland would produce this hormone naturally? What else does this hormone stimulate?

   _____

   _____

   _____

2. Why is it important to understand the laws of your state regarding individuals with diabetes who drive school buses and other forms of public transportation?

   _____

   _____

   _____

RESEARCH ACTIVITY

Use Internet search engines to research the following topic and write a brief description of what you find. It is important to use reputable websites.

1. Visit www.diabetes.org. Research information as to how diabetes plays an ethnic and cross-cultural role. What facts do you find most surprising regarding this topic? How prevalent is diabetes within your ethnic race or culture?

   _____

   _____

   _____

   _____

   _____

CHAPTER 33
The Reproductive System

STUDENT STUDY GUIDE

Use the following guide to assist in your learning of the concepts from the chapter.

I. The Female Reproductive System

   1. Ovaries

      A. The ovaries are located on both sides of the _____.

      B. They are attached to the _____ by the _____ ligament.

      C. They are controlled by the hormones from the _____ gland.

      D. The microscopic structure includes the _____ (the outer layer) and the _____.

   2. The Uterus

      A. The uterus is a hollow, _____-shaped organ.

      B. It is located in the anterior _____ cavity between the _____ and the symphysis _____, above the bladder and in front of the _____.

      C. Functions of the Uterus

         i. _____

        ii. _____

       iii. _____

   3. Layers of the Uterine Wall

         i. _____

        ii. _____

       iii. _____

   4. Fallopian Tubes

      A. The fallopian tubes are also called the _____ tubes or the _____.

      B. Functions include moving _____ from the _____ to the uterus.

      C. The Three Layers of the Fallopian Tubes

         i. _____

        ii. _____

       iii. _____

   5. Features of the Fallopian Tubes

         i. _____

        ii. _____

       iii. _____

       iv. _____

   6. The Vagina

      A. The vagina is a(n) _____ tube.

      B. It extended from the _____ to the uterus.

      C. It is located between the _____ and the _____.

7. The Five Organs of the Vulva That Make Up the External Female Genitalia
   i. _____
   ii. _____
   iii. _____
   iv. _____
   v. _____

8. Breasts
   A. Breasts are also called _____ glands.
   B. They are composed of fatty, _____ and _____ tissue.
   C. The _____ is the dark, pigmented circular area of skin found on each breast.
   D. The _____ is the elevated area in the center of the _____.

9. Prolactin
   A. Prolactin is the _____ produced by the anterior lobe of the pituitary gland.
   B. It stimulates the _____ glands to produce _____.

10. An Overview of the Menstrual Cycle
    A. _____ is the onset of the menstrual cycle.
    B. _____ is the cessation of the menstrual cycle.
    C. The menstrual cycle is normally _____ days.
    D. It has _____ phases.

II. The Pathology of the Female Reproductive System
   1. Disorders of the Female Reproductive System (briefly explain each of the following disorders)
      A. Abruptio placentae: _____
      B. Amenorrhea: _____
      C. Breech presentation: _____
      D. Cervical polyps: _____
      E. Condyloma: _____
      F. Cystocele: _____
      G. Ectopic pregnancy: _____

   2. Cancers of the Female Reproductive System (list the three types and briefly explain each)
      i. _____
      ii. _____
      iii. _____

   3. Types of Ovarian Cancer (list the three types and briefly explain each)
      i. _____
      ii. _____
      iii. _____

   4. Signs and Symptoms of Early-Stage Ovarian Cancer
      i. _____
      ii. _____
      iii. _____
      iv. _____
      v. _____
      vi. _____
      vii. _____
      viii. _____
      ix. _____
      x. _____
      xi. _____
      xii. _____
      xiii. _____
      xiv. _____

5. Signs and Symptoms of Advanced Ovarian Cancer
   i. _____
   ii. _____
   iii. _____
   iv. _____
   v. _____
   vi. _____

6. Treatment for Ovarian Cancer
   A. Treatment is based on the type, _____, and _____ of the cancer.
   B. Treatment can include _____, _____ therapy, _____, and _____ therapies.
   C. _____ therapies, such as traditional Chinese medicines or special diets, are sometimes used.

7. Uterine Cancer (Endometrial Cancer)
   A. Uterine cancer generally develops in the _____ tissues of the _____.
   B. If detected and _____ early, treatment is usually very successful.

8. Factors That Can Increase the Risk of Uterine Cancer
   i. _____
   ii. _____
   iii. _____
   iv. _____
   v. _____
   vi. _____

9. Signs and Symptoms of Uterine Cancer
   i. _____
   ii. _____
   iii. _____
   iv. _____
   v. _____
   vi. _____
   vii. _____
   viii. _____

10. Uterine Fibroids
    A. Uterine fibroids are _____ growths or tumors.
    B. They are made up of _____ cells and other tissues that grow within the wall of the _____.
    C. They can occur as a(n) _____ growth or as a(n) _____ of _____.
    D. They are common in women of _____ age.
    E. _____ women are the most susceptible of all racial groups.
    F. There is a higher risk of fibroids among women who are _____.

11. Signs and Symptoms of Uterine Fibroids
    i. _____
    ii. _____
    iii. _____
    iv. _____
    v. _____
    vi. _____
    vii. _____

12. Treatment for Uterine Fibroids
    A. _____ medications for mild symptoms
    B. _____ hormone agonists to decrease the size of the fibroids
    C. _____ agents to stop or slow the growth of fibroids

13. Pelvic Inflammatory Disease (PID)

    A. PID is an infection of the upper _____ area.
    B. It is caused by disease-carrying _____.
    C. It can affect the _____, ovaries, and _____ tubes.
    D. If untreated, it can cause _____.

14. Signs and Symptoms of and Treatment for Pelvic Inflammatory Disease

    A. Signs and Symptoms of PID
        i. _____
        ii. _____
        iii. _____
        iv. _____
        v. _____
        vi. _____
    B. Treatment for PID involves treating the underlying _____.

15. Ovarian Cysts

    A. Ovarian cysts are _____ filled with _____ or a semisolid material that develops on or within the ovary.
    B. Functional cysts are relatively common and usually disappear within _____ days without treatment.

16. Signs and Symptoms of Ovarian Cysts

    A. A constant, dull _____ pain
    B. Abdominal _____ or _____

17. Treatment for Ovarian Cysts

    A. Oral _____ may be prescribed.
    B. If larger than _____ cm or persisting for longer than _____ weeks, the cyst may require surgical removal.

18. Preeclampsia

    A. Preeclampsia is _____ during pregnancy.
    B. If untreated, it can result in true _____.
    C. Symptoms of Preeclampsia
        i. _____
        ii. _____
        iii. _____
        iv. _____

19. Premenstrual Syndrome (PMS)

    A. PMS is also called _____ _____ disorder.
    B. It is estimated to affect _____% of women who menstruate.
    C. Only _____ to _____% of menstruating women are severely impaired by PMS.
    D. It is believed that PMS is associated with the amount of _____ produced.

20. Signs and Symptoms of Premenstrual Syndrome

        i. _____
        ii. _____
        iii. _____
        iv. _____
        v. _____
        vi. _____
        vii. _____
        viii. _____
        ix. _____

x. _____

xi. _____

xii. _____

xiii. _____

xiv. _____

xv. _____

xvi. _____

21. Treatment for Premenstrual Syndrome

   i. _____

   ii. _____

   iii. _____

   iv. _____

   v. _____

   vi. _____

22. Disorders of the Female Reproductive System (briefly explain each)

   A. Prolapsed uterus: _____

   B. Rh factor: _____

   C. Salpingitis: _____

   D. Spontaneous abortion: _____

   E. Toxic shock syndrome: _____

23. Breast Cancer

   A. Breast cancer affects women primarily and about _____% of men.

   B. _____ % of breast cancers develop in the tiny _____ that extend from the _____ of the mammary glands to the nipple.

   C. Cancer may also develop in the _____.

   D. The most serious cancers are _____ cancers, which spread from their origin into other tissues.

24. Risk Factors for Breast Cancer

   A. _____ history

   B. Women who begin _____ at an early age or experience a late menopause

25. Signs and Symptoms of Breast Cancer

   A. A(n) _____ in the breast, under the arm, or above the collarbone

   B. _____ discharge

   C. Nipple _____

26. Factors to Be Considered When Treating Breast Cancer

   i. _____

   ii. _____

   iii. _____

   iv. _____

   v. _____

27. Surgical Treatment for Breast Cancer (list the four types of surgery)

   i. _____

   ii. _____

   iii. _____

   iv. _____

28. Cervicitis

   A. Cervicitis is an inflammation of the _____.

   B. Symptoms include _____ or _____ vaginal discharge; frequent and _____ urination; pain during _____; and _____ bleeding after intercourse, between menstrual periods, or after menopause.

29. Treatment for Cervicitis

   A. _____ are used to treat an underlying _____ infection.
   B. If the infection is _____, such as genital herpes, a(n) _____ medication is given.
   C. The person's sexual partner may also be treated to prevent _____.

30. Dysmenorrhea

   A. Signs and symptoms include dull or throbbing pain, usually centered in the _____ abdomen and radiating toward the _____ back or _____.
   B. Some women may also experience nausea and vomiting, _____, irritability, _____, or dizziness.

31. Treatment for Dysmenorrhea

   A. Dysmenorrhea is controlled by treating the _____ disorder.
   B. _____, such as acetaminophen and ibuprofen, are used to relieve pain.
   C. Aromatherapy and _____ are helpful for some women.

32. Endometriosis

   A. Endometriosis occurs when _____ tissue is found _____ the uterus.
   B. One theory as to the cause of endometriosis is that during menstruation, some of the _____ tissue backs up through the _____ tubes into the abdomen.

33. Signs and Symptoms of Endometriosis

   i. _____
   ii. _____
   iii. _____
   iv. _____
   v. _____
   vi. _____
   vii. _____
   viii. _____

34. Treatment for Endometriosis

   A. Early diagnosis and treatment may limit _____ growth and help prevent _____.
   B. Pregnancy, _____, and other hormones appear to delay the onset of endometriosis.
   C. Treatment with medication focuses on treating the _____.
   D. _____ is generally reserved for women with severe endometriosis.

35. Fibrocystic Breast Disease

   A. Fibrocystic breast disease involves common, _____ changes in the tissues of the breast.
   B. It is common in _____ breasts.
   C. The condition usually subsides with _____.
   D. It is estimated to affect more than _____ % of all women.

36. Signs and Symptoms of Fibrocystic Breast Disease

   i. _____
   ii. _____
   iii. _____
   iv. _____
   v. _____

37. Treatment for Fibrocystic Breast Disease

   i. _____
   ii. _____
   iii. _____
   iv. _____
   v. _____

38. Sexually Transmitted Disease (STDs).

    A. STDs are transmitted via the exchange of _____, _____, and other bodily fluids, or by direct contact with the affected areas of people with STDs.

    B. STDs are also called _____ diseases.

39. The Most Common Sexually Transmitted Disease (STDs) in the United States

    i. _____

    ii. _____

    iii. _____

    iv. _____

    v. _____

    vi. _____

40. Reducing the Risk of Contracting a Sexually Transmitted Disease (STDs)

    i. _____

    ii. _____

    iii. _____

41. Sexually Transmitted Infections (list and briefly explain each)

    i. Acquired immune deficiency syndrome (AIDS): _____
_____

    ii. Candidiasis: _____

    iii. Chancroid: _____

    iv. Chlamydial infection: _____

    v. Genital herpes: _____

    vi. Genital warts: _____

    vii. Gonorrhea: _____

    viii. Hepatitis: _____

    ix. Syphilis: _____

    x. Trichomoniasis: _____

42. Vaginitis

    A. Vaginitis is an inflammation of the vagina that can result in discharge, _____, or _____.

    B. The most common cause is a change in the normal balance of vaginal _____ or a(n) _____.

    C. Reduced _____ levels after menopause are another contributing factor.

    D. The most common types of vaginitis are as follows:

       i. _____

       ii. _____

       iii. _____

       iv. _____

III. The Male Reproductive System

  1. The Scrotum

    A. The scrotum is a pouch-like structure behind the _____.

    B. It is suspended from the _____ region.

    C. It is divided into _____ sacs by a septum.

  2. The Penis

    A. The penis is composed of _____ tissue covered by skin.

    B. The size and shape of the penis vary; the average erect penis is about _____ to _____ cm in length.

    C. The penis is covered with a loose fold of skin called the _____, or _____.

3. The Epididymis

   A. The epididymis is a coiled tube lying on the posterior aspect of the _____.

   B. It is between _____ and _____ feet in length.

   C. It is coiled into a space that is less than _____ cm in length and ends at the _____.

      _____.

   D. Its function is to serve as the storage site for maturing _____.

4. The Ductus Deferens

   A. The ductus deferens is a slim, muscular tube about _____ cm in length that is continuous with the _____.

   B. It is the excretory duct of the _____.

   C. It extends from a point adjacent to the _____ and enters the abdomen at the _____ canal.

5. The Two Seminal Vesicles

   A. The vesicles are connected by a narrow _____ to the _____.

   B. They form the _____ duct.

   C. They produce a(n) _____ fluid that becomes part of the seminal fluid, or semen.

6. The Prostate Gland

   A. The prostate gland lies behind the _____ bladder.

   B. It wraps around the first _____ cm of the urethra.

   C. It is about _____ cm wide.

   D. It secretes a(n) _____ fluid that aids in maintaining the viability of the _____.

7. The Male Urethra

   A. The male urethra is approximately _____ inches long.

   B. It is divided into three sections: _____, _____, and _____.

   C. It extends from the bladder to the _____ orifice at the end of the _____.

IV. The Pathology of the Male Reproductive System

   1. Disorders of the Male Reproductive System (briefly explain each)

      A. Anorchism: _____

      B. Aspermia: _____

      C. Azoospermia: _____

      D. Carcinoma of the testes: _____

      E. Cryptorchidism: _____

      F. Phimosis: _____

      G. Prostatitis: _____

      H. Varicocele: _____

   2. Benign Prostatic Hyperplasia (BPH)

      A. BPH is also known as _____.

      B. It may occur in men _____ years of age and older.

      C. By age _____, four out of five men have an enlarged _____.

   3. Signs and Symptoms of Benign Prostatic Hyperplasia

      i. _____

      ii. _____

      iii. _____

      iv. _____

      v. _____

      vi. _____

      vii. _____

      viii. _____

4. Treatment for Benign Prostatic Hyperplasia

    i. _____

    ii. _____

    iii. _____

    iv. _____

5. Epididymitis

    A. Epididymitis is an inflammation or _____ of the epididymis.

    B. The most severe pain and swelling are usually associated with the _____ form.

    C. Symptoms may last for more than _____ weeks after treatment begins.

    D. It can occur any time after the onset of puberty, but is most common between the ages of _____ and _____.

6. Risk Factors for Epididymitis

    A. Infection of the _____, _____, _____, or _____ _____

    B. A narrowing of the _____

    C. Use of a(n) _____ catheter

7. Causes of Epididymitis

    A. Epididymitis can be caused by the same organisms that cause some ____ or can result from _____ surgery.

    B. It is generally caused by _____-generating _____ associated with infections in other parts of the body.

    C. It can also be caused by an injury to or _____ of the scrotum.

8. Signs and Symptoms of Epididymitis

    A. Sudden redness and swelling of the _____

    B. The affected _____ is hard and sore.

    C. Enlarged _____ nodes in the groin that may cause scrotal pain

9. Treatment for Epididymitis

    A. Because it can cause _____, _____ therapy must be initiated as soon as symptoms appear.

    B. Patients are advised to wear _____ _____ when they resume normal activities.

10. Erectile Dysfunction

    A. Erectile dysfunction is the inability to achieve or _____ a(n) _____.

    B. Is not a(n) _____ part of aging.

    C. It occurs when not enough blood is supplied to the _____.

11. Risk Factors for Erectile Dysfunction

    i. _____

    ii. _____

    iii. _____

    iv. _____

    v. _____

    vi. _____

    vii. _____

    viii. _____

    ix. _____

    x. _____

    xi. _____

    xii. _____

    xiii. _____

    xiv. _____

    xv. _____

12. Treatment for Erectile Dysfunction

    i. _____

    ii. _____

    iii. _____

    iv. _____

    v. _____

13. Hydrocele

    A. Hydrocele is a painless buildup of _____ fluid around one or both _____ that causes swelling in the _____ or groin area.

    B. It can be _____ or acquired.

14. Signs and Symptoms of Hydrocele

    A. The scrotum may have a(n) _____ tinge.

    B. The swelling is _____, may be soft or firm, and cannot be reduced by changing its position or gently pushing it up.

    C. The swelling may change in _____.

15. Prostate Cancer

    A. Prostate cancer is a(n) _____ tumor that grows in the _____ gland.

    B. It is the second-leading cause of cancer _____ in men.

    C. By age 50, _____ in _____ American men has some _____ cells in the prostate gland.

    D. The average age of diagnosis is _____.

16. Risk Factors for Prostate Cancer

    i. _____

    ii. _____

    iii. _____

    iv. _____

    v. _____

17. Signs and Symptoms of Prostate Cancer

    i. _____

    ii. _____

    iii. _____

    iv. _____

    v. _____

    vi. _____

    vii. _____

    viii. _____

    ix. _____

18. Treatment for Prostate Cancer

    i. _____

    ii. _____

    iii. _____

    iv. _____

    v. _____

    vi. _____

    vii. _____

    viii. _____

APPLIED PRACTICE

1. Label the uterus, ovaries, and associated structures.

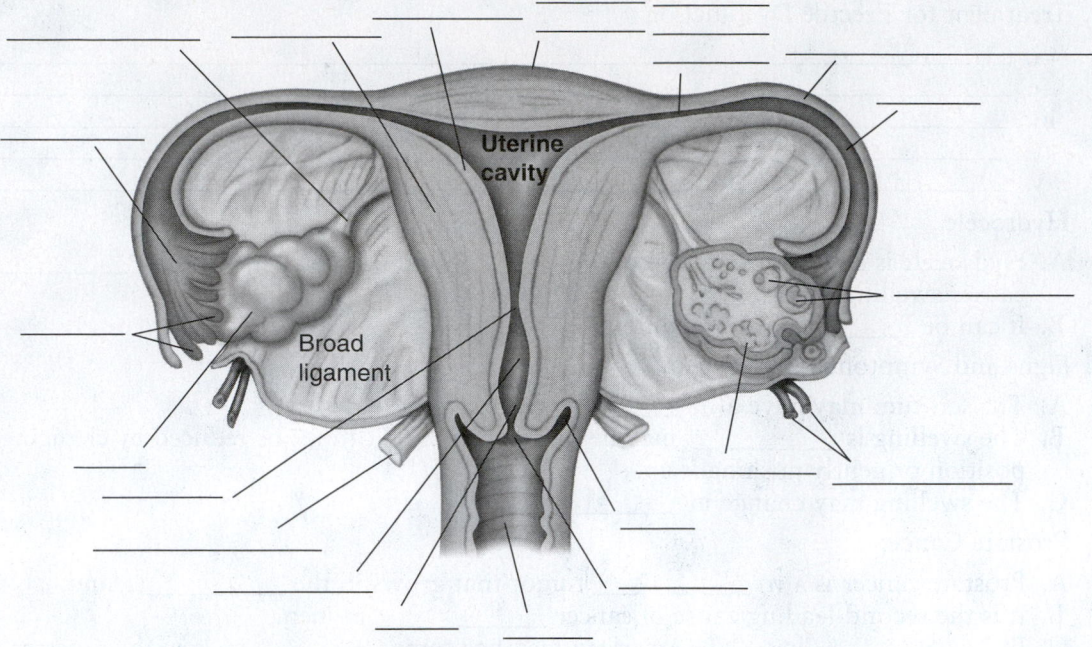

Uterine cavity

Broad ligament

2. Label the structures of the male reproductive system.

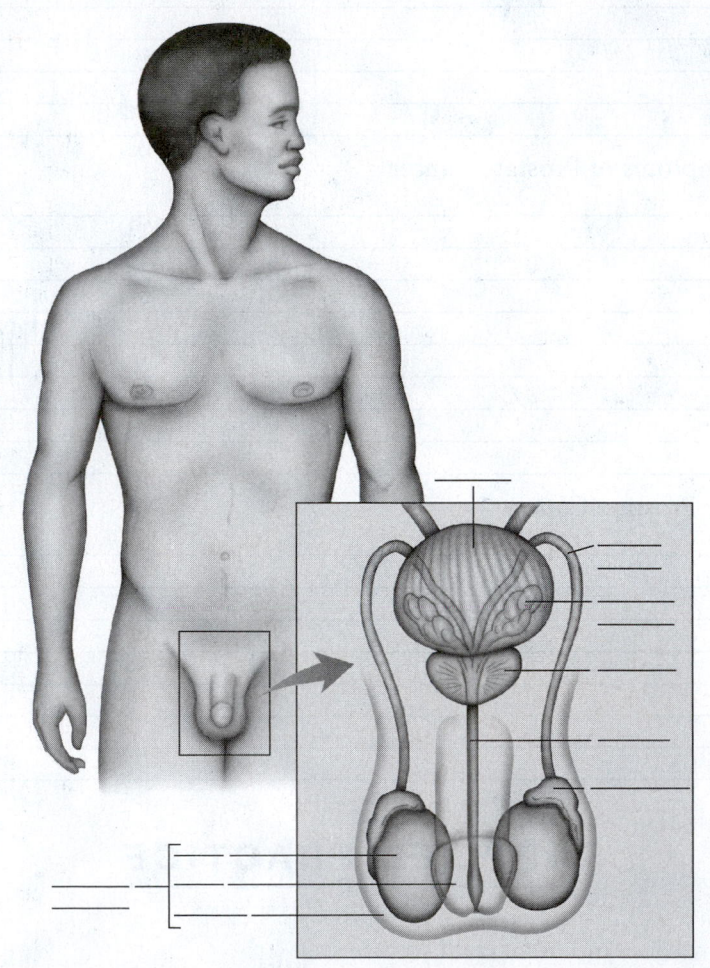

LEARNING ACTIVITY: FILL IN THE BLANK

Using words from the list below, fill in the blanks to complete the following statements.

benign prostatic hyperplasia	ovarian cysts
cervical cancer	pelvic inflammatory disease (PID)
circumcision	perineum
dysmenorrhea	premenstrual syndrome (PMS)
endometriosis	scrotum
hydrocele	testes
hysterectomy	urethritis
menarche	uterine fibroids
ovarian cancer	vaginitis

1. Phimosis is typically treated by performing a(n) _____.
2. Anorchism is a congenital absence of one or both _____.
3. _____ occurs at the age of puberty.
4. The main symptom of a(n) _____ is a swollen scrotum or groin area.
5. The _____ is between the vulva and the anus.
6. _____ is an enlargement of the prostate gland.
7. Symptoms of epididymitis include chills, fever, and acute _____.
8. To test for _____, a pap test is typically performed.
9. A genitourinary infection caused by a parasite that is usually asymptomatic (without symptoms) in both males and females; can produce itching and/or burning and a foul-smelling discharge and result in _____ in women.
10. Typically, by the time _____ is diagnosed, the cancer is usually at an advanced stage.
11. _____ is defined as the symptoms that develop just prior to the onset of a menstrual period.
12. _____ are not disease related and typically disappear on their own.
13. _____ is described as painful cramping associated with menstruation.
14. A(n) _____ involves the removal of the uterus.
15. _____ is the most common and serious complication of STIs among women.

CRITICAL THINKING

Answer the following questions to the best of your ability. Use the textbook as a reference.

1. A patient asks you if you think that her infant son should be circumcised. How do you respond?

   _____

   _____

   _____

2. How can you ensure a patient's privacy when you are calling to talk with the patient by phone?

_____

_____

_____

RESEARCH ACTIVITY

Use Internet search engines to research the following topic and write a brief description of what you find. It is important to use reputable websites.

1. Visit www.cdc.gov. As you navigate through the site, what information do you find that would be helpful to provide a patient who has a sexually transmitted disease?

_____

_____

_____

_____

_____

CHAPTER 38
Assisting with Reproductive and Urinary Specialties

STUDENT STUDY GUIDE

Use the following guide to assist in your learning of the concepts from the chapter.

I. Assisting with Specialty Examinations of the Female Reproductive System

 1. Examination of the Female Reproductive Organs

   i. _____

   ii. _____

   iii. _____

   iv. _____

 2. The Importance of the Clinical Breast Examination (CBE)

   A. Over a lifetime, _____ in _____ women will develop breast cancer.

   B. _____, _____ _____ _____ (CBE), _____ _____ _____ (BSE), and MRIs are tools for early detection.

   C. Women who are at a greater risk of developing breast cancer should have a(n) _____ and a(n) _____ every year.

 3. Steps for the Breast Examination

   A. The patient lies in the _____ position.

   B. The patient is typically asked to place her hand behind her _____ on the side that is being examined first.

   C. This position allows the physician to examine the _____ nodes under the _____.

   D. The physician _____ the breast using his or her fingertips in a(n) _____ manner around all of the breast tissue to search for lumps, tenderness, or inflammation.

   E. In addition, any _____ or _____ of the skin around the breast and nipple is noted.

   F. The nipples are checked for _____, _____, or discharge.

 4. The Health Benefits of Breast Self-Examination (BSE)

   A. The overall goal should be for the patient to be _____ with her own breasts and to report any _____ immediately to her physician.

   B. The physician may advise the patient to perform BSE every _____, usually _____ week after the menstrual period ends.

   C. Women who have reached _____ should examine their breasts on the same day each month.

 5. Correct Application of Fingertips for a Breast Self-Examination in the Shower

   A. Raise the right _____.

   B. Use the left hand to examine the _____ _____.

   C. Then raise the left arm and use the right hand to examine the _____ _____.

   D. Using flat _____, check breast tissue and _____ tissue, gently feeling for any lump or thickening.

6. Correct Application of Fingertips for a Breast Self-Examination in Front of a Mirror

   A. Inspect the breasts for any _____ in shape while the arms are at the side of the body.
   B. Look for _____, _____, or _____ of the skin; lumps; or changes in the _____, such as inversion.
   C. Gently squeeze both nipples and look for _____.
   D. Raise the arms _____ and look for size, shape, and _____ changes in each breast.
   E. With palms resting on _____, flex chest muscles, looking for any obvious differences in the breasts.

7. Correct Application of Fingertips for a Breast Self-Examination Lying Down

   A. To examine the right breast, place a(n) _____ or folded towel behind the right shoulder and place the right hand _____ the head.
   B. Using the hand with fingers flat, gently press the breast tissue, using small _____ motions starting at the _____ _____ of the breast at the 12 o'clock position and spiraling toward the _____.
   C. Gently squeeze the nipple of each breast between the thumb and index finger, noting any _____ or _____.

8. Recommendations from the American Cancer Society for Breast Examinations

   A. A baseline mammogram should be done at age _____.
   B. Women older than age _____ should have a yearly breast examination by a physician and a mammogram every 1 to 2 years.
   C. Women older than age _____ should have a yearly breast examination by a physician and a yearly mammogram.

9. Instructions for a Patient Prior to a Pap Test

   A. Avoid sexual intercourse for at least _____ hours before the examination.
   B. The patient should not schedule a Pap test during a time when she may have her _____.
   C. Schedule the Pap test for at least _____ days after the last day of menstruation.

10. The Pelvic Examination

   A. The pelvic examination begins with an examination of the external genitalia for _____, _____, or _____.
   B. Next, the vaginal _____ is inserted into the vagina to inspect the vagina and cervix for _____, _____, _____, or discharge.
   C. Vaginal specula may be either _____, and need to be sanitized and sterilized after each use, or disposable, and meant for one use only.

11. The Importance of the Pap Smear

   i. _____
   ii. _____
   iii. _____

12. Human Papilloma Viruses (HPVs)

   A. HPVs are responsible for the majority of _____ cancer cases and for genital warts.
   B. Women who become sexually active at an early age, as well as those who have had _____ _____, are at higher risk of infection from HPV.
   C. A new vaccine, _____, prevents infection.
   D. _____ of cervical cancers and _____ of genital warts will not be prevented by these vaccines.

13. The Older "Dry" Method of Pap Smear Collection

   A. Separate slides are made by the _____.
   B. The medical assistant (MA) labels the slides C, V, and E (_____, _____, and _____ canal) based on the source of the cells.
   C. The MA then sprays them with a(n) _____ spray to preserve the cells.

14. The Newer, More Accurate "Liquid" Method of Pap Smear Collection

    A. This method requires the _____ to be collected in a manner similar to that used in the dry method.

    B. The plastic vaginal _____ or _____ that is used is swirled in a liquid _____ medium in order to suspend and preserve the sample.

15. Prenatal Care and Postnatal Care

    A. _____ _____ is provided to pregnant women before delivery, including a series of visits and specific tests to promote the health of both the mother and the fetus.

    B. _____ _____ covers the time from the delivery of the infant through the mother's _____-week _____ follow-up appointment.

16. The First Trimester of Pregnancy

    A. The first trimester includes the period of time from _____ of the embryo in the uterus through the _____ week.

    B. This is the period in which the embryo is most _____ to substances that may cause birth defects.

    C. After the _____ week, the embryo is referred to as a(n) _____.

17. The Second Trimester of Pregnancy

    A. The second trimester begins at the end of the _____ week and continues to the end of the _____ month.

    B. It is the stage at which the refinement of all the _____ takes place.

    C. Fetal movement, also called _____, may be felt.

18. The Third Trimester of Pregnancy

    A. The period from the end of the _____ month to birth is marked by an increase in the size and _____ the fetus.

    B. During this stage, the fetus usually assumes a(n) _____-_____ position.

    C. It is said to have reached the age of _____ (able to sustain life on its own) at 7 months.

19. Elements of the First Prenatal Visit (list the procedures that are typically performed and ordered during this visit)

    i. _____

    ii. _____

    iii. _____

    iv. _____

    v. _____

    vi. _____

20. The Contents of the Prenatal History

    i. _____

    ii. _____

    iii. _____

    iv. _____

    v. _____

    vi. _____

21. The Contents of the Past Obstetrical History

    A. _____, or the number of times that the patient has been pregnant (not necessarily delivered)

    B. _____, or births after 20 weeks of gestation, regardless of whether the infant was born alive or dead

    C. The number of _____ or the number of fetuses that did not reach the age of viability

22. Information Requested for the Present Pregnancy History

    i. _____

    ii. _____

    iii. _____

    iv. _____

    v. _____

23. Follow-Up Prenatal Visits

    A. Every _____ weeks through the _____ week

    B. Every _____ weeks up to the _____ week, and then every week until delivery

    C. During a prenatal visit, the physician will typically do the following:

        i. _____

        ii. _____

        iii. _____

        iv. _____

        v. _____

24. The Medical Assistant's Role During Follow-Up Visits

    i. _____

    ii. _____

    iii. _____

    iv. _____

    v. _____

    vi. _____

    vii. _____

25. Amniocentesis

    A. Amniocentesis is the puncturing of the _____ _____ using a needle and syringe for the purpose of withdrawing _____ fluid for testing.

    B. It can assist in determining fetal _____, _____, and _____ disorders.

26. Procedures and Diagnostic Tests for the Female Reproductive System (briefly explain each type)

    A. Chorionic villus sampling (CVS): _____

    B. Colposcopy: _____

    C. Conization: _____

    D. Culdoscopy: _____

    E. Human chorionic gonadotropin (HCG): _____

    F. Hysterosalpingography: _____

    G. Hysteroscopy: _____

    H. Kegel exercises: _____

    I. Laparotomy: _____

    J. Laparoscopy: _____

    K. Oophorectomy: _____

    L. Panhysterectomy: _____

    M. Panhysterosalpingo-oophorectomy: _____

    N. Pelvimetry: _____

    O. Salpingo-oophorectomy: _____

27. Screening Tests Performed During Pregnancy

    A. The _____-_____ (AFP) test is a blood test taken between the 15th and 18th week of pregnancy to detect _____ _____ defects.

    B. The _____ _____ _____ is a special ultrasound test of the fetus to screen for the risk of Down syndrome and other birth defects.

28. Amniocentesis

   A. Amniocentesis is performed between the _____ and _____ week of gestation.
   B. It involves using a fine needle to take a sample of _____ _____ from the sac around the fetus.
   C. Fluid containing _____ _____ is cultured, grown in a laboratory, and screened to detect _____ defects such as Down syndrome.
   D. It is used to assess fetal _____, _____, and _____.
   E. It is recommended for women older than _____ and those who have a family history of genetic defects.

29. Glucose Tolerance Test

   A. The glucose tolerance test is performed to test for gestational _____.
   B. It is performed between the _____ and _____ week of pregnancy.
   C. After fasting, the patient is given a specific dosage of _____ and blood is taken 1 hour later.
   D. An elevated test result requires an additional, more comprehensive 3-hour _____ test.
   E. A diet that is low in _____, moderate in carbohydrates, and high in _____, as well as regular exercise, is recommended.

30. Group B *Streptococcus*

   A. Group B *Streptococcus* is commonly found in the _____ and _____ tract; it normally does not cause illness.
   B. A vaginal culture at _____ to _____ weeks is recommended.
   C. One to _____ % of infants may be infected, and the infection may be life threatening.
   D. A patient who tests positive will be treated with _____ during labor to prevent fetal infection.

31. Ultrasound

   A. Ultrasound is used to determine the _____, _____ _____, _____ of the fetus, and obvious birth defects.
   B. It is generally performed at _____ to _____ weeks, and is generally painless.

32. The Process of Birth

   A. The first stage of labor varies in length and ends with _____ _____ (widening of the cervix) and _____ (thinning of the cervical walls).
   B. Stage two, the pushing stage, occurs from the period of complete _____ and _____ through the birth of the fetus.
   C. Stage three is the period from the birth of the fetus to the _____ of the _____.

33. Possible Complications During Birth

   A. _____ _____ is a complication in which the placenta develops in the lower portion of the uterus, blocking the opening of the cervix.
   B. _____ _____ is a complication that occurs when the placenta tears away from the uterine wall, resulting in hemorrhaging and fetal distress.
   C. Hypertension during pregnancy, or _____ _____, occurs in roughly 10% of pregnancies.
   D. _____ is when protein in the urine and edema occur.

34. Postpartum Visit

   A. The postpartum visit should be scheduled approximately _____ weeks after delivery.
   B. It provides time to evaluate the overall _____ _____ of the patient and provide contraceptive information if desired.
   C. The postpartum visit includes the following:
      i. _____
      ii. _____

iii. _____

iv. _____

35. Methods of Contraception

A. Barrier contraceptive methods include use of male and female _____, _____, shields, _____, sponges, and _____ caps.

B. Hormonal methods use hormones to change the levels of female hormones in the body to prevent _____ or _____ of the fertilized ovum.

C. An intrauterine device (IUD) is a small device with _____ that is placed in the uterus by the physician.

D. Natural family planning is also known as the _____ _____ or, most recently, fertility-awareness-based birth control, a method in which intercourse is avoided around the time of ovulation.

E. _____ _____ involves the withdrawal of the male's penis before ejaculation in the vagina.

II. Assisting with Specialty Examinations of the Male Reproductive System

1. Circumcision

A. Circumcision is surgical removal of the end of the _____, or _____, of the penis.

B. The primary reason for this procedure is ease of _____.

C. Circumcision is also a(n) _____ practiced in some religions.

2. Procedures and Diagnostic Tests for the Male Reproductive System (briefly explain each type)

A. Castration: _____

B. Epididymectomy: _____

C. Erickson Sperm Separation: _____

D. Fluorescent treponemal antibody absorption: _____

E. Orchidopexy: _____

F. Orchiectomy: _____

G. Prostatectomy: _____

H. Testosterone toxicology: _____

I. Transurethral resection of the prostate (TURP): _____

J. Venereal disease research laboratory (VDRL): _____

3. Steps for Instructing a Male Patient to Perform a Testicular Exam

A. _____ the patient and introduce yourself.

B. Explain to the patient that he or she should perform the examination in the _____ or right after a warm shower, which causes the _____ _____ to relax.

C. Using the testicular model or illustration, explain that he should place his middle and index fingers underneath the _____ and thumb on top and use a gentle motion to roll the _____ between the fingers.

D. Indicate on the model or illustration the location of the _____, a soft tubular cord behind the testis that stores and carries sperm.

4. Vasectomy

A. A vasectomy involves cutting the _____ _____ and tying off the ends to prevent sperm from being transported out of the testes.

B. After a vasectomy, the man still achieves a(n) _____ and ejaculates, but without the presence of _____.

C. Another birth control method should be used for _____–_____ weeks afterward or until a sample taken after the vasectomy confirms the absence of sperm.

D. In some cases, the procedure is _____, but a vasectomy should be considered a(n) _____ form of birth control.

5. Sexually Transmitted Infections (STIs)

    A. STIs are transmitted by sexual contact from _____ to person or _____ to child.

    B. They are caused by _____.

    C. They are generally treated successfully with _____.

    D. Viral STDs, such as _____, _____ _____, _____, and _____, are incurable.

6. Symptoms of a Sexually Transmitted Infection

    i. _____

    ii. _____

    iii. _____

    iv. _____

7. Bacterial Vaginosis (BV)

    A. BV is the most common _____ _____ in women of childbearing age.

    B. Certain behaviors increase the risk of infection, such as _____ _____ and douching.

    C. Symptoms include a thin _____ or _____ discharge with an unpleasant fishy odor.

    D. BV increases susceptibility to other _____.

    E. Treatment is important for _____ women.

8. Chlamydia Infections

    A. Chlamydia infections are caused by the bacterium _____ _____.

    B. In males, chlamydia is characterized by _____ and _____.

    C. Chlamydia may lead to _____ _____ _____ in women.

    D. Infected females have an increased risk of _____ pregnancy and sterility.

    E. Infants born to infected mothers may develop _____ or _____.

    F. Chlamydia can be successfully treated with _____ or _____.

9. Genital Human Papilloma Virus Infection

    A. _____ _____, or _____, are found in clusters on the external sexual organs of both males and females, and internally in the female in the vagina and cervix and in the anus and rectum of the male.

    B. They can be discovered in the female by a(n) _____ _____, although the patient may not have visible signs of warts.

    C. Genital warts increase a female's risk of developing _____ _____.

10. Genital Herpes

    A. Genital herpes is caused by _____ _____ _____ _____ (HSV-1) and type 2 (HSV-2).

    B. There is no known cure for herpes, but _____ may lessen the duration of symptoms.

    C. _____ are usually self-limiting, but may reoccur during stressful situations.

11. Gonorrhea

    A. Gonorrhea is an STI that is caused by the organism _____ _____, a bacterium that grows well under warm, moist conditions.

    B. It can grow in the _____, _____ _____, and uterus in the female.

    C. It can grow in the _____, _____, _____, and _____ of both males and females.

    D. In the male, gonorrhea is characterized by _____ _____, clear at first, and then becoming thick and milky, burning, itching, and producing pain upon urination.

    E. Females are often _____, and then they develop a yellowish-green discharge.

    F. Other symptoms include _____ _____, _____ _____, anal discharge, and fever.

12. Treatment for Gonorrhea

    A. Treatment includes large doses of _____ or _____ with follow-up examinations.

    B. If left untreated, gonorrhea can cause _____ in males and females.

    C. Gonorrhea can be diagnosed by _____ and _____ _____.

    D. Many people who have gonorrhea also have _____ and must be treated for both.

13. Human Immunodeficiency Virus (HIV)

    A. Causes _____ _____ _____ (AIDS), the final stage of HIV infection.

    B. It is a very delicate virus that cannot survive _____ of the body.

    C. It is not spread by casual contact or day-to-day activities such as _____ _____, _____, or sitting on toilet seats.

14. Methods of Transmission of Human Immunodeficiency Virus

    A. _____, _____, or anal sex with someone who is infected

    B. Sharing _____ or _____ with someone who is infected

    C. Being exposed as a(n) _____ or infant to HIV before or during birth or breastfeeding

    D. Coming in contact with _____ that is infected

15. Preventing the Transmission of Human Immunodeficiency Virus

    i. _____

    ii. _____

    iii. _____

    iv. _____

    v. _____

    vi. _____

    vii. _____

16. Lymphogranuloma Venereum (LGV)

    A. LGV is an STI that is caused by three strains of the bacterium _____ _____.

    B. It is difficult to diagnose because the symptoms are _____ to that of other conditions.

    C. It can be mistaken for _____ STIs like syphilis and genital herpes.

    D. Untreated, LGV may cause _____ obstruction and _____ (massive swelling of the scrotum).

17. Pelvic Inflammatory Disease (PID)

    A. *PID* is the term used to describe inflammation of the vagina, cervix, uterus, and _____ _____ in the female.

    B. If left untreated, _____ _____ may develop in the fallopian tube, which then blocks the movement of the ovum in the tubes.

    C. If the tubes are completely blocked, _____ cannot reach the ovum to cause fertilization.

    D. If partially blocked, a fertilized ovum may begin to grow in the _____ _____ instead of in the uterus.

    E. It is diagnosed by _____ _____ and an ultrasound of the abdomen.

    F. It can result in _____ _____, _____, and even death if untreated.

    G. _____ can cure PID.

    H. Treatment does not correct any damage already done to the _____ organs.

18. Syphilis

    A. Syphilis is an STD that is caused by the bacterium _____ _____.

    B. It is spread by direct person-to-person contact with a(n) _____ _____, or sore.

    C. Sores may occur on the genitals, anus, _____, _____, and _____.

    D. It may be transmitted to a newborn by an infected mother, resulting in _____ or developmental delays or death after birth.

E. A primary chancre occurs in about _____ weeks or up to _____ months after exposure.

F. Secondary-stage signs are a(n) _____ on the palms of the hands, the soles of the feet, and elsewhere on the body, along with fever, swollen glands, _____ _____, and fatigue.

G. The latent stages occur _____ to _____ years after the first two stages have disappeared.

H. The disease will damage the brain, heart, liver, and other internal organs, causing _____, _____, blindness, and death.

I. It is diagnosed by _____-_____ microscopic examination of chancre material or by blood tests for the presence of syphilis antibodies (RPR, VDRL).

J. During the primary stage, a single, large dose of _____ may cure the patient.

19. Trichomoniasis

A. Trichomoniasis is a protozoal infection caused by the organism _____ _____, resulting in an infection of the lower genitourinary tract.

B. It causes a white or yellow, _____ _____ discharge with a foul odor in females.

C. The male is usually _____, except for _____ itching.

D. A diagnosis is made by obtaining a sample of vaginal _____ and preparing a slide with normal saline solution.

E. Treatment for both males and females is a course of the antibiotic _____ or _____ taken orally.

20. Symptoms of Urinary Tract Disorders

A. Increased urine production is seen in _____.

B. Frequent urination is seen in _____ _____ infections.

C. Swelling and weight gain are seen in _____ _____ _____ (CHF) and renal dysfunction.

D. Decreased urinary output is seen in urinary _____.

21. Procedures and Diagnostic Tests for the Urinary System (briefly describe each)

A. Creatinine clearance: _____

B. Cystography: _____

C. Cystoscopy: _____

D. Extracorporeal shockwave lithotripsy (ESWL): _____

E. Excretory urography: _____

F. Hemodialysis: _____

G. Intravenous pyelogram (IVP): _____

H. Kidney, ureters, bladder (KUB): _____

I. Meatotomy: _____

J. Peritoneal dialysis: _____

K. Retrograde pyelogram: _____

L. Sound: _____

M. Urography: _____

N. Ultrasonography of the kidneys: _____

22. Benign Prostate Hyperplasia (BPH)

A. As the _____ enlarges, it presses on the urethra and causes restriction of the flow of urine.

B. Restricted urinary flow can result in _____ _____, interruption of the _____ _____, and difficulty starting to urinate.

23. Prostate Cancer

    A. Prostate cancer is a slow-growing _____ tumor of the prostate gland.

    B. It may spread to the adjacent _____ _____ and male reproductive organs, as well as to the lymph nodes and bones.

    C. It is the _____ most common form of cancer in men, with one in eight males affected.

    D. Its cause is unknown, but age, heredity, and a(n) _____-_____ diet increase the risk of developing it.

24. Symptoms of Prostate Cancer

    i. _____

    ii. _____

    iii. _____

    iv. _____

    v. _____

25. Screening for Prostate Cancer

    A. Prostate-specific antigen (PSA) _____ _____ and a(n) _____ rectal examination

    B. The PSA test checks for a(n) _____ released by the prostate.

    C. If levels are elevated, then a(n) _____ of prostate tissue is done, usually in the office.

    D. If the results are positive for cancer cells, then a(n) _____ _____ is done to detect possible spread of the disease.

    E. PSA results of under _____ are considered to be normal.

26. Treatment for Prostate Cancer

    i. _____

    ii. _____

    iii. _____

    iv. _____

    v. _____

27. Acute and Chronic Renal Failure

    A. Kidney failure is the inability of the kidneys to adequately _____ _____ waste products from the blood.

    B. Acute kidney failure has a rapid onset of a few days to a few _____.

    C. Causes of Acute Renal Failure

        i. _____

        ii. _____

        iii. _____

28. Symptoms of Acute Renal Failure

    i. _____

    ii. _____

    iii. _____

    iv. _____

    v. _____

    vi. _____

29. Diagnosing Acute Renal Failure (list the types of tests and diagnostic procedures used)

    i. _____

    ii. _____

    iii. _____

    iv. _____

    v. _____

30. Chronic Renal Failure

   A. Chronic renal failure is a slow _____, decline in kidney function over a period of months to several years.

   B. Acute kidney failure can become chronic if, after treatment, the kidneys do not _____ recover.

   C. Any condition that can cause acute renal failure can cause _____ _____ failure.

31. Common Causes of Chronic Renal Failure

   i. _____

   ii. _____

   iii. _____

   iv. _____

   v. _____

32. Symptoms of Chronic Renal Failure

   A. Patient may experience mild symptoms, including _____ and elevated _____ _____ nitrogen.

   B. As the condition progresses, _____, lack of _____ _____, anemia, loss of appetite, and shortness of breath affect the patient's quality of life.

33. Diagnosing Chronic Renal Failure

   A. Diagnosis is based on patient _____, _____, and blood tests for the levels of _____ and blood urea nitrogen.

   B. Chronic renal failure is _____ if not treated.

   C. Survival for patients with end-stage renal disease is a(n) _____ _____.

34. Treatment for Chronic Renal Failure

   A. Treatment involves various medications to adjust _____ _____, regulate _____ _____, and counteract anemia.

   B. Treatment includes restriction of _____ and _____ in the diet.

   C. When these treatments are no longer effective, kidney _____ or _____ are the alternatives.

   D. Most patients with advanced kidney failure die within _____ to _____ years even with dialysis.

KEY TERMINOLOGY REVIEW

Write a sentence using each of the selected key terms in the correct context.

1. *amenorrhea:*

   _____

   _____

2. *chorionic villus sampling (CVS):*

   _____

   _____

3. *dysplasia:*

   _____

   _____

4. *lochia:*

_____

_____

5. *puerperium:*

_____

_____

APPLIED PRACTICE

Follow the directions as instructed for each question.

1. Sometimes patients are not ready either physically or emotionally to fully understand their medical diagnosis. The medical assistant must be able to clearly explain, in simple language, any terms that are confusing to the patient. The medical assistant must use many teaching methods to facilitate the patient's comprehension of his or her diagnosis and treatment plan. List three teaching methods that the medical assistant can use to help the patient.

_____

_____

2. Many states mandate that suspicions of abuse be reported. How would you go about reporting any suspicion you may have?

_____

_____

_____

LEARNING ACTIVITY: FILL IN THE BLANK

Using your text as necessary, fill in the blanks in the following questions.

1. The ACS suggests that women in their 20s and 30s have a(n) _____ as part of a periodic regular health exam by a health professional every 3 years.

2. Females develop breast cancer 100 times more frequently than males, probably due to the effects of _____.

3. Prior to the patient scheduling a Pap test, the medical assistant should advise her not to douche for _____-_____ hours before the examination.

4. The pelvic examination begins with an examination of the _____.

5. Women who become sexually active at an early age, as well as those who have multiple partners, are at _____ risk of infection from HPV.

6. The Pap smear is _____% accurate in detecting cervical carcinoma.

7. The third trimester is the period from the end of the _____ month to birth.

8. The normal FHT is _____-_____ beats per minute.

9. Condoms have an effectiveness rate of about _____%.

10. Women are fertile for about _____ years of their adult lives.

11. An alternative birth control method should be used for _____-_____ weeks after a vasectomy or until a sample confirms the absence of sperm.

12. The symptoms of gonorrhea do not appear in females until _____ months after exposure.

13. _____ has no known cause and is the most common vaginal infection in women of childbearing age.

14. Untreated, gonorrhea can cause _____ in both males and females and can spread to the blood or joints.

15. Benign prostate hyperplasia (BPH) is an enlargement of the prostate gland that may occur after age _____.

CRITICAL THINKING

Answer the following questions to the best of your ability. Use the textbook as a reference.

1. Imagine the following scenario: You are a female. You have completed your externship and have been hired by a urology clinic for your first full-time medical assistant position. You are directed by the physician to instruct a patient in how to perform a testicular self-exam. You are suddenly nervous about doing this with a real patient even though you have practiced this in your medical assisting program with other students. Describe in one or two paragraphs how you would feel and what you would do or calm yourself to bolster your own comfort and confidence.

_____

_____

_____

2. A patient, 18-year-old Maria Riojas, has come in with a chief complaint of bleeding between her periods. This will be her third GYN visit since menarche, and she is still quite apprehensive about the examination and getting undressed. She says that she hopes that the doctor won't have to do a pelvic examination today; she just wants a stronger or different birth control pill. Her friend told her that she has breakthrough bleeding because she is on the wrong pill. What would you say to the patient?

_____

_____

_____

3. A patient comes in with her husband, and she asks that he be allowed to come into the examination room with her. When you ask her to disrobe, she looks hesitant, then looks at her husband and doesn't move to take the gown and drape. What do you anticipate is happening? What should you do?

_____

_____

_____

4. A patient who is 6 months, pregnant calls in saying that she has been bleeding a little (just spotting) all morning and wanted to let the doctor know. She wants an appointment for Thursday and today is Monday. What would you say?

_____

_____

_____

RESEARCH ACTIVITY

Use Internet search engines to research the following topic and write a brief description of what you find. It is important to use reputable websites.

1. Select one procedure and diagnostic test for the female reproductive system and one procedure and diagnostic test for the male reproductive system. Conduct research on each using online resources and/or your school or local library. Write a paragraph on what you learned about each procedure/diagnostic test, including why the test is done, how the test is done, and what type of treatment might be available if the test result is positive. Be sure to cite your sources.

   _____

   _____

   _____

   _____

   _____

CHAPTER 39
Assisting with Eye and Ear Care

STUDENT STUDY GUIDE

Use the following guide to assist in your learning of the concepts from the chapter.

I. The Study of the Eye

1. The Ophthalmologist

   A. The ophthalmologist performs eye _____ and eye _____.
   B. The ophthalmologist prescribes medications, _____, and contact lenses.

2. The Doctor of Optometry (OD)

   A. The OD is also referred to as a(n) _____.
   B. The OD performs eye examinations, prescribes medications, and write prescriptions for _____ and contact lenses.

3. The Optician

   A. The optician _____ and _____ prescription lenses and contacts.
   B. The optician completes a _____ to _____-year apprenticeship.

4. The Ophthalmoscope

   A. The ophthalmoscope is used to view the _____ parts of the _____.
   B. The physician positions the ophthalmoscope so that _____ penetrates the _____ of the patient's eye and screens for _____ damage and _____ problems.

5. Evaluating the Status of the Patient's Pupils

   A. PERRLA is an acronym that stands for _____ _____, _____, _____ to _____, and _____ and focus on objects at different _____.
   B. Injuries to the brain may result in the patient having pupils of _____ size.

6. Visual Acuity

   A. Normal visual acuity, or clearness of vision, is referred to as _____ vision.
   B. Causes of Errors in Refraction
      i. The eyeball is too _____.
      ii. The eyeball is too _____.
      iii. The lens has _____ its _____.
      iv. The _____ or _____ has an irregular _____.

7. Myopia

   A. Myopia is a condition in which the eye sees _____ objects well but _____ objects appear _____.
   B. It occurs either because the eyeball is too _____ or because the _____ is too _____, and the light _____ do not reach the _____.

8. Strabismus

    A. Children with strabismus appear _____ and may need to wear a(n) _____ over the _____ _____ to _____ the weaker eye.

    B. If the _____ and _____ are ineffective, surgery on the eye _____ may be necessary.

9. The Snellen Chart

    A. A person with normal vision can read the top line at _____ feet.

    B. To the _____ of each line is a(n) _____ indicating that a person with normal vision can read the lines at decreasing distances of _____, _____, _____, _____, _____, and _____ feet.

    C. For preschool children or patients who are _____ or have a(n) _____ barrier, the Snellen E, the _____, or pictorial charts are used.

10. Eye Abbreviations

    A. The abbreviation for the right eye is _____.

    B. The abbreviation for the left eye is _____.

    C. The abbreviation for both eyes is _____.

11. Steps for Using the Snellen Chart

    A. Determine the patient's ability to recognize _____.

    B. Place the patient _____ feet from the chart, either seated or standing, as long as the Snellen chart is at _____ level.

    C. Following office policies (regarding which eye to test first), have the patient cover the other eye with a(n) _____.

    D. Instruct the patient to keep both eyes _____ even though one eye is covered.

    E. Use a pointer and point to the letters or appropriate symbols in _____ order.

    F. Starting with the _____ line, ask the patient to identify the letters on each line, and then proceed down the chart to the last line that the patient can read without _____.

    G. Observe for signs of _____ or _____ the head, which indicate difficulty identifying letters.

    H. Record the _____ numbers adjacent to the line that the patient can read without _____.

    I. Following testing of both eyes, clean the _____ with _____ and _____.

12. Steps for Testing for Near-Vision Acuity Using the Jaeger Card

    A. The patient reads the card held at a normal reading distance (_____ to _____ inches).

    B. The card has a series of paragraphs in decreasing _____ of _____ with a(n) _____ above each.

    C. Number one (_____) is next to the paragraph with the _____ _____, and as the text becomes larger, the number _____.

    D. Paragraph _____ represents 20/20 vision.

13. Color Vision Impairment

    A. Defects in color vision are _____, _____, or acquired through disease or injury.

    B. Changes in color vision may indicate diseases of the _____, _____ _____, or _____.

14. The Ishihara Test

    A. The Ishihara test screens for color vision _____.

    B. The patient is shown _____ color plates or pages and must correctly identify _____ to be considered to have color vision within a normal range.

15. Contrast Sensitivity

    A. Contrast sensitivity is used to measure the patient's ability to distinguish faint _____ in shades of _____.

    B. Several new testing procedures have been used to test for contrast sensitivity, including the _____ _____ _____ and the _____ _____ _____.

16. Procedures and Diagnostic Tests Related to the Eye

    A. _____

    B. _____

    C. _____

    D. _____

    E. _____

    F. _____

    G. _____

    H. _____

    I. _____

    J. _____

    K. _____

    L. _____

    M. _____

    N. _____

17. Fluorescein Angiography

    A. This is the process of injecting _____, followed by a series of _____ of the _____ through dilated pupils.

    B. It provides diagnostic information about the blood flow in the _____.

    C. It detects _____ changes in diabetics and _____ _____.

    D. It identifies _____ in the macular area of the _____, determining whether there is _____ of the _____.

18. Radial Keratotomy

    A. Radial keratotomy is a surgical procedure that may be performed to correct _____.

    B. Incisions are made in the _____ to flatten it, thereby shortening the _____ so that _____ reaches the _____.

    C. Complications of surgery can lead to _____.

19. Steps for Irrigating the Eye

    A. The label of the irrigating solution must be checked _____ times to ensure that it is the correct _____ and _____ as ordered by the physician.

    B. The solution is brought to room temperature by _____ the bottle in a(n) _____ _____ or by standing the bottle in a(n) _____ water _____.

    C. If both eyes are to be irrigated, then _____ separate sets of equipment must be used to prevent _____.

    D. Hold the syringe _____ inch from the eye.

    E. Gently irrigate from the inner to the outer _____, or _____ of the eye, aiming at the _____ _____.

20. The Instillation of Eye Medication

    A. Only _____ or _____ medications can be used in the eye and they must be _____.

    B. Encourage patients to discard eye medications when the prescribed treatment time has been _____.

21. Steps for the Instillation of Eye Medication
   A. Check the _____ of the medication, the _____ date, and the _____ three times.
   B. Ask the patient if he or she has any known _____ to the medication.
   C. Position the patient with his or her headed tilted _____, with eyes looking _____.
   D. Pull down the _____ _____, exposing the _____.
   E. Place the dropper about _____ inch above the _____ with your dominant hand.
   F. Insert the proper number of drops into the _____ of the conjunctiva. If ointment is used, apply as a thin strip from _____ to _____ canthus.
   G. Ask the patient to gently _____ the eye and _____ the eyeball.
   H. Dry the excess medication from the _____ canthus to the _____ canthus using _____ gauze.
   I. Explain to the patient that his or her vision may be _____.

II. The Study of the Ear

   1. Steps for Irrigating the Ear
      A. Check the name, _____, and _____ date of the irrigating solution _____ times.
      B. Have the patient sit with the affected ear tilted slightly _____.
      C. Place a towel over the patient's _____ and ask the patient to hold the _____ basin.
      D. Clean the _____ ear with a(n) _____ cotton ball.
      E. Pour the warmed solution into a(n) _____ basin and fill the syringe with _____ cc of solution.
      F. Aim the stream of flow toward the _____ of the _____.

   2. Steps for Instilling Ear Medication
      i. _____
      ii. _____
      iii. _____
      iv. _____
      v. _____
      vi. _____
      vii. _____
      viii. _____
      ix. _____
      x. _____
      xi. _____
      xii. _____

   3. Steps for Performing Audiometric Testing
      i. _____
      ii. _____
      iii. _____
      iv. _____
      v. _____
      vi. _____
      vii. _____
      viii. _____
      ix. _____
      x. _____

xi. _____

xii. _____

xiii. _____

xiv. _____

4. Tests and Procedures for the Ear (briefly explain each of the following)

A. Audiometric test: _____

B. Electrochochleography: _____

C. Falling test: _____

D. Mastoid antrotomy: _____

E. Myringoplasty: _____

F. Otoplasty: _____

G. Stapedectomy: _____

H. Tympanoplasty: _____

I. Rinne test: _____

J. Weber test: _____

5. Examination of the Nose and Throat

A. The physician uses a nasal _____ to inspect the _____ lining of the nose for signs of _____ and _____.

B. Examination includes the use of a tongue _____ to examine the _____ for signs of _____, enlarged _____, and abnormalities of the tongue or _____ _____.

6. Signs and Symptoms of Nasal Problems

i. _____

ii. _____

iii. _____

iv. _____

7. Steps for Instilling Nasal Medication

i. _____

ii. _____

iii. _____

iv. _____

v. _____

vi. _____

vii. _____

viii. _____

ix. _____

x. _____

xi. _____

xii. _____

xiii. _____

xiv. _____

xv. _____

xvi. _____

xvii. _____

xviii. _____

xix. _____

xx. _____

KEY TERMINOLOGY REVIEW

Match the each of the following vocabulary terms to the correct definition.

a. astigmatism

b. frequencies

c. myopia

d. myringa

e. strabismus

1. _____ The medical term for the eardrum.

2. _____ An eye disorder caused by weakness in the external eye muscles, resulting in the eyes looking in different directions.

3. _____ A refractive disorder in which irregularities in the curvature of the cornea cause light not to focus on the retina but instead to spread out over an area, causing overall blurring of vision.

4. _____ Also known as nearsightedness.

5. _____ Number of fluctuations per second of energy in the form of sound waves.

APPLIED PRACTICE

Follow the directions as instructed for each activity.

Activity 1: *Read the following scenario and then answer the questions.*

Shawn Collins, RMA, is working as a medical assistant at a local family practice. Rajan Avuri, a 17-year-old patient, is being seen for a driver's license eye examination. As part of the exam, Shawn tests Rajan's vision with a Snellen eye chart similar to the Snellen eye chart below. Shawn asks Rajan to cover his right eye and read line 8. Rajan reads the following letters from left to right: "D, E, F, P, O, T, E, C." Shawn asks Rajan to continue on and read line 9. Rajan reads the following letters from left to right: "L, E, P, O, D, R, O, T."

Shawn then asks Rajan to uncover his right eye and cover his left eye for assessment. Beginning with line 8, Rajan reads the following letters from left to right: "D, E, F, R, O, T, E, C." Rajan is not able to distinguish any letters on the lines below line 8.

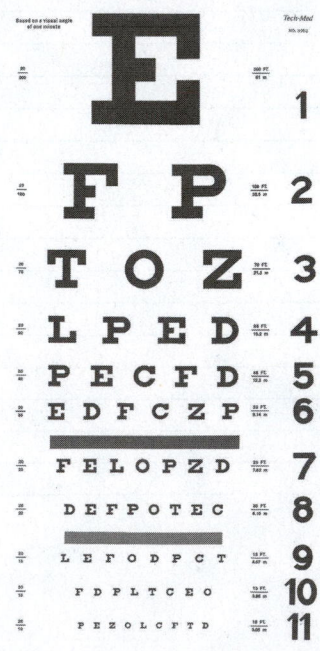

1. How should Shawn record Rajan's vision in his left eye? Explain your answer.

_____

_____

_____

2. How should Shawn record Rajan's vision in his right eye? Explain your answer.

_____

_____

_____

Activity 2

1. A 2-year-old child must have a myringotomy performed because the child has had reoccurring ear infections. Explain to the parents what this procedure entails.

_____

_____

_____

LEARNING ACTIVITY: MULTIPLE CHOICE

Circle the correct answer to each of the following questions.

1. Which of the following specialists is not a medical doctor?

    A. Ophthalmologist
    B. Otorhinolaryngologist
    C. Optometrist
    D. None of the above

2. Which instrument measures intraocular pressure?

    A. Ophthalmoscope
    B. Tonometer
    C. Slit lamp
    D. Otoscope

3. The ability to distinguish colors depends on the cones of the _____, which react to light and permit us to see shades of red, green, and blue.

    A. choroid
    B. cornea
    C. retina
    D. iris

4. Which of the following surgical procedures may be performed to correct myopia?

    A. Keratoplasty
    B. Radial keratotomy
    C. Phacoemulsification
    D. None of the above

5. To be declared legally blind, a person must only be able to see at _____ feet what a normal person would see at 200 feet.

    A. 20
    B. 40
    C. 50
    D. 100

6. The most common type of color vision defect, which is inherited, is the inability to distinguish

    A. blue and yellow.
    B. blue and black.
    C. red and green.
    D. All of the above

7. The abbreviation AD (aurus dextra) is for

    A. both ears.
    B. the left ear.
    C. the right ear.
    D. None of the above

8. Which of the following instrument(s) is used in the office for ear examinations?

    A. Otoscope
    B. Tuning fork
    C. Audiometer
    D. All of the above

9. Sensorineural hearing loss is due to

    A. nerve damage.
    B. obstruction of sound waves.
    C. old age.
    D. None of the above

10. When instilling ear medication into a child's ear, the ear should be pulled

    A. up and back.
    B. down and back.
    C. up.
    D. Any of the above

CRITICAL THINKING

Answer the following questions to the best of your ability. Use the textbook as a reference.

1. You need to perform a Snellen visual acuity test and an Ishihara color vision test per the physician's orders. You do not have an occluder or the Ishihara plates. Which of the tests, if any, could you still perform using a different item and what replacement item(s) can you use?

   _____

   _____

   _____

C. Sensation of pain _____

D. _____ sleep is shortened; there is more awakening during the night.

E. Brain cells are lost, but intelligence is intact unless a(n) _____ condition is present.

F. Decreased sensitivity of _____ for heat, cold, pain, and pressure

8. Physical Changes That Accompany Aging: The Sensory System

   A. It is more difficult to see _____ objects.

   B. Night vision may _____.

   C. _____ (clouding of the lens) are more common.

   D. Peripheral vision and depth perception _____.

   E. Smell and taste receptors are less _____.

9. Physical Changes That Accompany Aging: The Musculoskeletal System

   A. There is less muscle _____ and _____.

   B. Arthritis and _____ are more common.

   C. The body is more _____.

10. Physical Changes That Accompany Aging: The Urinary System

    A. The kidneys _____ in size.

    B. Urine production is less _____.

    C. _____ incontinence may develop.

11. Physical Changes That Accompany Aging: The Digestive System

    A. The primary _____ sensations of salty, sweet, and sour decrease.

    B. _____ increases; flatulence increases.

    C. Movement of food through the digestive tract _____.

12. Physical Changes That Accompany Aging: The Cardiovascular System

    A. Blood vessels are less _____ and more _____.

    B. The heart may not pump as _____.

    C. Decreased _____ output and circulation

13. Physical Changes That Accompany Aging: The Endocrine System

    A. Decrease in _____ and progesterone

    B. Hot _____, _____ feelings

    C. Higher levels of _____ and thyroid-stimulating hormone

    D. _____ gain

    E. _____ production is less efficient.

    F. Diabetes _____ is more likely.

14. Physical Changes That Accompany Aging: The Reproductive System

    A. Females: Ovulation and menstruation cease; the vaginal walls are _____ and _____.

    B. Males: The scrotum is less _____; the prostate gland may _____.

15. Diseases and Conditions That Affect the Elderly (briefly explain each disease and condition)

    A. Alzheimer's disease and other dementias: _____

    B. Aortic aneurysm: _____

    C. Atrophic urethritis and vaginitis: _____

    D. Decubitus ulcers (bedsores): _____

    E. Benign prostatic hyperplasia: _____

    F. Cataracts: _____

    G. Chronic lymphocytic leukemia: _____

    H. Diabetes mellitus type 2: _____

    I. Glaucoma: _____

    J. Hypothyroidism: _____

K. Osteoarthritis: _____

L. Osteoporosis: _____

M. Parkinson's disease: _____

N. Pneumonia: _____

O. Shingles (herpes zoster): _____

P. Stroke: _____

Q. Urinary incontinence: _____

16. Considerations When Treating Elderly Patients

A. Allow extra time for older patients to _____ and _____ to questions.

B. Do not _____ sentences for older patients or _____ a patient while talking about the patient to his or her family members or caregivers.

C. Offer your _____ to patients when walking, and _____ them on and off the examination table as needed.

D. Make sure that the _____ is secure as patients get on and off the examination table.

E. If you use a(n) _____ scale in your office, assist patients onto and off of the platform and provide wall-mounted _____ for additional support.

17. Sensory Changes in the Elderly (provide the word for each given definition)

A. _____ is an impairment of hearing that is associated with aging.

B. _____ is the inability to focus on objects at close range, which reduces the ability of the elderly to interact with the environment around them.

18. Inquiring About Sensory Abilities

i. _____

ii. _____

iii. _____

iv. _____

19. Addressing Issues Associated with Aging

A. Provide information on exercises that the elderly can perform at home while seated to increase _____ strength.

B. Encourage eating proper amounts of _____ products to supply needed _____.

C. Discuss _____ issues at home that can put the elderly patient at risk.

20. Mental Health is the capacity to:

i. _____

ii. _____

iii. _____

21. Mental Deterioration

A. Mental deterioration is not a(n) _____ part of aging.

B. As people age, the risk of mental _____ increases.

C. Mental health is the capacity to cope _____ with life changes, manage life's _____, and achieve a state of _____ balance.

D. Brain _____ slows with aging.

E. For optimal mental health, the elderly should have a sense of _____ and feel that they are of _____ to society.

22. Cognitive Ability

A. Cognitive ability is the ability to think _____.

B. The _____ status of the mind is altered by health status, genetics, social factors, educational accomplishments, and physical activity.

C. Normally, an individual's personality does not change with age unless there is a(n) _____ problem.

23. Three Types of Memory (briefly describe each type of memory)
    A. Short-term memory:_____
    B. Long-term memory:_____
    C. Sensory memory:_____

24. Memory
    A. Aging does not necessarily mean a loss of _____ or _____ ability in the elderly.
    B. With age, the ability to retrieve information from _____-_____ memory may be slower.
    C. Physical exercise increases _____ flow and helps maintain blood supply to the brain, improving memory _____.

25. Learning
    A. The ability to learn is not _____ by aging.
    B. _____ memory (the ability to retain information while using other information) slows with age.
    C. Keeping the brain active with games, puzzles, and other types of stimulation helps maintain _____.

26. Sleep
    A. Studies have shown that memories and information are _____ during sleep.
    B. _____ physical rest delays the brain's response time.

27. The Four Areas of Memory Loss
    i. _____
    ii. _____
    iii. _____
    iv. _____

28. Suggestions for Dealing with Memory Loss
    A. Encourage recalling distant memories.
        i. Caregivers can review with patients _____, _____, and _____.
    B. Retaining New Information
        i. Keep new information _____ and _____ it frequently.
        ii. If the information has more than _____ steps, break these steps down into smaller _____ so that they can be learned individually.
    C. Remembering Names
        i. Consistently _____-_____ yourself and what your intentions are.
    D. Separating Fact from Fiction
        i. It is important to correct the patient in a(n) _____ manner.

29. Addressing the Effects of Medications on Mental Abilities
    A. Provide the patient or caregiver with a(n) _____ organizer and a printed list of the _____ that he or she is taking and why he or she is taking them.
    B. Warn the patient about possible food or drug _____ with written and _____ information.

30. Confusion in the Elderly
    A. "Confusion" is the term used by physicians and health care providers to indicate that the person cannot:
        i. _____
        ii. _____

iii. _____

iv. _____

B. Acute confusion is characterized by symptoms that last for less than _____ months.

C. Chronic confusion is characterized by symptoms that persist for longer than _____ months.

31. The Three Categories of Confusion (briefly explain each category)

A. Systemic confusion: _____

B. Mechanical confusion: _____

C. Psychosocial/environmental confusion: _____

32. Common Causes of Confusion

A. The most common cause of acute confusion is a(n) _____ (UTI).

B. The confusion will be resolved with no _____ damage as soon as the infection has cleared.

33. Sundowners Syndrome

A. This is a type of confusion that occurs after sundown or at night in patients with _____ or other forms of _____.

B. It tends to be more common in persons with _____ impairments.

C. Factors that may increase the incidence of Sundowners syndrome include:

i. _____

ii. _____

iii. _____

iv. _____

v. _____

34. Characteristics of Depression

i. _____

ii. _____

iii. _____

iv. _____

35. Facts About Depression

A. Depression in the elderly may be caused by _____ that seem overwhelming.

B. Depression can be worsened by some _____ interactions.

36. Dementia

A. Dementia is marked by a(n) _____ loss of memory and other _____ functions.

B. It can occur at any _____, but is more frequently found in the elderly.

C. Currently, there are more than _____ different types of dementia.

D. Dementia affects about _____ of people who are over age 65.

E. Onset is usually _____.

F. It is not a normal _____ of aging.

G. It is irreversible unless caused by a treatable condition such as a(n) _____ or a thyroid dysfunction.

H. Half of all persons over _____ years of age have no signs of dementia.

I. Approximately half of all dementia patients suffer from _____.

37. Causes of Dementia

i. _____

ii. _____

iii. _____

iv. _____

38. Symptoms of Dementia
    A. Dementia gradually worsens at different rates over _____ to _____ years.
    B. The first sign is usually _____.
    C. The person has difficulty learning new _____.
    D. The person may forget what he or she is _____.
    E. He or she may forget the correct _____ for _____ objects, have difficulty with time _____, and misplace items or put them in an inappropriate place.
    F. The person may show a lack of _____, have mood swings, and demonstrate lack of initiative or disinterest in something that he or she previously _____ to do.

39. Alzheimer's Disease
    A. Alzheimer's disease is a progressive disorder of the _____ system that eventually destroys mental capacities.
    B. It occurs more frequently in the _____.
    C. Scientists have pinpointed several _____ abnormalities that are linked to the type of Alzheimer's disease that tends to run in families.
    D. Although there is a normal loss of some memory as people age, the memory loss associated with Alzheimer's disease is _____.

40. Diagnosing Alzheimer's Disease
    A. Diagnoses of dementia and Alzheimer's disease are obtained by _____ other possibilities.
    B. After ruling out possible causes, the patient should be given the _____ _____ to evaluate recall, writing, and math skills.
    C. A significant portion of the Alzheimer's disease/dementia diagnosis depends on _____ revealed by the patient and family members or caregivers.

41. Symptoms of Alzheimer's Disease
       i. _____
      ii. _____
     iii. _____
      iv. _____
       v. _____
      vi. _____

42. Treatment of Alzheimer's Disease
    A. During the early stages, medications, such as _____, are purported to slow the progression of the disease.
    B. Patients should not drink _____, which can worsen the symptoms of Alzheimer's disease.
    C. Some depressed Alzheimer's patients may benefit from taking _____ in the early stages.
    D. Creating a soothing home environment, avoiding _____, and avoiding constantly correcting _____ all help to reduce the stress on Alzheimer's patients.

43. Caring for the Dementia Patient in the Medical Office
    A. Always tell the patient what you are going to _____ and what to _____ next.
    B. Follow a simple _____.
    C. The patient may not _____ your information.
    D. The dementia patient cannot control his or her _____.
    E. Use the tactics of _____ and _____ when necessary.
    F. Allow the patient to maintain _____.
    G. Take a(n) _____ stand with the patient when necessary.

44. Advanced Medical Directives
   A. Advance medical directives provide _____ or _____ formulated by the patient that express his or her desires with regard to terminal care.
   B. They may state whether or not _____ is desired.
   C. Other directives should spell out the wishes of the patient if he or she degrades into a persistent _____ state.
   D. These directives may indicate whether he or she wants medicine to be _____, except for pain relief, and whether he or she wants nutrition and _____ withheld.
   E. In most states, unless the physician writes a specific order restating what the patient has expressed, a directive is not _____ on the staff and facility.

45. Forms of Elder Abuse
   i. _____
   ii. _____
   iii. _____
   iv. _____
   v. _____
   vi. _____

KEY TERMINOLOGY REVIEW

Match each of the following vocabulary terms to the correct definition.

a. ageism
b. assisted-living facilities
c. cognitive ability
d. extended-care facilities
e. respite care

1. _____ Prejudice against and incorrect assumptions about an individual or individuals because of their age.

2. _____ The ability to think clearly, reason, and perceive is affected by many factors.

3. _____ Short-term care for the chronically ill.

4. _____ Facilities designed for residents who cannot live independently but do not require 24-hour care.

5. _____ Facilities that provide specialized care for the elderly.

APPLIED PRACTICE

Follow the directions as instructed for each question.

1. Read the scenario and answer the questions that follow.

Scenario

Fredrick Alamar, age 73, presents to your office today for a physical and a flu vaccination. Upon obtaining his weight, it is apparent that Mr. Alamar has lost 18 pounds since his last visit 2 months ago, which was shortly after his wife died. You make a note of this in his chart. Prior visits to the office have shown Mr. Alamar to be in fairly good health for his age. He only takes metoprolol succinate for hypertension. As you obtain his blood pressure, Mr. Alamar removes his sweater. You notice scratches and bruising on his lower back. He states, "I fell after stepping out of the bathtub. I have been falling down a lot more lately and I don't seem to have any strength." After noting this in his chart, you excuse yourself from the examination room and inform the doctor of Mr. Alamar's changes since his last visit.

---

a. What are the likely causes of Mr. Alamar's significant weight loss?

_____

_____

b. What could be the cause of his recent lack of strength?

_____

_____

c. What things could be done to help Mr. Alamar at home?

_____

_____

d. The doctor may recommend a form of permanent care for Mr. Alamar. What options may be available for Mr. Alamar?

_____

_____

LEARNING ACTIVITY: MULTIPLE CHOICE

Circle the correct answers to each of the following questions.

1. Which of the following characteristics do baby boomers have that will affect health care and your role as a provider of health care?
   a. They are considered to be the best-educated generational group.
   b. They will be receiving less family assistance as they age because of fewer children.
   c. They may be caring for an ailing parent and a young child at the same time.
   d. All of the above

2. Which of the following is *not* an assistive device to aid older individuals?
   a. Handrails and grab bars
   b. Throw rugs
   c. Cane
   d. Bedside commode

3. Life expectancy is increasing due to
   a. better living conditions.
   b. new medications.
   c. better nutrition.
   d. All of the above

4. Factors that affect how we age include
   a. genetics.
   b. sports cars.
   c. occupational hazards.
   d. All of the above

5. Musculoskeletal system aging is characterized by
   a. decrease in muscle strength.
   b. inability to see far distances.
   c. increased risk of falling.
   d. All of the above

6. Which of the following are true statements concerning aging?
   a. Changes in sensorimotor abilities improve how the elderly interact with their environment.
   b. The loss of hearing, taste, smell, and mobility can lead to depression.
   c. The nervous system begins to speed up.
   d. All of the above

7. Urinary system changes that can occur with aging include
   a. thyroid hypofunction.
   b. reduced ability to concentrate urine.
   c. faster waste removal by the kidneys.
   d. orthostatic hypotension.

8. According to your textbook, which of the following does *not* accelerate the aging process?
   a. Disease
   b. Stress
   c. Depression
   d. Lack of social interaction

9. What factors are related to the mental health of aging populations?
   a. Capacity to cope effectively with life changes
   b. Sleep 8–10 hours per night
   c. Achieve a state of emotional balance
   d. All of the above

10. What might you do to find out if elderly patients are receiving proper nutrition?
    a. Engage elderly patients in a discussion of favorite foods.
    b. Ask which restaurants are their favorites.
    c. Observe their teeth and oral hygiene.
    d. Ask when their last meal was.

CHAPTER 43
Assisting with Medical Emergencies and Emergency Preparedness

STUDENT STUDY GUIDE

Use the following guide to assist in your learning of the concepts from the chapter.

I. Responding to a Medical Office Emergency

    1. The Emergency Medical Services (EMS) System

        A. EMS was established to provide _____ care.
        B. EMS provides safe and prompt _____ to an emergency facility.

    2. Good Samaritan Laws

        A. These state laws protect a health care professional from _____ while giving emergency care to an accident victim.
        B. Once a healthcare professional has begun to provide care to the patient, she must remain with the patient as long as the scene i _____,

    3. The Chain of Survival

        i. _____
        ii. _____
        iii. _____
        iv. _____
        v. _____

    4. The Medical Assistant's Emergency Response Primary Assessment

        A. Determine the patient's name, _____, and gender.
        B. Determine the patient's need for _____.
        C. Obtain a history of the _____.
        D. Gather the patient's _____ information.
        E. Determine the patient's _____.
        F. Take the patient's _____.

    5. Items in an Emergency Crash Kit

        i. _____
        ii. _____
        iii. _____
        iv. _____
        v. _____
        vi. _____
        vii. _____
        viii. _____
        ix. _____

6. The Medical Assistant and the Crash Kit
   A. The medical assistant (MA) should do _____ checks of emergency supplies in the crash kit.
   B. Tasks involved in checking the crash kit include the following:
      i. _____
      ii. _____
      iii. _____
      iv. _____

II. Medical Emergencies
   1. Respond to an Adult with an Obstructed Airway
      A. Stand _____ the patient with your feet slightly apart, placing _____ _____ between the patient's feet and _____ to the outside.
      B. Place the _____ finger of one hand at the person's _____ or belt buckle.
      C. Make a(n) _____ with your other hand and place it, _____ side to the patient, above your other hand.
      D. Place your marking hand over your _____ fist and begin to give quick _____ and _____ thrusts.
      E. Continue to give thrusts until the object has been expelled or the patient becomes _____.
      F. Before administering the _____ breaths, open the airway with the _____- _____ chin lift and look for a foreign body in the patient's mouth and remove it if one is visible.
      G. _____ finger sweeps are no longer recommended and should not be performed.
      H. Continue with cycles of _____ compressions and _____ breaths until the foreign body is expelled or advanced medical personnel arrive to relieve you.

   2. Steps for Adult Rescue Breathing and One-Rescuer CPR
      A. _____ the patient and determine whether help is needed.
      B. Shout, "_____?" while gently shaking the patient's shoulders.
      C. If the adult patient is determined to be _____, activate EMS immediately by calling 911 and get a(n) _____ if one is available.

   3. Assessing CAB
      A. Airway: Perform a head-_____ chin _____, or, if a neck injury is suspected, a jaw _____.
      B. If you are alone, activate _____ immediately by calling _____.

   4. Performing Breaths
      A. If breathing is absent, put on a(n) _____ and administer _____ breaths.
      B. If your breaths do not cause the chest to _____, look in the patient's mouth and remove the object if one is seen.
      C. If no object is seen, make a second attempt to administer a(n) _____ breath.

   5. Performing Chest Compressions
      A. If you do not feel a pulse, begin _____.
      B. Kneel at the patient's side and place your hand in the center of the _____ on the lower half of the _____.
      C. Place your other hand on _____ of the first hand, using only the heels of your hands to administer compressions.
      D. Keep your shoulders directly over your _____.
      E. Compress the chest _____ to _____ inches; then allow the sternum to relax.
      F. Do not lift your hands off the _____.

G. Continue to compress the chest a total of _____ times; then administer _____ breaths.

H. Repeat this sequence for _____. Reassess the patient and continue CPR if necessary.

6. Steps for Infant or Young Child Rescue Breathing and One-Rescuer CPR

A. If the infant is determined to be _____, activate _____ by calling 911; get a(n) _____ if one is available.

B. Gently, with _____ or _____ fingers, tilt the patient's _____ and open the _____.

C. If breathing is absent, secure a(n) _____ over the patient's mouth and nose.

7. Administering Chest Compressions on a Child

A. Place _____ in the center of the chest just below the nipple line.

B. Compressions should be made _____ to _____ the depth of the chest. Perform 30 quick compressions.

C. Give two more rescue breaths followed by _____ more compressions. Continue the _____ compressions and breaths.

8. Automated External Defibrillation (AED)

A. AEDs are highly effective when used immediately after or within minutes of an adult _____.

B. An AED is not used on _____.

9. Symptoms of Respiratory Distress

    i. _____

    ii. _____

    iii. _____

    iv. _____

    v. _____

    vi. _____

    vii. _____

    viii. _____

10. Steps for Administering Oxygen

A. Check the _____ on the oxygen tank to make sure that it has enough oxygen in it.

B. Start the flow of oxygen by opening the _____.

C. Attach the _____ tubing to the flow meter.

D. Adjust the oxygen _____ according to the physician's order.

E. Hold the cannula tips over the _____ of your _____, without touching the skin, to determine whether oxygen is flowing.

F. Place the tips of the _____ into the patient's nostrils.

G. Wrap the tubing behind the patient's _____.

H. Instruct the patient to breathe normally through the _____ and _____.

I. Check the patient's oxygen level with a(n) _____.

J. Place the probe over the _____ finger and record the reading.

K. If necessary, have the patient take a short _____ to verify that the oxygen flow rate is sufficient for activity.

11. Symptoms of Hyperventilation

    i. _____

    ii. _____

    iii. _____

    iv. _____

    v. _____

    vi. _____

12. Treatment for Hyperventilation

   A. Inform the physician and encourage the patient to _____.

13. Chest Pain

   A. The primary complaint will be pain in the _____ or _____ side of the chest, described as _____, _____, _____, _____, or aching.
   B. The pain may radiate to the _____ arm, to the _____, or up the neck.
   C. Sometimes the pain is brought on by _____.

14. Care of Chest Pain

   A. Have the individual stop what he or she is doing and _____, feet _____ if possible.
   B. Ask a coworker to stay with the patient while you inform the _____ of the situation.
   C. If oxygen is available, administer it according to office protocol by _____ cannula at _____ to _____ liters per minute until the physician or emergency personnel arrive.
   D. If the patient has previously been diagnosed with angia and has nitroglycerin tablets, insert _____ tablet under the _____.
   E. If the _____ is not relieved, inform the _____ or EMS on the scene.

15. Shock

   A. Shock is the collapse of the _____ system caused by insufficient cardiac output.
   B. _____, shock can progress very rapidly to death.

16. Causes of Shock

   i. _____
   ii. _____
   iii. _____
   iv. _____
   v. _____
   vi. _____
   vii. _____
   viii. _____

17. General Signs of Shock

   i. _____
   ii. _____
   iii. _____
   iv. _____
   v. _____
   vi. _____
   vii. _____
   viii. _____
   ix. _____
   x. _____
   xi. _____
   xii. _____
   xiii. _____
   xiv. _____

18. Anaphylactic Shock

   A. Anaphylactic shock is a severe _____ to a foreign substance, such as medications, bug bites, and latex gloves.
   B. Inform the physician immediately and call _____.

C. The physician may order _____ and/or a(n) _____.

D. _____ is the most important factor in anaphylactic shock.

19. Signs of Diabetic Emergencies

    i. _____

    ii. _____

    iii. _____

    iv. _____

    v. _____

    vi. _____

    vii. _____

    viii. _____

20. Arterial Bleeding

A. Arterial bleeding is usually copious, rapid, and _____.

B. Blood often spurts, echoing the _____.

C. It must be brought _____ as soon as possible.

D. Apply pressure directly over the _____ and _____ of the injured part to help slow blood flow.

21. Bleeding from Veins and Capillaries

A. Venous blood can usually be controlled with _____.

B. Blood from the capillaries _____ rather than flows and can be halted with direct pressure.

22. Abrasions

A. An abrasion occurs when the _____ of skin is scraped away, leaving the underlying tissue exposed.

B. Common Terms for Abrasions

    i. _____

    ii. _____

    iii. _____

    iv. _____

23. Avulsions

A. An avulsion is a(n) _____ of skin or tissue.

B. It usually occurs on _____ and _____.

C. Cleanse minor avulsion wounds with _____ and _____ and return any skin flap to its normal position.

D. Apply direct pressure, and then apply a dressing after _____ is controlled.

24. Amputation

A. If body part has been _____, cleanse the _____ with sterile saline.

B. Wrap it with moist, sterile gauze. Seal it in a(n) _____; place the _____ in a container on ice.

C. Prompt medical attention and preservation of the _____ enhance the chances for successful reattachment.

25. Lacerations

A. A laceration is a(n) _____ in which the skin and underlying tissue are torn.

B. It usually has _____ edges that may interfere with the healing process.

C. If bleeding is _____, a physician should direct the cleansing process.

D. Lacerations over a joint may require joint _____ for a few days while healing progresses.

26. Incisions

A. An incision is a cut with smooth edges that is made with a knife or other _____ object.

B. It is treated in the same manner as any _____.

C. If there is damage to underlying _____, such as a tendon or ligament, surgical intervention is required.

27. Puncture Wounds

    A. A puncture wound is the result of a pointed _____ penetrating the skin and tissue.
    B. Often the wound edges close, trapping _____ and _____ in the tissue.
    C. Depending on the nature of the pointed object, cleansing may consist of simply soaking the area, or may require invasive _____.
    D. After cleansing, a(n) _____ is applied.

28. Impaled Objects

    A. The general rule is to leave the _____ in place until it can be safely removed by trained personnel.
    B. Control _____ and _____ the impaled object with a bulky dressing held in place with tape or bandages.
    C. _____ the area to prevent movement.

29. Soft Tissue Injuries

    A. Soft tissue injuries involve both the skin and _____ tissue.
    B. Avulsions, amputations, puncture wounds and _____ are considered soft tissue injuries because tissue, as well as skin, is involved.
    C. Damage to the underlying tissue may involve _____, _____, muscles, and _____ tissue.

30. Crush Injuries

    A. Crush injuries result when force is applied to the _____.
    B. Depending on the area involved, the crush may be similar to the _____ of tissue or it may be so severe as to involve _____ and _____.
    C. Elevating the body part above the _____ and applying _____ are often the only intervention needed.
    D. With a more severe injury, the body part should be _____.
    E. Monitoring vital signs and observing _____, _____, and _____ are essential to deciding whether more extensive intervention is needed.

31. Open Wounds (define each type)

    A. Superficial: _____
    B. Deep: _____

32. Open Wound Care

    A. Apply _____ to the wound.
    B. If necessary, use a(n) _____ dressing.
    C. Cleanse the wound from the _____, beginning with vigorous irrigation using a disinfecting solution prescribed by the physician.
    D. Wipe the edges of the wound with sterile gauze in all directions, _____ from the wound.
    E. Cover with a(n) _____ dressing and fasten the dressing in place.

33. Applying a Triangular Bandage

    A. Keep the injured arm as _____ as possible.
    B. Carefully slide the triangular bandage under the _____ to be held.
    C. The two shorter sides should be pointing toward the _____, and the remaining longer edge should be parallel to the _____.
    D. Bring the _____ side up and over the arm.
    E. Tie the ends of the bandage behind and slightly to the _____ of the neck.
    F. Tuck the peak of the bandage in toward the _____ of the bandage.

34. Applying a Figure 8 Bandage

    A. Place the _____ of one hand on one end of the bandage.

    B. Anchor the bandage with your _____, and then complete one _____ around the extremity or body part.

    C. Continue to alternate wrapping above and below the _____ or dressing, circling behind the _____ or dressing area until the injured area is covered adequately.

    D. If applying a bandage to a(n) _____, ensure that the _____ are exposed to evaluate circulation.

35. Applying a Tubular Bandage (list the steps for applying this type of bandage)

    i. _____

    ii. _____

    iii. _____

    iv. _____

    v. _____

    vi. _____

    vii. _____

    viii. _____

    ix. _____

    x. _____

36. Epistaxis (Nosebleeds)

    A. Epistaxis is usually _____-_____ threatening.

    B. It tends to occur more commonly in _____ weather or under dusty conditions.

37. Caring for a Patient with a Nosebleed

    A. The physician will twist a(n) _____ and pack the patient's nose.

    B. A(n) _____ pack should be held against the bridge of the patient's nose.

    C. A patient may need a(n) _____ procedure if the bleeding does not stop.

38. Classification of Burns (briefly explain each type)

    A. Superficial burns: _____

    B. Partial thickness burns: _____

    C. Full thickness burns: _____

39. Caring for a Patient with Superficial Burns

    A. _____ water.

    B. Use _____ and _____, if ordered by the physician.

40. Caring for a Patient with Partial Thickness Burns

    A. Cool the burn with water as long as there are no _____.

    B. _____ use analgesic creams and ointments.

    C. Cover with a(n) _____.

    D. Treat for _____, if necessary.

41. Caring for a Patient with Full Thickness Burns

    A. Transport the patient to a(n) _____.

    B. Cover burns with _____, _____.

    C. _____ the dead skin or damaged tissue (should be done only by a physician).

    D. Manage the pain with _____ as ordered by a physician.

42. Caring for a Patient with Upper Airway Burns

    A. Prompt _____ by the physician or EMS

    B. Transport to a(n) _____ center

    C. Listen for _____ (noisy breathing).

    D. Administer _____ as ordered by the physician.

43. Caring for a Patient with Large Surface Area Burns

    i. _____

    ii. _____

    iii. _____

44. Hyperthermia: Heat Exhaustion

    A. Heat exhaustion is extreme _____ due to heat.

    B. It occurs as the result of _____ and _____ depletion from the body.

    C. Strenuous _____ often preceded heat exhaustion.

45. Hyperthermia: Heat Stroke

    A. Heat stroke is advanced heat exhaustion; body temperature is _____.

    B. Many patients will not _____.

    C. No _____ takes place, so the body stores heat in increasing amounts.

    D. Eventually, the _____ cells begin to die and permanent damage or death may result.

46. Signs and Symptoms of Heat Exhaustion

    i. _____

    ii. _____

    iii. _____

    iv. _____

    v. _____

    vi. _____

    vii. _____

    viii. _____

47. Treating Heat Exhaustion

    A. Move to a(n) _____ environment.

    B. Encourage the patient to _____.

    C. Apply _____, _____ compresses and give sips of water.

48. Signs and Symptoms of Heat Stroke

    i. _____

    ii. _____

    iii. _____

    iv. _____

    v. _____

    vi. _____

    vii. _____

    viii. _____

    ix. _____

    x. _____

    xi. _____

    xii. _____

    xiii. _____

49. Treating Heat Stroke

    A. Remove the patient from _____ of heat.

    B. _____ the victim's clothing.

    C. _____ the body as quickly as possible by pouring _____ water over the patient.

    D. Contact _____ if physician is not available.

50. Hypothermia

    A. Hypothermia means the core body temperature is below _____ degrees.

    B. It results from prolonged exposure to _____ or _____ water.

51. Signs and Symptoms of Hypothermia

    i. _____

    ii. _____

    iii. _____

    iv. _____

    v. _____

52. Treating Hypothermia

    A. Remove _____ and _____ clothes.

    B. Wrap the patient in _____ blankets.

    C. _____ packs may be used, but not directly on the _____.

    D. Provide sips of _____ liquid.

    E. Arrange for _____ to treatment facility for assessment by a physician.

53. Convulsions (Seizures)

    A. Seizures are produced by _____ activity in the brain.

    B. They are characterized by _____ that alternate between the contraction and relaxation of muscles.

54. Caring for a Patient with Convulsions (Seizures)

    A. _____ spasms of the full body can restrict breathing.

    B. The patient may bite his or her _____, causing bleeding and swelling, which may obstruct the airway.

    C. Prevent _____.

    D. Pay close attention to what the patient is _____ so that you can _____ it later.

55. Fainting

    A. Fainting is a(n) _____ loss of consciousness.

    B. The patient usually _____ and becomes _____, but should awaken and return to normal functioning within a minute.

    C. Patients seldom become _____ or have _____ as a result of simple fainting, but may be injured in the course of a fall.

56. Caring for a Patient Who Has Fainted

    A. If the patient fainted and there is no response, provide _____ if the physician orders this.

    B. Check the _____ and call for help.

    C. If the patient is breathing well but will not wake up, place him or her on the _____ side and notify the physician.

    D. If the physician is unavailable, contact _____.

    E. Obtain a full set of _____ and obtain a _____ reading if possible.

57. Fractures (briefly explain both types)

    A. Closed (simple): _____

    B. Open (compound): _____

58. Splinting Injuries

    A. Fractures of long bones require _____ by splinting to prevent joint movement _____ and _____ the fracture.

59. Sprains

    A. Sprains occur when _____, _____, or ligaments are torn.

    B. They may be the result of trauma or cumulative _____ of the joint.

60. Strains

    A. A strain is often called a(n) _____.

    B. It occurs when a muscle or tendon is overextended by _____.

C. The patient may be unable to use the _____.

D. In the lower extremities, _____ is painful and sometimes impossible.

61. Dislocation

    A. In a dislocation, the bone is actually pulled away from the _____, stretching or tearing the _____ and tendons.

    B. A(n) _____ is generally noted.

    C. A dislocation must be reduced and the bone _____ into the joint.

    D. Injured body parts should be _____ to prevent additional damage and to reduce pain.

    E. The application of _____ also helps with the pain and slows edema.

III. Emergency Preparedness

  1. The Role of the Medical Assistant During an Emergency

    A. Be knowledgeable in the area of emergency _____.

    B. Know how to respond in the event of a(n) _____ disaster, such as a terrorist event, and to a(n) _____ disaster, such as a hurricane.

    C. Remaining _____ in the event of an emergency is paramount to the success of handling the emergency.

  2. Preparing for an Earthquake

    A. Check for _____ around the facility.

    B. Identify safe places both _____ and _____.

    C. Educate yourself and your _____.

    D. Have _____ supplies on hand.

    E. Develop an emergency _____ plan.

  3. Checking for Facility Hazards

    A. Make sure that _____ are fastened securely to walls.

    B. Do not place large or heavy objects on the _____.

    C. Store any breakable items in low, closed _____ equipped with locks.

    D. Avoid hanging _____ on walls above where patients will sit or lie.

    E. Secure overhead _____.

    F. Repair any defective _____ or leaky gas connections.

    G. _____ water heaters to wall studs bolted to the floor.

    H. Repair _____ in the ceilings or foundations.

    I. All _____ products should be stored in closed cabinets with locks, on the bottom shelf.

  4. Safe Places to Go During an Earthquake

    A. Under sturdy _____

    B. Against a(n) _____ wall

    C. Away from _____ that could shatter

    D. Away from _____ or furniture that could fall over

    E. If outside, stay away from _____, trees, telephone or _____ lines, overpasses, or elevated expressways.

  5. Disaster Supplies

    i. _____

    ii. _____

    iii. _____

    iv. _____

    v. _____

  6. Warning Signs of a Tornado

    i. _____

    ii. _____

    iii. _____

7. Safety During a Tornado

   A. Move to the basement of a building or the _____ of a structure.

   B. If a basement is not available, it is advisable to seek shelter in a(n) _____ or _____ hallway.

   C. Above all else, stay away from _____, _____, and outside walls.

   D. Avoid _____ and use the stairs to reach the lowest level of the facility.

8. Fire Preparedness

   A. Equip the office with properly working _____ placed on every level of the building on the ceiling or high on the walls.

   B. Equip every room with a(n) _____ detector and test and clean once per month.

   C. Know the _____ routes to use in the event of a fire.

   D. Ensure that _____ are available if the office is located above the first level.

   E. Store _____ items in well-ventilated areas.

   F. Repair any _____ wiring to avoid a fire hazard.

   G. Locate _____ throughout the office and train staff on their use.

9. Escaping a Fire

   A. If a person's clothes are on fire, that person should _____, _____, and _____ until the fire is extinguished.

   B. Check closed doors for _____ before opening.

   C. If the door is hot, it should not be _____, and another route of escape should be sought. If the door is cool, it should be _____.

   D. When escaping a fire, _____ under any smoke on the way to the exit and close doors as they are passed through to delay the spread of fire.

   E. Once out of the building, do not attempt to _____ until or unless the fire department declares that it is safe to do so.

10. In the Event of a Flood

   A. Listen to the radio for _____.

   B. Move to _____ ground.

   C. If there is time before evacuating, disconnect any _____ and shut off utilities at their main valves.

   D. When evacuating, be careful not to walk through _____ water.

11. Preparing for a Hurricane

   A. Secure the windows using _____.

   B. Trees and shrubs around the office should be well _____.

   C. If the medical office is to be evacuated before a hurricane, listen to the radio or television for information provided by local _____.

   D. During the hurricane, listen to the _____ or _____ for information and prepare for high winds and possible flooding.

12. Types of Terrorist Attacks

    i. _____

    ii. _____

    iii. _____

13. Questions to Ask If a Bomb Threat Is Made

    i. _____

    ii. _____

    iii. _____

    iv. _____

    v. _____

14. Biological Threats (list and briefly explain each type)
    i. _____
    ii. _____
    iii. _____
    iv. _____
    v. _____
    vi. _____

15. In the Event of a Biological Attack
    A. Be prepared to evacuate the area _____.
    B. Wash with _____ and _____.
    C. Contact the _____.
    D. Listen to the radio for _____.
    E. Remove and bag clothing if _____.

16. In the Event of a Nuclear Blast
    A. Take cover as quickly as possible, _____ if the building has a basement.
    B. Remain in a safe location, listening to the radio for _____.
    C. Do not look at the _____ or _____.
    D. Lie flat on the ground with your head _____.
    E. Seek _____ as quickly as possible.

17. The Role of the Medical Assistant in a Mock Environmental Exposure Event
    A. Aid in _____ planning.
    B. _____ patients to determine which patients require immediate attention.
    C. Assist in _____-_____ response for wounded individuals.
    D. Administer _____ and other vaccines under the direction of a physician.
    E. Facilitate order and organization in the midst of _____.
    F. Implement and follow through on a(n) _____ safety plan.

KEY TERMINOLOGY REVIEW

Match each of the following key terms to the correct definition.

a. anaphylactic shock

b. first responders

c. heat exhaustion

d. hyperglycemia

e. hypothermia

1. _____ EMS providers trained to recognize medical conditions, initiate basic life support, and access other parts of the system.

2. _____ High blood sugar level.

3. _____ A severe allergic reaction that causes respiratory distress because of swelling of the upper airways.

4. _____ A core temperature of below 95°F.

5. _____ Extreme fatigue caused by heat, which occurs as the result of sodium and water depletion from the body.

APPLIED PRACTICE

Read the scenarios and then answer the questions that follow.

Scenario A

Tasha Lopez, RMA, has recently been hired as a clinical medical assistant for a brand new family practice. She has been asked to stock the emergency medical box with drugs and make sure that it is ready in case of an emergency.

This is what she found:

- Atropine
- Diphenhydramine
- Furosemide
- Instant glucose
- Lidocaine
- Local anesthetics

- Normal saline
- Phenobarbital and diazepam
- Solu-Cortef
- Syrup of ipecac
- Verapamil

---

1. Based on the inventory list, what are some items that Tasha should add?

   _____

   _____

   _____

Scenario B

Sasha Daniels, CMA (AAMA), is employed at Community Urgent Care. A 47-year-old male patient has been brought to the facility. His right index finger was partially torn from his hand while he was working on a piece of farming machinery. His coworker has driven him to the medical facility.

---

1. What type of injury has this man sustained?

   _____

2. How should he be treated?

   _____

   _____

   _____

LEARNING ACTIVITY: TRUE/FALSE

Indicate whether the following statements are true or false by placing a T or an F on the line that precedes each statement.

_____ 1. An AED can be used on children ages 1 to 8 years old.

_____ 2. Lock jaw is also known as an avulsion.

_____ 3. A nosebleed that occurs after a head injury and does not stop should be considered a serious emergency until proven otherwise.

_____ 4. In general, perform "CPR first" for unresponsive children and infants.

_____ 5. Shock, the collapse of the cardiovascular system, is caused by insufficient cardiac output.

_____ 6. Arterial bleeding is usually slow and pale red.

_____ 7. Simple direct pressure with a dressing will usually stop bleeding from a soft tissue injury.

_____ 8. Nosebleeds may be messy and embarrassing and are usually life-threatening occurrences.

_____ 9. The severity of a burn depends on the amount and depth of tissue injury.

_____ 10. Once a seizure stops, especially a full-body seizure, it is normal for a patient to remain unconscious for as long as 2 hours.

CRITICAL THINKING

Answer the following questions to the best of your ability. Use the textbook as a reference.

1. A patient has presented to the front desk without an appointment and is obviously short of breath (SOB), her lips and fingertips appear a bit cyanotic. How would you assess her treatment?

    _____

    _____

    _____

2. Your first job out of school is in an emergency care facility that has had an unfortunate number of lawsuits brought against it and its staff. What are your legal responsibilities as a medical assistant?

    _____

    _____

    _____

3. An 85-year-old man is choking on a hot dog. How will his advanced age affect your treatment of him?

    _____

    _____

    _____

RESEARCH ACTIVITY

Use Internet search engines to research the following topic and write a brief description of what you find. It is important to use reputable websites.

1. There is much to learn about how to face various types of emergencies. Select two emergencies that you believe you may face on the job as a medical assistant. Then conduct research on these emergencies using the Internet. Write an essay on what you learned through your research. Be sure to cite your sources.

    _____

    _____

    _____

    _____

    _____

CHAPTER 44
The Clinical Laboratory

STUDENT STUDY GUIDE

Use the following guide to assist in your learning of the concepts from the chapter.

I. The Clinical Laboratory

  1. The Role of the Clinical Laboratory in Patient Care

      i. _____

      ii. _____

      iii. _____

      iv. _____

      v. _____

  2. The Outside Laboratory

    A. The outside laboratory handles specimens collected from many types of _____.

    B. It performs tests ranging from the _____ to the very _____.

  3. The Reference Laboratory

    A. The reference laboratory handles more _____ tests than an outside laboratory and those tests that are _____ requested.

    B. Tests performed on a regular basis at a reference laboratory may provide more _____ results than tests performed a few times a year in a(n) _____ laboratory.

  4. The Physician's Office Laboratory

    A. In the office laboratory, the doctor has the advantage of receiving the results more _____ than if the tests were done outside of the office.

    B. Disadvantages

      i. _____

      ii. _____

  5. Record management

    A. A _____ is a form that provides essential information about a test that is ordered.

    B. With _____ (EHRs), many offices can communicate with outside labs through the computer.

  6. The Agencies and Committees That Set and Review Laboratory Safety Guidelines

      i. _____

      ii. _____

      iii. _____

      iv. _____

      v. _____

  7. The Occupational Safety and Health Administration (OSHA)

    A. OSHA creates safeguards covering nearly every _____ in the United States.

    B. If no specific guidelines exist, then the "_____" must be followed.

8. Standard Precautions

   A. Standard precautions were developed by the _____.
   B. They combine the major features of _____ precautions and _____
      isolation precautions into one set of recommendations.
   C. The CDC's precautions are enforced by _____.

9. The Clinical Laboratory Improvement Amendments (CLIA)

   A. The CLIA were enacted by Congress in _____.
   B. States may have their own _____, but they must be at
      least as stringent as the federal government's regulations.
   C. Information regarding state _____ may be obtained from state health departments.

10. The Clinical Laboratory Improvement Amendments' Classification of Tests

    i. _____
    ii. _____
    iii. _____

11. Common Examples of Waived Tests

    i. _____
    ii. _____
    iii. _____
    iv. _____
    v. _____
    vi. _____
    vii. _____
    viii. _____
    ix. _____

12. Laboratory Safety Regulations

    i. _____
    ii. _____
    iii. _____
    iv. _____

13. Contents of the Material Safety Data Sheet (MSDS)

    i. _____
    ii. _____
    iii. _____
    iv. _____
    v. _____

14. Biohazards

    A. Biohazards have the potential to _____ others.
    B. Since 1992, all laboratories must have OSHA's _____ __
       _____ in place.
    C. The CDC's _____ must be employed when dealing
       with any infectious materials.

15. The Bloodborne Standards Requirements for Health Care Employers

    A. Review all new safety devices that lessen the risk of _____ to employees.
    B. Ask for safety input from employees on a(n) _____ basis.
    C. Keep a detailed report of all _____ incidents.

16. Addressing Fire and Safety Hazards in the Medical Office

    A. Have an awareness of the _____ plan and _____.

B. Know the location of safety devices such as _____,
_____, and safety blankets.

C. Remove _____ properly.

17. Equipment Generally Found in a Physician's Office Laboratory

   A. A(n) _____ is used to sterilize equipment or instruments that are used on patients or in certain test procedures.

   B. A(n) _____ is used to separate urine so that sediment can be examined under the microscope.

   C. A(n) _____ is used to separate whole blood samples into layers to measure a patient's hematocrit.

   D. A(n) _____ is a type of handheld photometer that is used to test glucose levels in patients.

18. Microscope

   A. A microscope is frequently used in the medical office to examine _____ and various types of smears.

   B. It is an optical instrument that magnifies structures that are unseen by the _____ eye for the purpose of counting, naming, or _____.

   C. Better microscopes have better _____.

19. The Process of Using and Cleaning a Microscope

   A. Always carry the microscope with one hand on the _____ and one hand under the _____.

   B. Make sure that the stage is in the _____ position before starting.

   C. Clean objectives with _____ starting with 10X and ending with oil immersion.

   D. Turn on the light and rotate the nosepiece until the _____ is directly over the slide.

   E. Place the prepared slide on the _____.

   F. Use the _____ knob to raise the stage until the objective is close to the slide on the stage.

   G. Look through the _____ and adjust the _____ knob until the microscope field is seen (it is a round circle of bright light).

   H. Use the _____ knob to obtain a clearer image.

   I. Open the _____ and adjust the _____ to focus if necessary.

   J. Raise or lower the _____ to alter light refraction.

   K. Change the objective to _____ and readjust as needed.

   L. Move the objective and place a(n) _____ of _____ on the slide before completing the turn to the oil immersion lens.

   M. When focusing and examination is complete, lower the _____ before removing the slide.

   N. Turn off the _____.

   O. Clean the _____ and objectives with _____ paper.

   P. Clean the oil immersion lens with _____ cleaner.

   Q. Unplug the _____ and wrap it around the base.

   R. Cover the microscope with a(n) _____.

   S. Clean the _____ and store it.

   T. Document _____ and _____ in the logbook.

KEY TERMINOLOGY REVIEW

Match each of the following vocabulary terms to the correct definition.

a. Certificate of Waiver Tests (WTs)   d. photometer

b. compound microscope   e. physician's office laboratory

c. outside laboratory

1. _____ A microscope with two sets of lenses, oculars, and objectives.

2. _____ The least complex and present the least risk if performed incorrectly.

3. _____ A laboratory in which some of the tests that the physician orders are performed right in the office.

4. _____ It is either hospital-based or independent and handles specimens collected from many types of facilities.

5. _____ An instrument that measures light intensity.

APPLIED PRACTICE

Follow the directions as instructed for each question.

1. Label the parts of the compound microscope.

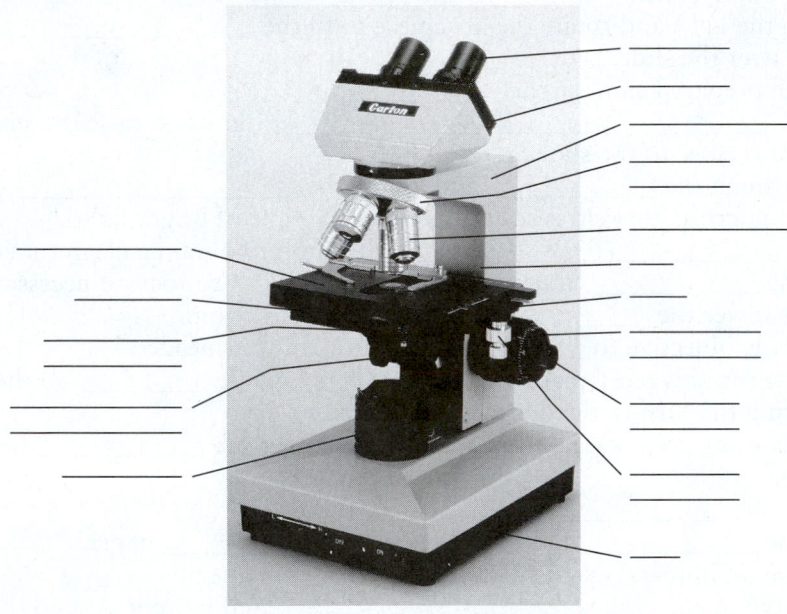

2. Read the scenario and then answer the following questions.

Scenario

On your first day of work at a clinical laboratory, you are ordered to clean up any hazardous waste after each procedure and at the end of each day. How does your training prepare you for this task? What is the definition of hazardous waste? Briefly explain what you would do.

_____

_____

_____

LEARNING ACTIVITY: TRUE/FALSE

Indicate whether the following statements are true or false by placing a T or an F on the line that precedes each statement.

_____ 1. A binocular microscope has one ocular lens.

_____ 2. The condenser is located on the substage of a microscope.

_____ 3. Oil immersion is used with the 10X lens to increase the power to 100X.

_____ 4. There are two focus knobs—one for low power and the other for high power.

_____ 5. When you are finished working with a microscope, you must clean the lenses with any soft cloth or paper.

CRITICAL THINKING

Answer the following questions to the best of your ability. Use the textbook as a reference.

1. The office is unusually busy, patients are crabby, and the doctor has repeatedly berated you for working too slowly. You have thought about cutting corners. Is this ever a good idea? Why or why not?

_____

_____

_____

2. Michelle Oswald's blood test has returned, and it is found to be abnormal. You were the medical assistant who took the test and felt especially close to Mrs. Oswald because she reminded you of your mother. Should you call the patient yourself? What is your responsibility in this case?

_____

_____

_____

RESEARCH ACTIVITY

Use Internet search engines to research the following topic and write a brief description of what you find. It is important to use reputable websites.

1. To learn more about the agencies and committees that set and review safety guidelines affecting clinical laboratories, go to the Internet to conduct further research. Write an essay on your findings and what more you learned beyond what is presented in the textbook about these agencies and committees and the guidelines established for laboratories. Be sure to cite your sources.

_____

_____

_____

_____

_____

CHAPTER 45

Microbiology

STUDENT STUDY GUIDE

Use the following guide to assist in your learning of the concepts from the chapter.

I. Introduction to Microbiology

1. Microorganisms: A Definition

    A. Microorganisms are also called _____.
    B. They are living organisms that can be seen only with a(n) _____.
    C. Normal flora on our bodies consists of _____ bacteria.
    D. Microorganisms include _____, viruses, _____, and bacteria.

2. Classification of Microorganisms

    A. Microorganisms are categorized by their ability to cause disease as either _____ or _____.

    B. bacteria are also characterized by their reactions to certain _____.

3. What Microorganisms Need in Order to Grow

    i. _____
    ii. _____
    iii. _____
    iv. _____

4. Microbiology and Microorganisms

    A. Microbiology is the study of _____ that cannot be seen with the naked eye.
    B. Microorganisms are the _____ that microbiology studies.

5. By correctly processing and testing of _____, early diagnosis and treatment of diseases can take place.

    i. _____
    ii. _____
    iii. _____
    iv. _____
    v. _____
    vi. _____

6. Classifications of Microorganisms (list the two classifications)

    i. _____
    ii. _____

7. Retention of Dyes

   A. Bacteria are _____ by how they react to stain or dye.
   B. _____ stain is used for most gram-positive and gram-negative bacteria.
   C. Others use _____-_____ stain.

8. Hemolytic Properties

   A. One way in which to classify bacteria is by the bacteria's ability to _____ red blood cells in blood _____.
   B. A microbiologist observes the characteristics of a(n) _____ of cells.
   C. The organism that causes _____ is beta hemolytic.

9. Diseases Caused by Pathogenic Microorganisms

   i. _____
   ii. _____
   iii. _____
   iv. _____
   v. _____
   vi. _____
   vii. _____
   viii. _____
   ix. _____
   x. _____

10. Bacterium/Bacteria

   A. Bacteria are small, _____ microorganisms that are capable of rapid _____.
   B. Their reproductive ability explains how some infections become _____ in a short time and can be dangerous.
   C. Bacteria may be named for their _____ (shape). Types of shapes are as follows:
      i. _____
      ii. _____
      iii. _____

11. Cocci

   A. Cocci are _____ bacteria that are arranged in various configurations.
   B. Staphylococci are _____-_____, grape-like clusters of _____, some of which are pathogenic.
   C. Nonpathogenic staphylococci are found on our _____ and in many of our body _____, or openings.

12. *Staphylococcus Aureus* (*S. Aureus*), or Staph

   A. *S. aureus* is the major pathogen of this genus and may be found as _____ in the nose and on the skin.
   B. Staph causes _____, especially when _____ is lowered by a break in the skin or in the mucous membranes.
   C. It is a common cause of _____ infections and may also cause _____, meningitis, and _____ in persons who have reduced resistance.

13. Methicillin-Resistant *Staphylococcus Aureus* (MRSA)

   A. MRSA is a form of _____.
   B. Tests are available to indicate the _____ or _____ of this enzyme and to help determine the most favorable treatment.

14. Streptococci

   A. Streptococci are round, _____-_____ bacteria that are arranged in chains.
   B. Some are _____ and others are dangerous to humans.
   C. They are part of the normal flora of the _____ tract and skin.

15. Group A Beta-hemolytic *Streptococcus Pyogenes*

    A. Group A beta-hemolytic *Streptococcus pyogenes* cause a variety of diseases, varying from
        _____ to _____.

    B. Diseases caused by group A beta-hemolytic *Streptococcus pyogenes* include the following:
        i. _____
        ii. _____
        iii. _____
        iv. _____
        v. _____
        vi. _____
        vii. _____
        viii. _____

16. Diplococci

    A. Diplococci occur in _____.
    B. Some diplococci are gram _____ and others are gram _____.
    C. Diseases Caused by Diplococci
        i. _____
        ii. _____
        iii. _____
        iv. _____

17. Bacillus/Bacilli

    A. _____-_____ bacilli may be pathogenic or nonpathogenic.
    B. Some bacilli are gram _____ and others are gram _____.
    C. Bacilli are responsible for a wide variety of illnesses. Some of these illnesses are as follows:
        i. _____
        ii. _____
        iii. _____
        iv. _____
        v. _____
        vi. _____

18. Gram-Negative Bacilli

    A. _____ are a large family of gram-negative bacilli that are found mainly in
        the intestinal tract.
    B. Many of them will cause infections in other _____ in the body.
    C. One type, _____, is most frequently associated with urinary tract infections.
    D. The group of _____ organisms is a major cause of foodborne illnesses worldwide.

19. *Helicobacter pylori* (*H. pylori*)

    A. *H. pylori* is a(n) _____-_____ bacillus.
    B. It was discovered in the early _____.
    C. The organism is found in about _____ of the population and causes _____
        symptoms in most individuals.
    D. It was discovered that *H. pylori* is the causative agent of _____ ulcers and a risk
        factor in _____ malignancy in some infected persons.
    E. The organism is responsive to a number of antibiotics, including _____.
    F. The discovery of *H. pylori* led to major breakthroughs in treatment for _____.

20. Gram-Positive Bacilli

    A. Gram-positive bacilli may be found in _____ or singly and are _____ forming
        or _____ forming.

B. Notable Gram-Positive Bacilli
 i. _____, which causes botulism
 ii. _____, which causes tetanus

21. Vibrios

A. Vibrios are _____-_____ bacilli.
B. The main pathogen is *Vibrio cholerae*, whose _____ causes cholera.
C. Cholera
 i. Cholera is characterized by profuse _____ stools, vomiting, leg cramps, _____, and shock.
 ii. It is caused by ingesting drinking water or eating _____ from water contaminated with infected urine, feces, or _____.

22. Spirilla and Spirochetes

A. Spirilla and spirochetes are _____-shaped or _____-shaped organisms.
B. They are _____ that are twisted in various shapes.
C. They are classified as a separate category of _____.
D. Some are nonpathogenic and are found in certain areas of the body and others, such as _____, cause the sexually transmitted infection syphilis.
E. *Borrelia burgdorferi*, a spirillum, was discovered in the mid-1970s to be the causative agent of _____.

23. Mycobacteria

A. Mycobacteria have a different type of material in the _____ and can be stained only with a(n) _____-_____ stain.
B. _____ is the causative agent of tuberculosis, and *Mycobacterium leprae* is the cause of _____.
C. These organisms do not stain well with a(n) _____ stain.
D. In a positive slide for _____-_____ (AFB), the slender bacilli will appear pink when exposed to an acid-fast stain.

24. Rickettsia and Chlamydia

A. Rickettsia is a bacterial parasite that lives in _____ and _____, which transmit the disease when they bite.
B. Chlamydia
 i. Chlamydia is a(n) _____ parasite, but it does not live in arthropod hosts.
 ii. It must invade _____ cells to reproduce.

25. Viruses

A. Viruses are the smallest known _____ organisms.
B. They depend on the _____ of other organisms for growth.

26. Diseases Caused by Viruses

 i. _____
 ii. _____
 iii. _____
 iv. _____
 v. _____
 vi. _____
 vii. _____
 viii. _____
 ix. _____

27. Types of Microorganisms: Protozoa

A. Protozoa are _____-_____ organisms.
B. Some are _____ and others are nonparasitic.

C. They move with _____, or _____ feet.

D. Diseases Caused by Protozoa

    i. _____

    ii. _____

28. Types of Microorganisms: Fungus/Fungi

A. Fungi include parasitic and nonparasitic _____ and _____.

B. They depend on other _____ for nutrition.

C. Reproduction occurs through _____.

D. They feed on _____.

II. Specimen Collection and Testing Procedures

1. Guidelines for specimin collection

A. Confirm the _____ of the patient by asking the patient to state his or her name and spell it, if necessary.

B. Use only _____ containers.

C. Ensure that the _____ is tightly closed and appropriately sealed.

D. Deliver specimen promptly to the laboratory and _____ it.

2. Information Required on a Specimen Label

    i. _____

    ii. _____

    iii. _____

    iv. _____

    v. _____

3. Information for the Laboratory Requisition

    i. _____

    ii. _____

    iii. _____

    iv. _____

    v. _____

    vi. _____

    vii. _____

    viii. _____

    ix. _____

    x. _____

    xi. _____

4. Collection Devices

A. The Culturette System (list the items included)

    i. _____

    ii. _____

    iii. _____

5. Microbiology Equipment and Procedures

A. Inoculating Equipment

    i. _____

    ii. _____

    iii. _____

B. Culture Media Classifications

    i. _____

    ii. _____

    iii. _____

    iv. _____

6. Common Culture Media
    i. _____
    ii. _____
    iii. _____
    iv. _____
    v. _____
    vi. _____

7. Microbiology Equipment and Procedures: Inoculating Media
    A. An inoculating _____ is used to create a(n) _____ culture.
    B. After inoculation, a(n) _____ dish is placed in a(n) _____ to allow the organism to grow.

8. Microbiology Equipment and Procedures: Sensitivity Testing
    A. Sensitivity testing determines which _____ will kill the _____.
    B. Tools include a(n) _____ dish and _____ agar.

9. Steps for Performing a Direct Smear
    A. Perform hand _____ and don gloves.
    B. _____ the equipment.
    C. _____ a clean slide.
    D. _____ a specimen sample.
    E. Allow the slide to air dry for _____ to _____ minutes.
    F. Hold the slide with _____ forceps and pass over the _____ flame.
    G. The slide is ready to be _____.

10. Steps for Preparing a Wet Mount Slide
    A. Perform _____ and don gloves.
    B. _____ a dry slide.
    C. _____ the dry slide.
    D. Place a drop of _____ solution on top of the specimen.
    E. Place a(n) _____ onto the smeared slide.

11. Gram Stain
    A. Gram stain is used to differentiate, or separate, bacteria into two groups: gram _____ and gram _____.
    B. Different bacteria stain differently, depending on the _____ in their walls.
    C. Gram-positive bacteria retain the crystal _____-_____ color and gram-negative bacteria retain only the _____ color.
    D. Gram stains must always be accompanied by a culture for _____ identification.

12. Throat swabs
    A. The throat specimen is one of the most _____ requested specimens in an office laboratory.
    B. Based on the _____ and _____ with which the patient presents, the physician will order a test to identify the pathogen involved and will begin treatment.
    C. Confirmation of _____ is important because of its virulence and possible complications.
    D. When performing a throat culture, it is important not to touch the _____ of the mouth or the tongue with the _____ to avoid contaminating it.

13. The Sputum Sample
    A. Sputum is the _____ that is expelled by coughing or clearing the bronchi.
    B. To obtain a sample, the patient must be carefully instructed to _____, spitting the coughed up material into a sterile container.
    C. Explain to the patient that this should not be _____ from the mouth.
    D. The purpose of obtaining a sputum specimen is to isolate and diagnose diseases such as _____, influenza, and _____.

14. The Urine Specimen
    A. For a culture, a urine specimen must be either a(n) _____ specimen or a(n) _____-_____ midstream sample (CCMS).
    B. Both methods provide _____ samples.
    C. Any other type of urine specimen would be contaminated by organisms in the container or on the _____ or _____ of the patient.
    D. In doctor's offices and smaller facilities, _____-_____ culture units are used.
    E. Often, urine cultures require a means to provide a(n) _____ result of the number of microorganisms in the sample.

15. The Stool Specimen
    A. A stool specimen may be tested for _____, _____, or _____ infections; for the presence of occult blood; and for excessive amounts of fat _____.
    B. The method of collection varies with the _____ of _____ ordered.
    C. Fecal specimens must be free of _____ or _____ from the toilet and toilet tissue.

16. Occult Blood
    A. Patients are instructed to write their _____, _____, and _____ on the label of the unit.
    B. Patients should close the unit and take it or _____ it to the doctor's office or the laboratory as requested.
    C. It is important to check the _____ of any test kit before giving it to the patient.

17. The Stool Specimen for Ova and Parasites
    A. The presence of _____ organisms, such as ova and parasites, may be determined by testing feces or stool.
    B. The presence of ova, or _____, or other forms of a parasite indicates parasitic _____.
    C. Identification of the parasite aids in the selection of the _____ treatment.
    D. Commercial kits are available that provide containers for fresh stool specimen and two additional vials for preserved specimens, one containing _____ and the other containing _____ alcohol.

18. Wound Specimens
    A. Sterile swabs are used to obtain a specimen from a wound, _____, or _____ to test for pathogenic microorganisms.
    B. The procedure is similar to obtaining a(n) _____ culture.
    C. Several specimens may be necessary from different _____.
    D. Be sure to _____ each specimen appropriately as to the source.

19. The Collection of Cerebrospinal Fluid (CSF)
    A. CSF collection is always treated as a(n) _____ procedure.
    B. The procedure is _____ for the patient, and the specimen must be handled with care.
    C. Usually _____ tubes are collected under sterile conditions and are sent for testing.
    D. The _____ and _____ test should be performed before chemical and other tests using the second of the three tubes.
    E. Tubes one and three are more likely to be _____ because of the entry and removal processes of collection.

20. The Group A Strep Screen
    A. The group A strep screen is performed frequently in _____.
    B. It is especially efficient in the _____ office because it is _____-_____ and can be done while the patient waits.
    C. The screen is a(n) _____ test for group A beta-hemolytic streptococci.
    D. There are many _____-_____ available that test for the extracted group A beta-hemolytic streptococcus antigen.

KEY TERMINOLOGY REVIEW

Without using any material from your textbook, write a sentence using each selected key term in the correct context as related to the topics presented in Chapter 45.

1. *enteritis*
   _____
   _____

2. *morphology*
   _____
   _____

3. *normal flora*
   _____
   _____

4. *spore*
   _____
   _____

5. *steatorrhea*
   _____
   _____

APPLIED PRACTICE

Follow the directions as instructed for each question.

1. Obtaining a stool specimen for ova and parasites versus for pinworms
   a. List the equipment and supplies needed for obtaining a stool specimen for ova and parasites.
      _____
      _____
      _____

   b. List the equipment and supplies needed for obtaining a stool specimen for examination for pinworms.
      _____
      _____
      _____

c. Discuss the differences and similarities between the two procedures.

_____

_____

_____

2. List the diseases that can occur from the following pathogens.

Body Location	Pathogen	Disease
Respiratory system	*Streptococcus pyogenes* *Corynebacterium diphtheriae* *Mycobacterium tuberculosis* *Haemophilus influenzae type B* *Streptococcus pneumoniae*	_____ _____ _____ _____ _____
Central nervous system	*Neisseria meningitides* Polioviruses Rabies virus	_____ _____ _____
Genitourinary system	Herpes simplex viruses 1 and 2 *Candida albicans (fungus)* *Chlamydia trachomatis* *Escherichia coli*	_____ _____ _____ _____
Integumentary system	*Staphylococcus aureus* Varicella zoster virus	_____ _____ _____ _____
Gastrointestinal system	Hepatitis A, B, and C viruses *Salmonella enteritidis* *Escherichia coli*	_____ _____ _____
Circulatory system and blood, immune system	*Streptococcus pyogenes* *Staphylococcus aureus* *Plasmodium falciparum, P. vivax, P. malariae, P. ovale* Human immunodeficiency virus Epstein-Barr virus *Borrelia burgdorferi*	_____ _____ _____ _____ _____ _____
Tissue	*Streptococcus pyogenes*	_____

LEARNING ACTIVITY: FILL IN THE BLANK

Using words from the following list, fill in the blanks to complete the following statements.

Note: Some terms are used in more than one statement.

agar	laboratory	prokaryotic
agglutination	lawn technique	seaweed
cephalosporins	methicillin-resistant	smear
colony	microorganisms	*Streptococci*
culture medium	motility	viable
eukaryotic	organelles	wet mount
feces	ova	

1. The Group A Strep Screen is an antigen detection test for group A beta-hemolytic _____ and follows the general procedure for antigen–antibody _____ tests, which produce a clumping of cells.

2. Differences such as cell structure and the presence or absence of _____ are used to classify organisms.

3. The "super bug" _____-_____ *Staphylococcus aureus* (MRSA) produces an enzyme that makes the organism resistant to penicillin and _____, which are normally used for treatment, and renders these antibiotics ineffective.

4. A _____ is a thin layer of _____ spread on a glass slide for identification purposes.

5. _____ is a gelatinous substance made from seaweed that is added to a(n) _____ to provide nutrition and a semisolid surface on which microbes can grow.

6. _____ cells have a nucleus and _____ in the cytoplasm, whereas _____ cells are simpler in structure, without a nucleus or organelles, such as bacteria.

7. A(n) _____ is a preparation in a liquid that will preserve the _____ of the microbe.

8. The Mueller–Hinton agar is inoculated with the pure culture specimen in overlapping strokes in a technique called the _____ or _____ count.

9. Microorganisms must remain _____ (capable of living) when they reach the _____.

10. The stool or _____ of the patient can be inspected for the presence of _____ and mature forms of the worm.

CRITICAL THINKING

Answer the following questions to the best of your ability. Use the textbook as a reference.

1. A patient has been instructed to collect stool specimens to be tested for occult blood. You ask him to refrain from eating red meat or taking vitamin C for 3 days prior to testing for occult blood. Why? What other instructions does this patient need to follow in order to obtain an accurate test result?

   _____

   _____

   _____

2. Mrs. Chen is a 70-year-old woman from mainland China who has come to the clinic because of recent, sudden constipation. Mrs. Chen is shy and very hesitant to speak with a male medical assistant about her condition. How can the clinic help Mrs. Chen?

_____

_____

_____

3. You are preparing a specimen smear for a microbiological examination by the doctor. You heat-fix the slide, but you realize that you have heated it too much because it has become hard to hold. What does this do to the specimen, and what would you do if this occurred?

_____

_____

_____

RESEARCH ACTIVITY

Use Internet search engines to research the following topic and write a brief description of what you find. It is important to use reputable websites.

1. Methicillin-resistant *Staphylococcus aureus* (MRSA) has become a very real threat, not only to health care workers but also to the general population. Visit www.cdc.gov and provide answers to the following questions:

   a. What is MRSA?
   b. What are some other multidrug-resistant organisms (MDROs)?
   c. In your opinion, what can be done to prevent the transmission of these organisms?

_____

_____

_____

_____

_____

CHAPTER 46
Urinalysis

STUDENT STUDY GUIDE

Use the following guide to assist in your learning of the concepts from the chapter.

I. Urinalysis

  1. An Overview of Urinalysis

    A. The Purpose of Performing a Urinalysis
      i. Provides the _____ clue of illness.
      ii. Provides information about the _____ of the urinary system and other _____ information.
    B. The properties of urine help detect:
      i. _____
      ii. _____
      iii. _____

  2. Types of Urinalyses: Routine Sample

    A. Collected in a(n) _____ container
    B. Collected in the office or brought from _____
    C. Used only for _____ screenings

  3. Types of Urinalyses: Morning Sample

    A. A morning sample is the most _____ urine.
    B. It is collected _____ upon on arising in the morning.
    C. It is used for _____ testing, urine _____, and _____ examination.
    D. The specimen should be brought in within _____ minutes to an hour after collection.
    E. Refrigerate the sample if an examination cannot be done within _____ hours, or add a preservative.

  4. Types of Urinalyses: Timed Specimen

    A. A timed specimen is necessary for _____ analysis of substances.
    B. It is used to analyze _____, _____, and _____.

  5. Types of Urinalyses: Twenty-Four Hour Specimen

    A. Collection begins after the patient _____ for the first time in the morning.
    B. Every drop of urine is collected in a container for _____ hours.
    C. It is used to determine _____ rate, check specific _____ levels, and check for _____ abnormalities.

  6. Types of Urinalyses: Two-Hour Postprandial

    A. The specimen is collected _____ hours after a meal has been eaten.
    B. It is used to screen for _____ that may be spilled into the urine once the blood levels exceed the _____ threshold.

  7. Types of Urinalyses: Catheterized Specimen

    A. This type is used to collect a(n) _____ urine specimen.
    B. Collecting urine with the use of a catheter ensures that the specimen is free of _____.

C. The _____ and its surrounding tissues are cleaned to create a(n) _____ field.

D. A small, _____ tube is inserted through the _____ to the _____.

8. Types of Urinalyses: Suprapubic Specimen

A. A suprapubic puncture is performed using a(n) _____ needle and syringe.

B. It is used for _____ examinations.

9. A Review of Urine Chemistry

A. Testing for Chemical Characteristics (list the substances for which urine is tested)

  i. _____

  ii. _____

  iii. _____

  iv. _____

  v. _____

  vi. _____

  vii. _____

  viii. _____

  ix. _____

10. Reagent Strips

A. The strip is dipped into the _____ sample.

B. Color changes indicate the presence and _____ of substances in the urine.

11. Clinitests®

A. Clinitests® are chemically treated tablets that are added to urine to determine the amount of _____ in the urine.

B. The tablets change color according to the _____ in the urine.

12. Steps for Preparing a Urine Sample for Microscopic Analysis

A. Perform the required _____ and chemical tests.

B. Place the urine in a(n) _____ tube and the tube into a(n) _____.

C. Pour off the _____.

D. Microscopically analyze the _____ material.

13. Microscopic Analysis (list the formed elements in urine that are evaluated)

  i. _____

  ii. _____

  iii. _____

  iv. _____

  v. _____

  vi. _____

  vii. _____

  viii. _____

KEY TERMINOLOGY REVIEW

Match each of the following vocabulary terms to the correct definition.

a. bacturia

b. hematuria

c. oliguria

d. sediment

e. urinalysis

1. _____ Blood in the urine.

2. _____ Bacteria in the urine.

3. _____ The solid material that settles at the bottom of a test tube after centrifugation.

4. _____ Provides valuable information about many functions in the body, including kidney function.

5. _____ Decreased amounts of urine production.

APPLIED PRACTICE

Follow the directions as instructed for each question.

1. Label the parts of the refractometer.

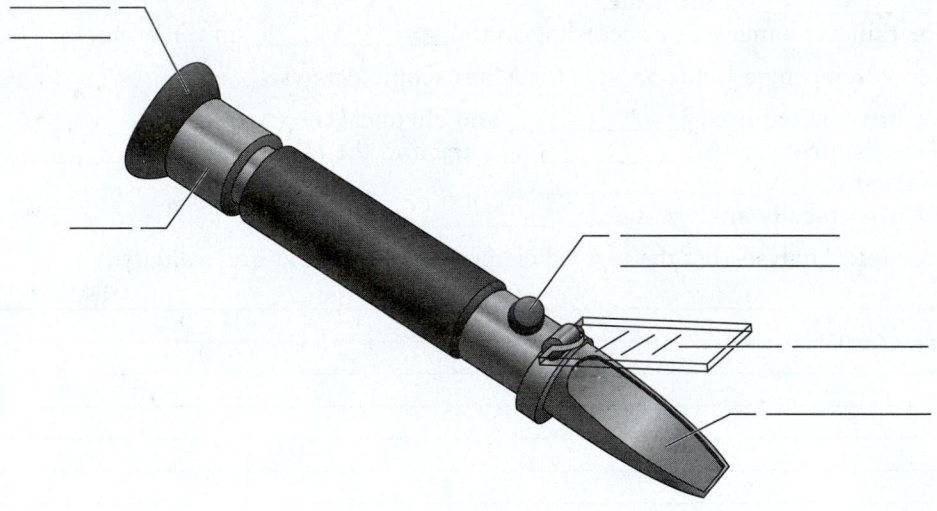

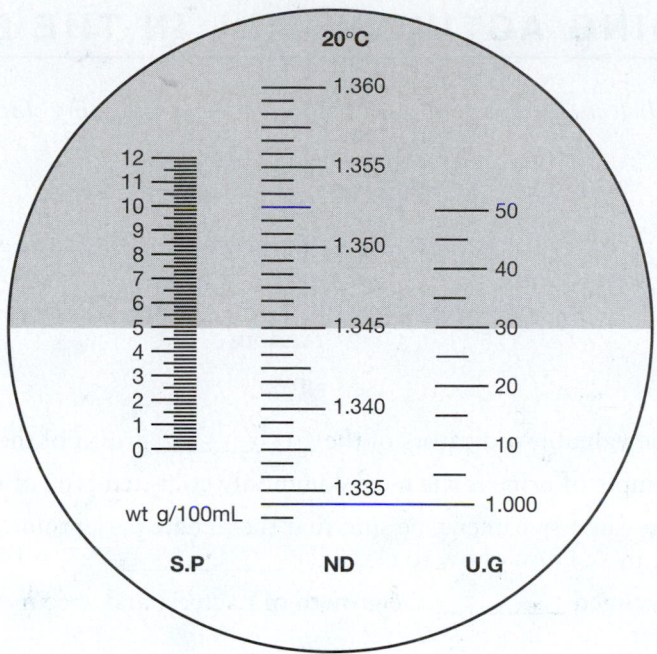

2. By each of the following microscopic images, note what is being seen in each urine sample.

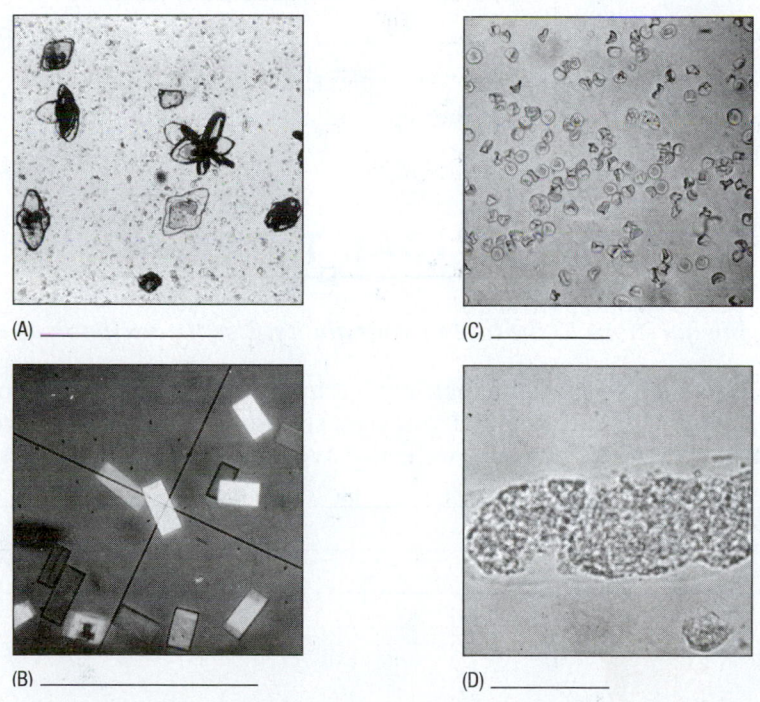

(A) _____

(C) _____

(B) _____

(D) _____

LEARNING ACTIVITY: FILL IN THE BLANK

Using words from the list below, fill in the blanks to complete the following statements.

acidity   organisms

alkalinity   overall

bile duct   physical

foreskin   positive

fruity   random

labia   slows

1. Urine samples provide valuable indicators of the _____ health of the patient.

2. A(n) _____ sample of urine is the most commonly collected type of urine specimen.

3. When collecting clean-catch specimens, be sure that the female patient understands how to clean the _____ and the male knows how to clean the _____.

4. Refrigeration of a specimen _____ the growth of bacteria and specimen deterioration, but does not stop it.

5. The _____ characteristics of urine may be important diagnostic tools for the physician.

6. Individuals testing positive for ketones may have a(n) _____ odor to their urine.

7. The pH of a solution indicates _____ and _____.

8. If urobilinogen is not present, a(n) _____ _____ obstruction may be present.

9. If a leukocyte test is positive, then a protein test should be _____.

10. Microscopic examination identifies the type and approximate number of _____ present in a urine specimen.

CRITICAL THINKING

Answer the following questions to the best of your ability. Use the textbook as a reference.

1. You are to instruct a 68-year-old female patient in the collection of a 24-hour urine specimen. Explain this, in your own words, as if you were speaking to the patient. Avoid medical terms that the patient may not understand very well; also avoid treating the patient as if she were a child.

   _____

   _____

   _____

2. You have collected a clean-catch urine specimen from Mrs. Gonzalez, a long-time patient, and you have already performed the physical assessment of the color, odor, and clarity. The following are the results of your chemical testing. Fill in the normal value for each, circle those that are abnormal as if you were flagging them for the physician, and then state the possible reasons for the abnormal results.

Tests	Your Results on Mrs. Gonzalez	Normal Value	Possible Causes
Color	orange-red		
Clarity	cloudy		
pH	7.8		
Specific gravity	1.026		
Protein	++ or positive		
Glucose	0		
Ketones	0		
Bilirubin	0		
Urobilinogen	4		
Blood	+		
Leukocytes	++++		
Nitrite	0		

RESEARCH ACTIVITY

Use Internet search engines to research the following topic and write a brief description of what you find. It is important to use reputable websites.

1. To learn more about the Clinical Laboratory Improvement Amendments (CLIA) waived test, consult the Internet and/or use school or local library resources. Write an essay on what you learned from your research regarding CLIA and waived tests.

_____

_____

_____

_____

_____

CHAPTER 47

Phlebotomy and Blood Collection

STUDENT STUDY GUIDE

Use the following guide to assist in your learning of the concepts from the chapter.

I. Phlebotomy and Blood Collection

1. Venipuncture

   A. Venipuncture and phlebotomy both refer to the collection of _____ through a tiny _____ in a(n) _____.

   B. Three methods are used:
      i. The vacuum tube method is used for a _____ _____.
      ii. A syringe and needle are used if there are no _____ _____.
      iii. A butterfly is used for a(n) _____ _____.

2. Vacuum Blood Tube Order for Filling

   i. _____
   ii. _____
   iii. _____
   iv. _____
   v. _____
   vi. _____
   vii. _____
   viii. _____
   ix. _____
   x. _____

3. Vacutainer® Color, Additive, and Function (briefly explain each additive and function)

   A. Yellow
      i. The additive is _____.
      ii. It prevents _____.
      iii. It is used for _____.

   B. Light blue
      i. The additive is _____.
      ii. It removes _____.
      iii. It is used for _____.

   C. Red
      i. This additive contains _____.
      ii. It is used for _____.

   D. Red Marbled
      i. The additive is _____.
      ii. It enhances _____.
      iii. It is used for _____.

   E. Green
      i. The additive is _____.
      ii. It prevents _____.
      iii. It is used for _____.

F. Light Green
    i. The additive is _____.
    ii. It aids in _____.
    iii. It is used for _____.
G. Lavender
    i. The additive is _____.
    ii. It removes _____.
    iii. It is used for _____.
H. Pink, White, or Royal Blue
    i. The additive is _____.
    ii. It prevents _____.
    iii. It is used for _____.
I. Gray
    i. The additive is _____.
    ii. It removes _____.
    iii. It is used for _____.
J. Dark Blue
    i. The additive is _____.
    ii. It detects _____.

4. Sites for Venipuncture

    i. _____
    ii. _____
    iii. _____

5. Patient Preparation

A. Competency can be demonstrated by having all the _____ _____ assembled before the blood draw.
B. Always ask if the patient has had any_____ during previous venipunctures.
C. A(n) _____ is a bruise.

6. Steps for Obtaining Venous Blood with a Sterile Syringe and Needle

A. Apply a tourniquet _____ to _____ inches above the antecubital space.
B. Clean the venipuncture site with a(n) _____ wipe, and then allow to _____ _____.
C. Have the patient make a(n) _____ and hold it shut until he or she is told to release it.
D. Make sure that there is no _____ in the syringe.
E. Remove the _____ _____ and insert the needle into the vein.
F. Slowly pull back the syringe _____ until the proper amount of blood has been obtained.
G. Instruct the patient to _____ his or her fist.
H. Release the _____ and withdraw the needle quickly.
I. Release the tourniquet and withdraw the _____ quickly. Immediately cover with gauze. Instruct the patient to keep _____ on the site and raise the arm to prevent hematomas from occurring.
J. Apply the _____ _____ _____ to the end of the syringe.

7. The Butterfly Method of Venipuncture

A. Uses a needle that is attached to _____- to _____-inch tubing.
B. The end of the tubing can be attached to the _____ or the _____ _____ tube holder.
C. The butterfly method is used for _____ veins that are difficult to draw from with the standard vacuum container method or syringe and needle method.
D. It is called the butterfly method because the needle on the end has a(n) _____ portion that keeps the needle from turning and _____ the needle into the small vein.

E. The needle used for the butterfly method is a small _____-, _____-, or _____-gauge needle.

F. The drawback to performing the butterfly method is the fact that it is more _____ than a standard needle.

8. Capillary Puncture

A. Capillaries are _____ _____.

B. _____ _____ and oxygen are exchanged at this level.

C. Use this method to collect _____ amounts of blood.

9. Steps for Performing a Capillary Puncture

A. Select the _____ or _____ finger on the nondominant hand; wipe with alcohol.

B. Remove the plastic protective tip of the _____.

C. Grasp the patient's hand and squeeze the finger gently 1 inch _____ the puncture site.

D. Puncture with a(n) _____ _____ motion to get a full blood drop.

E. Wipe away the _____ _____ with gauze.

F. Obtain the sample using a(n) _____ capillary tube.

G. Apply clean gauze over the site and ask the patient to apply _____.

KEY TERMINOLOGY REVIEW

Match each of the following vocabulary terms with the correct definition.

a. antecubital space

b. capillaries

c. heparin

d. platelets

e. serum

1. _____ Plasma without the fibrinogen.

2. _____ A depression in the front of the elbow; it is the most commonly used site for venipuncture.

3. _____ The smallest of the body's blood vessels.

4. _____ A substance that prevents clotting.

5. _____ The smallest cells found in the blood; they are formed in the bone marrow.

APPLIED PRACTICE

Follow the directions as instructed for each question.

1. Read the scenario on the next page and answer the following questions.

Scenario

Julie Turner is working as a clinical medical assistant. A patient, Hector Olanski, comes in for a blood draw. The physician's order reads as follows:

COOK FAMILY MEDICINE
(188) 555-1111

Patient: Hector Olanski

DOB: 7-3-1938
Date: 3-22-20XX

Rx PTT and CBC

Dx: (1) Heparin monitoring (E934.2)
    (2) Phlebitis of lower extremities (451.2)

Dr. Liam Cook

While gathering supplies, Julie grabs a lavender-topped tube, a red-topped tube, and a light-blue-topped tube.

a. Did Julie collect the correct tubes for Mr. Olanski's blood draw? Why or why not? Explain your answer based on each of the tubes of blood that Julie collected.

_____

_____

_____

b. What would be the correct order of draw?

_____

_____

_____

c. Are there any additives in the tubes that Julie is using for the blood draw? If so, explain which additives are used (based on the color) and the action of each additive.

_____

_____

_____

2. Fill in the label below according to how Julie should label each of Mr. Olanski's tubes of blood.

LEARNING ACTIVITY: TRUE/FALSE

Indicate whether the statement is true (T) or false (F).

_____ 1. Partially filled tubes, especially the light-blue-topped tube, can cause erroneous test results, resulting in the patient's blood needing to be redrawn.

_____ 2. Occasionally, uncontrollable bleeding can occur when the needle is withdrawn.

_____ 3. Capillary puncture is also called a fingerstick.

_____ 4. Wait until all of the blood tubes have been collected before asking the patient to release his or her fist.

_____ 5. The liquid component of blood is called plasma.

CRITICAL THINKING

Answer the following questions to the best of your ability. Utilize the textbook as a reference.

1. A patient needs to have blood drawn for an ESR and a glucose level. The patient is extremely nervous and worried about the pain that she will experience with a blood draw and asks if you can "stick her finger" instead. Will that work in this scenario? Why or why not?

   _____

   _____

   _____

2. You have drawn three tubes of blood (gray-topped, lavender-topped, and green-topped). You filled the lavender-topped tube first, the gray-topped tube second, and the green-topped tube last. Is this the correct order of draw? If not, what could possibly happen because of this?

   _____

   _____

   _____

3. A patient has come in today for a blood draw to check her cholesterol level. She is 78 years old, has fragile skin, and her veins are impossible to see. Which method of phlebotomy would you use on this patient and why?

   _____

   _____

   _____

4. Your next patient for phlebotomy today is a 6-year-old child. What special considerations are appropriate for this patient?

   _____

   _____

   _____

RESEARCH ACTIVITY

Use Internet search engines to research the following topic and write a brief description of what you find. It is important to use reputable websites.

1. Visit the Clinical and Laboratory Standards Institute at www.clsi.org. Navigate through the website and identify reasons why the website would be beneficial for medical assistants working in a clinical or physician's office laboratory.

   _____

   _____

   _____

   _____

   _____

CHAPTER 48
Hematology

STUDENT STUDY GUIDE

Use the following guide to assist in your learning of the concepts from the chapter.

I. The Formation and Components of Blood

1. Blood Formation and Blood Components

   A. Blood cells originate from the _____ _____ cell.
   B. Blood cells mature into one of _____ individual types of cells.

2. Red Blood Cells (RBCs)

   A. RBCs are formed in _____ _____.
   B. They contain _____.
   C. Formation is controlled somewhat by _____.
   D. They last for about _____ months and are continuously being reproduced in the body.
   E. The normal RBC range for a male adult is _____ to _____ million/mm^3.
   F. The normal RBC range for a female is _____ to _____ million/mm^3.

3. The Function of Hemoglobin

   A. Hemoglobin carries oxygen from the lungs to the _____ of the body.
   B. It carries _____ _____ from the body back to the lungs, where it can be expelled with exhalation.

4. White Blood Cells (WBCs)

   A. WBCs are also known as _____.
   B. They are produced in the bone marrow from _____ _____.
   C. They are larger than _____ blood cells.
   D. Their principal function is to _____ against infection.
   E. The range of WBCs in an adult is _____ to _____ thousand/mm^3.

5. Leukocyte Classification

   A. Granulocytes (briefly explain each type)
      i. Basophils: _____
      ii. Eosinophils: _____
      iii. Neutrophils: _____
   B. Agranulocytes (briefly explain each type)
      i. Monocytes: _____
      ii. Lymphocytes: _____

6. Basophils

   A. Basophils are thought to be produced by the _____ _____.
   B. They produce _____.
   C. Patients who have had excessive exposure to radiation may have _____ basophils.
   D. They appear in tissues where a(n) _____ _____ is occurring.

7. Eosinophils

    A. Eosinophils are assumed to be produced by the _____ _____.

    B. Detection of a large number of eosinophils can indicate a(n) _____ condition or the presence of certain _____ conditions.

    C. Eosinophils have granules that produce a(n) _____ color on the laboratory-stained slide.

8. Neutrophils

    A. Neutrophils are divided into two categories: _____ neutrophils and _____ neurophils.

    B. The body reproduces neutrophils on an ongoing basis, and they only survive for _____ days.

    C. Reproduction is increased when _____ _____ is occurring.

    D. Neutrophils combat infection by _____.

    E. Phagocytosis is the process in which the _____ surrounds, swallows, and digests the _____.

9. Monocytes

    A. Monocytes are formed in the _____ _____ from stem cells.

    B. They assist in _____.

    C. They ingest foreign particles or _____ that the neutrophils are unable to digest.

    D. They assist in cleaning up _____ debris that may have been left from the infection.

    E. An increase in monocytes is seen in patients who have certain diseases, such as tuberculosis, typhoid, and _____ _____ _____ fever.

10. Lymphocytes

    A. Lymphocytes are produced in the _____ _____ and in _____ _____ such as the spleen and lymph nodes.

    B. They produce _____ against foreign substances such as bacteria, viruses, and pollens.

    C. Lymphocytes are small and large and can proliferate into _____ and _____ cells.

    D. Lymphocytes do not have _____ and are nonsegmented.

11. Platelets (Thrombocytes)

    A. Thrombocytes are formed in the _____ _____.

    B. Their main function is to assist in the _____ of blood.

    C. Thrombocytes lead to the formation of thrombin, which converts _____ to _____.

    D. The typical range is between _____ and _____ platelets/mm^3.

II. Tests

    1. List the 14 tests that make up the comprehensive metabolic panel.

        i. _____

        ii. _____

        iii. _____

        iv. _____

        v. _____

        vi. _____

        vii. _____

        viii. _____

        ix. _____

        x. _____

        xi. _____

        xii. _____

        xiii. _____

        xiv. _____

2. Normal Values for Common Laboratory Tests

   A. Total cholesterol: _____

   B. Glucose: _____

   C. Triglycerides: _____

   D. Creatinine: _____

   E. Uric acid: _____

   F. BUN: _____

   G. Sodium: _____

   H. Potassium: _____

   I. Chloride: _____

   J. CO_2: _____

   K. White blood cells: _____

   L. Red blood cells: _____

   M. Hemoglobin: _____

   N. Hematocrit: _____

   O. Sedimentation rate: _____

   P. Platelets: _____

3. Microhematocrit

   A. Provides the physician with information about the patient's _____ _____ cell volume.

   B. A(n) _____ hematocrit indicates anemia or hemorrhaging.

   C. A(n) _____ hematocrit indicates dehydration or polycythemia.

   D. A(n) _____ hematocrit is 40–50% in males and 35–45% in females.

4. Performing a Microhematocrit

   A. Fill _____ capillary tubes three-quarters full.

   B. Seal one end with the _____ _____.

   C. Place the capillary tubes in the _____ with the sealed ends against the _____ _____.

   D. If more than one patient's blood is being tested, write down the _____ of the _____ that the patient's tube is in.

   E. Spin for 3 to 5 minutes at _____ rpms.

   F. After centrifuging, the sample will be separated into three layers.

      i. The top layer is _____.

      ii. The middle layer, or the buffy coat, is made up of _____ and _____.

      iii. The bottom layer is _____ _____.

   G. Remove the tubes immediately after the centrifuge _____. If the tubes are not removed immediately, the blood may begin to _____ _____.

   H. Use the _____ _____ by placing the sealing clay just below the zero line on both tubes. Then, on both tubes, match the _____ of the _____ with the 100 line.

   I. Read the results on both tubes directly below the _____ _____. Then add those results together and divide by _____.

   J. Discard the tubes into the _____ container.

   K. Record the value as a(n) _____ on the patient's medical record.

5. Hemoglobin

   A. Low hemoglobin may indicate _____-_____ _____.

   B. Elevated readings are present in patients with _____ and in extreme situations, such as burns.

   C. Normal values for adult females are _____ to _____ g/dL, and for males, _____ to _____ g/dL.

D. Levels can either be measured by an automated blood analyzer or manually by using a(n) _____.

E. Typically, the _____ _____ _____ is less accurate and not as reliable as the automated blood analyzer.

6. Equipment Used to Measure Hemoglobin

    i. _____

    ii. _____

7. Methods for Determining Hemoglobin Values

    i. _____

    ii. _____

8. White Blood Cells (WBCs)

A. There are _____ types of WBCs, each with distinct characteristics.

B. Count _____ WBCs, and then express each cell type as a(n) _____.

C. Values may differ between _____ and _____ analyses.

9. Normal White Blood Cell Values for Adults

A. Neutrophils: _____

B. Eosinophils: _____

C. Basophils: _____

D. Lymphocytes: _____

E. Monocytes: _____

10. Red Blood Cells (RBCs)

A. RBCs are _____ colored.

B. They appear _____ with slightly _____ centers.

C. They have no _____ or _____.

D. RBCs with nuclei are called _____.

E. Normal-looking RBCs are recorded as _____.

11. Differential White Blood Cell Count

A. This test determines the _____ of each type of WBC, RBC morphology, and platelet estimation.

B. Performing this test _____ is a skill that requires practice to achieve proficiency.

C. Testing is done using a microscope with a bright light and _____ magnification with a(n) _____ _____ slide.

D. Focus near the edge of the stained slide where the cells are _____ and where the cells are _____ layer thick.

E. The test can also be performed by the _____ analyzer.

12. Preparing Slides for a Differential White Blood Cell Count

A. Obtain a whole-blood sample using _____ as the anticoagulant of choice. Blood must be _____ thoroughly before testing.

B. Using a dropper, place one drop of _____ _____ blood on the end of a clean, glass slide.

C. Using the short side of another _____, _____ slide, back the slide to the drop of blood.

D. Allow the blood to spread across the _____ side of the slide.

E. Holding the spreader slide at a(n) _____-_____ angle, spread the blood across the length of the slide.

F. Use gentle, continuous pressure and a smooth gliding motion to create a(n) _____.

G. Notice that the smear has a(n) _____ side that gradually changes to a(n) _____ side.

H. The thin side has a(n) _____ edge, and the blood covers _____-_____ to _____-_____ the length of the slide.

I. Allow the slide to air dry on a(n) _____.
J. Label the _____ edge of the slide with the patient's name and the date.
K. Stain the slide using _____ staining method.
L. Flood the slide with stain for exactly _____ seconds or the amount of time indicated by the manufacturer.
M. Rinse with _____ water until the water runs clear.
N. Allow the slide to _____ _____ before examining it under the microscope.
O. _____ findings may need to be referred to a laboratory technician for analysis.

13. Platelets

    A. Platelets are about _____ the size of RBCs.
    B. They stain _____ and tend to appear in a clump.
    C. They appear to have a(n) _____ _____ edge and contain small granules.
    D. There are typically between _____ and _____ platelets in one field of view.

14. The Erythrocyte Sedimentation Rate (ESR)

    A. The ESR is also called the _____ rate.
    B. Drawing a patient's ESR can be done using either the _____ or _____ method.
    C. When performing the _____ method, the _____ tube is calibrated in millimeters per hour.
    D. Depending on the type of method used, the _____ values may vary.
    E. The Wintrobe method indicates that the normal ESR in an adult female is _____ to _____ mm/hr; in an adult male, it is 0 to 9 mm/hr.
    F. Increased values may indicate a(n) _____.
    G. A person's ESR may also be elevated because of a variety of reasons, including _____, _____, and malignant tumors.
    H. The sed rate is related to the condition of the red blood cells and the amount of _____ in the plasma.
    I. When a sed rate test is conducted on a patient, the rate at which the RBCs _____ indicates the existence of possible conditions.

15. Phenylketonuria (PKU)

    A. PKU is a(n) _____ disease.
    B. The unmetabolized portion of the _____ _____ phenylalanine accumulates in the bloodstream.
    C. If undetected, it results in _____ _____.
    D. The PKU test is always performed on _____ to determine the presence of the _____ protein phenylalanine.

16. Equipment and supplies for Performing a Phenylketonuria Test

    i. _____
    ii. _____
    iii. _____
    iv. _____
    v. _____

17. Testing for Mononucleosis (Mono)

    A. The test is called the mononucleosis _____ test.
    B. The test is used to help determine whether a patient has _____ _____.
    C. The test is ordered with a(n) _____ and a strep test.
    D. Mono is common in _____ patients who show symptoms of fever, headache, swollen glands, and fatigue.
    E. If a patient has a positive mono test, an increased number of white blood cells, _____ _____, and symptoms, then the patient is diagnosed with infectious mononucleosis.
    F. If the mono test is _____, but other symptoms exist, it may be too early to detect mono.

KEY TERMINOLOGY REVIEW

Match each of the following vocabulary terms with the correct definition.

a. anemia

b. basophils

c. lymphocytes

d. phenylketonuria

e. serum

1. _____ Deficiency of hemoglobin caused by a lack of RBCs.

2. _____ Plasma without the fibrinogen.

3. _____ A congenital disease caused by a defect in the metabolism of an amino acid.

4. _____ Like other white cells, these are thought to be produced by the bone marrow; they produce heparin.

5. _____ The smallest cells found in the blood, they are formed in the bone marrow.

APPLIED PRACTICE

Follow the directions as instructed for each question.

1.

> **Scenario:**
>
> Lorraine Spencer is working as a medical assistant. She has been asked to perform a Glycoslated Hemoglobin A1C test. Describe what equipment she will use, what supplies she will need, and the method and steps she will take in performing this test. Show an example of the chart notation for this test. Lorraine
>
> Date: 3-22-20XX

_____

_____

_____

2. Fill in the label below according to how Julie should label each of Mr. Olanski's tubes of blood.

LEARNING ACTIVITY: TRUE/FALSE

Indicate whether the following statements are true or false by placing a T or an F on the line that precedes each statement.

_____ 1. Blood analysis is not considered to be a routine tool of medicine.

_____ 2. MCV, MVHV, and MCV are used to differentiate specific types of anemia.

_____ 3. The functions of blood are transportation and hydration.

_____ 4. The liquid component of blood is called plasma.

_____ 5. BUN is the abbreviation for blood urea nitrogen.

CRITICAL THINKING

Answer the following questions to the best of your ability. Use the textbook as a reference.

1. Name five common blood chemistry tests. Include the full name and the purpose of the test.

   _____

   _____

   _____

2. Describe how diabetes is monitored and managed through blood tests.

   _____

   _____

   _____

RESEARCH ACTIVITY

Use Internet search engines to research the following topic and write a brief description of what you find. It is important to use reputable websites.

1. Visit the U.S. Bureau of Labor Statistics website and look up the job of a medical laboratory technician. Describe the responsibilities of a med lab tech, the education requirements, and the projected need for people in this kind of job over the next several years.

   _____

   _____

   _____

   _____

   _____

CHAPTER 49
Radiology

STUDENT STUDY GUIDE

Use the following guide to assist in your learning of the concepts from the chapter.

I. Introduction to Radiology

    1. Radiology

        A. Radiology is the branch of medicine that uses _____ substances, or matter that gives off _____.
        B. Radiology uses various techniques for visualizing the _____ structures of the body for the diagnosis and treatment of disease.
        C. Divided into Three Specialties
            i.   _____
            ii. _____
            iii. _____

    2. Radiology Personnel

        A. A(n) _____ is a physician who specializes in radiology.
        B. A(n) _____, or _____ technologist, makes diagnostic radiographs, or X-rays.

    3. The Duties of a Radiological Technologist

        A. _____ patients for radiographic procedures
        B. Determines the proper _____, _____, and _____ time for each X-ray
        C. _____ radiographic equipment
        D. Develops the _____
        E. Assists the _____ with special procedures

    4. The Principles of X-rays

        A. X-rays were developed in 1895 by _____ _____ _____.
        B. X-rays are produced in a(n) _____ _____ when electrons collide.
        C. This collision produces _____ rays.
        D. X-rays coming from the tube form an X-ray _____.
        E. The radiation field is a cross section of the X-ray beam and the _____ of _____.
        F. The patient is placed between the tube that produces the X-ray _____ and the _____.

    5. Characteristics of X-rays

        A. X-rays penetrate substances of different _____ to varying _____.
        B. They cause _____ of the substances through which they pass.
        C. They cause certain substances to _____.
        D. They travel in a(n) _____ _____.
        E. They can _____ body cells.

6. Diagnostic Imaging

   A. Diagnostic imaging involves the use of the following:

      i. _____

      ii. _____

      iii. _____

      iv. _____

      v. _____

7. The Contrast Medium

   A. The contrast medium is a(n) _____ substance.

   B. It does not allow the _____ of X-rays.

   C. Types include _____ (barium), _____, air, and gas.

   D. It is administered orally, by _____ (parenterally), or by _____.

   E. It acts to convert a(n) _____ or structure into a(n) _____ area.

8. Contrast Medium Materials

   A. Barium Sulfate

      i. Barium sulfate is a positive _____ _____.

      ii. It consists of a(n) _____ compound mixed with water.

      iii. It is used for _____ examination.

   B. Iodine Contrast Compounds

      i. Iodine contrast compounds are used to form _____ compounds.

      ii. They cannot be used on patients who are allergic to _____ or _____.

      iii. They interfere with _____ medicine.

   C. Negative Contrast

      i. Negative contrast appears _____ on X-rays.

      ii. It is used to visualize the _____.

9. The Role of the Medical Assistant During Radiology Exams

   A. Schedules the _____

   B. _____ the patient about the procedure

   C. Explains to the patient any _____ required

   D. Ensures that the patient is provided with a(n) _____-_____ gown and drape

   E. Requests that the patient remove all _____ materials

   F. Assists the patient _____ and _____ the procedure

   G. Provides _____-_____ instructions

   H. Informs the patient about _____ to _____ the results

10. X-ray Procedures That Require Special Preparation

   A. Angiogram: No _____ if the examination is in the morning or _____ if the examination is in the afternoon.

   B. Barium Enema (Lower GI)

      i. Enemas are administered until the bowel return is _____ on the evening before the examination.

      ii. The doctor may order a rectal _____ in the morning or a(n) _____ such as 2 oz. of castor oil or citrate of magnesia at 4:00 P.M. the day before the procedure.

      iii. The patient is to have clear liquids and _____ for dinner.

      iv. Nothing may be taken by mouth (NPO) after _____.

   C. Barium Meal (Upper GI): NPO after _____.

   D. Cholecystogram (GB Series)

      i. The patient may have a light supper of non-fatty food, such as _____ and _____ without _____ or oil, the evening before the procedure.

      ii. _____ tablets (prescribed by the physician) are taken with water after supper.

      iii. NPO except for water until after the _____ the following day.

E. Computerized Tomography (CT): NPO for _____ hours before the procedure if a(n) _____ medium is used.

F. Intravenous Pyelogram (IVP)
   i. Three _____ tablets or 2 oz. of _____ _____ at 4:00 P.M. the day before the procedure.
   ii. Eat a(n) _____ supper.
   iii. _____ after midnight.

G. Retrograde Pyelogram
   i. Enemas are administered or _____ are taken on the _____ before the procedure.
   ii. NPO for _____ hours before the procedure.

H. Ultrasound: May require a full _____ or _____, depending on the type of ultrasound.

11. Steps for Assisting with a Radiological Procedure

    A. Check the X-ray examination _____.
    B. Check the necessary X-ray _____ as needed.
    C. Identify the patient and determine whether the patient has complied with the _____ _____.
    D. Explain the procedure to the patient, and then instruct the patient to remove _____ as necessary for the procedure.
    E. Ask the patient to remove all _____ and _____.

12. Anteroposterior (AP)

    A. The X-ray beam is directed from _____ to _____.
    B. The patient may be standing or _____.
    C. The patient's front will face the X-ray _____ and the patient's back will be near the _____ _____.

13. Posterioanterior (PA)

    A. The X-ray beam is directed from _____ to _____.
    B. The patient will be standing _____.
    C. The patient's _____ will face the X-ray equipment and his or her _____ will be near the film plate.

14. The Oblique Position

    A. The patient is turned at an angle to the film plate so that the X-ray beam can be directed at an area that would be hidden on a(n) _____, _____, or _____ X-ray.

15. The Lateral Position

    A. The X-ray beam is directed toward _____ _____ of the body.
    B. In the right lateral (RL) position, the patient's right side is near the _____ _____ and the left side is near the _____ _____.
    C. In the left lateral (LL) position, the patient's _____ side is near the film plate.

16. The Axial Position

    A. The X-ray tube is angled to direct the X-ray beam along the _____ of the body or body part.
    B. With _____ angulation, the X-ray beam is directed at an angle from the feet toward the head.
    C. With _____ angulation, the X-ray beam is directed from the head toward the feet.

17. Information Required for Scheduling a Radiological Procedure

    i. _____
    ii. _____
    iii. _____

iv. _____

v. _____

18. Beverages That May Be Restricted on an All-Liquid Diet

    i. _____

    ii. _____

    iii. _____

    iv. _____

    v. _____

    vi. _____

    vii. _____

    viii. _____

19. Guidelines for Sequencing Multiple Diagnostic Procedures

  A. Schedule all radiographic examinations and tests that do not require a(n) _____ _____ and iodine intake first.

  B. Do CT scans of the _____ and _____ before performing procedures that require barium.

  C. CT procedures that require an IV contrast medium may be done _____ blood is drawn for the iodine uptake series.

II. Diagnostic Imaging Procedures

  1. General Categories of Diagnostic Imaging

    i. _____

    ii. _____

    iii. _____

    iv. _____

  2. Methods for Administering Contrast Media

    i. _____

    ii. _____

    iii. _____

    iv. _____

  3. Radiological Imaging Procedures That Require Contrast Media

    i. _____

    ii. _____

    iii. _____

  4. Fluoroscopy Procedures

  A. Fluoroscopy is a(n) _____ examination of a portion of the body or the functioning of an organ using a fluoroscope.

  B. It allows the radiologist to have _____ images.

  C. It is a(n) _____ image that is seen on the fluoroscope and can be filmed using a radiograph (X-ray) to obtain a(n) _____ record.

  D. _____ _____ are often used to better visualize organ functioning and abnormalities.

  5. Gastrointestinal Series

  A. A gastrointestinal series is a(n) _____ study of the _____ _____.

  B. It uses a(n) _____ medium.

  C. It can involve an upper or lower _____ _____.

  6. Patient Instructions for the Upper GI Series

  A. NPO after _____.

  B. No _____.

C. Drink _____ _____ during the procedure.

D. The procedure can last _____ hours.

E. _____ eating can be resumed after the procedure.

F. Drinking _____ after the procedure is important.

G. Stool may be _____ for a few days.

7. Patient Instructions for the Lower GI Series

   A. _____-_____ diet a few days before the procedure

   B. _____-_____ diet the morning before the procedure.

   C. A(n) _____ may be needed the day before the procedure.

   D. A(n) _____ or barium sulfate is given, which the patient retains during the procedure.

   E. Prior to the end of the procedure, the enema is _____ and an X-ray of the _____ _____ is taken.

   F. A regular diet can be resumed, including a lot of _____.

   G. The patient may have _____ stools for 1 or 2 days following the procedure.

8. Intravenous Pyelogram (IVP)

   A. An IVP is an examination of the kidneys, _____, and bladder.

   B. The procedure takes about _____ to _____ hours.

   C. _____ is used.

   D. _____-_____ diet, including a lot of water the day before the procedure.

   E. _____ after midnight.

   F. A(n) _____ with an enema the night before the procedure may be ordered.

9. Cholecystogram

   A. A cholecystogram is an examination of the _____.

   B. It requires a(n) _____ medium.

   C. It is utilized when _____ has not provided a definitive diagnosis.

   D. _____-_____ meal the night before the procedure with contrast medium pills.

   E. _____ after midnight.

   F. After the procedure, the patient is asked to eat a(n) _____ meal; _____ hour later, another X-ray is taken.

   G. _____ may occur after the procedure.

10. Myelography

    A. Myelography is a fluoroscopic procedure used to visualize the _____ _____.

    B. It involves a(n) _____ puncture.

    C. It is used to detect _____ of the spinal cord or _____ disks.

    D. It is typically done if a(n) _____ or a(n) _____ has not provided enough detail.

11. Pneumoencephalograph

    A. A pneumoencephalograph is performed by injecting _____ instead of a contrast medium after some cerebral spinal fluid has been removed.

    B. It allows visualization of the _____ of the brain.

12. Angiography

    A. Angiography provides a visualization of the _____ _____ of blood vessels after a(n) _____ material has been injected into the blood vessels.

    B. A contrast medium is injected into a(n) _____ or _____ by way of a catheter, which is threaded through the vessel until it reaches the correct site.

    C. Because iodine is used as the contrast medium, the patient should be tested for a(n) _____ to iodine before the procedure begins.

    D. The patient is monitored for a few hours after the procedure for any signs of _____ from the puncture site.

13. Cardiac Catheterization

   A. Cardiac catheterization is a form of _____.
   B. It is frequently performed to assess the status of the _____ _____.
   C. The catheter is inserted into the _____ artery and fed through the arteries until it reaches the heart.
   D. If obstructions are discovered, therapeutic interventions such as _____ _____ or stent insertion can take place to relieve a blockage of the coronary arteries.

14. Arthrography

   A. Arthrography is used to produce an arthrogram, or image, of the inside of a(n) _____.
   B. It helps diagnose abnormalities of the _____, tendons, _____, and cartilage of the knee, hip, or shoulder.
   C. The procedure involves injecting a local _____ followed by a contrast medium or _____, or both, into the joint.
   D. A(n) _____ is used to evaluate the functioning of the joint.
   E. The procedure usually takes about 1 hour, and the patient should be advised to expect some slight _____ and _____ for a day or two.
   F. The patient should be advised to _____ the joint during that time.

15. Procedures That Do Not Require Contrast Media Films (list the portions of the anatomy that do not require contrast media)

   i. _____
   ii. _____
   iii. _____
   iv. _____
   v. _____
   vi. _____
   vii. _____

16. Mammography

   A. Mammography is a radiological examination of the _____ _____ of the breast.
   B. It identifies benign and malignant _____ (tumors).

17. Patient Instructions for Mammography

   A. Because of the effects that these products can have on the clarity of the test, prior to the procedure patients should be instructed not to use the following:
      i. _____
      ii. _____
      iii. _____
      iv. _____

18. The Mammography Procedure

   A. The patient stands in _____ of the X-ray equipment.
   B. The technician positions the patient carefully in order to have all _____ _____ examined.
   C. The patient should be instructed to follow the technician's directions regarding the placement of _____, _____, and _____ position.
   D. Patients of _____ _____ are given a lead apron to wear during the procedure.
   E. Each breast is _____ compressed by the equipment to spread the tissue for better viewing.
   F. X-rays are directed at _____ into the breast tissue.

G. The procedure takes a(n) _____ _____ for each view, with the entire procedure lasting about a half hour.

H. Patients may feel discomfort because of _____ during the breast compression.

19. Addressing Breast Lumps

   A. If a(n) _____ is detected, the patient should follow up immediately with further testing and not wait to see if the _____ disappears over time.

   B. Many abnormalities detected on mammograms are _____ and present no danger to the patient.

   C. Once a mammogram reveals _____ tissue, a breast biopsy should be done to confirm the type of mass detected.

20. Stereotactic Breast Biopsy

   A. This technique is less _____ and less _____ than previous types of biopsies.

   B. The procedure is done with the patient lying _____ _____ with the breast compressed between two _____ with the suspicious mass centered in the window of a paddle.

   C. A computer determines the precise positioning of the _____ _____.

   D. A small sample of _____ is taken and sent for review by a pathologist.

21. Tomography

   A. Tomography allows for the penetration of _____ areas.

   B. Tomography produces _____.

   C. Computed tomography produces _____ scans.

22. Computed Tomography (CT)

   A. CT combines radiography with computer analysis of _____ _____.

   B. An X-ray camera _____ completely around the patient, and the computer accumulates _____-_____ slices from each rotation of the camera.

   C. The CT scanner consists of a(n) _____ table with a remote control; the circular structure, or _____, that houses the X-ray equipment; and a(n) _____ _____ with monitor and computer equipment.

23. The CT Procedure

   A. The patient lies on a(n) _____ table that slides into the scanner.

   B. The procedure is painless, is _____, and requires no special preparation.

   C. The computer calculates various factors to detect _____ _____, such as tumors; _____ displacement; and _____ accumulation.

24. Positron Emission Tomography (PET)

   A. PET examines the _____ _____ of the body.

   B. The patient is injected with or inhales a(n) _____ substance.

   C. PET is used to assist in treating the following conditions:

       i. _____

       ii. _____

       iii. _____

       iv. _____

25. Magnetic Resonance Imaging (MRI)

   A. MRIs provide a visual of internal _____, _____, and structures.

   B. The image is _____-_____.

   C. The hard portion of _____ _____ cannot be viewed.

   D. It cannot be used on patients who have _____ or _____ clips on blood vessels.

   E. No _____ radiation is used.

   F. MRIs allow for the observation of organ _____.

26. Patient Instructions for Magnetic Resonance Imaging
    A. Remove all _____, _____ _____, and metallic objects, such as watches, belts, hearing aids, and hairpins.
    B. Identify which devices, if any, have been inserted into the patient's body, such as the following:
        i. _____
        ii. _____
        iii. _____
        iv. _____
    C. Leave _____ _____ or devices that contain metallic or _____ _____ strips outside the MRI chamber.
    D. Use a patient gown if patient's clothing has _____ or metal snaps.

27. Digital Radiology
    A. Digital radiology uses standard _____.
    B. An image is projected onto a TV or _____ _____ screen.
    C. Digital angiography is used for the cardiac and _____ arteries and head and neck angiograms.

28. Ultrasound/Sonography
    A. Ultrasound is used _____-_____ _____ to view internal structures.
    B. It provides _____ monitoring and the detection of abnormalities of the heart, liver, and kidneys.

29. Patient Preparation for the Ultrasound Examination
    A. The patient should wear _____-fitting garments or clothing that is easy to remove because the procedure is performed over bare skin.
    B. During a fetal ultrasound or pelvic ultrasound, the patient is instructed not to _____ right before the test because a full _____ displaces the intestines and allows for a better view of the uterus.
    C. The patient may be asked to drink a(n) _____ or more of water just prior to either of these examinations.
    D. For an ultrasound of the _____ or _____, the patient may be asked not to eat for several hours before the procedure.

30. Radiation Therapy
    A. Radiation therapy uses a specific dose of radiation to kill _____ cells.
    B. Normal cells are altered, but will naturally _____.
    C. Radiation therapy is also known by the following names:
        i. _____
        ii. _____
        iii. _____

31. Types of Rays Used in Radiation Therapy (briefly explain each type)
    A. Alpha Rays
        i. _____
        ii. _____
    B. Beta Rays
        i. _____
        ii. _____
    C. Gamma Rays
        i. _____
        ii. _____

32. Conditions That Are Treated with Radiation Therapy
    i. _____
    ii. _____
    iii. _____
    iv. _____
    v. _____
    vi. _____

33. Methods for Administering Radiation (provide the name of each of the methods described)
    A. _____ _____ _____ (ERT): Administering calculated doses of radiation to a specific site.
    B. _____ _____ _____ (IRT): Administering radiation through a sealed container that houses radioactive material, administering radiation through a liquid form via the patient's mouth or bloodstream, or administering radiation by instilling it into a body cavity.

34. Nuclear Medicine
    A. Nuclear medicine is also known as _____ imaging.
    B. It uses radioactive _____ to treat and diagnosis diseases.
    C. It involves the use of radioactive isotopes of _____, _____, and other elements.

35. Units of Radiation (provide the name of each type of unit)
    A. _____: Unit used to measure the amount of ionizing radiation absorbed.
    B. _____: Unit used to measure occupational exposure.
    C. Units used to measure the effects of radiation:
       i. _____
       ii. _____
       iii. _____

36. The Effects of Overexposure to Radiation
    i. _____
    ii. _____
    iii. _____
    iv. _____
    v. _____
    vi. _____
    vii. _____

37. Primary Radiation
    A. Primary radiation strikes the patient either for _____ reasons or for an X-ray examination.
    B. Once the primary _____ strikes the patient, it can then become _____ radiation as it bounces off the patient.

38. Guidelines for Maintaining the Personal Safety of the Medical Assistant and the Patient
    A. Wear a(n) _____ _____ on outer clothing when exposed to any form of radiation.
    B. Ensure that the _____ is never covered.
    C. Stay behind the _____ _____ in a(n) _____-_____ room when X-ray equipment is being used.
    D. Note the _____ or lighted display indicating that X-ray equipment is in use.
    E. _____ personnel should leave the X-ray room.
    F. Wear _____ devices if you are in the room when an X-ray is being taken.
    G. Have periodic testing to ensure that there are no _____ _____ from radiation exposure.

H. Ask the _____ if he or she has had any recent exposure to X-rays.

I. Place a(n) _____ _____ over the patient's abdominal and reproductive organs for patients who are of childbearing age or are pregnant.

39. Storage of X-ray Films

A. X-ray films are kept in containers that protect film from light, heat, _____ _____, and moisture.

B. They are stored in a dry, cool place in a(n) _____ _____.

C. They are stored on end to prevent _____ _____ and where expiration dates can be viewed.

D. Films should only be _____ with one hand.

E. Processed films should be stored in _____ _____ and filed in film cabinets.

40. Ownership of the Film

A. _____ reports can be sent to other physicians at the patient's request.

B. Films can be loaned to _____ physicians if necessary.

C. Films are a(n) _____ _____ of the patient.

KEY TERMINOLOGY REVIEW

Match each of the following vocabulary terms with the correct definition.

a. angiography

b. fluoroscopy

c. Gantry

d. radiolucent

e. radiopaque

1. _____ Procedure using a contrast medium whereby the actual function of a particular organ or structure can be visualized.

2. _____ A radiological procedure that involves the use of a contrast medium.

3. _____ Permitting greater penetration of X-rays.

4. _____ A circular structure that houses the X-ray equipment.

5. _____ Allows fewer X-rays to pass through.

APPLIED PRACTICE

Use information from the patient's chart listed below to answer the following questions.

Epley, Marguerite V.
11-24-1941

3/18/20XX, 2:15 P.M.

Ht: 5'5"Wt: 115 lbs.   T: 98.6°F   P: 90 bpm   BP: 136/88

cc: Pt. presents to office with rt. lower leg pain, after falling while getting out of her bathtub.
Pt. rates the pain as a 6 on a scale of 1 to 10. Rt. lower leg appears to be swollen and without
bruising at this time.

Jerry Li, CMA (AAMA)

Scenario: Dr. Jefferson wants Jerry, the CMA (AAMA), to perform an X-ray of Ms. Epley's lower rt. leg.
The order reads as follows:

PT: Marguerite Epley DOB: 11/24/1941
Rt. lower leg X-ray. AP and lateral views.
Dx: R/O Fx *(Diagnosis: Rule out fracture)*

1. Dr. Jefferson ordered an AP view. What does this mean?

    _____

    _____

2. How do you think Jerry should position the patient for the lateral view?

    _____

    _____

3. List some of the protective barriers that Jerry would implement during the X-ray.

    _____

    _____

LEARNING ACTIVITY: FILL IN THE BLANK

Using words from the list below, fill in the blanks to complete the following statements.

allergic	front to back	safety precautions
carbon dioxide	high-frequency	sonography
childbearing age	iodine	stomach
contrast medium	liquid	ultrasound
dietary	negative	ultraviolet
education	pregnant	upper GI series

1. In preparation for a(n) _____, the patient should not eat or drink after midnight because the _____ must be empty for this procedure.

2. The field of radiology uses X-rays, radioactive substances, and other forms of radiant energy such as _____ rays.

3. A(n) _____ is a radiopaque substance that facilitates radiographic imaging of internal structures.

4. _____ contrast media include air, _____, and other gases.

5. In the anteroposterior view (AP), the central ray is directed from _____.

6. Before an X-ray, any female must be asked whether she could be _____.

7. With regard to patient preparation and instructions for an IVP: This procedure should not be performed on a patient who is _____ to _____.

8. _____, or _____, is the use of _____ sound waves to image internal structures.

9. Special _____ restrictions in preparation for radiographic procedures often call for an all-_____ diet on the day before the procedure.

10. The medical assistant's role in medical imaging may involve patient preparation and _____, scheduling, and following _____.

CRITICAL THINKING

Answer the following questions to the best of your ability. Use the textbook as a reference.

1. You have placed a patient on the table for an X-ray and notice that the lead strip around the table has a few very small cracks in it. What should you do?

   _____

   _____

   _____

2. Mr. Abdul has come in for a cholecystogram. As you put the patient into the room, you ask him if he has followed the preparation instructions of taking iodine the day before and then NPO this morning. He looks surprised and then admits that he forgot to take the iodine. What would you do?

   _____

   _____

   _____

3. A patient comes to the front desk and does not have an appointment. She wants to get her original mammogram because she is moving to another state. What can you tell this patient?

   _____

   _____

   _____

8. Prefilled Cartridge Injection Systems

   A. These systems use a prefilled, _____-dose cartridge that fits in a special cartridge holder.

   B. The system is convenient because medications do not have to be _____ up prior to injection.

   C. The cartridge holders are _____ and long lasting.

9. OSHA

   A. OSHA stands for _____.

   B. OSHA provides guidelines for the _____ of contaminated needles and syringes.

   C. OSHA outlines follow-up procedures for health care workers who are stuck with _____ needles.

10. The Biohazard Sharps Container

    A. All medical offices must have a(n) _____ proof, rigid, _____ container labeled with a(n) _____ biohazard sticker for the disposal of sharps.

    B. These containers should be replaced and disposed of properly when _____ full.

11. Charting Medications

    A. Parenteral medications and oral medications are charted using the same documentation, as follows (list the information that should be provided):
       i. _____
       ii. _____
       iii. _____
       iv. _____
       v. _____
       vi. _____

II. Injection Methods

   1. The Deltoid Muscle

      A. This injection site works well for _____-volume injections only.

      B. The muscle is found by measuring _____ finger widths _____ the _____ process of the shoulder.

      C. Do not give shots in the _____ of the arm.

      D. Use a(n) _____-gauge needle.

      E. For smaller arms, use a(n) _____-gauge, _____-inch needle.

   2. The Vastus Lateralis Muscle

      A. In infants, the vastus lateralis muscle lies _____ the greater _____ of the _____.

      B. In adults, the vastus lateralis muscle extends from the _____ of the anterior _____ to the middle of the lateral _____ one handbreadth above the _____.

   3. The Dorsogluteal Muscle

      A. Patient should lie _____ and point toes _____.

      B. Draw an imaginary line from the greater trochanter of the _____ to the posterior superior _____ spine.

   4. The Ventrogluteal Muscle

      A. Place the palm of the _____ hand on the greater trochanter and the _____ finger on the superior _____ crest.

      B. Inject in the space between the _____ and _____ fingers.

      C. Give the injection at a(n) _____-degree angle.

5. Subcutaneous Injections

   A. Subcutaneous injections are used for _____ doses of _____ medications.

   B. They are used in the _____, the upper back, the _____, and the thighs.

   C. They are given at a(n) _____-degree angle.

6. Intradermal Injections

   A. Common sites for giving an intradermal injection include the _____ chest and _____ back, as well as the _____ forearm.

   B. Because just the top level of skin is entered, a small _____, or bubble, that contains the injection fluid appears on the skin.

   C. Do not _____ the area after giving the injection.

7. The Tuberculin Skin Test

   A. This test is administered _____.

   B. It is performed to determine whether a patient has developed an immune response to the bacterium that causes _____.

   C. The test cannot tell if the infection is _____ or _____.

8. Tuberculin Skin Test Results

   A. Redness alone at the skin test site is a(n) _____ reaction.

   B. A firm _____ is a(n) _____ reaction to the skin test.

9. Intravenous (IV) Therapy

   A. This process involves administering fluids and solutions directly into a patient's _____.

   B. Medical assistants must consult their state _____ act before attempting any IV procedure.

10. How to Prepare an IV Tray (list the steps)

    i. _____
    ii. _____
    iii. _____
    iv. _____
    v. _____
    vi. _____
    vii. _____
    viii. _____
    ix. _____
    x. _____

III. Immunization

   1. Antibodies and Immunity

      A. Antibodies are _____ substances that are produced by _____ in the spleen, lymph nodes, and tissues.

      B. Antibodies respond to defend against _____ or foreign substances.

   2. Childhood and Adolescent Immunizations

      A. Every year, a new recommended childhood and adolescent immunization schedule is produced by the _____, the CDC's _____ _____, and the American Academy of Family Physicians.

      B. The schedule indicates the recommended _____ for immunizations.

3. The Hepatitis B Vaccine

   A. Hepatitis B is spread by the _____ virus.
   B. It is transmitted by contaminated _____ in blood.
   C. A child will receive a total of _____ doses before he or she is 24 weeks old.

4. The Diphtheria Vaccine

   A. This vaccine is given to children in _____ doses.
   B. The _____ dose is given between _____ and _____ years of age.
   C. Diphtheria is diagnosed through a(n) _____ culture.
   D. The symptoms are _____, _____, and _____ _____.

5. The Pertussis Vaccine

   A. Pertussis is caused by _____, directly and indirectly transmitted.
   B. Only _____ vaccination is needed before the child is immune to the disease.

6. The Haemophilus Influenzae Type B Conjugate Vaccine

   A. _____ out of _____ children in the United States under 5 years of age gets Hib disease.
   B. It is caused by a(n) _____ that is spread through the _____.

7. The Hepatitis A Vaccine

   A. Hepatitis A affects the _____.
   B. It spreads through personal contact or by eating _____ food or drinking water.
   C. The vaccine is given to children over _____ years old.

8. The Poliovirus Vaccine

   A. This vaccine has been available since _____.
   B. Polio is caused by a(n) _____.
   C. It spreads through contact with _____.

9. Reconstituting a Powdered Medication for Administration

   A. Medications supplied in a powdered form generally have a(n) _____ shelf life.
   B. In order to be injected, these powdered medications must be reconstituted with diluents, usually _____.

10. Steps for Reconstituting a Powdered Medication for Administration (list the steps)

    i. _____
    ii. _____
       _____
    iii. _____
        _____
    iv. _____
    v. _____
    vi. _____
    vii. _____
    viii. _____
         _____

KEY TERMINOLOGY REVIEW

Complete the following sentences using the key terms found at the beginning of the chapter.

1. The _____ site is most commonly used for large volume, deep intramuscular injections or irritating, viscous (thick) medications.

2. _____ are used for dispensing oral medication into the respiratory tract.

3. Meningitis is a result of _____.

4. _____ administration means administering a medication through an injection.

5. An alcohol pad or cotton pad must be used to hold the vial to prevent glass cuts when opening _____.

APPLIED PRACTICE

Complete the following exercises.

1. On the figure below, label each part of the syringe.

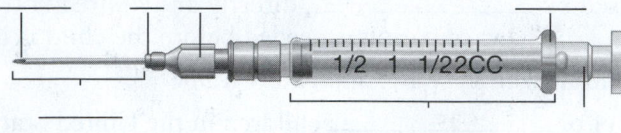

2. To demonstrate your knowledge regarding the angle of insertion for intramuscular, subcutaneous, and interdermal injections, indicate on the figure provided which angles represent each type of injection. In addition, provide the names of each of the layers of the skin.

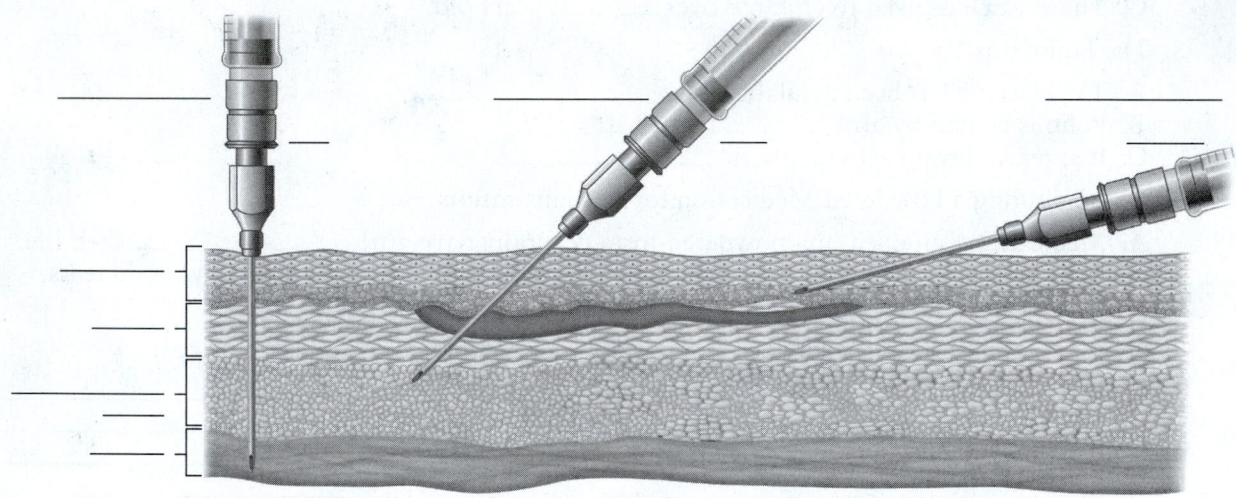

LEARNING ACTIVITY: TRUE/FALSE

Indicate whether the following statements are true or false by placing a T or an F on the line that precedes each statement.

_____ 1. Artificially acquired active immunity develops in response to receiving vaccinations with active organisms.

_____ 2. The deltoid muscle is located on the lower outer surface of the upper arm.

_____ 3. Transmission of diphtheria is by direct and indirect contact.

_____ 4. Hepatitis B, a form of viral hepatitis, is highly contagious and can be fatal.

_____ 5. Immunity can be either genetic or acquired.

_____ 6. Intramuscular injections are usually given with 25- or 26-gauge needles.

_____ 7. Many liquid medications are prescribed for the pediatric patient because of the ease of administration.

_____ 8. The MMR is given in three doses.

_____ 9. Oral medication is swallowed; it enters the body through the tissues of the gastrointestinal system and is then slowly absorbed into the body.

_____ 10. When giving a medication using the Z-track method, you need to pull the skin upwards prior to inserting the needle.

CRITICAL THINKING

Answer the following questions to the best of your ability. Use the textbook as a reference.

1. Explain why IV infusion of medication is the most dangerous method used to administer medication and MUST be the right medication, strength, and amount. Errors with this route can cause serious problems. All routes of medication administration MUST be done accurately, but there are specific reasons why this route is riskier than the others.

   _____

   _____

   _____

2. Although a very small of amount of bubbles or air injected into the muscle or the subcutaneous tissue would not be harmful, the medical assistant must never let this happen. Explain why it is not acceptable to have even tiny bubbles within the medication inside the syringe.

   _____

   _____

   _____

RESEARCH ACTIVITY

Use Internet search engines to research the following topic and report what you find. It is important to use reputable websites.

1. Some parents believe that it is not necessary to immunize their children. To learn more about this issue, conduct research online and then write an essay on your findings. Conclude with a synopsis of what you believe about the necessity of immunizations for children. Be sure to cite your sources.

   _____

   _____

   _____

   _____

CHAPTER 56
Patient Education

STUDENT STUDY GUIDE

Use the following guide to assist in your learning of the concepts from the chapter.

I. Teaching Methods and Strategies

1. Patient Centered Education

   A. The education process begins with _____, or evaluation of the patient's needs.
   B. _____ the plan involves teaching the patient specifically what to do.
   C. Document the teaching you have done by _____ it in the patient's health record.
   D. Educate the patient about his or her own _____ behaviors.

2. List 5 teaching methods

   i. _____
   ii. _____
   iii. _____
   iv. _____
   v. _____

3. Guidelines for Creating a Community Resource Brochure

   A. Identify _____ _____ that are available to help patients with disease prevention or health promotion, such as smoking cessation or weight loss.
   B. Research information found in a(n) _____ _____, newspaper, or website.
   C. Create an attractive _____ for distribution to patients that includes the name, location, telephone number, and services offered by the resources.
   D. After the brochure has been polished, obtain approval from the _____ _____ or physician before distributing the brochure to patients.

4. Information to Be Included in a Public Relations Brochure

   i. _____
   ii. _____
   iii. _____
   iv. _____
   v. _____
   vi. _____
   vii. _____
   viii. _____

5. Motivational Incentives for Adult Patients

   i. _____
   ii. _____
   iii. _____
   iv. _____
   v. _____

6. Roadblocks to Effective Patient Learning
    i. _____
    ii. _____
    iii. _____

7. Communication and Language Roadblocks
    i. _____
    ii. _____
    iii. _____
    iv. _____
    v. _____
    vi. _____
    vii. _____
    viii. _____
    ix. _____
    x. _____
    xi. _____

8. The Effects of Cultural Influences
    i. _____
    ii. _____
    iii. _____
    iv. _____
    v. _____
    vi. _____

9. The Effects of the Patient's Stage of Development
    A. Attitudes and _____ have a powerful impact on learning readiness.
    B. Some patients may _____ education because of previous negative experiences.
    C. In addition, illness affects people in different ways; _____ and _____ can be obstacles to learning.

10. Ways to Overcome Roadblocks
    A. Create a learning _____ that encourages patient readiness.
    B. Consider _____ the session if the patient is not feeling well at the time.

11. Lecture
    A. The advantages of lecturing include efficiency and the absence of limits on the _____ of patients.
    B. The disadvantage of lecturing is that there is no _____ in which to handle an individual patient's confusion.

12. Role-Playing
    A. Definition: The patient participates in a(n) _____ _____ in which he or she acts out a story.
    B. Advantages
        i. _____
        ii. _____
    C. Disadvantages
        i. _____
        ii. _____

13. Case Problems
    A. Definition: Apply _____ to real situations.
    B. Advantages: They are believable and concrete instead of _____.
    C. Disadvantages: Significant _____ may be missing, and effectiveness depends on the _____.

14. Demonstration/Return Demonstration
    A. Definition: _____ patients how to do something, and then _____ has them do the same procedure.
    B. Advantages
        i. _____
        ii. _____
    C. Disadvantages
        i. _____
        ii. _____
    D. Usefulness
        i. _____
        ii. _____

15. Contracting
    A. Definition: Sets up goals with clear _____ and _____ for the patient.
    B. Advantages
        i. _____
        ii. _____
        iii. _____
    C. Disadvantages
        i. _____
        ii. _____
        iii. _____
    D. Usefulness
        i. _____
        ii. _____

16. The Use of a Significant Other
    A. Definition: Teaches a close _____/_____ the same information that the patient is being taught.
    B. Advantages
        i. _____
        ii. _____
    C. Disadvantages
        i. _____
        ii. _____
        iii. _____
    D. Usefulness
        i. _____
        ii. _____
        iii. _____

17. Past Experiences
    A. Definition: Build on what has been _____ in the past instead of creating a new set of knowledge.
    B. Advantages
        i. _____
        ii. _____
    C. Disadvantages
        i. _____
        ii. _____
    D. Usefulness
        i. _____
        ii. _____

18. Group Teaching
    A. Definition: Brings together patients who have common _____ needs.
    B. Advantages
        i. _____
        ii. _____
        iii. _____
    C. Disadvantages
        i. _____
        ii. _____
        iii. _____
        iv. _____
    D. Usefulness
        i. _____

19. Programmed Instruction
    A. Definition: _____
    B. Advantages
        i. _____
        ii. _____
        iii. _____
        iv. _____
    C. Disadvantages
        i. _____
        ii. _____
        iii. _____
        iv. _____
    D. Usefulness
        i. _____
        ii. _____

20. Simulations (Games)
    A. Definition: Create a(n) _____ _____ for learning purposes.
    B. Advantages
        i. _____
        ii. _____
        iii. _____
    C. Disadvantages
        i. _____
        ii. _____
        iii. _____

21. Tests of Knowledge
    A. Definition: The patient is given _____ _____ that are related to his or her knowledge of the subject.
    B. Advantages
        i. _____
        ii. _____
        iii. _____
    C. Disadvantages
        i. _____
        ii. _____
        iii. _____

22. Printed Handouts

    A. Definition: Brochures or instruction sheets are printed for the purpose of _____ knowledge to the patient.

    B. Advantages

        i. _____

        ii. _____

    C. Disadvantages

        i. _____

        ii. _____

23. Diagrams

    A. Definition: Diagrams are _____ of concepts in _____ form.

    B. Advantages

        i. _____

        ii. _____

        iii. _____

    C. Disadvantages

        i. _____

        ii. _____

24. Models

    A. Definition: Models are _____ _____ of an object that is produced in a substance such as clay or plaster.

    B. Advantages

        i. _____

        ii. _____

    C. Disadvantage: _____

25. Film

    A. Definition: In this context, a film is considered to be a video, _____ _____, or moving picture.

    B. Advantages

        i. _____

        ii. _____

    C. Disadvantages

        i. _____

        ii. _____

        iii. _____

26. Helpful Materials to Use When Teaching Children

    A. Children may need to see a treatment or procedure performed on a(n) _____ before tolerating it well.

    B. Many children like to _____ equipment that will be used on them, such as a(n) _____ or a blood pressure cuff.

    C. Older children may wish to see videos about their upcoming _____ or other treatments.

27. Considerations for Teaching the Visually Impaired

    A. Visually impaired patients may not be able to read written instructions unless the type is _____ _____, and some may not be able to read it at all.

    B. The medical assistant may need to make _____-_____ instructions of information that is usually written.

    C. Be sure to clear _____ from the office that might impede the patient, and make sure to hold the patient's hand to lead him or her to examinations and procedures.

28. Considerations for Teaching Non-English-Speaking Patients
    A. When the appointment is made, ask the patient if he or she would like to have a(n) _____ present.
    B. The patient may prefer to bring a relative who _____ _____.
    C. Be sure to get the patient's permission to discuss _____ _____ with relatives.
    D. Send _____ _____ home with the patient.
    E. If a large percentage of patients in the office speaks a particular language other than English, it may be helpful to create brochures in _____ _____.
    F. Consider _____ and _____, as well as the patient's likes and dislikes, to promote compliance.

29. Changes That Affect the Elderly Learner
    i. _____
    ii. _____
    iii. _____
    iv. _____

30. Methods to Be Considered When Teaching the Elderly
    A. Use handouts with _____ _____, and use video and audiovisual displays.
    B. _____-_____ slides are preferable to a fast video or movie because the slide can be stopped to reinforce learning.
    C. _____-_____ can be useful as long as the patient's energy level can be maintained.
    D. _____ _____ should be included in the teaching process whenever possible.
    E. The elderly person is accustomed to being in _____ and may not wish to learn anything new if he or she does not see the _____ of doing so.

31. Considerations for Creating a Teaching Plan
    A. Patients may not be honest and open in a busy place where they lack _____.
    B. It is ideal if patient education can take place in a(n) _____-_____ room with privacy.
    C. Sometimes placing patient education materials in racks in examining rooms allows patients to take brochures _____.
    D. If a medical assistant is teaching a patient how to use equipment, then that equipment should be _____ for the patient.
    E. If the patient asks a question that the medical assistant (MA) cannot answer, the MA should admit that he or she does not know the answer and _____ _____ to the patient with the answer to the question.
    F. Teaching resources are available for _____, or the MA can develop _____ for the office.
    G. Patients have different _____ styles, and the teaching should match the patient's preferred style.

32. Ways to Help Patients Be More Compliant
    A. Ensure a(n) _____ relationship is formed between the patient and the health care provider, physician, and other staff such as the medical assistant.
    B. Convey to the patient the knowledge that he or she needs to make _____ decisions about health care.
    C. Reinforce learning and reduce _____ by working out a(n) _____-_____ plan with regular evaluation of progress.
    D. This plan should include a(n) _____ stating what the patient should be able to do, as well as a(n) _____ indicating when the objective should be accomplished.

KEY TERMINOLOGY REVIEW

Complete each sentence by selecting the correct key term from the textbook. A few of the sentences will use more than one key term.

1. The education process begins with _____, or _____ of the patient's needs.

2. If a patient is unable to complete a teaching plan, be sure to _____ this in the patient's chart.

3. _____ the plan involves actually teaching the patient what to do.

4. Some procedures that require small-muscle _____, such as flossing the teeth and opening medication bottles, are almost impossible for elderly persons with arthritis.

5. _____ are the goals of patient education.

APPLIED PRACTICE

Explain how you would handle the following scenario.

Scenario

Ethan is an RMA working at a pain management clinic. He often conducts patient education seminars on proper medication administration and methods of pain management. Today, Ethan is working with Aidan Baker, a child who had a below-the-knee right leg amputation, and who is also deaf. Explain how you would approach a child with special needs.

_____

_____

_____

_____

LEARNING ACTIVITY: MULTIPLE CHOICE

Circle the correct answer to each of the following questions.

1. What is the main difference between adult and child learning?

   a. The child expects milk and cookies afterward.
   b. The adult needs self-directed learning.
   c. The adult is stubborn and will tend to refuse most new knowledge.
   d. The child is likely to cry throughout most of the teaching session.

2. Which of the following should be part of an effective teaching plan?

   a. Understanding desired outcomes
   b. Behaving in a commanding, authoritative way
   c. Using sarcasm and ironic comments when the patient is slow
   d. Offering private lessons

3. Which of the following should *not* be an aspect of teaching older adults?

    a. Understanding that older adults may take longer to process new information
    b. Keeping instructions to the point and providing clear written materials
    c. Not talking down to an adult
    d. Keeping a bowl of favorite candies nearby for reinforcement

4. Which of the following is conducive to a proper learning environment?

    a. The reception area
    b. A private examination room
    c. The hallway
    d. The front desk

5. Which of the following is *not* an appropriate teaching resource?

    a. Audiocassettes
    b. Videos
    c. Pamphlets
    d. Personal websites

CRITICAL THINKING

Answer the following questions to the best of your ability. Use the textbook as a reference.

1. Scenario

    You are a new medical assistant, and the physician has asked you to go into the examination room and give patient teaching to Mrs. McCarty about her rheumatoid arthritis pain management plan. The physician has written in the chart what the plan is but you are not very familiar with rheumatoid arthritis. Would you (a) try to do the best you can, (b) ask another MA to tell you what to do or how to do it, or (c) ask the patient to wait while you research office policy manuals and information on the Internet to figure it out? Choose one of the options and then explain your reasoning.

    _____

    _____

    _____

2. Scenario

    You are a medical assistant at an OB/GYN office. The physician has recently put you in charge of creating a list of resources and materials to be used in a patient education library. What patient education topics would you include in an OB/GYN resource library? List at least three topics and explain why you chose them.

    _____

    _____

    _____

RESEARCH ACTIVITY

Use Internet search engines to research the following topic and write a brief description of what you find. It is important to use reputable websites.

1. Choose a topic for patient education and search the Internet for reputable information. List at least five reputable websites that could be used for patient education. Also, list at least five items of special interest that you learned.

   _____

   _____

   _____

   _____

   _____

CHAPTER 57

Nutrition

STUDENT STUDY GUIDE

Use the following guide to assist in your learning of the concepts from the chapter.

I. Nutrition

1. Diet and Nutrition (provide the name of the professional who is described)

    A. _____: A professional who provides advice on nutrition.
    B. _____: A professional who promotes good health through proper diet and the use of diet in the treatment of disease.

2. Digestion

    A. Digestion is the actual process the body undergoes when it converts food into _____ _____ that can be absorbed into the blood and used by the body tissues and organs.
    B. The actual digestive process is accomplished by physically breaking down, diluting, dissolving, and chemically splitting into _____ _____, the food substance we consume.

3. Major Nutrient Classes

    i.   _____
    ii. _____
    iii. _____
    iv. _____
    v.   _____
    vi. _____

4. Carbohydrates

    A. Carbohydrates include the following:

        i.   _____
        ii. _____
        iii. _____

    B. Carbohydrates are stored in the body as _____.

5. Carbohydrates for Health

    A. _____ carbohydrates are ideal foods for a healthy diet.
    B. They are generally low in _____, high in _____, and a good source of vitamins and minerals.
    C. Excess carbohydrates are stored as _____ (after the small amount of glycogen stores fill up).

6. Carbohydrate Consumption Recommendations

    A. Only _____ of calories from refined sugar
    B. Approximately _____ to _____ of calories from carbohydrates

7. Sources of Carbohydrates
   i. _____
   ii. _____

8. Fats
   A. Fats are also called _____.
   B. They do not dissolve in _____.
   C. Some fat is needed in the diet for _____ _____.
   D. Fats are a major _____ source for the body.
   E. Fats are found in animal and _____ food products.
   F. Fats provide taste, consistency, and _____ to foods.

9. Saturated Fats
   A. Saturated fats are produced by _____ sources.
   B. They have many _____ effects on the body.
   C. No more than _____ of the daily caloric intake should come from saturated fat.
   D. Reducing intake of these fats can help _____ the risk of disease.

10. Unsaturated Fats
    A. Polyunsaturated fat is found in _____ and fish oils.
    B. Monounsaturated fat can lower _____ levels and _____.

11. How Fats Benefit the Body
    A. Fats serve as a(n) _____ energy source.
    B. They help _____ fat-soluble vitamins.
    C. They provide some _____ to foods.
    D. They satisfy the _____.
    E. _____ the skin and internal tissues.
    F. They are _____ for energy use after the meal.

12. Fat Consumption Recommendations
    A. Only _____ of calories should come from saturated fat.
    B. Less than _____ of total calories should come from fat.

13. Sources of Fats (list the sources for each of the following fats)
    A. Saturated Fats: _____
    B. Polyunsaturated Fats: _____
    C. Monounsaturated Fats: _____

14. Protein
    A. Protein forms the _____ of every cell.
    B. It is formed from _____ of amino acids.
    C. Protein is needed by the body to accomplish the following:
       i. _____
       ii. _____
       iii. _____

15. Reading Food Labels
    A. Complete proteins provide all nine of the essential _____.
    B. Combining certain _____ proteins can add up to a complete protein.

16. Water
    A. Water has no _____ value.
    B. The human body is _____ to _____ water.
    C. _____ holds more water.

D. _____ holds less water.

E. The water content is _____ in males than in females and _____ with age.

17. Sources of Water

   i. _____

   ii. _____

   iii. _____

18. The Functions of Water

   A. Water carries _____ and nutrients to cells.

   B. It regulates body _____.

   C. It prevents _____.

   D. It replaces water lost through perspiration, respiration, _____, and _____.

   E. It removes waste products from _____.

   F. It protects _____ and tissues.

19. The Amount of Water Needed Varies Because of the Following Factors

   i. _____

   ii. _____

   iii. _____

   iv. _____

   v. _____

   vi. _____

   vii. _____

20. Vitamin Classifications

   A. Water-Soluble Vitamins (provide examples of water-soluble vitamins)

      i. _____

      ii. _____

      iii. _____

      iv. _____

      v. _____

   B. Fat-Soluble Vitamins (provide examples of fat-soluble vitamins)

      i. _____

      ii. _____

      iii. _____

      iv. _____

21. Requirements for Vitamins

   A. Several conditions increase the requirement for vitamins beyond the usual recommended amounts:

      i. _____

      ii. _____

      iii. _____

      iv. _____

22. Sources of Vitamins: Vitamin B_1 (Thiamine)

      i. _____

      ii. _____

      iii. _____

      iv. _____

v. _____

vi. _____

23. Sources of Vitamins: Vitamin B$_2$ (Riboflavin)

    i. _____

    ii. _____

    iii. _____

    iv. _____

    v. _____

    vi. _____

24. Sources of Vitamins: Vitamin B$_6$

    i. _____

    ii. _____

    iii. _____

    iv. _____

    v. _____

    vi. _____

25. Sources of Vitamins: Vitamin B$_{12}$

    i. _____

    ii. _____

    iii. _____

    iv. _____

    v. _____

26. Sources of Vitamins: Niacin

    i. _____

    ii. _____

    iii. _____

    iv. _____

    v. _____

27. Sources of Vitamins: Biotin

    i. _____

    ii. _____

    iii. _____

28. Sources of Vitamins: Folacin (Folic Acid)

    i. _____

    ii. _____

29. Sources of Vitamins: Pantothenic Acid

    i. _____

    ii. _____

30. Sources of Vitamins: Vitamin C

    i. _____

    ii. _____

    iii. _____

31. Sources of Vitamins: Vitamin A

    i. _____

    ii. _____

    iii. _____

    iv. _____

32. Sources of Vitamins: Vitamin D

    i. _____

    ii. _____

    iii. _____

    iv. _____

    v. _____

    vi. _____

33. Sources of Vitamins: Vitamin E

    i. _____

    ii. _____

    iii. _____

34. Sources of Vitamins: Vitamin K

    i. _____

    ii. _____

    iii. _____

    iv. _____

35. Minerals

    A. Minerals are _____ substances that are of neither plant nor animal origin.

    B. They are found throughout the body, but mainly in _____ and _____.

36. Mineral Classifications

    A. Macrominerals (list the minerals that are classified as macrominerals)

        i. _____

        ii. _____

        iii. _____

        iv. _____

        v. _____

        vi. _____

        vii. _____

    B. Microminerals (list the minerals that are classified as microminerals)

        i. _____

        ii. _____

        iii. _____

        iv. _____

        v. _____

        vi. _____

        vii. _____

        viii. _____

        ix. _____

        x. _____

        xi. _____

        xii. _____

37. Sources of Minerals: Calcium

    i. _____

    ii. _____

    iii. _____

    iv. _____

    v. _____

    vi. _____

38. Sources of Minerals: Copper

    i. _____

    ii. _____

    iii. _____

    iv. _____

    v. _____

39. Sources of Minerals: Fluorine

    i. _____

    ii. _____

    iii. _____

40. Sources of Minerals: Iodine

    i. _____

    ii. _____

    iii. _____

41. Sources of Minerals: Iron

    i. _____

    ii. _____

    iii. _____

    iv. _____

    v. _____

    vi. _____

42. Sources of Minerals: Magnesium

    i. _____

    ii. _____

    iii. _____

    iv. _____

    v. _____

    vi. _____

    vii. _____

43. Sources of Minerals: Phosphorus

    i. _____

    ii. _____

    iii. _____

    iv. _____

    v. _____

    vi. _____

44. Sources of Minerals: Potassium

    i. _____

    ii. _____

    iii. _____

    iv. _____

    v. _____

45. Sources of Minerals: Sodium

    i. _____

    ii. _____

    iii. _____

    iv. _____

    v. _____

    vi. _____

46. Cholesterol

  A. Cholesterol is normally found in and is _____ by the body.
  B. It is _____ for the _____ of bodily systems, such as the nervous system, and for the formation of cell membranes and many hormones.

47. Sources of Cholesterol

  A. The _____ body
  B. Animal _____
  C. Your _____ produces most of the cholesterol in your body (1000 mg/day).

48. Cholesterol in the Body

  A. Cholesterol moves into and out of the body cells within _____.
  B. _____-_____ _____ (HDLs) carry cholesterol away from the bloodstream.
  C. _____-_____ _____ (LDLs) carry most of the cholesterol into the bloodstream.

49. Cholesterol and Disease

  A. An increase in cholesterol is linked to an increase in the following diseases:
      i. _____
      ii. _____

50. Dietary Guidelines for Americans

      i. _____
      ii. _____
      iii. _____
      iv. _____
      v. _____

51. Calories

  A. Food intake is measured in terms of the _____ that food produces.
  B. Calorie: A measurement of a unit of _____ that provides _____.

52. Caloric Requirements

  A. All food (except water) generates _____ in the body.
  B. The daily caloric requirement is based on the following:
      i. _____
      ii. _____
      iii. _____
      iv. _____
  C. Men generally need more _____ than women.
  D. Women require more calories during _____ and _____.

53. Patient Education

  A. Diet _____ should be carefully explained to the patient.
  B. Patients are often referred to a(n) _____ _____ (RD) who will discuss the therapeutic diet with the patient.
  C. The medical assistant will often provide _____ education for patients in the medical office.
  D. _____ _____ are often associated with dietary modification and should be included in patient education.

54. The Clear Liquid Diet

  A. A clear liquid diet contains no _____ _____ or milk products.
  B. It is frequently required before certain _____ _____, examinations, or surgery.
  C. The patient must not remain on a clear liquid diet for _____ periods.

D. Foods Included in a Clear Liquid Diet
    i. _____
    ii. _____
    iii. _____
    iv. _____
    v. _____

55. The Full Liquid Diet

  A. Prescribed for patients who are unable to chew and/or digest solid food because of the following conditions:
    i. _____
    ii. _____
    iii. _____
  B. Often prescribed as the next step after a(n) _____ _____ diet.
  C. Foods Included in a Full Liquid Diet
    i. _____
    ii. _____
    iii. _____
    iv. _____
    v. _____
    vi. _____

56. The Mechanical Soft Diet

  A. This diet is recommended for patients who have _____ _____ or difficulty swallowing.
  B. It is recommended for patients who are recovering from _____.
  C. Foods Included in a Mechanical Soft Diet
    i. _____
    ii. _____
    iii. _____
    iv. _____
    v. _____
    vi. _____
    vii. _____

57. The Bland Diet

  A. This diet contains no seasonings or _____ that are irritating.
  B. It is prescribed for patients who have _____ problems or allergies.
  C. It eliminates foods that are _____ _____ (e.g., cabbage).
  D. It eliminates _____ and spices.
  E. It eliminates foods that are high in _____.
  F. Foods Included in a Bland Diet
    i. _____
    ii. _____
    iii. _____
    iv. _____
    v. _____

58. The BRAT Diet

  A. BRAT stands for _____, _____, _____, and _____.
  B. This diet is prescribed for _____ _____ who are experiencing vomiting, nausea, and diarrhea.

59. The High-Protein Diet

    A. This diet is recommended for patients who are recovering from _____ _____.

    B. It aids in _____.

60. The Diabetic Diet

    A. Considerations for placing a patient on a diabetic diet include the following:

        i. _____

        ii. _____

        iii. _____

        iv. _____

        v. _____

    B. This diet often uses a(n) _____ _____ system to allow patients to select preferred foods.

    C. Foods are grouped into the Food Pyramid categories, which are the following:

        i. _____

        ii. _____

        iii. _____

        iv. _____

        v. _____

        vi. _____

61. The High-Residue/Fiber Diet

    A. This diet is used to treat patients with _____ _____.

    B. Dietary fiber may provide protection against the following diseases or conditions:

        i. _____

        ii. _____

        iii. _____

        iv. _____

        v. _____

        vi. _____

        vii. _____

        viii. _____

    C. This diet may _____ cholesterol.

    D. The recommended daily intake of fiber is _____ to _____ grams per day.

    E. Fiber is not found in _____ products or _____ products.

62. The Low-Residue Diet

    A. The low-residue diet is often called a(n) _____-_____ diet.

    B. It is useful for patients with the following conditions:

        i. _____

        ii. _____

        iii. _____

        iv. _____

    C. Foods Included in a Low-Residue Diet

        i. _____

        ii. _____

        iii. _____

        iv. _____

        v. _____

        vi. _____

        vii. _____

63. The Low-Fat/Cholesterol Diet

    A. This diet is aimed at keeping fat content between _____ and _____ grams of fat per day.

    B. The average American diet contains between _____ and _____ grams of fat per day.

C. This diet may reduce the risk of colon, breast, and _____ cancer; _____ _____; and _____.

D. Foods Included in a Low-Fat/Cholesterol Diet

   i. _____

   ii. _____

   iii. _____

   iv. _____

   v. _____

64. The Low-Sodium/Salt Diet

A. This diet is used for patients with _____ and heart or kidney disease.

B. It is recommended for patients on _____-_____ diets in order to reduce water retention.

65. Guidelines for a Low-Sodium/Salt Diet

A. Mild Restriction: _____ to _____ mg of sodium per day

   i. Allow _____ _____ of table salt per day.

   ii. Limit foods that contain salt, including _____ foods.

B. Moderate Restriction: _____ to _____ mg of sodium per day

   i. Allow _____ _____ of table salt per day.

   ii. No processed and _____ foods with salt

   iii. No salt in food _____

   iv. This is the most _____ low-sodium/salt diet.

C. Severe Restriction: _____ mg of sodium per day

   i. Limit _____ _____ _____, including salt in cooking.

   ii. Use only _____-_____ products.

   iii. Increase the intake of _____ _____ and _____.

   iv. Read _____ carefully.

66. The Caloric Content Diet

A. This diet is often prescribed as a(n) _____-_____ _____ for persons affected by excess weight.

B. It helps to prevent and control the following diseases or conditions:

   i. _____

   ii. _____

   iii. _____

C. The _____-_____ diet uses a balance of the five food groups and low-fat foods.

D. Guidelines for a Low-Calorie-Content Diet

   i. _____

   ii. _____

   iii. _____

   iv. _____

   v. _____

   vi. _____

E. Caloric intake should total _____ calories.

F. Keep a(n) _____ _____.

67. Healthy Food Choices: Eat Less Fat

A. Eat _____ and fish more often.

B. Prepare all meats by roasting, broiling, or _____.

C. Trim off all _____ fat.

D. Remove the _____ from all poultry.

E. Avoid adding _____ during cooking.

F. Eat fewer _____-_____ foods.

G. Drink skim or _____-_____ milk.

68. Healthy Food Choices: Eat More High-Fiber Foods

A. Choose dried beans, _____, and _____ more often.

B. Eat whole-_____ _____, cereals, and crackers.

C. Eat more _____, both raw and cooked.

D. Try _____-_____ foods such as oat bran, barley, brown rice, bulgur, and wild rice.

69. Healthy Food Choices: Use Less Salt

A. Reduce the amount of _____ that you use in cooking.

B. Try not to put _____ on food at the table.

C. Eat fewer _____-_____ foods such as canned soups, ham, hot dogs, pickles, sauerkraut, and foods that taste salty.

70. Healthy Food Choices: Eat Less Sugar

A. Avoid _____ _____, syrup, honey, jam, jelly, candy, sweet rolls, fruit canned in syrup, regular gelatin, desserts, pie, cake with icing, and other sweets.

B. Avoid _____ soft drinks.

C. Choose fresh fruit or fruit canned in _____ _____ or water.

D. If desired, use non-caloric _____ instead of sugar.

KEY TERMINOLOGY REVIEW

Match each of the following vocabulary terms with the correct definition.

a. calorie

b. lactose

c. lipids

d. minerals

e. Recommended Dietary Allowances (RDAs)

1. _____ Recommendations for the amount of protein, vitamins, and minerals that Americans should try to eat for good nutrition (developed by the Food and Nutrition Board of the National Academy of Sciences).

2. _____ Fatty acids that can be chemically classified as saturated or unsaturated.

3. _____ Inorganic elements that are of neither animal nor plant origin.

4. _____ A measurement of a unit of heat that provides energy.

5. _____ The combination of glucose and galactose that is found in animal milk.

APPLIED PRACTICE

Follow the directions as instructed for each question.

> **Scenario**
>
> Emily is a medical assistant working for Dr. Wynn. Melody Hoffstettler is the first patient of the day. Melody has been unable to control her eating for most of her life and has come for help with this issue. Dr. Wynn suggests that Emily start by explaining the revised Food Guide Pyramid as a way to begin the conversation.

1. Pretend that you are Emily and write as if you were talking to Melody.

   _____

   _____

   _____

2. Draw and explain MyPyramid in such a way that Emily will understand and feel encouraged and confident.

LEARNING ACTIVITY: TRUE/FALSE

Indicate whether the following statements are true or false by placing a T or an F on the line that precedes each statement.

_____ 1. Energy released from the metabolization of proteins, fats, and carbohydrates is measured in units of kilograms.

_____ 2. The key to a balanced diet is to eat a variety of foods in the correct amount.

_____ 3. Reducing the intake of fat can also reduce the risk of certain types of cancer.

_____ 4. A good postoperative diet is the full liquid diet.

_____ 5. Children are placed on the BRAT diet when they behave like one.

_____ 6. A person's religion can play a role in his or her nutrition.

_____ 7. In a heart-healthy diet, avoid tuna packed in oil.

_____ 8. Carbohydrates are the body's primary source of energy and are found primarily in breads, cereals, pasta products, rice, fruit, and potatoes.

_____ 9. Vitamins are not sources of energy, but they are required for good health.

_____ 10. Minerals constitute 11% percent of the body.

CHAPTER 59
Professionalism

STUDENT STUDY GUIDE

Use the following guide to assist in your learning of the concepts from the chapter.

I. Professionalism

  1. Office Systems

    A. A system is a(n) _____ interacting group of people who function with an organized set of doctrines and _____ typically recorded in a formal policy and procedures manual.

    B. Having a clear understanding of managers' expectations makes the system function _____.

    C. If a medical assistant does not know how to perform a procedure, an admission must be made to his or her _____ in order that the medical assistant can receive the needed training.

  2. Communication

    A. Communication is perhaps the most important _____ skill.

    B. Many problems can be solved by having effective communication _____ among team members.

  3. Active Listening

    A. While a patient is speaking, if the medical assistant is already beginning to formulate an answer instead of listening, some _____ information may not be heard.

    B. If the physician is giving an order and the medical assistant is thinking of something else, the results can be _____.

    C. Instead of making _____ about what is being said, a medical assistant with good professional skills will focus on the _____ and will ask for clarification if needed.

  4. The Key to Presenting Difficult Concepts

    A. Seek _____ from the listener to make sure that he or she understands.

    B. When communicating with a patient, always take into account the _____ and _____ of the patient.

    C. Use a different _____ depending on the age and mental capacity of the patient.

  5. Critical Thinking

    A. For proper decision making, the medical assistant needs to retrieve _____ facts and events, add _____ to the thinking process, and act in the appropriate manner.

    B. Critical thinking involves differentiating _____ from _____ or opinion.

  6. Insurance Billing and Critical Thinking

    A. The medical assistant must advocate for the patient with the patient's _____ company through a maze of complicated rules for _____.

    B. Thinking critically can improve _____ from the _____ company to the medical practice and greatly relieve the burden on the patient.

7. Laboratory Results and Critical Thinking
    A. Although the medical assistant should never diagnose a patient, it is the medical assistant's responsibility to bring _____ results to the physician's attention.
    B. A critically thinking medical assistant will take in all information before forming a(n) _____.

8. Value Judgments
    A. A medical assistant must make value judgments on a(n) _____ basis.
    B. Critical thinking should become so _____ that the medical assistant is comfortable with value judgments.

9. Teamwork in the Medical Setting
    A. Teamwork is a critical workplace _____.
    B. All medical assistants need to understand how the team functions and be prepared to share _____.
    C. The medical assistant should practice only within his or her own _____ of practice.

10. Diversity in the Medical Office
    A. It is in everyone's best interest that _____, stereotypes, and prejudices be put aside.
    B. Holding grudges or _____ beliefs can prevent the team from functioning smoothly.

11. Managing Priorities
    A. Patient priorities may be managed by a combination of an efficient _____ and a(n) _____ system.
    B. Because the medical assistant is versatile, he or she may be asked to do _____ tasks over a short length of time.
    C. If a medical assistant is distracted by family issues or other personal problems, it can be detrimental and have a(n) _____ impact on job performance.

12. Stress Management (explain how each of the following techniques helps with stress management)
    A. Aromatherapy: _____
    B. Biofeedback: _____
    C. Deep breathing: _____
    D. Distraction: _____
    E. Exercise: _____
    F. Guided imagery: _____
    G. Hypnosis: _____
    H. Humor: _____
    I. Meditation and prayer: _____
    J. Music: _____
    K. Relaxation: _____
    L. Slow breath counting: _____
    M. Water therapy: _____
    N. Heat: _____
    O. Cold: _____
    P. Pressure: _____

13. Time Management
    A. Time management requires the ability to _____ what the important tasks are and to complete them on _____.
    B. One of the main responsibilities of the office manager or medical assistant is to manage all of the _____ office functions.

C. Before establishing a time management system, it is important to define office
_____ with the physician.

14. Professional Dress (list what constitutes professional attire)

    i. _____

   ii. _____

  iii. _____

  iv. _____

   v. _____

  vi. _____

 vii. _____

viii. _____

KEY TERMINOLOGY REVIEW

Match each of the following vocabulary terms with the correct definition.

a. Affective

b. Biofeedback

c. Lifelong learning

d. Psychomotor

e. System

1. _____ is a type of therapy that utilizes biological information in order to relieve stress.

2. _____ skills are behaviors that come from feelings and emotions and are truly important in the medical office.

3. _____ refers to coordination of mind and body.

4. A(n) _____ is a regularly interacting group of people who function with an organized set of doctrines and principles.

5. _____ is the process of continuing to learn throughout one's life.

APPLIED PRACTICE

Read the scenario and answer the following questions.

Scenario

John Summers is an office manager at Hillcrest Family Medicine. The physicians at the office have voiced concern to John regarding the lack of professionalism among the office staff. They have asked John to conduct a staff meeting to focus on the importance of professionalism. The physicians have asked that John highlight five qualities of a professional in a health care setting. The physicians have also asked John to decide upon appropriate consequences for unprofessional behavior.

1. What five qualities do you think John should choose to discuss during the staff meeting? Explain why.

_____

_____

_____

2. How do you think John should handle this request by the physicians for him to decide on consequences for unprofessional behavior? What consequences do you think would be appropriate for unprofessional behavior?

_____

_____

_____

LEARNING ACTIVITY: TRUE/FALSE

Indicate whether the following statements are true or false by placing a T or an F on the line that precedes each statement.

_____ 1. It is very important that the medical assistant always engage in active listening.

_____ 2. When communicating in the health care environment, accuracy is more important than brevity.

_____ 3. Critical thinking involves differentiating fact from fiction or opinion.

_____ 4. The first step in resolving conflicts is to seek to understand the situation.

_____ 5. If two workers are in conflict, it may be wise to ask a peer to resolve the conflict.

_____ 6. The office manager generally has most of the control over the tasks presented in the office.

_____ 7. Urgent tasks are not necessarily important tasks.

_____ 8. Stress can be caused by pain.

_____ 9. In the busy medical office, many tasks may have to be deferred to a later time.

_____ 10. It is not the medical assistant's job to question laboratory results that do not seem to be consistent with the patient's presentation.

CRITICAL THINKING

Answer the following questions to the best of your ability. Use the textbook as a reference.

1. In preparation for his externship, Stefan Marquise has been assigned to write an essay on barriers to professionalism in the health care setting. What information should Stefan include in his essay?

_____

_____

_____

2. A very angry patient asks to talk with the office manager. The patient explains to the office manager that she overheard two staff members discussing the test results of another patient, who happens to be her sister-in-law. How should the office manager handle this situation?

_____

_____

_____

3. Karen, the office manager, has noticed that a medical assistant, Charles, has been answering his cell phone while at work, as well as checking his e-mail between patients. Today, Charles's wife came to the office to talk with Charles during the busy morning hours. How should Karen address Charles's unprofessional behavior?

_____

_____

_____

RESEARCH ACTIVITY

Use Internet search engines to research the following topic and write a brief description of what you find. It is important to use reputable websites.

1. Type the word "professionalism" into an Internet search engine. What are some of the most interesting and helpful results that are returned with your search?

_____

_____

_____

_____

CHAPTER 60
Externship and Career Opportunities

STUDENT STUDY GUIDE

Use the following guide to assist in your learning of the concepts from the chapter.

I. Preparing for the Externship and Certification Examination

   1. The Externship Experience

      A. An externship is a situation in which one leaves the classroom and works, without _____, in a health care setting under the supervision of someone at the site.

      B. It offers the student an opportunity to get _____-_____-_____ experience.

      C. It can be as short as _____ weeks or as long as one semester of school.

      D. Schools that are accredited by the Council on Accreditation of Allied Health Education Programs (CAAHEP) in conjunction with the AAMA require an externship of a minimum of _____ hours.

      E. The American Medical Technologists require a similar experience, which is known as a(n) _____.

      F. Both professional organizations expect the graduates to have had actual _____ experiences in a real-world medical office in order to be certified.

      G. The externship experience should provide the medical assistant with ample experience in both _____ and _____ skills.

      H. Ideally, the practicum or externship experience is carefully monitored by the clinical instructor or _____/_____ coordinator so that any problems that may arise can be addressed.

   2. The Benefits of Participating in an Externship

      A. Having the opportunity to see how a physician's office, _____ _____, or clinic operates on a day-to-day basis

      B. Being exposed to a variety of different _____ in a work setting

      C. Gaining additional experience using skills such as the following:

         i. _____

         ii. _____

         iii. _____

      D. Learning how to budget your _____ and _____ your workday, school day, and home life

   3. Areas Evaluated in the Externship

         i. _____

         ii. _____

         iii. _____

         iv. _____

         v. _____

         vi. _____

         vii. _____

         viii. _____

4. The Role of the Preceptor
   A. The preceptor provides additional _____ and _____ for the student by observing the performance of particular skills.
   B. He or she provides a(n) _____, _____ _____ for the student, usually at the midpoint and end point.
   C. The preceptor looks for continual _____ in skills as the student gains confidence.
   D. The student should make every attempt to establish a(n) _____, or a comfortable working relationship, with the preceptor.

5. Areas Covered on a Typical Evaluation Form
   i. _____
   ii. _____
   iii. _____
   iv. _____
   v. _____
   vi. _____
   vii. _____
   viii. _____
   ix. _____
   x. _____
   xi. _____
   xii. _____
   xiii. _____
   xiv. _____
   xv. _____

6. Evaluating the Externship Experience (What questions could you ask yourself in order to evaluate your externship experience?)
   i. _____
   ii. _____
   iii. _____
   iv. _____

7. The AAMA Certification Exam
   A. This exam is given at numerous _____ _____ throughout the United States.
   B. It is available only to medical assistants who have completed a(n) _____-_____ program in medical assisting.
   C. The Certified Medical Assistant (CMA) examination is a comprehensive test that includes the following:
      i. _____
      ii. _____
      iii. _____

8. Major Areas Tested on the CMA (AAMA) and RMA (AMT) Examinations
   A. General
      i. _____
      ii. _____
      iii. _____
      iv. _____
   B. Administrative
      i. _____
      ii. _____
      iii. _____
      iv. _____
      v. _____

C. Clinical

    i. _____

    ii. _____

    iii. _____

    iv. _____

    v. _____

9. Taking the (RMA) (AMT) and CMA Certification Exams

  A. Examinations are available at numerous computer centers throughout the _____.

  B. Students should _____ while answering the sample test questions, because the actual examination is timed.

II. Getting Hired

  1. Preparing for Your Job Search

    i. _____

    ii. _____

    iii. _____

    iv. _____

  2. The Six Most Common Job Search Mistakes

    i. _____

    ii. _____

    iii. _____

    iv. _____

    v. _____

    vi. _____

  3. Where to Search for Jobs

    i. _____

    ii. _____

    iii. _____

    iv. _____

    v. _____

    vi. _____

    vii. _____

    viii. _____

    ix. _____

    x. _____

    xi. _____

  4. Writing a Résumé

  A. A résumé should be typed on 8½" × 11", good-quality _____ or off-_____ paper.

  B. Do not use _____ colored paper.

  C. A résumé should be neatly typed and _____ free.

  D. Always use a(n) _____ _____ to prepare your résumé so that you can easily update it.

  E. Always have a backup copy of your résumé stored on a disk, _____ _____, or other type of storage device.

  F. _____ your résumé to make sure that it is error free.

  5. Standard Items on a Résumé

    i. _____

    ii. _____

iii. _____

iv. _____

v. _____

vi. _____

vii. _____

6. The Heading

   A. Your name, address, and telephone number are prepared as a(n) _____ _____ at the top of the page.

   B. If you have a cellular phone number and a(n) _____ _____, this information can also be included.

   C. When this information is printed in slightly _____ type than the rest of the text, it stands out and provides an easy reference for the reader.

7. The Objective

   A. Listing an objective lets the reader know your _____ goals.

   B. When you write your objective, it should be _____ and to the point with regard to what you want in a career.

   C. Your objective may need to be _____, depending on where you are sending your résumé.

8. Education

   A. If you are still a student or are a recent graduate with limited work experience, list your education first, in _____ _____ order, beginning with the most recent school/program.

   B. Add any educational experiences that you have had, such as _____, _____, and courses.

9. Employment

   A. List your work experience in the _____ chronological order.

   B. Include externship or practicum experience with a brief description of your _____.

10. Professional Organizations and Memberships

   A. Belonging to a professional organization can be a wonderful experience. It helps you to stay _____ on topics related to your career.

   B. Being a member and participating in a(n) _____ shows your dedication, commitment, and loyalty to your chosen career field.

   C. Many schools have organized a(n) _____ _____ _____.

   D. For a yearly fee, students or graduates can also obtain membership in the _____ or the _____ _____ _____.

11. Credentials

   A. Include information about your professional credentials, such as _____ (AAMA) certification or _____ (AMT) registration.

   B. If you do not have any credentials, _____ _____ include this section on your résumé.

12. References

   A. The references section should never include the name, address, and phone number of the _____ you will be using.

   B. You need to indicate only that references are _____ _____ _____.

13. Items NOT to Be Included on a Résumé

   i. _____

   ii. _____

iii. _____

iv. _____

v. _____

vi. _____

vii. _____

viii. _____

14. Considerations Regarding Your References

    A. State at the _____ of your résumé that references will be furnished upon request.

    B. Type on a separate piece of paper a list of at least _____ references with their addresses and phone numbers.

    C. Names of references are generally not included on the _____ _____.

    D. Obtain permission to use a(n) _____ as a reference.

    E. It is wise to include the names of _____, as well as personal references.

15. Characteristics of the Cover Letter

    A. The cover letter should be _____.

    B. It is not a(n) _____ of everything that is in your résumé.

    C. Explain what you can do for the employer and why your qualifications are a good _____ for the employer's requirements.

    D. Be sure to include an address and _____ _____ where you can be reached.

    E. Do not add _____ comments or additional information to your cover letter.

    F. Always review the _____ of the employer's name and address carefully for accuracy.

    G. If you have word processing capability, you may wish to _____ several _____ cover letters that you can then access from your computer and add the appropriate heading.

16. Common Mistakes to Avoid When Writing a Cover Letter

    A. Failing to _____ the letter to a specific person in the organization

    B. Failing to clearly state the _____ for which you are applying

    C. Sending a cover letter that is too long; _____ _____ works best.

    D. Sending a letter that is poorly _____ has spelling or typographical errors

    E. Always send the _____ cover letter, never a copy.

17. Reference Materials for Interviewing (list some reference materials that you can use to prepare for an interview)

    i. _____

    ii. _____

    iii. _____

    iv. _____

18. Dressing for the Interview: What to Avoid

    i. _____

    ii. _____

    iii. _____

    iv. _____

    v. _____

    vi. _____

    vii. _____

    viii. _____

    ix. _____

    x. _____

    xi. _____

19. Dressing for the Interview: What to Wear

    i. _____

    ii. _____

    iii. _____

    iv. _____

    v. _____

    vi. _____

    vii. _____

    viii. _____

20. Guidelines for the Interview

    A. Provide a copy of your résumé and references to the _____.

    B. Never give dishonest or _____ answers.

    C. Know what questions are _____ from being asked in an interview.

    D. Do not make _____ or _____ the focus of the first interview.

    E. Be _____ when the interview is over.

21. The Ten Most Common Errors Committed When Interviewing

    i. _____

    ii. _____

    iii. _____

    iv. _____

    v. _____

    vi. _____

    vii. _____

    viii. _____

    ix. _____

    x. _____

22. Documentation for Completing an Application

    i. _____

    ii. _____

    iii. _____

    iv. _____

    v. _____

23. After the Interview

    A. Always send a letter thanking the interviewer for his or her _____.

        i. It is a good opportunity to again express your _____ in the position.

        ii. Be meticulous about proofreading your letter for mistakes. It may be your final _____ _____ with the interviewer before the decision to hire is made.

    B. You may wish to call the office a few days later to ask about the _____ made on filling the position.

    C. If you are offered a position and decide not to accept it, you would use the same _____ when turning down an offer as you would use when accepting one.

24. Six Basic Skills That Employers Want

    i. _____

    ii. _____

    iii. _____

    iv. _____

    v. _____

    vi. _____

25. Characteristics That Employers Want to See in a Medical Assistant
    i. _____
    ii. _____
    iii. _____
    iv. _____
    v. _____

KEY TERMINOLOGY REVIEW

Match each of the following vocabulary terms with the correct definition.

a. blind ad
b. personal assessment
c. preceptor

d. professional reference
e. proofread

1. _____ Does not identify the institution or facility that placed the ad.

2. _____ Statement of someone who has either worked with you or has known you for a period of time.

3. _____ Making sure that your résumé and cover letter are error free in content and typing.

4. _____ Self-evaluation of strengths and weaknesses.

5. _____ Provides additional instruction and guidance for a student by observing the performance of particular skills.

APPLIED PRACTICE

Assume that you are a recent medical assistant graduate preparing to enter the workforce.

1. You have recently received a phone call for an interview for Mountain View Health Care Center. How will you research the medical facility prior to your interview, and why is this important?

   _____
   _____
   _____

2. Considering your current wardrobe, which outfit would you choose to wear to your interview and why?

   _____
   _____
   _____

3. Practice writing a cover letter to go along with your application. Submit your letter with your completed workbook materials.

LEARNING ACTIVITY: MULTIPLE CHOICE

Circle the correct answer to each of the following questions.

1. The _____ is a fellow medical assistant who will serve as a resource for the student medical assistant during the externship.

   a. office manager
   b. mentor
   c. physician
   d. None of the above

2. Which of the following is a responsibility of the student medical assistant during the externship?

   a. Be on time.
   b. Dress appropriately.
   c. Act in a professional manner.
   d. All of the above

3. Which of the following should *not* be part of an interview?

   a. Have a specific job in mind when you interview so that you project self-assurance.
   b. Prepare responses should the interviewer ask you difficult questions or ask you to describe yourself.
   c. Show off your legs.
   d. Carry extra copies of your résumé.

4. When a student medical assistant has a concern about something at the externship site, to whom should the student bring the problem?

   a. The medical assisting program director
   b. A coworker
   c. The student's spouse
   d. The dean of the college

5. Which of the following may be a reason that a medical assistant may not be called for an interview?

   a. The résumé contains typographical errors.
   b. The résumé contains grammatical errors.
   c. The résumé contains crossed-out words and handwritten corrections.
   d. All of the above

6. A résumé should ideally be _____ pages in length.

   a. two to three
   b. one to two
   c. three to four
   d. four to five

7. A thank-you note should be sent to the potential employer after an interview within _____ days.

   a. 1–2
   b. 2–3
   c. 3–5
   d. 6–8

8. Which of the following are places that a medical assistant might look for employment?

    a. The newspaper
    b. The local medical assisting program
    c. An employment agency
    d. All of the above

9. Which of the following is an interview "don't"?

    a. Requesting parking validation
    b. Arriving a bit early
    c. Taking notes
    d. All of the above

10. Which of the following is an appropriate dress code for an applicant going to a job interview?

    a. Casual attire
    b. Business suit
    c. Scrubs
    d. Any of the above

CRITICAL THINKING

Answer the following questions to the best of your ability. Use the textbook as a reference.

1. Willie Harrison is finishing his medical assisting training and is preparing for his externship experience. Willie's wife asks him what he will be doing during his externship. How might Willie answer her question?

    _____

    _____

    _____

2. Joann Felmer is a student in an administrative medical assisting course. She has been given an assignment to describe the benefits of the externship experience for the student medical assistant. How might Joann answer this question?

    _____

    _____

    _____

3. Corey Rubatino, CMA (AAMA), has recently been hired to work for Dr. Joe Cresanti. On Corey's first day, he has been asked by Dr. Cresanti to describe what is meant by practicing within his scope of practice. How might Corey answer this question?

    _____

    _____

    _____

4. Maggie Levinski, RMA, is the program director in an accredited medical assisting program. She is attempting to add new externship sites to the program roster. When Maggie meets with someone from a potential site, she is asked to explain the benefits of the externship to the site. How might Maggie answer this question?

    _____

    _____

    _____

RESEARCH ACTIVITY

Use Internet search engines to research the following topic and write a brief description of what you find. It is important to use reputable websites.

1. Using the Internet and other sources, locate prospective job opportunities for medical assistants in your area. Which jobs interest you most? Explain why.

    _____

    _____

    _____

    _____

    _____

Competency Check-Offs

Affective Behaviors

Affective behaviors are very important to the role of medical assisting. These behaviors display sensitivity to the patient, convey an understanding of laws and regulations, and also provide an overall professional component to the medical assisting profession.

The weighed competencies that are found in the student workbook vary slightly from the competencies found in the textbook. The competencies within the student workbook have placed an emphasis on these affective behaviors by showing them in a **bold and _italicized_** font. Not all procedures will have affective behaviors; affective behaviors will primarily be addressed during a procedure that involves direct patient contact.

Your instructors will be expecting to see these behaviors demonstrated during the performance of a procedure, as necessary. Failure to exhibit these affective behaviors will result in a loss of points associated with the point value of the given step. It is essential to review the weighted competencies found in the workbook prior to being tested and graded.

Procedure 5-1:

Effective Listening Skills

Objective: Use effective listening skills to obtain chief complaint from patient.

Supplies: Patient history form

Affective Behaviors: Affective behaviors provide a professional approach to a skill that enhances the patient encounter. These behaviors may also display sensitivity to a patient's rights and enhance communication. Pay close attention to these skills, which will be in ***bold, italicized*** font.

Notes to the Student

_____

_____

_____

_____

_____

_____

Skills Assessment Requirements

Read and familiarize yourself with the procedure; complete the minimum practice requirements (MPRs). Document each MPR using proper charting technique. Complete each procedure within a reasonable amount of time, with a minimum of 85% accuracy.

Name: _____

Date: _____

POINT VALUE ✦ = 3–6 points ✳ = 7–9 points		PRACTICE TRIAL	GRADED TRIAL # 1	GRADED TRIAL # 2	NOTES
1. ✦	Identify patient.				
2. ✳	**Smile and establish eye contact.** *Explain why this is important.*				
3. ✦	Seat the patient in the appropriate area.				
4. ✳	**Focus full attention on patient.**				
5. ✦	Ask the patient the reason for the appointment.				
6. ✦	Ask open-ended questions.				
7. ✳	Do not interrupt the patient.				
8. ✳	**Provide feedback by paraphrasing what the patient said.**				
9. ✳	**Observe the patient for signs of needing to give more information.**				
10. ✦	**Restate the chief complaint before leaving the patient.**				
11. ✳	**Conclude the patient interview in an appropriate manner.**				
12. ✳	Document the chief complaint.				

Name: _____

Date: _____

Document: Enter the appropriate information in the chart below.

Grading

Points Earned	_____		
Points Possible	_____	90	90
Percent Grade (Points Earned/Points Possible)	_____		
PASS:	_____	❏ YES ❏ NO ❏ N/A	❏ YES ❏ NO ❏ N/A

Instructor Sign-Off

Instructor: _____   **Date:** _____

Procedure 5-2:

Assisting the Hearing-Impaired Patient

Objective: Use effective communication skills to assist a hearing-impaired patient prepare for a physical examination.

Supplies: Paper and pencil

Affective Behaviors: Affective behaviors provide a professional approach to a skill that enhances the patient encounter. These behaviors may also display sensitivity to a patient's rights and enhance communication. Pay close attention to these skills, which will be in ***bold, italicized*** font.

Notes to the Student

_____

_____

_____

_____

_____

_____

Skills Assessment Requirements

Read and familiarize yourself with the procedure; complete the minimum practice requirements (MPRs). Document each MPR using proper charting technique. Complete each procedure within a reasonable amount of time, with a minimum of 85% accuracy.

Competency Check-Offs **513**

Name: _____

Date: _____

POINT VALUE ✦ = 3–6 points ✳ = 7–9 points		PRACTICE TRIAL	GRADED TRIAL # 1	GRADED TRIAL # 2	NOTES
1. ✦	Identify patient.				
2. ✦	Reduce external noise as much as possible.				
3. ✳	**Smile, establish eye contact, and face the patient.**				
4. ✦	**Speak slowly and do not shout.**				
5. ✦	Provide careful explanation of the procedure.				
6. ✦	**Provide paper and pen for the patient to use if desired.**				
7. ✦	Use written information to reinforce the message for the patient.				
8. ✦	If possible, have the patient repeat your response to ensure that the message was received accurately.				
9. ✦	**Give directions using actions as well as words.**				
10. ✦	**Be sensitive to the patient's needs.**				
11. ✦	**Employ an empathetic, professional attitude.**				
12. ✳	Notify physician of any patient concerns.				

Name: _____

Date: _____

Document: Enter the appropriate information in the chart below.

Grading

Points Earned	_____		
Points Possible	_____	78	78
Percent Grade (Points Earned/Points Possible)	_____		
PASS:	_____	❑ YES ❑ NO ❑ N/A	❑ YES ❑ NO ❑ N/A

Instructor Sign-Off

Instructor: _____ **Date:** _____

Procedure 6-1:

Handling a Fire in the Medical Office

Objective: To respond to a fire in the medical office.

Supplies: Policy and procedures manual; evacuation maps of the office

Affective Behaviors: Affective behaviors provide a professional approach to a skill that enhances the patient encounter. These behaviors may also display sensitivity to a patient's rights and enhance communication. Pay close attention to these skills, which will be in **bold, *italicized*** font.

Notes to the Student

_____

_____

_____

_____

_____

_____

Skills Assessment Requirements

Read and familiarize yourself with the procedure; complete the minimum practice requirements (MPRs). Document each MPR using proper charting technique. Complete each procedure within a reasonable amount of time, with a minimum of 85% accuracy.

Name: _____

Date: _____

Note: Planned fire drills should be executed at least annually and preferably more frequently so that all employees know their role and expectations in the event of an actual disaster.

POINT VALUE ✦ = 3–6 points ✳ = 7–9 points		PRACTICE TRIAL	GRADED TRIAL # 1	GRADED TRIAL # 2	NOTES
1. ✳	As soon as a fire is discovered, call 911 or the local fire department, following the same procedure as practiced during fire drills.				
2. ✦	Activate the established mechanism for signaling fire within the office. This may mean pulling the alarm, calling a code over the intercom, or taking other action.				
3. ✦	All staff should calmly and quickly assist in getting all patients out of the office in an orderly manner, following the exit routes on the posted evacuation maps, and using the stairs, if applicable.				
4. ✦	If the fire is contained, attempt to extinguish it using the fire extinguisher. However, if the fire is not contained, valuable time should not be spent attempting to extinguish it. Instead, evacuation should promptly begin.				
5. ✦	The individual charged with ensuring that all rooms are cleared should quickly go through the office to confirm that no one is left behind.				
6. ✦	After each room is evacuated, the door is to be closed.				
7. ✦	Staff and patients should gather away from the building at the predetermined area.				

Name: _____

Date: _____

Document: Enter the appropriate information in the chart below.

Grading

Points Earned	_____		
Points Possible	_____	45	45
Percent Grade (Points Earned/Points Possible)	_____		
PASS:	_____	❏ YES ❏ NO ❏ N/A	❏ YES ❏ NO ❏ N/A

Instructor Sign-Off

Instructor: _____ **Date:** _____

Name: _____

Date: _____

Procedure 6-2:

Proper Use of an Eyewash Device

Objective: To effectively use an eyewash station to remove hazardous materials from the eyes.

Supplies: Eyewash station attached to a sink faucet; drying towel

Affective Behaviors: Affective behaviors provide a professional approach to a skill that enhances the patient encounter. These behaviors may also display sensitivity to a patient's rights and enhance communication. Pay close attention to these skills, which will be in ***bold, italicized*** font.

Notes to the Student

_____

_____

_____

_____

_____

_____

Skills Assessment Requirements

Read and familiarize yourself with the procedure; complete the minimum practice requirements (MPRs). Document each MPR using proper charting technique. Complete each procedure within a reasonable amount of time, with a minimum of 85% accuracy.

POINT VALUE ✦ = 3–6 points ✳ = 7–9 points		PRACTICE TRIAL	GRADED TRIAL # 1	GRADED TRIAL # 2	NOTES
1. ✳	When an irritant has entered the eye(s), immediately notify a coworker and go to the eyewash station.				
2. ✦	Remove glasses and/or contact lenses. DO NOT RUB THE EYES.				
3. ✦	Remove the caps or covers from the eyewash device and start the flow of water.				
4. ✦	Place head over the stream of water, holding both eyes open. Even if only one eye was affected, both eyes should be washed. Be careful that the contaminant from the affected eye does not get in the unaffected eye.				
5. ✦	For a mild irritation, 5 minutes of flushing with water should be sufficient. However, if the irritant was a corrosive material, it is recommended to flush for up to 60 minutes to ensure the chemical is thoroughly rinsed from the eyes.				
6. ✦	Seek medical attention to have the eyes examined.				
7. ✦	Complete an incident report.				

Name: _____

Date: _____

Document: Enter the appropriate information in the chart below.

Grading

Points Earned	_____		
Points Possible	_____	45	45
Percent Grade (Points Earned/Points Possible)	_____		
PASS:	_____	❏ YES ❏ NO ❏ N/A	❏ YES ❏ NO ❏ N/A

Instructor Sign-Off

Instructor: _____   **Date:** _____

Procedure 6-3:

Housekeeping Using OSHA Guidelines

Objective: Safely clean and disinfect contaminated surfaces.

Supplies: Prepared spill kit; gloves; 1:10 bleach/water solution; dustpan; broom; sharps container; biohazard bag or container

Affective Behaviors: Affective behaviors provide a professional approach to a skill that enhances the patient encounter. These behaviors may also display sensitivity to a patient's rights and enhance communication. Pay close attention to these skills, which will be in **bold, *italicized*** font.

Notes to the Student

_____

_____

_____

_____

_____

_____

Skills Assessment Requirements

Read and familiarize yourself with the procedure; complete the minimum practice requirements (MPRs). Document each MPR using proper charting technique. Complete each procedure within a reasonable amount of time, with a minimum of 85% accuracy.

POINT VALUE ✦ = 3–6 points ✳ = 7–9 points		PRACTICE TRIAL	GRADED TRIAL # 1	GRADED TRIAL # 2	NOTES
1. ✳	Before performing any housekeeping procedures, ensure the appropriate PPE has been applied. See Figure A in text.				
2. ✦	For any wet spills, use the prepared spill kit according to package directions.				
3. ✳	Immediately after exposure to infectious materials, clean and disinfect contaminated surfaces with a 1:10 bleach/water solution. All surfaces must be decontaminated on a regular schedule. This schedule must be posted, signed by the person who performs the decontamination, and kept with OSHA records.				
4. ✦	Properly bag contaminated clothing and laundry in leak-proof labeled biohazard bags. Contaminated laundry should not be handled or washed at the medical office or with any uncontaminated clothing.				
5. ✦	Replace a damaged biohazard bag by placing a second bag around the first. Do not remove infectious material from the damaged bag.				
6. ✦	Biohazardous waste must be removed by a licensed waste disposal service and incinerated or autoclaved before it is placed in a designated landfill area.				
7. ✦	Use puncture-proof, sealable, biohazard sharps containers for all needles and sharps, such as razors and glass pipettes.				

Name: _____

Date: _____

POINT VALUE ✦ = 3–6 points ✶ = 7–9 points		PRACTICE TRIAL	GRADED TRIAL # 1	GRADED TRIAL # 2	NOTES
8. ✦	Place each sharps container close to the work area, and ensure that each container remains upright.				
9. ✦	Replace a sharps container when it is two-thirds full.				
10. ✦	Seal and label each sharps container before placing it with the biohazardous waste for removal by the disposal service.				
11. ✦	In the event of broken glass, use a dustpan or other mechanical device, such as a hemostat or another type of forceps, to pick it up. Never pick up broken glass with hands.				
12. ✦	Properly dispose of any PPE used during housekeeping. Failure to do so may result in an OSHA citation.				
13. ✶	Perform hand hygiene both before and after using gloves.				

Name: _____

Date: _____

Document: Enter the appropriate information in the chart below.

Grading

Points Earned	_____		
Points Possible	_____	84	84
Percent Grade (Points Earned/Points Possible)	_____		
PASS:	_____	❑ YES ❑ NO ❑ N/A	❑ YES ❑ NO ❑ N/A

Instructor Sign-Off

Instructor: _____   Date: _____

Procedure 7-1:

Answering the Telephone and Placing Calls on Hold

Objective: Ensure that the telephone is answered in a professional manner and that, if necessary, patients are placed on hold appropriately.

Supplies: Telephone; message pad; pen; notepad

Affective Behaviors: Affective behaviors provide a professional approach to a skill that enhances the patient encounter. These behaviors may also display sensitivity to a patient's rights and enhance communication. Pay close attention to these skills, which will be in **bold, italicized** font.

Notes to the Student

_____

_____

_____

_____

_____

_____

Skills Assessment Requirements

Read and familiarize yourself with the procedure; complete the minimum practice requirements (MPRs). Document each MPR using proper charting technique. Complete each procedure within a reasonable amount of time, with a minimum of 85% accuracy.

POINT VALUE ✦ = 3–6 points ✶ = 7–9 points		PRACTICE TRIAL	GRADED TRIAL # 1	GRADED TRIAL # 2	NOTES
1. ✶	Answer the telephone by at least the third ring, with the mouthpiece 1 to 2 inches from your mouth.				
2. ✦	**Smile and speak clearly, using inflection, a pleasant tone, and a moderate rate of speech.**				
3. ✦	Answer using the greeting your office prefers (e.g., "Thank you for calling Dr. Smith's office. This is Carlos. How may I help you?").				
4. ✶	At this point, callers will typically identify themselves. If not, ask callers to identify themselves and then verify the information against the patient's medical record.				
5. ✶	Listen to the caller closely to verify the reason for the call, which may include, but is not limited to, the following: • a patient calling to schedule an appointment • a patient calling to request a prescription refill • another physician's office calling about a mutual patient • an insurance company calling regarding a patient's claim • a relative or friend of an office employee or physician				
6. ✶	Once you have determined the reason for the call, act accordingly while providing excellent customer service.				
	In busy offices, you may need to answer more than one incoming telephone line. When this occurs, you will combine the procedure just described with the following steps.				

Name: _____

Date: _____

POINT VALUE ✦ = 3–6 points ✶ = 7–9 points		PRACTICE TRIAL	GRADED TRIAL # 1	GRADED TRIAL # 2	NOTES
7. ✶	When you are speaking with one caller and another incoming line rings, you must notify the current caller that another line is ringing and ask if the current caller can hold. Wait for the caller's response, and then place the first call on hold.				
8. ✦	Answer the second call following the procedures described, ask the second caller if he or she can hold, wait for a response, and then place the second call on hold.				
	(If the second call is an emergency, do not ask the person to hold and assist the caller immediately.)				
9. ✦	Return to the first call, **thank the caller for holding, and continue assisting the person**. When you return to that caller, do not ask "Who are you waiting for?" because it conveys the impression that you have forgotten about that person.				
10. ✦	Once the first call is completed, return to the second call, **thank the person for holding,** and continue assisting that caller.				
11. ✦	If the caller asks to speak with another employee who is not readily available and it is necessary to place the call on hold, check back with the caller approximately every 30 seconds. This lets the caller know you are actively working on his or her behalf, and it also provides an opportunity for the caller to leave a message instead of continuing to hold.				

Document: Enter the appropriate information in the chart below.

Grading

Points Earned	_____		
Points Possible	_____	81	81
Percent Grade (Points Earned/Points Possible)	_____		
PASS:	_____	❏ YES ❏ NO ❏ N/A	❏ YES ❏ NO ❏ N/A

Instructor Sign-Off

Instructor: _____ **Date:** _____

Name: _____

Date: _____

Procedure 7-2:

Taking a Telephone Message

Objective: Ensure that the correct and relevant information is retrieved when taking a telephone message.

Supplies: Message form or pad with carbon or carbonless for duplicates; pen; electronic health record if available

Affective Behaviors: Affective behaviors provide a professional approach to a skill that enhances the patient encounter. These behaviors may also display sensitivity to a patient's rights and enhance communication. Pay close attention to these skills, which will be in **_bold, italicized_** font.

Notes to the Student

_____

_____

_____

_____

_____

_____

Skills Assessment Requirements

Read and familiarize yourself with the procedure; complete the minimum practice requirements (MPRs). Document each MPR using proper charting technique. Complete each procedure within a reasonable amount of time, with a minimum of 85% accuracy.

Name: _____

Date: _____

POINT VALUE ✦ = 3–6 points ✳ = 7–9 points		PRACTICE TRIAL	GRADED TRIAL # 1	GRADED TRIAL # 2	NOTES
1. ✦	***Smile before answering the telephone and, in a warm voice, properly answer the telephone.***				
2. ✦	Use a message form to keep record of the message, or document it directly in the electronic health record.)				
3. ✦	Record the date and time of the call.				
4. ✳	Record the caller's full name and a callback number with area code for use during office hours. (Always ask the caller to spell his or her name and provide another identifier, such as date of birth or Social Security number.) If recording the message in an electronic health record, verify that you have the correct patient record.				
5. ✳	Document for whom the message is intended.				
6. ✳	Document the complete message. Avoid using abbreviations, other than accepted medical abbreviations. Include symptoms, such as temperature, rash, and emesis, as well as duration of symptoms.				
7. ✳	***Thank the patient for calling and, before hanging up the telephone, ask if he or she has any other questions.***				
8. ✳	To indicate that you took a handwritten message, either write out your first and last name or record the initial of your first name and your last name spelled out. If using an electronic health record, save the message and forward it to the intended recipient.				

Name: _____

Date: _____

Document: Enter the appropriate information in the chart below.

Grading

Points Earned	_____		
Points Possible	_____	54	54
Percent Grade (Points Earned/Points Possible)	_____		
PASS:	_____	❏ YES ❏ NO ❏ N/A	❏ YES ❏ NO ❏ N/A

Instructor Sign-Off

Instructor: _____   **Date:** _____

Procedure 7-3:

Taking a Prescription Refill Message

Objective: Ensure that correct information is acquired when refilling a patient's prescription.

Supplies: Message pad or paper; pen

Affective Behaviors: Affective behaviors provide a professional approach to a skill that enhances the patient encounter. These behaviors may also display sensitivity to a patient's rights and enhance communication. Pay close attention to these skills, which will be in **_bold, italicized_** font.

Notes to the Student

_____

_____

_____

_____

_____

_____

Skills Assessment Requirements

Read and familiarize yourself with the procedure; complete the minimum practice requirements (MPRs). Document each MPR using proper charting technique. Complete each procedure within a reasonable amount of time, with a minimum of 85% accuracy.

Name: _____

Date: _____

POINT VALUE ✦ = 3–6 points ✳ = 7–9 points		PRACTICE TRIAL	GRADED TRIAL # 1	GRADED TRIAL # 2	NOTES
1. ✳	Document the name of the patient. (This name may be different from the name of the caller.) Always ensure the proper spelling of the name because many names can be similar.				
2. ✦	Document the patient's telephone number or callback number.				
3. ✳	Document the name and dosage of the medication. Ask the caller to spell the name of the medication if you are unclear about what the caller is saying.				
4. ✦	Document how long the patient has been on the medication.				
5. ✦	Document the patient's symptoms and why the prescription is still needed.				
6. ✳	Ask for the patient's date of birth and weight (if the patient is a child).				
7. ✦	Ask for the name and telephone number of the pharmacy and the prescription number.				
8. ✦	Let the caller know you will give the message to the physician and you will call back if the prescription cannot be refilled.				
9. ✦	Attach the telephone message to the patient's medical record and give both to the physician to review.				
10. ✳	If the office uses an electronic health record (EHR) system, the refill request may be documented in the patient's EHR and the physician would be notified to review the message in the EHR.				

Name: _____

Date: _____

Document: Enter the appropriate information in the chart below.

Grading

Points Earned	_____		
Points Possible	_____	81	81
Percent Grade (Points Earned/Points Possible)	_____		
PASS:	_____	❏ YES ❏ NO ❏ N/A	❏ YES ❏ NO ❏ N/A

Instructor Sign-Off

Instructor: _____   **Date:** _____

Procedure 7-4:

Placing a Conference Call

Objective: Allow for a discussion over the telephone among three or more parties from various locations.

Supplies: Telephone numbers of participating parties

Affective Behaviors: Affective behaviors provide a professional approach to a skill that enhances the patient encounter. These behaviors may also display sensitivity to a patient's rights and enhance communication. Pay close attention to these skills, which will be in **bold, *italicized*** font.

Notes to the Student

_____

_____

_____

_____

_____

_____

Skills Assessment Requirements

Read and familiarize yourself with the procedure; complete the minimum practice requirements (MPRs). Document each MPR using proper charting technique. Complete each procedure within a reasonable amount of time, with a minimum of 85% accuracy.

Name: _____

Date: _____

POINT VALUE ✦ = 3–6 points ✱ = 7–9 points		PRACTICE TRIAL	GRADED TRIAL # 1	GRADED TRIAL # 2	NOTES
1. ✦	Gather the telephone numbers of all participants before beginning the call.				
2. ✱	Determine the time that everyone will be available for the conference call. You may have to call people in advance to determine a convenient time. Be aware of time zone differences when arranging conference calls.				
3. ✦	Dial "0" for operator and give the operator the name and telephone number (area code first) for each person to be called.				
4. ✦	The operator will then place a call to each party. When all the participants are on the line, the operator will come back to the original caller (you) and the conversation can begin. If you are placing this call for your physician, he or she will pick up on your line.				
5. ✦	If you are setting up the conference call ahead of time, tell the operator when you wish the conference call to begin.				

Name: _____

Date: _____

Document: Enter the appropriate information in the chart below.

Grading

Points Earned	_____		
Points Possible	_____	33	33
Percent Grade (Points Earned/Points Possible)	_____		
PASS:	_____	❏ YES ❏ NO ❏ N/A	❏ YES ❏ NO ❏ N/A

Instructor Sign-Off

Instructor: _____ Date: _____

Procedure 8-1:

Opening the Office

Objective: Prepare and set up the office to receive patients and operate efficiently.

Supplies: Checklist of opening office procedures; office keys for rooms and files; message forms or pad; master list of scheduled patients

Affective Behaviors: Affective behaviors provide a professional approach to a skill that enhances the patient encounter. These behaviors may also display sensitivity to a patient's rights and enhance communication. Pay close attention to these skills, which will be in ***bold, italicized*** font.

Notes to the Student

_____

_____

_____

_____

_____

_____

Skills Assessment Requirements

Read and familiarize yourself with the procedure; complete the minimum practice requirements (MPRs). Document each MPR using proper charting technique. Complete each procedure within a reasonable amount of time, with a minimum of 85% accuracy.

Name: _____

Date: _____

POINT VALUE ✦ = 3–6 points ✳ = 7–9 points		PRACTICE TRIAL	GRADED TRIAL # 1	GRADED TRIAL # 2	NOTES
1. ✦	Arrive at least 30 minutes prior to the first scheduled appointment.				
2. ✦	Turn on the lights in the patient reception area before the first patient arrives.				
3. ✦	Check that the heating or air conditioning and computers are working properly.				
4. ✳	Turn on office equipment such as computers, copiers, printers, and fax machines. Fill all machines with paper.				
5. ✦	Check the reception room for safety hazards such as frayed electrical cords, slippery floor, or torn carpeting. Place a warning sign near any safety hazard and report it immediately to the office manager.				
6. ✦	Check magazines and recycle or discard any that are torn, damaged, or outdated.				
7. ✦	Check for cleanliness and report inadequate housekeeping services.				
8. ✦	Unlock file rooms or cabinets where records are kept.				
9. ✳	Take calls from the answering machine or answering service. Handle any that need immediate attention.				
10. ✦	Unlock any money that may be used for the day. Count and balance the money to make sure that the amount is the same as it was when closing the office the day before.				
11. ✦	Unlock the outer office door.				

POINT VALUE ✦ = 3–6 points ✳ = 7–9 points	PRACTICE TRIAL	GRADED TRIAL # 1	GRADED TRIAL # 2	NOTES
12. ✳ Queue up each physician's appointment schedule on the appropriate computer device and verify that electronic charts for scheduled patients are accessible. Verify that all paper charts have been pulled and collated, together with a printout of each physician's master appointment list, if using paper records. If a patient has been added to the schedule after the records were pulled, pull, review, and add this patient's record to the other records.				
13. ✳ Make phone calls to gather any laboratory test information that is missing from the record. Provide the physician(s) and nurse(s) with a copy of the list of any laboratory test information that you have called for but that has not yet been received.				
14. ✦ Print the day's patient schedule and place it on the physician's desk or other designated area.				

Name: _____

Date: _____

Document: Enter the appropriate information in the chart below.

Grading

Points Earned	_____		
Points Possible	_____	93	93
Percent Grade (Points Earned/Points Possible)	_____		
PASS:	_____	❏ YES ❏ NO ❏ N/A	❏ YES ❏ NO ❏ N/A

Instructor Sign-Off

Instructor: _____ **Date:** _____

Procedure 8-2:

Registering a New Patient

Objective: Accurately complete a registration form for a new patient.

Supplies: For paper-based charts: Registration form; pen; clipboard; private area

For electronic health records: Computer and possibly online access

Affective Behaviors: Affective behaviors provide a professional approach to a skill that enhances the patient encounter. These behaviors may also display sensitivity to a patient's rights and enhance communication. Pay close attention to these skills, which will be in **bold, *italicized*** font.

Notes to the Student

_____

_____

_____

_____

_____

_____

Skills Assessment Requirements

Read and familiarize yourself with the procedure; complete the minimum practice requirements (MPRs). Document each MPR using proper charting technique. Complete each procedure within a reasonable amount of time, with a minimum of 85% accuracy.

Note: If the patient has not completed a registration form before the appointment, the receptionist may need to assist the patient.

POINT VALUE ✦ = 3–6 points ✳ = 7–9 points	PRACTICE TRIAL	GRADED TRIAL # 1	GRADED TRIAL # 2	NOTES
1. ✦ Gather the supplies.				
2. ✦ Verify that the patient has not been seen in the office before.				
3. ✳ Obtain and record the following information from the patient: • Full name spelled correctly • Date of birth • Home address, including zip code • Telephone number, including area code • Cell phone number, including area code • Marital status • Employer • Employer address • Employer telephone number • Social Security number • Insurance information, including group number • Insurance subscriber's name • Insurance copayment amount (Photocopy both sides of the insurance card.) • Name of the patient's guardian, if applicable • Name of the person responsible for payment • Address of the person responsible for payment • Telephone number of the person responsible for payment • Photocopy of the patient's photo ID, such as a driver's license or military ID				

POINT VALUE ✦ = 3–6 points ✶ = 7–9 points		PRACTICE TRIAL	GRADED TRIAL # 1	GRADED TRIAL # 2	NOTES
4. ✦	After the preceding information has been documented, *review everything with the patient to ensure accuracy.*				
5. ✦	For patients who are unable to complete the form themselves, document within the record that the patient verbally provided the documented demographic information, verify everything for accuracy, and have the patient sign in the appropriate area. The receptionist completing the form should also sign and date it.				
6. ✶	Ask the patient to read and sign the HIPAA Notice of Privacy Practices. *If the patient declines to sign the form, write a note on the form indicating that the patient refused to sign and, if possible, the reason.* The receptionist writing the note should sign and date it. Remember that HIPAA requires that patients be notified of the privacy practices and *asked* to sign the form, but does not *require* a signature. This form is a consent, not an authorization. Patients who do not sign the form can be seen by the physician and their information can be processed and used.				

Name: _____

Date: _____

Document: Enter the appropriate information in the chart below.

Grading

Points Earned	_____		
Points Possible	_____	45	45
Percent Grade (Points Earned/Points Possible)	_____		
PASS:	_____	❏ YES ❏ NO ❏ N/A	❏ YES ❏ NO ❏ N/A

Instructor Sign-Off

Instructor: _____ **Date:** _____

Procedure 8-3:

Collecting Copayments

Objective: Accurately collect a copayment from a patient.

Supplies: Computer or ledger card; cash box; credit card terminal

Affective Behaviors: Affective behaviors provide a professional approach to a skill that enhances the patient encounter. These behaviors may also display sensitivity to a patient's rights and enhance communication. Pay close attention to these skills, which will be in **_bold, italicized_** font.

Notes to the Student

_____

_____

_____

_____

_____

_____

Skills Assessment Requirements

Read and familiarize yourself with the procedure; complete the minimum practice requirements (MPRs). Document each MPR using proper charting technique. Complete each procedure within a reasonable amount of time, with a minimum of 85% accuracy.

Name: _____

Date: _____

POINT VALUE ✦ = 3–6 points ✳ = 7–9 points		PRACTICE TRIAL	GRADED TRIAL # 1	GRADED TRIAL # 2	NOTES
1. ✦	Gather the supplies.				
2. ✦	Access the patient's computerized or paper-based financial account.				
3. ✦	Verify the patient's identity.				
4. ✳	Verify that the insurance information on file is current, or obtain updated insurance card and policy information.				
5. ✳	Look up the amount of the copay for the type of visit the patient has scheduled. Some insurance plans have different copays for different types of visits. The copay for a preventive care visit may be $0 and the copay for a problem-oriented visit $10 or $20.				
6. ✳	Say to the patient, "Your copay today is $ _____. How would you like to make payment? We accept cash, check, credit card, or debit card."				
7. ✳	Accept the payment. a. If the patient pays in cash, count the money to be certain it is the correct amount. If the patient requires change, lay the patient's payment next to the cash box, remove the amount of change, and count it out to the patient. After the patient accepts the change, place the original money in the cash box. Enter the payment amount and form of payment (cash) on the patient's financial record.				

POINT VALUE ✦ = 3–6 points ✳ = 7–9 points		PRACTICE TRIAL	GRADED TRIAL # 1	GRADED TRIAL # 2	NOTES
	b. If the patient pays by check, verify that the name and address on the check are correct. Verify that the payment amount is correct and that the check has been signed. Some offices allow the patient to leave the "Pay To" field blank, then use a rubber stamp to apply the office's name in the appropriate place. Enter the payment amount, form of payment (check), and check number on the patient's financial record. Place the check in the cash box or other designated place.				
	c. If the patient pays by credit or debit card, verify that the name on the card is correct. Ask the patient if he or she prefers to use debit or credit. Swipe the card in the credit card terminal, select debit or credit, and enter the payment amount. Follow instructions for your specific terminal to complete the transaction. Patients paying by debit need to enter their PIN number. Ask the patient to sign the electronic signature pad or paper slip. If required by your system, verify the last four digits of the card number and the three-digit security code on the back of the card. Enter the payment amount, form of payment (credit or debit card), and credit card transaction number on the patient's financial record. Place the charge card receipt in the cash box or other designated place.				

Name: _____

Date: _____

POINT VALUE ✦ = 3–6 points ✷ = 7–9 points		PRACTICE TRIAL	GRADED TRIAL # 1	GRADED TRIAL # 2	NOTES
8. ✦	Generate a receipt for the patient showing today's visit and the amount paid. Patients paying with a credit card should receive two receipts, one from the credit card terminal that documents the charge to the card and one from the patient's financial account showing the amount posted to the account.				
9. ✷	Thank the patient for the payment and give instructions on what to do next, such as, "Thank you. You may have a seat and someone will call you back in a few minutes, when the doctor is ready to see you."				

Name: _____

Date: _____

Document: Enter the appropriate information in the chart below.

Grading

Points Earned	_____		
Points Possible	_____	69	69
Percent Grade (Points Earned/Points Possible)	_____		
PASS:	_____	❏ YES ❏ NO ❏ N/A	❏ YES ❏ NO ❏ N/A

Instructor Sign-Off

Instructor: _____ **Date:** _____

Procedure 8-4:

Closing the Office

Objective: Secure the office properly during nonoperating hours.

Supplies: Checklist of office closing procedures; blank deposit forms and envelope/pouch; office keys for rooms and files

Affective Behaviors: Affective behaviors provide a professional approach to a skill that enhances the patient encounter. These behaviors may also display sensitivity to a patient's rights and enhance communication. Pay close attention to these skills, which will be in **bold, *italicized*** font.

Notes to the Student

_____

_____

_____

_____

_____

_____

Skills Assessment Requirements

Read and familiarize yourself with the procedure; complete the minimum practice requirements (MPRs). Document each MPR using proper charting technique. Complete each procedure within a reasonable amount of time, with a minimum of 85% accuracy.

POINT VALUE ✦ = 3–6 points ✳ = 7–9 points		PRACTICE TRIAL	GRADED TRIAL #1	GRADED TRIAL #2	NOTES
1. ✦	Allow at least 15 to 30 minutes at the end of the day to close the office.				
2. ✦	Check all records used during the day for any orders that may have been missed. In addition, make sure that every visit is posted and billed.				
3. ✳	Check the appointment schedule and verify that there is an encounter form or posted visit for every patient who came in. Make a list of no-shows and cancellations that did not reschedule.				
4. ✳	Balance the cash box in the presence of another staff member. Ensure that the total amount of cash and checks matches the amounts recorded by the computer system. Prepare a deposit of the day's receipts. Place the deposit in the office safe unless you will make the bank deposit on your way home. It is wise to have the person designated to make the daily bank deposit vary the time of deposit. Many offices now use a courier for this task. For purposes of accounting controls, the person preparing the bank deposit and the person actually making the deposit should be different. Both people should be bonded.				
5. ✳	Queue up or pull records for patients who will be seen the next day. Place the collated records with the encounter forms attached and the master list of the next day's scheduled patients together in the appropriate place. Also, make a copy of this master list of patients for each physician.				

POINT VALUE ✦ = 3–6 points ✶ = 7–9 points		PRACTICE TRIAL	GRADED TRIAL # 1	GRADED TRIAL # 2	NOTES
6. ✦	Lock all files and file rooms, physician offices, and other individual offices within the medical practice.				
7. ✦	Turn off electrical equipment and appliances. *Note:* Some equipment such as an incubator, fax machine, and computer may require 24-hour operation and should not be turned off.				
8. ✦	Check all examination rooms to make sure they are clean and supplied for the next day. *Note:* This step may be done by the medical assistant who was in charge of rooming patients that day.				
9. ✦	Straighten the reception room. Put away all magazines and pick up toys.				
10. ✦	Leave any instructions for nighttime cleaning personnel in a designated place.				
11. ✦	Activate the answering service before leaving. Know the name of the physician who is accepting emergency calls, or is on call, until morning. Remind the physician who is on call.				
12. ✶	Lock all doors except the one you will use to exit.				
13. ✶	Activate the security system if there is one. Turn off the lights per the office policy.				
14. ✶	Lock the door after you exit. Take two steps away, then step forward again to double-check that the door is locked.				

Document: Enter the appropriate information in the chart below.

Grading

Points Earned	_____		
Points Possible	_____	102	102
Percent Grade (Points Earned/Points Possible)	_____		
	_____	❑ YES ❑ NO ❑ N/A	❑ YES ❑ NO ❑ N/A

Instructor Sign-Off

Instructor: _____   **Date:** _____

Procedure 9-1:

Scheduling Established Patients

Objective: Use an appointment scheduling system to schedule patients with efficiency.

Equipment and Supplies: Pencil or pen (if preferred by office management); appointment schedule book or computerized scheduling system

Affective Behaviors: Affective behaviors provide a professional approach to a skill that enhances the patient encounter. These behaviors may also display sensitivity to a patient's rights and enhance communication. Pay close attention to these skills, which will be in **bold, *italicized*** font.

Notes to the Student

_____

_____

_____

_____

_____

_____

Skills Assessment Requirements

Read and familiarize yourself with the procedure; complete the minimum practice requirements (MPRs). Document each MPR using proper charting technique. Complete each procedure within a reasonable amount of time, with a minimum of 85% accuracy.

Name: _____

Date: _____

POINT VALUE ✦ = 3–6 points ✱ = 7–9 points		PRACTICE TRIAL	GRADED TRIAL # 1	GRADED TRIAL # 2	NOTES
1. ✦	Understand the scheduling system used in your office.				
2. ✦	If using computerized scheduling, log in to the scheduling system with your user name and password that have been previously established. When scheduling manually, use a pencil so appointments can be erased to make changes as needed. *Please note:* Some offices prefer the use of black or blue ink instead of pencil.				
3. ✦	Before scheduling patients, set up a matrix by blocking out all time periods when the physician is not available (hospital rounds, vacation, etc.) for appointments.				
4. ✱	Schedule appointments by beginning with the first empty appointment in the morning or early in the afternoon, and then fill in the day. Do not schedule appointments at the end of the day with large open gaps in between.				
5. ✦	For computerized scheduling, access the menu that enables you to search for the correct patient. Some systems allow searching by the patient's birth date or medical record number. This decreases the chances of pulling up the wrong patient if you have more than one patient with the same name. For manual scheduling, print the patient's full first and last name next to the appropriate time on the schedule. Add Jr. for *Junior* and Sr. for *Senior* if two patients in a family have the same name.				

POINT VALUE ✦ = 3–6 points ✷ = 7–9 points		PRACTICE TRIAL	GRADED TRIAL # 1	GRADED TRIAL # 2	NOTES
6. ✦	For computerized scheduling, verify that the telephone numbers in the system are correct. If they are incorrect, take the time right then to update them. Correct contact information is necessary if the office needs to get in touch with the patient before the appointment. For manual scheduling, ask the patient for a current work and home telephone number, including the area code. Include a cell phone number if the patient has one. Write these numbers next to the patient's name.				
7. ✦	**Record the reason for the visit on the schedule,** using accepted medical abbreviations only.				
8. ✷	Allow the correct amount of time for the appointment. If an appointment will take more than the minimum time allotted on the schedule, be sure to adjust the length of time as needed. For computerized scheduling, you may specify the length of the appointment by entering the number of minutes, such as 15, 30, or 60 minutes. Some systems may allow you to highlight the time blocks on the screen. For manual scheduling, draw an arrow to indicate that the patient requires two or three blocks of time. In some offices, a line is drawn across the time blocks.				

POINT VALUE ✦ = 3–6 points ✷ = 7–9 points	PRACTICE TRIAL	GRADED TRIAL # 1	GRADED TRIAL # 2	NOTES
9. ✦ **After the appointment is recorded, repeat to the patient the date, time, and any special instructions.**				
10. ✦ If the patient is in the office while you are scheduling the appointment, **record the appointment on a reminder card and hand it to the patient.**				

Note: In offices where scheduling is done by computer, follow any on-screen prompts in addition to the steps suggested above.

Document: Enter the appropriate information in the chart below.

Grading

Points Earned	_____		
Points Possible	_____	72	72
Percent Grade (Points Earned/Points Possible)	_____		
PASS:	_____	❏ YES ❏ NO ❏ N/A	❏ YES ❏ NO ❏ N/A

Instructor Sign-Off

Instructor: _____   **Date:** _____

Procedure 9-2:

Scheduling a New Patient Appointment

Objective: Schedule the first visit for a new patient.

Equipment and Supplies: Pencil or pen (if preferred by office management); computerized scheduling system or appointment book.

Affective Behaviors: Affective behaviors provide a professional approach to a skill that enhances the patient encounter. These behaviors may also display sensitivity to a patient's rights and enhance communication. Pay close attention to these skills, which will be in **bold, *italicized*** font.

Notes to the Student

_____

_____

_____

_____

_____

_____

Skills Assessment Requirements

Read and familiarize yourself with the procedure; complete the minimum practice requirements (MPRs). Document each MPR using proper charting technique. Complete each procedure within a reasonable amount of time, with a minimum of 85% accuracy.

Name: _____

Date: _____

POINT VALUE ✦ = 3–6 points ✶ = 7–9 points		PRACTICE TRIAL	GRADED TRIAL # 1	GRADED TRIAL # 2	NOTES
1. ✦	Assemble the necessary appointment scheduling equipment.				
2. ✶	Obtain the patient's full legal name and correct spelling, birth date, full address, telephone contacts (home, office, cell), and e-mail address.				
3. ✦	Record the patient's chief complaint and symptoms.				
4. ✶	Request the name of the patient's insurance carrier and insurance policy number.				
5. ✦	Ask how the patient was referred to the medical office (physician referral, friend, colleague, insurance company, etc.).				
6. ✦	Ask the patient if he or she has a preference for morning or afternoon appointments.				
7. ✦	Attempt to accommodate the new patient's request for a preferred appointment time.				
8. ✦	Confirm the day, date, and time of the appointment, and **have the new patient repeat the information for verification and mutual understanding.**				
9. ✦	Advise the patient of any need to arrive early, before the official appointment time, in order to complete paperwork such as the patient history form and HIPAA content.				
10. ✦	Provide the new patient with directions to the office.				

Name: _____

Date: _____

POINT VALUE ✦ = 3–6 points ✴ = 7–9 points		PRACTICE TRIAL	GRADED TRIAL # 1	GRADED TRIAL # 2	NOTES
11. ✴	Inform the new patient of all materials to bring for the first visit (i.e., insurance card, photo identification, list of current medications, past medical records, current lab, X-rays, and other medical reports, as available).				
12. ✦	**Welcome and thank the new patient by name for selecting your medical office.**				
13. ✦	Forward all information as discussed with the new patient via e-mail or, if time allows, regular mail.				
14. ✦	Document the new patient information in a new medical record.				

Name: _____

Date: _____

Document: Enter the appropriate information in the chart below.

Grading

Points Earned	_____		
Points Possible	_____	93	93
Percent Grade (Points Earned/Points Possible)	_____		
PASS:	_____	❑ YES ❑ NO ❑ N/A	❑ YES ❑ NO ❑ N/A

Instructor Sign-Off

Instructor: _____   Date: _____

Name: _____

Date: _____

Procedure 9-3:

Arranging a Referral Appointment

Objective: Schedule a referral appointment for a patient.

Equipment and Supplies: Patient chart; telephone; paper; pen; Rolodex or physician directory; physician request for referral information

Affective Behaviors: Affective behaviors provide a professional approach to a skill that enhances the patient encounter. These behaviors may also display sensitivity to a patient's rights and enhance communication. Pay close attention to these skills, which will be in **bold, *italicized*** font.

Notes to the Student

_____

_____

_____

_____

_____

_____

Skills Assessment Requirements

Read and familiarize yourself with the procedure; complete the minimum practice requirements (MPRs). Document each MPR using proper charting technique. Complete each procedure within a reasonable amount of time, with a minimum of 85% accuracy.

Name: _____

Date: _____

POINT VALUE ✦ = 3–6 points ✳ = 7–9 points		PRACTICE TRIAL	GRADED TRIAL # 1	GRADED TRIAL # 2	NOTES
1. ✦	Gather supplies.				
2. ✦	Open patient chart for insurance information and physician request for referral.				
3. ✦	Place call to physician's office to which the patient is being referred.				
4. ✦	***Identify yourself and the physician on whose behalf you are calling.*** Let the office know you are calling to schedule a referral appointment.				
5. ✦	First, verify that the practice accepts the patient's medical insurance. If so, continue with the call and provide necessary patient information. If the office does not accept the patient's insurance, ***thank the practice for its time and notify the physician.*** The physician will then recommend another physician for the patient referral.				
6. ✳	If the office accepts the patient's insurance, provide the following information: patient's name, address, telephone number, and reason for referral.				
7. ✳	The office may or may not ask how soon the patient needs to be seen and then schedule the patient.				
8. ✦	Record the referral appointment information in the patient's chart as well as on an appointment reminder card for the patient.				
9. ✦	Be sure also to record the name of the individual with whom you spoke and the creation of the reminder card.				

Name: _____

Date: _____

POINT VALUE ✦ = 3–6 points ✶ = 7–9 points		PRACTICE TRIAL	GRADED TRIAL # 1	GRADED TRIAL # 2	NOTES
10. ✦	**_Notify the patient of the date and time of the appointment and provide the reminder card._**				
11. ✦	**_Verify that the patient knows the office location. If not, provide clearly written directions._**				
12. ✶	Forward any pertinent information such as laboratory tests or X-rays to the physician's office and record them in the patient's chart. If faxing information, be sure to place the fax confirmation in the patient's chart.				
13. ✶	If precertification is required, contact the patient's insurance company and request authorization. Depending on the insurance carrier, this may be done either by computer, telephone, or fax. The insurance company will require the following information: specialist's name, telephone number, and reason for the visit or request.				
14. ✦	If completing the precertification by telephone, document the precertification number and the name and telephone number of the individual who provides the number.				
15. ✶	Provide the precertification number and pertinent information to the physician's office to which the patient is being referred.				

Name: _____

Date: _____

Document: Enter the appropriate information in the chart below.

Grading

Points Earned	_____		
Points Possible	_____	108	108
Percent Grade (Points Earned/Points Possible)	_____		
PASS:	_____	❏ YES ❏ NO ❏ N/A	❏ YES ❏ NO ❏ N/A

Instructor Sign-Off

Instructor: _____   Date: _____

Procedure 9-4:

Scheduling Inpatient Surgical Procedures

Objective: Perform proper procedure to schedule inpatient surgical procedures.

Equipment and Supplies: Patient's chart; patient's insurance card; notepad and pen; written instructions for patient (if required)

Affective Behaviors: Affective behaviors provide a professional approach to a skill that enhances the patient encounter. These behaviors may also display sensitivity to a patient's rights and enhance communication. Pay close attention to these skills, which will be in **bold, *italicized*** font.

Notes to the Student

_____

_____

_____

_____

_____

_____

Skills Assessment Requirements

Read and familiarize yourself with the procedure; complete the minimum practice requirements (MPRs). Document each MPR using proper charting technique. Complete each procedure within a reasonable amount of time, with a minimum of 85% accuracy.

POINT VALUE ✦ = 3–6 points ✱ = 7–9 points		PRACTICE TRIAL	GRADED TRIAL # 1	GRADED TRIAL # 2	NOTES
1. ✦	Review the patient's chart for the most current information. Make sure the chart contains the physician's notes and orders regarding the surgical procedure.				
2. ✦	Verify with the physician the type of procedure that you are scheduling for the patient, and gather the following information from the physician: Category the surgical procedure falls under (routine, elective, urgent) Name of the surgeon to perform the procedure The surgeon's scheduling preference for this type of procedure Estimated length of time for the procedure Estimated length of stay				
3. ✦	Gather the following information from the patient and patient's chart: Patient's full name, age, sex, and any other pertinent identification or information Physician's current diagnosis Any allergies Special preoperative orders and patient instructions Patient's insurance information				
4. ✱	Obtain pre-authorization from the patient's insurance company, if required.				

Name: _____

Date: _____

POINT VALUE ✦ = 3–6 points ✶ = 7–9 points	PRACTICE TRIAL	GRADED TRIAL #1	GRADED TRIAL #2	NOTES
5. ✦ Contact the surgery scheduler at the facility and relay the requested surgery information. The surgery scheduler is the person in the hospital or surgery center who schedules the procedure, including the necessary preoperative appointments (e.g., blood work, chest X-ray, etc.), the actual surgery, and postoperative appointments, if necessary.				
6. ✦ The surgery scheduler will confirm the date and time of surgery and any special instructions to be relayed to the patient.				
7. ✦ Record the surgery scheduling information in the patient's chart.				
8. ✶ Record the surgery information on the appropriate physician's schedule.				
9. ✦ Follow office procedure and the surgeon's request for contacting other members of the surgical team.				
10. ✶ *Instruct the patient on special preparation and admission procedures. Provide written instructions, if available.*				

Document: Enter the appropriate information in the chart below.

Grading

Points Earned	_____		
Points Possible	_____	69	69
Percent Grade (Points Earned/Points Possible)	_____		
PASS:	_____	❏ YES ❏ NO ❏ N/A	❏ YES ❏ NO ❏ N/A

Instructor Sign-Off

Instructor: _____   **Date:** _____

Procedure 9-5:

Scheduling Outpatient Surgical Procedures

Objective: Demonstrate the ability to schedule outpatient procedures in the health care setting.

Equipment and Supplies: Telephone, patient's insurance card, notepad, pen, written instructions for patient

Affective Behaviors: Affective behaviors provide a professional approach to a skill that enhances the patient encounter. These behaviors may also display sensitivity to a patient's rights and enhance communication. Pay close attention to these skills, which will be in **_bold, italicized_** font.

Notes to the Student

_____

_____

_____

_____

_____

_____

Skills Assessment Requirements

Read and familiarize yourself with the procedure; complete the minimum practice requirements (MPRs). Document each MPR using proper charting technique. Complete each procedure within a reasonable amount of time, with a minimum of 85% accuracy.

POINT VALUE ✦ = 3–6 points ✱ = 7–9 points		PRACTICE TRIAL	GRADED TRIAL # 1	GRADED TRIAL # 2	NOTES
1. ✦	Review the patient's chart for the most current information. Make sure the chart contains the physician's notes and orders regarding the surgical procedure.				
2. ✦	Verify with the physician the type of procedure for which you are to schedule the patient and gather the following information from the physician: Category under which the surgical procedure falls (i.e., routine, elective, urgent) Name of the surgeon who will perform the procedure The surgeon's scheduling preference for this type of procedure Estimated length of time for the procedure				
3. ✦	Gather the following information from the patient and the patient's chart: Patient's full name, age, sex, and any other pertinent identification or information Physician's current diagnosis for the patient Any existing allergies Special preoperative orders and patient instructions Patient's insurance information Days/times patient is available for surgery				
4. ✱	Obtain pre-authorization from the patient's insurance company, if required.				

POINT VALUE ✦ = 3–6 points ✶ = 7–9 points		PRACTICE TRIAL	GRADED TRIAL # 1	GRADED TRIAL # 2	NOTES
5. ✦	According to the facility policy, **contact the outpatient scheduler at the local hospital or clinic and identify yourself and your office.**				
6. ✦	**Instruct the facility about the type of procedure and the amount of time the physician expects to need the operating room.**				
7. ✶	**Determine available days at the facility.**				
8. ✶	If possible, offer options to the patient and have the patient choose the best option.				
9. ✦	Notify the facility of the time and date chosen.				
10. ✶	Create a patient instruction sheet that includes the date and time of the procedure and any necessary preoperative instructions.				
11. ✦	Document the conversation in the patient's chart.				
12. ✶	Document the scheduled surgery on the appropriate physician's schedule.				

Document: Enter the appropriate information in the chart below.

Grading

Points Earned	_____		
Points Possible	_____	81	81
Percent Grade (Points Earned/Points Possible)	_____		
PASS:	_____	❏ YES ❏ NO ❏ N/A	❏ YES ❏ NO ❏ N/A

Instructor Sign-Off

Instructor: _____   Date: _____

Procedure 10-1:

Maintaining Equipment

Objective: Perform routine maintenance of office equipment with documentation.

Equipment and Supplies: Equipment maintenance log; access to desired piece of equipment; user manual; pen or pencil

Affective Behaviors: Affective behaviors provide a professional approach to a skill that enhances the patient encounter. These behaviors may also display sensitivity to a patient's rights and enhance communication. Pay close attention to these skills, which will be in **bold, *italicized*** font.

Notes to the Student

_____

_____

_____

_____

_____

_____

Skills Assessment Requirements

Read and familiarize yourself with the procedure; complete the minimum practice requirements (MPRs). Document each MPR using proper charting technique. Complete each procedure within a reasonable amount of time, with a minimum of 85% accuracy.

Name: _____

Date: _____

POINT VALUE ✦ = 3–6 points ✱ = 7–9 points	PRACTICE TRIAL	GRADED TRIAL # 1	GRADED TRIAL # 2	NOTES
1. ✦ Plan a time to perform equipment inspection and maintenance when it will not interfere with patient reception and care, such as before or after office hours.				
2. ✦ Refer to the equipment maintenance log to determine which pieces of equipment are scheduled for inspection and maintenance. Access the user manual or service instructions for each piece of equipment.				
3. ✦ Note that for certain aspects of inspection and maintenance, the equipment may need to be turned off and unplugged. For other tasks, such as calibration, the equipment may need to be turned on.				
4. ✦ Visually inspect the equipment, paying special attention to items identified in the user manual. Also check for frayed electrical cords, loose connections, missing screws or fasteners, and loose parts.				
5. ✦ Perform performance and calibration tests recommended by the manufacturer. Adjust equipment, as needed, according to manufacturer instructions.				
6. ✦ Clean equipment and replace lightbulbs, batteries, ink/toner, paper, and other supplies as needed. Always follow manufacturer instructions.				

POINT VALUE ✦ = 3–6 points ✳ = 7–9 points		PRACTICE TRIAL	GRADED TRIAL # 1	GRADED TRIAL # 2	NOTES
7. ✦	In the maintenance log, enter the date of the inspection and your name or initials. Note any problems that require further attention.				
8. ✦	If the equipment is not operating properly, unplug it and place a sign on it that states, "NOT IN SERVICE. DO NOT USE." **Inform the office manager of such.** Telephone the service company to schedule a service call.				

Name: _____

Date: _____

Document: Enter the appropriate information in the chart below.

Grading

Points Earned	_____		
Points Possible	_____	48	48
Percent Grade (Points Earned/Points Possible)	_____		
PASS:	_____	❏ YES ❏ NO ❏ N/A	❏ YES ❏ NO ❏ N/A

Instructor Sign-Off

Instructor: _____ **Date:** _____

Procedure 10-2:

Performing an Office Inventory and Ordering Office Supplies

Objective: Perform an inventory of office supplies.

Equipment and Supplies: Inventory sheets; pen or pencil; computer; supply catalogs or website addresses; order form

Affective Behaviors: Affective behaviors provide a professional approach to a skill that enhances the patient encounter. These behaviors may also display sensitivity to a patient's rights and enhance communication. Pay close attention to these skills, which will be in **bold, italicized** font.

Notes to the Student

_____

_____

_____

_____

_____

_____

Skills Assessment Requirements

Read and familiarize yourself with the procedure; complete the minimum practice requirements (MPRs). Document each MPR using proper charting technique. Complete each procedure within a reasonable amount of time, with a minimum of 85% accuracy.

Name: _____

Date: _____

POINT VALUE ✦ = 3–6 points ✳ = 7–9 points		PRACTICE TRIAL	GRADED TRIAL # 1	GRADED TRIAL # 2	NOTES
1. ✦	Plan a time to review inventory when it does not interfere with patient reception and care, such as before or after office hours.				
2. ✦	Collect and review inventory sheets from all supply storage locations. Highlight items that have reached or are very near the reorder point. Physically check the remaining supply of any items for which the inventory sheets are unclear.				
3. ✳	Refer to the catalog, website, or previous order form of each vendor with whom an order needs to be placed.				
4. ✦	Enter the item number, quantity, and price of each item. Double-check all numbers for accuracy.				
5. ✦	Prepare a purchase order, if required, and wait for approval before placing the order. Enter the purchase order on the supply order form or attach it to the order (manually or electronically).				
6. ✦	Submit the order to the vendor using an order form, website, or telephone order line. Verify when delivery can be expected.				

Name: _____

Date: _____

Document: Enter the appropriate information in the chart below.

Grading

Points Earned	_____		
Points Possible	_____	45	45
Percent Grade (Points Earned/Points Possible)	_____		
PASS:	_____	❑ YES ❑ NO ❑ N/A	❑ YES ❑ NO ❑ N/A

Instructor Sign-Off

Instructor:_____ **Date:** _____

Procedure 11-1:

Composing a Business Letter

Objective: Compose a business letter using proper guidelines.

Equipment and Supplies: Computer or typewriter; office stationery

Affective Behaviors: Affective behaviors provide a professional approach to a skill that enhances the patient encounter. These behaviors may also display sensitivity to a patient's rights and enhance communication. Pay close attention to these skills, which will be in *bold, italicized* font.

Notes to the Student

_____

_____

_____

_____

_____

_____

Skills Assessment Requirements

Read and familiarize yourself with the procedure; complete the minimum practice requirements (MPRs). Document each MPR using proper charting technique. Complete each procedure within a reasonable amount of time, with a minimum of 85% accuracy.

POINT VALUE ✦ = 3–6 points ✱ = 7–9 points		PRACTICE TRIAL	GRADED TRIAL # 1	GRADED TRIAL # 2	NOTES
1. ✦	Gather all necessary information and supplies.				
2. ✦	Determine the reason for the correspondence. Write down the main purpose of the letter.				
3. ✦	Make a list of all points you need to cover in the letter. Prepare a rough draft.				
4. ✱	Arrange the items in a logical manner. Make sure that the letter has all parts—a beginning, a middle, and an end. • The beginning or introduction should be appropriate for the intended reader. Use appropriate greetings and titles. • The middle should contain the supporting facts and details. Make sure the content relates to the purpose of the letter. • The end should be brief and pleasant and indicate any action that is to be taken by the reader or writer.				
5. ✱	Use a natural style of writing. Avoid showy language, and avoid medical terms when writing to the layperson. Also avoid inflated phrases				
6. ✱	Use a positive tone. Negative writing should always be avoided.				
7. ✦	Pay particular attention to spelling, punctuation, and grammar.				
8. ✱	When the rough draft is satisfactory, compose the final draft of the letter. Proofread for mistakes.				
9. ✦	Obtain necessary signatures. Include any enclosures as indicated.				

Name: _____

Date: _____

Document: Enter the appropriate information in the chart below.

Grading

Points Earned	_____		
Points Possible	_____	69	69
Percent Grade (Points Earned/Points Possible)	_____		
PASS:	_____	❏ YES ❏ NO ❏ N/A	❏ YES ❏ NO ❏ N/A

Instructor Sign-Off

Instructor: _____   **Date:** _____

Procedure 11-2:

Proofreading Written Documents

Objective: To draft grammatically correct correspondence with no spelling errors.

Equipment and Supplies: Ruler; pencil; piece of paper; computer; rough draft of document

Affective Behaviors: Affective behaviors provide a professional approach to a skill that enhances the patient encounter. These behaviors may also display sensitivity to a patient's rights and enhance communication. Pay close attention to these skills, which will be in ***bold, italicized*** font.

Notes to the Student

_____

_____

_____

_____

_____

_____

Skills Assessment Requirements

Read and familiarize yourself with the procedure; complete the minimum practice requirements (MPRs). Document each MPR using proper charting technique. Complete each procedure within a reasonable amount of time, with a minimum of 85% accuracy.

Name: _____

Date: _____

POINT VALUE ✦ = 3–6 points ✶ = 7–9 points		PRACTICE TRIAL	GRADED TRIAL #1	GRADED TRIAL #2	NOTES
1. ✦	Access the rough draft of the document you are working on.				
2. ✶	Read the document to ensure all points are covered and that thoughts flow logically.				
3. ✦	Run the computer program spelling and grammar checks and consider the suggestions made.				
4. ✶	Save the document, and then print it.				
5. ✦	Use a ruler, pencil, or edge of a piece of paper to follow each line as you proofread.				
6. ✦	Check for missing and repeated words.				
7. ✦	Verify the spelling of proper names and titles.				
8. ✶	Check where the word breaks occur.				
9. ✦	Verify numbers in dates, figures, and time (hours of the day).				
10. ✦	Read the opening and closing very carefully.				
11. ✶	Proofread at least twice. If still unsure, ask a coworker to review the document.				
12. ✶	Check the general appearance of the letter for spacing and format.				
13. ✦	Make the needed corrections, save, and print the document.				

Document: Enter the appropriate information in the chart below.

Grading

Points Earned	_____		
Points Possible	_____	99	99
Percent Grade (Points Earned/Points Possible)	_____		
PASS:	_____	❏ YES ❏ NO ❏ N/A	❏ YES ❏ NO ❏ N/A

Instructor Sign-Off

Instructor: _____   **Date:** _____

Procedure 11-3:

Opening and Sorting the Daily Mail

Objective: Sort and distribute the medical office's daily mail.

Equipment and Supplies: Date stamp; stamp with the name of the medical office; inkpad; paper clips; pencil

Affective Behaviors: Affective behaviors provide a professional approach to a skill that enhances the patient encounter. These behaviors may also display sensitivity to a patient's rights and enhance communication. Pay close attention to these skills, which will be in **bold, *italicized*** font.

Notes to the Student

_____

_____

_____

_____

_____

_____

Skills Assessment Requirements

Read and familiarize yourself with the procedure; complete the minimum practice requirements (MPRs). Document each MPR using proper charting technique. Complete each procedure within a reasonable amount of time, with a minimum of 85% accuracy.

POINT VALUE ✦ = 3–6 points ✶ = 7–9 points		PRACTICE TRIAL	GRADED TRIAL # 1	GRADED TRIAL # 2	NOTES
1. ✦	Gather the supplies needed to process the mail. Process the mail as soon as possible after it arrives, because it often contains time-sensitive documents and information that physician and staff members are waiting for.				
2. ✦	Sort the unopened mail into piles for first-class, personal or confidential, advertising circulars, and magazines.				
3. ✦	Discard and recycle unwanted advertising mail.				
4. ✶	Stamp the current date and time of arrival on each piece of mail. Purchase a rubber stamp and pad from an office supply store so that the date can be changed each day.				
5. ✦	Stamp the name of the medical office on all periodicals and newspapers.				
6. ✶	Set aside and do not open mail marked "Personal" or "Confidential." Place it unopened in the physician's inbox unless otherwise instructed.				
7. ✦	Lay all the envelopes with flaps down to reduce the motions involved in opening a large amount of mail. Use a letter opener to cut open the top edge of each envelope.				

POINT VALUE ✦ = 3–6 points ✳ = 7–9 points	PRACTICE TRIAL	GRADED TRIAL #1	GRADED TRIAL #2	NOTES
8. ✦ Remove enclosures from the envelope and attach them to the envelope with a paper clip. Place the envelope on top of the enclosures. Do not staple anything because staples would have to be removed later and could damage sensitive materials, such as X-rays. If an enclosure is noted in the correspondence but is not in the envelope, next to mention of the enclosure write "No" with your initials to indicate it was not included. Clip the opened envelope to the mail until the mail is completely processed. In some cases, a return address is only on the envelope and not on the inside correspondence.				
9. ✦ Annotate the mail. An annotation consists of writing a short comment in pencil to indicate the purpose of the letter and underlining the critical portions of the letter. If another document is referred to in the letter, then take initiative by pulling it from the file and attaching it to this correspondence.				

POINT VALUE ✦ = 3–6 points ✶ = 7–9 points	PRACTICE TRIAL	GRADED TRIAL # 1	GRADED TRIAL # 2	NOTES
10. ✦ The office should have a separate policy for opening mail that contains checks in payment of bills, such as those from insurance companies and patients. Usually this requires the following steps: • Stamp the back of the check in the designated area with the endorsement stamp for the medical office's bank account. • Make a photocopy of each check. • Attach the copy of the check to the paperwork that was included with the check, such as an explanation of insurance benefits or patient statement. • Enter the amount of the check and the payer in the daily cash log, which may be maintained either as a computer document or as a physical logbook. • Place the original check in the daily cash box. • Route the copy of the check and attachments to the appropriate person in the patient accounting department.				
11. ✶ Route the mail immediately after opening it. Another department or physician may be waiting for the document.				

Name: _____

Date: _____

Document: Enter the appropriate information in the chart below.

Grading

Points Earned	_____		
Points Possible	_____	81	81
Percent Grade (Points Earned/Points Possible)	_____		
PASS:	_____	❏ YES ❏ NO ❏ N/A	❏ YES ❏ NO ❏ N/A

Instructor Sign-Off

Instructor: _____   **Date:** _____

Procedure 12-1:

Installing Computer Hardware

Objective: Follow a general process for installing computer hardware components.

Equipment and Supplies: Computer on which hardware is to be installed; new hardware and all packaging; office equipment inventory log

Affective Behaviors: Affective behaviors provide a professional approach to a skill that enhances the patient encounter. These behaviors may also display sensitivity to a patient's rights and enhance communication. Pay close attention to these skills, which will be in **bold, *italicized*** font.

Notes to the Student

_____

_____

_____

_____

_____

_____

Skills Assessment Requirements

Read and familiarize yourself with the procedure; complete the minimum practice requirements (MPRs). Document each MPR using proper charting technique. Complete each procedure within a reasonable amount of time, with a minimum of 85% accuracy.

POINT VALUE ✦ = 3–6 points ✳ = 7–9 points		PRACTICE TRIAL	GRADED TRIAL # 1	GRADED TRIAL # 2	NOTES
1. ✦	Plan a time to install hardware when it does not interfere with patient reception and care and when you are not likely to be interrupted, such as before or after office hours.				
2. ✦	Check the make, model, and compatibility to ensure the device meets your expectations of what was to be purchased.				
3. ✦	Open the box that contains the hardware, being careful to not cut anything inside the package. Do not throw anything away.				
4. ✦	Locate the installation manual and/or parts list.				
5. ✦	Unpack the box and check off each item on the parts list as you locate it. Thoroughly check all packing materials. Look for small items that may have dropped to the bottom of the box or that may be packaged in a small envelope or plastic bag. When you think you are done, review the parts list one more time, and again check off every item to be certain you have it. Set the packing materials to one side, but do not throw anything away. If any parts are missing, call the manufacturer at the phone number usually located on the parts list.				
6. ✦	Read through the installation instructions one time, without performing any of the tasks. This helps you become familiar with the overall installation process, because the details for installing each piece of hardware are unique to that component.				

Name: _____

Date: _____

POINT VALUE ✦ = 3–6 points ✷ = 7–9 points	PRACTICE TRIAL	GRADED TRIAL # 1	GRADED TRIAL # 2	NOTES
7. ✦ Collect any additional materials or information the installation instructions refer to, including tools, such as a screwdriver, or any special information, such as existing passwords, equipment codes, or similar items of information.				
8. ✷ If installing an internal component, such as a new internal drive or memory chips, turn the computer off, unplug it, and open the case. If installing an external component, note if the computer is to be turned off or left on. If instructions state to turn off the computer, also unplug it from the wall. This protects both you and the hardware.				
9. ✷ Follow the manufacturer's installation instructions, checking off each step as you complete it. Do not skip or change the order of any steps. Reread each step to be sure you follow it correctly.				
10. ✷ If required, install any software that may accompany the hardware. Some components require you to install a device driver (software instructions needed for the component to communicate with the central processing unit [CPU]). You may need to access the manufacturer's website to download the most recent version of the driver.				

POINT VALUE ✦ = 3–6 points ✱ = 7–9 points		PRACTICE TRIAL	GRADED TRIAL # 1	GRADED TRIAL # 2	NOTES
11. ✱	Follow the manufacturer's instructions to test the operation of the newly installed component. This may require starting or restarting the computer.				
12. ✱	If the component does not function properly, read the troubleshooting instructions or frequently asked questions (FAQ) information usually included in the installation guide.				
13. ✦	Complete the required registration and warranty forms. These may be included in the package or you may be able to do this online.				
14. ✦	Record the addition of the equipment on the office's equipment inventory log.				
15. ✦	Locate the component's user manual or operating manual and file it in the appropriate location, per office policy. Sometimes the manual must be downloaded from the manufacturer's website.				
16. ✦	Retain all packing materials for at least 30 days in the event that the product needs to be returned or exchanged.				

Name: _____

Date: _____

Document: Enter the appropriate information in the chart below.

Grading

Points Earned	_____		
Points Possible	_____	111	111
Percent Grade (Points Earned/Points Possible)	_____		
PASS:	_____	❏ YES ❏ NO ❏ N/A	❏ YES ❏ NO ❏ N/A

Instructor Sign-Off

Instructor: _____   **Date:** _____

Procedure 12-2:

Installing Computer Software

Objective: Follow a general process for installing computer software.

Equipment and Supplies: Computer on which software is to be installed; new software and all packaging; office equipment inventory log

Affective Behaviors: Affective behaviors provide a professional approach to a skill that enhances the patient encounter. These behaviors may also display sensitivity to a patient's rights and enhance communication. Pay close attention to these skills, which will be in **_bold, italicized_** font.

Notes to the Student

_____

_____

_____

_____

_____

_____

Skills Assessment Requirements

Read and familiarize yourself with the procedure; complete the minimum practice requirements (MPRs). Document each MPR using proper charting technique. Complete each procedure within a reasonable amount of time, with a minimum of 85% accuracy.

POINT VALUE ✦ = 3–6 points ✱ = 7–9 points	PRACTICE TRIAL	GRADED TRIAL # 1	GRADED TRIAL # 2	NOTES
1. ✦ Plan a time to install software when it does not interfere with patient reception and care and when you are not likely to be interrupted, such as before or after office hours.				
2. ✦ Check the name, version, and compatibility printed on the software package to ensure it meets your expectations of what was to be purchased.				
3. ✦ Open the box that contains the software, being careful to not cut anything inside the package. Do not throw anything away.				
4. ✦ Locate the installation manual and/or parts list.				
5. ✦ Unpack the package and check off each item on the parts list as you locate it. Thoroughly check all packing materials. Recheck the parts list to be certain you have everything. Set the packing materials to one side, but do not throw anything away. If any items are missing, call the manufacturer at the phone number usually located on the parts list.				
6. ✦ Read through the installation instructions one time, without performing any of the tasks. This helps you become familiar with the overall installation process.				
7. ✱ Collect any additional materials or information the installation instructions refer to, including any existing passwords, equipment codes, or similar items of information.				

POINT VALUE ✦ = 3–6 points ✳ = 7–9 points		PRACTICE TRIAL	GRADED TRIAL # 1	GRADED TRIAL # 2	NOTES
8. ✳	Unless otherwise instructed by the manufacturer's instructions, turn on or reboot the computer to clear its memory. Verify that all software programs and Internet browsers are closed.				
9. ✳	In most cases, you will be instructed to insert a disk or CD into the DVD drive. The setup program or installation wizard usually starts automatically. If it does not start, refer to the installation instructions regarding how to start it.				
10. ✦	In some cases, you may be installing a program that was downloaded from the Internet. If this is the case, you will probably need to unzip a compressed file and click on the installation program (usually setup.exe) to begin the installation process. NOTE: Download software only if approved by office policy and only if authorized for office use. Do not download software for personal use under any circumstances.				
11. ✳	Respond to the prompts that appear on the screen. The first prompt usually asks you to accept the software licensing agreement. Then you usually need to enter the name of the user and the company. Accept the program's default suggestions for installation location (folder) and file locations unless your office computer policy provides other guidelines.				

POINT VALUE ✦ = 3–6 points ✳ = 7–9 points		PRACTICE TRIAL	GRADED TRIAL # 1	GRADED TRIAL # 2	NOTES
12. ✳	When installation is complete, you usually will be asked to restart the computer. Verify that the software functions as expected, following manufacturer's instructions. If there are none, start the program and test its major functions by performing sample tasks.				
13. ✳	If the software does not function properly, read the troubleshooting instructions or frequently asked questions (FAQs) included in the installation guide. Some companies provide a technical support phone number to call should there be problems.				
14. ✦	Complete the required registration and warranty forms. These may be included in the package or you may be able to do this online.				
15. ✦	Record the addition of the equipment on the office's software inventory log.				
16. ✦	Locate the software user manual and file it in the appropriate location, per office policy. Sometimes the manual must be downloaded from the manufacturer's website.				
17. ✦	Retain all packing materials for at least 30 days, in the event that the product needs to be returned or exchanged.				

Name: _____

Date: _____

Document: Enter the appropriate information in the chart below.

Grading

Points Earned	_____		
Points Possible	_____	120	120
Percent Grade (Points Earned/Points Possible)	_____		
PASS:	_____	❏ YES ❏ NO ❏ N/A	❏ YES ❏ NO ❏ N/A

Instructor Sign-Off

Instructor: _____ **Date:** _____

Procedure 12-3:

Using the Internet to Access Health Information

Objective: Use the World Wide Web to locate reliable health information related to the medical office.

Equipment and Supplies: Computer (powered on) with Internet browser

Affective Behaviors: Affective behaviors provide a professional approach to a skill that enhances the patient encounter. These behaviors may also display sensitivity to a patient's rights and enhance communication. Pay close attention to these skills, which will be in **bold, italicized** font.

Notes to the Student

_____

_____

_____

_____

_____

_____

Skills Assessment Requirements

Read and familiarize yourself with the procedure; complete the minimum practice requirements (MPRs). Document each MPR using proper charting technique. Complete each procedure within a reasonable amount of time, with a minimum of 85% accuracy.

POINT VALUE ✦ = 3–6 points ✳ = 7–9 points		**PRACTICE TRIAL**	**GRADED TRIAL # 1**	**GRADED TRIAL # 2**	**NOTES**
1. ✦	Open the Internet browser (a software program designed to access the Internet and World Wide Web) on the computer. Examples of Internet browsers are Internet Explorer, Chrome, Mozilla, and Firefox.				
2. ✦	If you have a preferred website, such as one of those listed in Table 12-4, you may navigate directly to the site by keying the website address into the address bar. Press ENTER to navigate to the website. Skip to step 8 below.				
3. ✦	Navigate to a search engine (an Internet-based application that searches websites for information) using one of the following methods: • Many Internet browsers use a particular search engine by default and open the search page when you open the browser. • If you have a preferred search engine, type its address in the address bar at the top of the browser (such as www.google .com or www.bing.com). • Type the words "search engine" in the address bar. The screen will display a list of popular search engines from which you can select.				
4. ✦	Locate the search window on the search engine screen. The search bar is usually a white box with button displaying the words "Search," or "Go," or the image of a small magnifying glass next to it.				

POINT VALUE ✦ = 3–6 points ✳ = 7–9 points		PRACTICE TRIAL	GRADED TRIAL # 1	GRADED TRIAL # 2	NOTES
5. ✦	In the search bar, key in a few specific keywords or phrases to describe your topic. Press ENTER or click the button next to the search bar to activate the search. Examples would be *influenza*, to locate general information about the flu; *children flu*, to locate information about how the flu affects children; or *flu 2014*, to locate information about flu strains in the year 2014.				
6. ✦	Review the search results on the screen. The screen will display a list of topics, each with a brief excerpt. The website address usually appears immediately under the topic title.				
7. ✦	Left-click on the topic title to navigate to the desired website.				
8. ✳	Upon arriving at the website, identify the organization or sponsor of the website, to ensure the information is reliable. The name may appear at the top of the screen. You can also look for a menu bar that contains the link "About Us." If the website address ends in *.com* and does not identify the sponsor, it is most likely a commercial site established to attract users who generate advertising revenue. Avoid such sites.				

Name: _____

Date: _____

POINT VALUE ✦ = 3–6 points ✻ = 7–9 points		PRACTICE TRIAL	GRADED TRIAL # 1	GRADED TRIAL # 2	NOTES
9. ✻	Determine if the page has the information you need. Read the title of the screen you have arrived at. Also read the menu choices, which may appear near the top of the page or on the left-hand side of the screen. Often, search engine results are very specific and the link takes you directly to the specific information you need. Other times, you may need to navigate through the menus to find the desired information or to conduct a second search within the site itself.				
10. ✻	If necessary, search for more information on the website using one of the following methods: • Explore the menu options by moving the mouse over each item and clicking on it, if necessary. • If a menu bar containing letters of the alphabet is present, click on the letter of the term you wish to search for. • Locate an internal search box near the top or left-hand side of the screen that enables you to search within the site. Enter keywords or a phrase related to the topic you are searching for.				

Name: _____

Date: _____

POINT VALUE ✦ = 3–6 points ✶ = 7–9 points	PRACTICE TRIAL	GRADED TRIAL # 1	GRADED TRIAL # 2	NOTES
11. ✶ Decide how to save the information using one of the following methods: • To print the page, click a printer icon that appears on the page, if available. Or, you may be able to right-click your mouse to bring up a menu that provides a print option. • Bookmark or save the link to the bookmark manager or favorites list in your browser. This stores the link so that you can return at a later time. The steps to do this vary slightly for each browser. • To e-mail a copy or link for the page, click an envelope icon that appears on the page, if available. You may e-mail it to yourself or to the person who requested the information.				
12. ✦ Repeat the steps as necessary. When done, close the browser. Tip for conducting an Internet search: • Conduct multiple searches using slightly different keywords or synonyms such as *flu* and *influenza*, or *bird flu* and *avian flu*.				

Name: _____

Date: _____

Document: Enter the appropriate information in the chart below.

Grading

Points Earned	_____		
Points Possible	_____	84	84
Percent Grade (Points Earned/Points Possible)	_____		
PASS:	_____	❏ YES ❏ NO ❏ N/A	❏ YES ❏ NO ❏ N/A

Instructor Sign-Off

Instructor: _____ Date: _____

Procedure 13-1:

Adding or Changing Items on a Patient's Record

Objective: Add an item to a patient's record and correctly change an error in documentation.

Equipment and Supplies: Medical record to be added to or changed; black pen; correct information or documentation to be added or changed

Affective Behaviors: Affective behaviors provide a professional approach to a skill that enhances the patient encounter. These behaviors may also display sensitivity to a patient's rights and enhance communication. Pay close attention to these skills, which will be in **bold, italicized** font.

Notes to the Student

_____

_____

_____

_____

_____

_____

Skills Assessment Requirements

Read and familiarize yourself with the procedure; complete the minimum practice requirements (MPRs). Document each MPR using proper charting technique. Complete each procedure within a reasonable amount of time, with a minimum of 85% accuracy.

POINT VALUE ✦ = 3–6 points ✳ = 7–9 points		PRACTICE TRIAL	GRADED TRIAL # 1	GRADED TRIAL # 2	NOTES
	Adding items to a record				
1. ✦	An item is added to a patient record as soon as it is discovered that the item was omitted.				
2. ✦	Locate the last entry in the medical record.				
3. ✦	Using a pen with black ink, on the next line of the record, immediately after the last entry, place the current date.				
4. ✦	On the same line, after the date, place the statement "late entry."				
5. ✦	Note the date on which the information to be added was gathered.				
6. ✦	Enter the information that was originally omitted.				
7. ✦	Sign the entry with your full name and credentials.				
	Changing items in the record				
1. ✦	If an incorrect entry was made in the medical record, or the entry was made in the wrong record, it must be corrected by the person who made the original entry.				
2. ✳	Locate the incorrect information.				
3. ✳	Using a pen with black ink, draw one single line through the incorrect information so that the incorrect information is not obscured and can still be read.				
4. ✳	Never erase entries in a medical record. Never use correction fluid in a medical record. NEVER mark through information so heavily that it cannot be read.				

POINT VALUE ✦ = 3–6 points ✱ = 7–9 points		PRACTICE TRIAL	GRADED TRIAL # 1	GRADED TRIAL # 2	NOTES
5. ✦	Place the date of the correction, your initials, and "Error" above the incorrect information.				
6. ✱	Enter the correct information.				

Document: Enter the appropriate information in the chart below.

Grading

Points Earned	_____		
Points Possible	_____	42 48	42 48
Percent Grade (Points Earned/Points Possible)	_____		
PASS:	_____	❏ YES ❏ NO ❏ N/A	❏ YES ❏ NO ❏ N/A

Instructor Sign-Off

Instructor: _____   **Date:** _____

Procedure 13-2:

Organizing a Patient's Medical Record

Objectives: To update a patient's medical record, to verify that the correct record is in use, and to place the information in the correct place in the record.

Equipment and Supplies: Patient medical record; assorted documents for filing in record

Affective Behaviors: Affective behaviors provide a professional approach to a skill that enhances the patient encounter. These behaviors may also display sensitivity to a patient's rights and enhance communication. Pay close attention to these skills, which will be in **_bold, italicized_** font.

Notes to the Student

_____

_____

_____

_____

_____

_____

Skills Assessment Requirements

Read and familiarize yourself with the procedure; complete the minimum practice requirements (MPRs). Document each MPR using proper charting technique. Complete each procedure within a reasonable amount of time, with a minimum of 85% accuracy.

POINT VALUE ✦ = 3–6 points ✳ = 7–9 points		PRACTICE TRIAL	GRADED TRIAL # 1	GRADED TRIAL # 2	NOTES
1. ✳	Verify that you have the right records for the patient record you have been given.				
2. ✳	File documents in chronological order in the correct areas of the file, according to your facility policy, for consistency. For example, file laboratory reports with other laboratory reports within the lab section, and with the most recent report on top.				
3. ✦	Return medical record to correct place in alphabetical order with other files.				

Name: _____

Date: _____

Document: Enter the appropriate information in the chart below.

Grading

Points Earned	_____		
Points Possible	_____	24	24
Percent Grade (Points Earned/Points Possible)	_____		
PASS:	_____	❏ YES ❏ NO ❏ N/A	❏ YES ❏ NO ❏ N/A

Instructor Sign-Off

Instructor: _____ **Date:** _____

Procedure 13-3:

Collating Records

Objective: Prepare medical records of scheduled patients for review by the physician.

Equipment and Supplies: Master list of scheduled patients; charts and records of scheduled patients

Affective Behaviors: Affective behaviors provide a professional approach to a skill that enhances the patient encounter. These behaviors may also display sensitivity to a patient's rights and enhance communication. Pay close attention to these skills, which will be in **_bold, italicized_** font.

Notes to the Student

_____

_____

_____

_____

_____

_____

Skills Assessment Requirements

Read and familiarize yourself with the procedure; complete the minimum practice requirements (MPRs). Document each MPR using proper charting technique. Complete each procedure within a reasonable amount of time, with a minimum of 85% accuracy.

Name: _____

Date: _____

POINT VALUE ✦ = 3–6 points ✳ = 7–9 points		PRACTICE TRIAL	GRADED TRIAL # 1	GRADED TRIAL # 2	NOTES
1. ✦	Print or copy the day's appointment schedule.				
2. ✦	Pull all the medical records of patients scheduled to be seen.				
3. ✳	In each record, review the patient's last appointment and make note of any results that should have been received, including laboratory tests, X-ray results, consultation notes, and other tests.				
4. ✳	If any of the results are not in the patient's chart, call the appropriate facilities to retrieve the results. In the patient's chart, document the date, time, the name of person with whom you spoke, and the expected action regarding the requested information. You may take oral results and record them as a verbal report, but request that the hard-copy results be faxed to the office as soon as possible.				
5. ✳	Make a list of all results that have been received by phone and any that are outstanding. Let the physician know what remains outstanding.				
6. ✦	Add all received information to each chart for the physician to review and sign off on.				

Name: _____

Date: _____

Document: Enter the appropriate information in the chart below.

Grading

Points Earned	_____		
Points Possible	_____	45	45
Percent Grade (Points Earned/Points Possible)	_____		
PASS:	_____	❏ YES ❏ NO ❏ N/A	❏ YES ❏ NO ❏ N/A

Instructor Sign-Off

Instructor: _____ **Date:** _____

Procedure 13-4:

Filing a Record Alphabetically

Objective: File a patient record in the correct order, using the alphabetical method for filing.

Equipment and Supplies: Patient record, alphabetic files

Affective Behaviors: Affective behaviors provide a professional approach to a skill that enhances the patient encounter. These behaviors may also display sensitivity to a patient's rights and enhance communication. Pay close attention to these skills, which will be in **_bold, italicized_** font.

Notes to the Student

_____

_____

_____

_____

_____

_____

Skills Assessment Requirements

Read and familiarize yourself with the procedure; complete the minimum practice requirements (MPRs). Document each MPR using proper charting technique. Complete each procedure within a reasonable amount of time, with a minimum of 85% accuracy.

Name: _____

Date: _____

POINT VALUE ✦ = 3–6 points ✱ = 7–9 points		PRACTICE TRIAL	GRADED TRIAL #1	GRADED TRIAL #2	NOTES
1. ✦	Locate the medical record files or medical record room.				
2. ✦	Observe the name on the medical record to be filed.				
3. ✦	Records are filed in alphabetic order by last name first, then first name, then middle name or initial. Each letter in the name is a separate unit. Locate the set of records containing the same last name as the record to be filed.				
4. ✦	Within the set of records containing the same last name as the record to be filed, locate the records with the same letter of the first name as the record to be filed.				
5. ✦	Using the alphabet as a guide, place the record to be filed after the record that comes before it in the alphabet but before the record that comes after it in the alphabet.				
6. ✱	A name with only an initial first name is filed before a full name. (Brown, H. is filed before Brown, Henry.) The filing rule "Nothing before something" is a useful tool here.				
7. ✱	Hyphenated names are treated as one unit. (Mary Freeman-Smith is indexed as Freemansmith, Mary.)				
8. ✦	Disregard apostrophes. (Megan O'Connor is indexed as Oconnor, Megan.)				

POINT VALUE ✦ = 3–6 points ✶ = 7–9 points		PRACTICE TRIAL	GRADED TRIAL # 1	GRADED TRIAL # 2	NOTES
9. ✶	Titles and initials are disregarded for filing, but placed in parentheses after the name. (Dr. Beth Ann Williams is indexed as Williams, Beth Ann, [Dr.].)				
10.✶	Married women are indexed using their legal name. The husband's name can be used for cross-referencing.				
11.✶	Seniority units, such as Jr. and Sr., are filed in numeric order from first to last.				
12.✶	Numeric seniority terms are filed before alphabetic terms.				
13.✦	After placing the file between the two records before and after it in the alphabet, check once more to be sure the file is properly placed.				
14.✦	If there is a marker or out-guide in place of the removed record, then take out the marker when replacing the file.				

Name: _____

Date: _____

Document: Enter the appropriate information in the chart below.

Grading

Points Earned	_____		
Points Possible	_____	102	102
Percent Grade (Points Earned/Points Possible)	_____		
PASS:	_____	❏ YES ❏ NO ❏ N/A	❏ YES ❏ NO ❏ N/A

Instructor Sign-Off

Instructor: _____ **Date:** _____

Procedure 13-5:

Filing a Record Numerically Using the Terminal-Digit Filing System

Objective: File a patient record in the correct order, using the terminal-digit method for filing.

Equipment and Supplies: Patient record, numeric file

Affective Behaviors: Affective behaviors provide a professional approach to a skill that enhances the patient encounter. These behaviors may also display sensitivity to a patient's rights and enhance communication. Pay close attention to these skills, which will be in **_bold, italicized_** font.

Notes to the Student

_____

_____

_____

_____

_____

_____

_____

Skills Assessment Requirements

Read and familiarize yourself with the procedure; complete the minimum practice requirements (MPRs). Document each MPR using proper charting technique. Complete each procedure within a reasonable amount of time, with a minimum of 85% accuracy.

POINT VALUE ✦ = 3–6 points ✶ = 7–9 points		PRACTICE TRIAL	GRADED TRIAL # 1	GRADED TRIAL # 2	NOTES
1. ✦	Locate the medical record file or the medical record room.				
2. ✦	Observe the numbers on the record to be filed.				
3. ✦	Locate the set of files with the same tertiary numbers as the record to be filed (these are the first two numbers on the record).				
4. ✦	Within the set of records with the same tertiary numbers, locate the row of records with the same secondary numbers as the record to be filed (the secondary numbers are the second two numbers on the record).				
5. ✦	Within the set of records with the same tertiary and secondary numbers as the record to be filed, place the record to be filed in numeric order by primary numbers (last two numbers on the record).				
6. ✦	After placing the file in numeric order by primary numbers, check once more to be sure the file is properly placed.				
7. ✦	If there is a marker or out-guide in place for the removed record, then take out the marker when replacing the file.				

Name: _____

Date: _____

Document: Enter the appropriate information in the chart below.

Grading

Points Earned	_____		
Points Possible	_____	42	42
Percent Grade (Points Earned/Points Possible)	_____		
PASS:	_____	❏ YES ❏ NO ❏ N/A	❏ YES ❏ NO ❏ N/A

Instructor Sign-Off

Instructor: _____ **Date:** _____

Procedure 13-6:

Locating Missing Files

Objective: Locate misfiled records.

Equipment and Supplies: Patient records

Affective Behaviors: Affective behaviors provide a professional approach to a skill that enhances the patient encounter. These behaviors may also display sensitivity to a patient's rights and enhance communication. Pay close attention to these skills, which will be in **_bold, italicized_** font.

Notes to the Student

_____

_____

_____

_____

_____

_____

Skills Assessment Requirements

Read and familiarize yourself with the procedure; complete the minimum practice requirements (MPRs). Document each MPR using proper charting technique. Complete each procedure within a reasonable amount of time, with a minimum of 85% accuracy.

Name: _____

Date: _____

POINT VALUE ✦ = 3–6 points ✱ = 7–9 points	PRACTICE TRIAL	GRADED TRIAL # 1	GRADED TRIAL # 2	NOTES
1. ✦ Begin by looking for a file with a sound-alike or look-alike name (e.g., Smith or Smits).				
2. ✱ If the patient has a first name that might be considered as a last name (e.g., Samuel Jacob), look in the section where you would find the first name (e.g., Samuel).				
3. ✦ If using a color-coded system, look for a folder that is out of place based on the color-coded label.				
4. ✦ If using a numeric system, look for a transposition of numbers (e.g., 236984 for 263984).				
5. ✦ Look for a transposition of letters.				
6. ✱ Look for an alternative spelling (e.g., Keane for Kane).				
7. ✱ Look at the folders that were filed before and after the missing record (e.g., pull out the schedule of all patients who were seen on the same day as the patient whose file is missing).				
8. ✱ Look on the physician's desk and through in and out baskets. Also, ask other staff members, such as the billing clerk, to examine their desks.				
9. ✱ Ask others in the office to assist you. Many times a set of fresh eyes can spot the misfiled chart immediately.				

Name: _____

Date: _____

Document: Enter the appropriate information in the chart below.

Grading

Points Earned	_____		
Points Possible	_____	69	69
Percent Grade (Points Earned/Points Possible)	_____		
PASS:	_____	❏ YES ❏ NO ❏ N/A	❏ YES ❏ NO ❏ N/A

Instructor Sign-Off

Instructor: _____   Date: _____

© 2015 Pearson Education, Inc.

Procedure 14-1:

Correcting an Entry in the Electronic Medical Record

Objective: Appropriately correct an entry in the electronic health record in an accurate manner following legal protocol.

Equipment and Supplies: Computer with electronic health record software

Affective Behaviors: Affective behaviors provide a professional approach to a skill that enhances the patient encounter. These behaviors may also display sensitivity to a patient's rights and enhance communication. Pay close attention to these skills, which will be in **_bold, italicized_** font.

Notes to the Student

_____

_____

_____

_____

_____

_____

Skills Assessment Requirements

Read and familiarize yourself with the procedure; complete the minimum practice requirements (MPRs). Document each MPR using proper charting technique. Complete each procedure within a reasonable amount of time, with a minimum of 85% accuracy.

Name: _____

Date: _____

POINT VALUE ✦ = 3–6 points ✳ = 7–9 points	PRACTICE TRIAL	GRADED TRIAL # 1	GRADED TRIAL # 2	NOTES
1. ✦ Log in with your assigned user identification name and the password you previously created.				
2. ✦ Identify the correct patient electronic health record (EHR) in which the error was made.				
3. ✦ Locate the error within the record.				
4. ✦ Review the rules associated with the software you are using for correcting or making an addendum to a patient's record.				
5. ✳ Make the appropriate correction within the EHR, according to the steps required within the software program.				
6. ✳ Complete the signature process, according to the steps required within the software program.				
7. ✳ Verify that the change made is correct and reflects the change you intended.				
8. ✳ Save the changes.				
9. ✦ Close the patient's EHR.				
10. ✦ Log off the system.				

Name: _____

Date: _____

Document: Enter the appropriate information in the chart below.

Grading

Points Earned	_____		
Points Possible	_____	72	72
Percent Grade (Points Earned/Points Possible)	_____		
PASS:	_____	❏ YES ❏ NO ❏ N/A	❏ YES ❏ NO ❏ N/A

Instructor Sign-Off

Instructor: _____ **Date:** _____

Procedure 14-2:

Recording Vital Signs

Objective: Appropriately correct an entry in the electronic health record in an accurate manner following legal protocol.

Equipment and Supplies: Computer with electronic health record software; blood pressure cuff designed to work with the data capture device for the EHR system and appropriately sized for the patient; blood pressure monitor (a box with controls and a read-out screen that is connected to the EHR system)

Affective Behaviors: Affective behaviors provide a professional approach to a skill that enhances the patient encounter. These behaviors may also display sensitivity to a patient's rights and enhance communication. Pay close attention to these skills, which will be in **_bold, italicized_** font.

Notes to the Student

_____

_____

_____

_____

_____

_____

Skills Assessment Requirements

Read and familiarize yourself with the procedure; complete the minimum practice requirements. Document each MPR using proper charting technique. Complete each procedure within a reasonable amount of time, with a minimum of 85% accuracy.

POINT VALUE ✦ = 3–6 points ✳ = 7–9 points	PRACTICE TRIAL	GRADED TRIAL # 1	GRADED TRIAL # 2	NOTES
1. ✦ Check to be sure the system is turned on and that the blood pressure monitor is properly connected, according to the steps required by the equipment manufacturer.				
2. ✦ Log in with your assigned user identification name and the password you previously created.				
3. ✳ Identify the correct patient EHR according to clinic policies.				
4. ✳ Determine appropriately sized blood pressure cuff, according to clinical procedures.				
5. ✦ Attach the blood pressure cuff to the blood pressure monitor.				
6. ✳ Position the patient properly and apply the blood pressure cuff according to clinical procedures.				
7. ✦ Push the button on the blood pressure (BP) monitor to start the reading.				
8. ✦ Access the patient's record according to the steps required within the software program.				
9. ✦ Locate the vital signs screen in the EHR.				
10. ✳ Confirm and record the BP reading according to the steps required within the software program.				
11. ✦ Follow clinical procedures to verify the reading with the patient.				
12. ✳ Key in data for vital signs taken manually, as appropriate.				

Name: _____

Date: _____

POINT VALUE ✦ = 3–6 points ✶ = 7–9 points		PRACTICE TRIAL	GRADED TRIAL # 1	GRADED TRIAL # 2	NOTES
13. ✶	Complete the signature process, according to the steps required within the software program.				
14. ✶	Verify that the entry is correct and reflects the data intended.				
15. ✦	Save the data.				
16. ✦	Close the patient's record.				
17. ✶	Log off the system.				
18. ✶	Remove cuff from patient.				

Name: _____

Date: _____

Document: Enter the appropriate information in the chart below.

Grading

Points Earned	_____		
Points Possible	_____	126	126
Percent Grade (Points Earned/Points Possible)	_____		
PASS:	_____	❏ YES ❏ NO ❏ N/A	❏ YES ❏ NO ❏ N/A

Instructor Sign-Off

Instructor: _____ Date: _____

Name: _____

Date: _____

Procedure 14-3:

Sending Automated Orders

Objective: Send an automated order to the lab using an EHR.

Equipment and Supplies: Computer with electronic health record software; orders from the physician

Affective Behaviors: Affective behaviors provide a professional approach to a skill that enhances the patient encounter. These behaviors may also display sensitivity to a patient's rights and enhance communication. Pay close attention to these skills, which will be in **bold, italicized** font.

Notes to the Student

_____

_____

_____

_____

_____

_____

Skills Assessment Requirements

Read and familiarize yourself with the procedure; complete the minimum practice requirements (MPRs). Document each MPR using proper charting technique. Complete each procedure within a reasonable amount of time, with a minimum of 85% accuracy.

Name: _____

Date: _____

POINT VALUE ✦ = 3–6 points ✱ = 7–9 points		PRACTICE TRIAL	GRADED TRIAL # 1	GRADED TRIAL # 2	NOTES
1. ✦	Be sure the system is turned on.				
2. ✦	Log in with your assigned user identification name and the password you previously created.				
3. ✱	Identify the correct patient EHR following clinic policies.				
4. ✱	Ask the patient where the lab order should be sent. Verify that the facility can accept electronic orders.				
5. ✦	Locate the order entry screen, according to the steps required within the software program.				
6. ✱	Select laboratory procedures, type of procedure, and specific type of test based on software.				
7. ✱	Enter all required parameters for test selected.				
8. ✱	Select the laboratory facility that is to receive the order.				
9. ✱	Complete the signature process, according to the steps required within the software program.				
10. ✱	Verify that the entry is correct, reflects the test intended, and agrees with the physician order. This may require navigating to a new location within the software, such as "order management."				
11. ✱	Save the order.				

POINT VALUE ♦ = 3–6 points ✶ = 7–9 points		PRACTICE TRIAL	GRADED TRIAL # 1	GRADED TRIAL # 2	NOTES
12. ✶	Activate or send the order according to the steps required within the software program.				
13. ♦	Close the patient's EHR.				
14. ♦	Log off the system.				

Name: _____

Date: _____

Document: Enter the appropriate information in the chart below.

Grading

Points Earned	_____		
Points Possible	_____	108	108
Percent Grade (Points Earned/Points Possible)	_____		
PASS:	_____	❏ YES ❏ NO ❏ N/A	❏ YES ❏ NO ❏ N/A

Instructor Sign-Off

Instructor: _____ Date: _____

Procedure 15-1:

Calculating Patient Financial Responsibility

Objective: Accurately calculate the patient's financial responsibility using the charges, deductible, coinsurance, and allowed amounts.

Equipment and Supplies: Pen; paper; insurance verification of benefits form; patient's insurance identification card; Explanation of Benefits form; calculator

Affective Behaviors: Affective behaviors provide a professional approach to a skill that enhances the patient encounter. These behaviors may also display sensitivity to a patient's rights and enhance communication. Pay close attention to these skills, which will be in ***bold, italicized*** font.

Notes to the Student

_____

_____

_____

_____

Skills Assessment Requirements

Read and familiarize yourself with the procedure; complete the minimum practice requirements (MPRs). Document each MPR using proper charting technique. Complete each procedure within a reasonable amount of time, with a minimum of 85% accuracy.

Name: _____

Date: _____

POINT VALUE ✦ = 3–6 points ✱ = 7–9 points		PRACTICE TRIAL	GRADED TRIAL # 1	GRADED TRIAL # 2	NOTES
1. ✦	After the patient's insurance coverage has been verified, locate the information on the verification form regarding the deductible and coinsurance amount.				
2. ✦	*Inform the patient of the deductible amount that needs to be paid after the beginning of the calendar or fiscal year, before insurance payments become effective.*				
3. ✦	*Explain to the patient that the amount charged for any particular procedure in the medical office will likely be reduced to a lower amount, called the allowed amount, when processed by the insurance carrier.*				
4. ✦	After the insurance payment is received, use the Explanation of Benefits (EOB) form to identify the amount the insurance carrier allowed on the claim.				
5. ✱	Calculate the total allowed amount by adding together the allowed amount for each service.				
6. ✱	Subtract the deductible from the total of the allowed charges.				
7. ✱	Multiply the remaining allowed amount by the coinsurance percentage to determine the patient's coinsurance amount.				
8. ✱	Add the deductible to the coinsurance amount to determine the amount the patient needs to pay out of pocket for the visit.				
9. ✱	*Explain the figures to the patient and collect the fees.*				

Document: Enter the appropriate information in the chart below.

Grading

Points Earned	_____		
Points Possible	_____	66	66
Percent Grade (Points Earned/Points Possible)	_____		
PASS:	_____	❏ YES ❏ NO ❏ N/A	❏ YES ❏ NO ❏ N/A

Instructor Sign-Off

Instructor: _____   **Date:** _____

Procedure 15-2:

Verifying Eligibility

Objective: Verify a patient's insurance eligibility in order to determine the covered services and patient's financial responsibility.

Equipment and Supplies: Insurance identification card; patient's registration form; insurance verification of benefits worksheet; telephone or computer; paper; pen

Affective Behaviors: Affective behaviors provide a professional approach to a skill that enhances the patient encounter. These behaviors may also display sensitivity to a patient's rights and enhance communication. Pay close attention to these skills, which will be in **bold, italicized** font.

Notes to the Student

_____

_____

_____

Skills Assessment Requirements

Read and familiarize yourself with the procedure; complete the minimum practice requirements (MPRs). Document each MPR using proper charting technique. Complete each procedure within a reasonable amount of time, with a minimum of 85% accuracy.

POINT VALUE ✦ = 3–6 points ✳ = 7–9 points	PRACTICE TRIAL	GRADED TRIAL #1	GRADED TRIAL #2	NOTES
1. ✦ Look at the patient's registration form to locate the patient's birth date and the patient's relationship to the insured.				
2. ✦ Look at the patient's insurance identification card to locate the name of the insured (policyholder), the insured's member identification number, and the telephone number of the insurance company.				
3. ✦ Call the insurance company at the provider customer service telephone number listed on the insurance identification card or access the insurance company's secure website, if available.				
4. ✦ When the customer service representative answers the call, write down the name of the customer service representative and the date and time of the call.				
5. ✦ *Verify spelling of policyholder's name and birth date.*				
6. ✦ *Verify patient's name and birth date.*				
7. ✳ *Verify coverage for type of service to be rendered, including frequency or number of visits.*				
8. ✳ *Verify when pre-authorization is needed.*				
9. ✳ *Verify patient's financial responsibility for deductible, copayment, or coinsurance amounts.*				

POINT VALUE ✦ = 3–6 points ✱ = 7–9 points		PRACTICE TRIAL	GRADED TRIAL # 1	GRADED TRIAL # 2	NOTES
10. ✦	Verify coordination of benefits rules if more than one policy covers the patient.				
11. ✦	Verify provider's participating or non-participating status.				
12. ✦	Verify the address to which insurance claims are to be mailed or the payer number needed for electronic billing.				

Name: _____

Date: _____

Document: Enter the appropriate information in the chart below.

Grading

Points Earned	_____		
Points Possible	_____	81	81
Percent Grade (Points Earned/Points Possible)	_____		
PASS:	_____	❏ YES ❏ NO ❏ N/A	❏ YES ❏ NO ❏ N/A

Instructor Sign-Off

Instructor: _____ Date: _____

Procedure 15-3:

Obtaining Insurance Company Authorizations

Objective: Obtain authorization from an insurance company for a procedure.

Equipment and Supplies: Patient insurance information (i.e., ID number, birth date of the insured, name and telephone number for provider customer service at the insurance company); paper and pen; description of the procedure the doctor has prescribed, including:

Current Procedural Terminology (CPT) code

Patient's diagnosis pertaining to the needed procedure

Location where procedure is to be performed (e.g., office, outpatient surgery, inpatient hospitalization)

Date by which the procedure must be performed

Affective Behaviors: Affective behaviors provide a professional approach to a skill that enhances the patient encounter. These behaviors may also display sensitivity to a patient's rights and enhance communication. Pay close attention to these skills, which will be in **bold, italicized** font.

Notes to the Student

_____

_____

_____

_____

Skills Assessment Requirements

Read and familiarize yourself with the procedure; complete the minimum practice requirements (MPRs). Document each MPR using proper charting technique. Complete each procedure within a reasonable amount of time, with a minimum of 85% accuracy.

POINT VALUE ✦ = 3–6 points ✶ = 7–9 points		PRACTICE TRIAL	GRADED TRIAL #1	GRADED TRIAL #2	NOTES
1. ✦	Write down the date and time of the call, the name of the insurance company, and the name of the insurance company representative on the phone.				
2. ✦	Give the insurance company representative your name and your office's/physician's name.				
3. ✦	Give the insurance company representative the name of the patient, the name of the insured, and the insured's ID number.				
4. ✦	Let the representative know what the procedure is your doctor has prescribed for the patient and the date by which the procedure must be performed.				
5. ✦	Provide the representative any other requested information (e.g., procedure code, diagnosis code, and place where the procedure is to be performed).				
6. ✶	Write down the authorization number the representative provides.				
7. ✦	Ask the representative if any supporting documentation (e.g., chart notes, operative report, laboratory report, or pathology report) is needed with the CMS-1500 billing form. If so, write down the required documentation.				
8. ✦	Keep all preceding information in the patient's file for reference in case the claim is not paid by the insurance carrier.				

Document: Enter the appropriate information in the chart below.

Grading

Points Earned	_____		
Points Possible	_____	51	51
Percent Grade (Points Earned/Points Possible)	_____		
PASS:	_____	❏ YES ❏ NO ❏ N/A	❏ YES ❏ NO ❏ N/A

Instructor Sign-Off

Instructor: _____   **Date:** _____

Procedure 15-4:

Obtaining Managed Care Referrals

Objective: Obtain a referral authorization from a managed care company.

Equipment and Supplies: Telephone; patient's medical chart; name and telephone number of patient's primary care provider

Affective Behaviors: Affective behaviors provide a professional approach to a skill that enhances the patient encounter. These behaviors may also display sensitivity to a patient's rights and enhance communication. Pay close attention to these skills, which will be in **bold, italicized** font.

Notes to the Student

_____

_____

_____

Skills Assessment Requirements

Read and familiarize yourself with the procedure; complete the minimum practice requirements (MPRs). Document each MPR using proper charting technique. Complete each procedure within a reasonable amount of time, with a minimum of 85% accuracy.

Name: _____

Date: _____

POINT VALUE ✦ = 3–6 points ✳ = 7–9 points		PRACTICE TRIAL	GRADED TRIAL # 1	GRADED TRIAL # 2	NOTES
1. ✦	*Call the patient's primary care provider's office, and ask for the person in charge of referrals.*				
2. ✳	Give the referral assistant the patient's information, including name and birth date.				
3. ✳	*Inform the referral assistant of the need for a referral to the physician, including the reason for the patient's visit in the medical office.*				
4. ✳	*Ask the referral assistant if any information from the patient's file is needed to process the referral.*				
5. ✳	*Ask the referral assistant when to expect the referral. If needed, provide the office fax number for information transmittal.*				
6. ✦	Document the content of the telephone call in the patient's file.				
7. ✦	Notify the physician and the patient of the content of the telephone call.				

Name: _____

Date: _____

Document: Enter the appropriate information in the chart below.

Grading

Points Earned	_____		
Points Possible	_____	54	54
Percent Grade (Points Earned/Points Possible)	_____		
PASS:	_____	❏ YES ❏ NO ❏ N/A	❏ YES ❏ NO ❏ N/A

Instructor Sign-Off

Instructor: _____ **Date:** _____

Procedure 15-5:

Completing a CMS-1500 Claim Form

Objective: Identify required data and accurately complete a paper-based CMS-1500 claim form.

Equipment and Supplies: New Patient Registration Form for Theresa Andrews; Encounter Form for Theresa Andrews; Table 15-5: Instructions on Completing the CMS-1500 Claim Form; Blank CMS-1500 form (photocopy Figure 15-8 or obtain from instructor); black ink pen; calculator

Affective Behaviors: Affective behaviors provide a professional approach to a skill that enhances the patient encounter. These behaviors may also display sensitivity to a patient's rights and enhance communication. Pay close attention to these skills, which will be in **bold, *italicized*** font.

Notes to the Student

_____

_____

_____

Skills Assessment Requirements

Read and familiarize yourself with the procedure; complete the minimum practice requirements (MPRs). Document each MPR using proper charting technique. Complete each procedure within a reasonable amount of time, with a minimum of 85% accuracy.

Name: _____

Date: _____

POINT VALUE ✦ = 3–6 points ✶ = 7–9 points		PRACTICE TRIAL	GRADED TRIAL #1	GRADED TRIAL #2	NOTES
1. ✦	Enter the insurance company name and mailing address in the Carrier Area. You will find all insurance information on the New Patient Registration Form.				
2. ✶	Check the correct box in Item 1.				
3. ✦	Enter the insured's ID number in Item 1a.				
4. ✦	Enter the patient's name in Item 2, if different from the insured.				
5. ✶	Complete Item 3, using MMDDYYYY date format.				
6. ✶	Complete Item 4.				
7. ✶	Leave Item 5 blank because it is the same as Item 7.				
8. ✶	Complete Item 6.				
9. ✶	Complete Item 7. Note that there are three lines of information to complete.				
10. ✶	Leave Item 8 blank.				
11. ✶	Leave Item 9a to 9d blank because there is no secondary insurance.				
12. ✶	Complete Item 10a, 10b, and 10c.				
13. ✶	Leave Item 10d blank.				
14. ✶	Enter the group number in Item 11.				
15. ✶	Complete Item 11a, using MMDDCCYY date format.				
16. ✶	Leave Item 11b blank.				
17. ✶	Enter the insurance plan name in Item 11c.				

Name: _____

Date: _____

POINT VALUE ✦ = 3–6 points ✱ = 7–9 points		PRACTICE TRIAL	GRADED TRIAL #1	GRADED TRIAL #2	NOTES
18. ✱	Mark NO in Item 11d.				
19. ✱	Enter "SOF" in Item 12.				
20. ✱	Enter "SOF" in Item 13.				
21. ✱	Leave Item 14 to Item 19 blank.				
22. ✱	Enter the first diagnosis code in Item 21, line A. You will find all information related to the visit on the encounter form.				
23. ✱	Enter the second diagnosis code in Item 21, line B.				
24. ✱	Enter the 1 to identify the ICD-10-CM code set in the top right corner of Item 21, next to the label "ICD Ind."				
25. ✱	Leave Item 22 and Item 23 blank.				
26. ✱	In Item 24A, line 1, enter the date of service in both the FROM and TO fields.				
27. ✱	Enter the place of service code in Item 24B.				
28. ✱	Leave Item 24C blank.				
29. ✱	Enter the CPT for the office visit code in Item 24D.				
30. ✱	In Item 24E, enter "A B" to designate that both diagnoses on lines 21A and 21B relate to this service.				
31. ✱	Enter the fee for the office visit in Item 24F.				
32. ✱	Enter 1 for units in Item 24G.				
33. ✱	Leave blank Item 24H and Item 24I.				

POINT VALUE ✦ = 3–6 points ✶ = 7–9 points		PRACTICE TRIAL	GRADED TRIAL # 1	GRADED TRIAL # 2	NOTES
34. ✶	Enter the physician's national provider identification (NPI) number on the unshaded portion of Item 24J. You will find this on the Encounter Form next to the physician's signature.				
35. ✶	Repeat these steps for Item 24A, line 2 for the chest X-ray.				
36. ✶	Enter the EIN in Item 25 and mark X in the appropriate box. You will find this at the bottom of the Encounter Form.				
37. ✶	Enter the patient's account number in Item 26. You will find this on the New Patient Registration Form.				
38. ✶	Mark YES in Item 27.				
39. ✶	Add up the total charges in column 24F. Write the total in Item 28.				
40. ✶	Leave Item 29 and Item 30 blank.				
41. ✶	Enter the physician's signature, credentials, and the date in Item 31. Be certain to stay within the lines of the box.				
42. ✶	Enter the name and address of the clinic in Item 32. You will find the clinic information at the bottom of the Encounter Form.				
43. ✶	Enter the clinic's group NPI number in 32a.				
44. ✶	Leave Item 32b blank.				

Name: _____

Date: _____

	POINT VALUE ✦ = 3–6 points ✶ = 7–9 points	PRACTICE TRIAL	GRADED TRIAL # 1	GRADED TRIAL # 2	NOTES
45. ✶	In Item 33, enter the clinic's phone number in the top right corner.				
46. ✶	Enter the clinic's name and address in Item 33.				
47. ✶	Enter the clinic's NPI number in Item 33a.				
48. ✶	Leave Item 33b blank.				
49. ✶	Proofread your work. Check spelling and numbers against your source documents.				
50. ✶	Check your claim against the sample CMS-1500 form in Figure A.				

Name: _____

Date: _____

Document: Enter the appropriate information in the chart below.

Grading

Points Earned	_____		
Points Possible	_____	441	441
Percent Grade (Points Earned/Points Possible)	_____		
PASS:	_____	❏ YES ❏ NO ❏ N/A	❏ YES ❏ NO ❏ N/A

Instructor Sign-Off

Instructor: _____   **Date:** _____

Procedure 15-6:

Electronic Insurance Claims

Objective: Identify required data and accurately complete computer screens needed to create and submit an electronic insurance claim.

Equipment and Supplies: Computer with medical billing software; patient medical chart; fee slip for patient's visit

Affective Behaviors: Affective behaviors provide a professional approach to a skill that enhances the patient encounter. These behaviors may also display sensitivity to a patient's rights and enhance communication. Pay close attention to these skills, which will be in **_bold, italicized_** font.

Notes to the Student

_____

_____

_____

Skills Assessment Requirements

Read and familiarize yourself with the procedure; complete the minimum practice requirements (MPRs). Document each MPR using proper charting technique. Complete each procedure within a reasonable amount of time, with a minimum of 85% accuracy.

POINT VALUE ✦ = 3–6 points ✶ = 7–9 points		PRACTICE TRIAL	GRADED TRIAL # 1	GRADED TRIAL # 2	NOTES
1. ✦	Log in to the patient accounting software with the user name and password previously created.				
2. ✦	Choose the patient's account ledger in the computer billing software.				
3. ✦	Verify that the fee slip is for the patient with the account opened on the computer.				
4. ✦	Enter the charges and coding as appropriate.				
5. ✦	Complete the patient insurance information field.				
6. ✦	Enter the patient's information, including address, telephone number, and birth date.				
7. ✦	Enter the insured's information, including address, telephone number, and birth date.				
8. ✦	Enter the patient's relationship to the insured.				
9. ✦	Enter the insured's identification and group number.				
10. ✶	Check the appropriate box to indicate the patient has authorized the release of information to the insurance company.				
11. ✶	Check the appropriate box to indicate the patient has assigned the benefits (payment) to the provider.				
12. ✶	Check the appropriate boxes to indicate if the visit was related to an accident.				

Name: _____

Date: _____

POINT VALUE ✦ = 3–6 points ✱ = 7–9 points		PRACTICE TRIAL	GRADED TRIAL # 1	GRADED TRIAL # 2	NOTES
13. ✱	If the visit was a result of an accident, enter the accident's date.				
14. ✱	Enter information regarding a referring physician, if applicable.				
15. ✱	Enter information regarding the dates of hospitalization for these charges, if applicable.				
16. ✱	Enter the treating provider's name, address, telephone number, national provider identification (NPI) number, and Internal Revenue Service (IRS) tax identification number.				
17. ✱	Enter information regarding the facility where the services were performed if not performed in the provider's office.				
18. ✱	Check the appropriate box to indicate the provider accepts assignment.				
19. ✱	Review all information on the screen for accuracy and completeness.				
20. ✱	Following the instructions for the software application, select the menu item to transmit electronic claims. Usually, all claims entered into the computer during the day (or week) can be sent at the same time.				

POINT VALUE ✦ = 3–6 points ✱ = 7–9 points		PRACTICE TRIAL	GRADED TRIAL # 1	GRADED TRIAL # 2	NOTES
21. ✱	Following the instructions for the software application, select the menu item to download a transmission report that lists all claims sent in the current batch. Review the report to verify that all claims were received.				
22. ✱	Identify the reason for any claims that did not transmit. These claims are flagged as "failed" or "did not transmit" or with similar wording. A code or abbreviation for the failure is provided. Look up the meaning of the code or abbreviation in the manual provided by the claims clearinghouse or software vendor. Correct the error(s) and resubmit.				

Name: _____

Date: _____

Document: Enter the appropriate information in the chart below.

Grading

Points Earned	_____		
Points Possible	_____	141	141
Percent Grade (Points Earned/ Points Possible)	_____		
PASS:	_____	❏ YES ❏ NO ❏ N/A	❏ YES ❏ NO ❏ N/A

Instructor Sign-Off

Instructor: _____ **Date:** _____

Competency Check-Offs **687**

Procedure 16-1:

Performing ICD-10-CM Diagnostic Coding

Objective: Perform accurate diagnostic coding using the ICD-10-CM coding manual.

Equipment and Supplies:
- Patient's medical chart
- Current ICD-10-CM coding manual
- Superbill with doctor's written diagnosis

Affective Behaviors: Affective behaviors provide a professional approach to a skill that enhances the patient encounter. These behaviors may also display sensitivity to a patient's rights and enhance communication. Pay close attention to these skills, which will be in **bold, italicized** font.

Notes to the Student

_____

_____

_____

Skills Assessment Requirements

Read and familiarize yourself with the procedure; complete the minimum practice requirements (MPRs). Document each MPR using proper charting technique. Complete each procedure within a reasonable amount of time, with a minimum of 85% accuracy.

POINT VALUE ✦ = 3–6 points ✳ = 7–9 points		PRACTICE TRIAL	GRADED TRIAL # 1	GRADED TRIAL # 2	NOTES
1. ✦	Locate the patient's diagnostic code(s) or description on the encounter form or in the chart notes.				
2. ✳	Verify that the diagnostic code(s) or description on the encounter form also appears in the patient's chart in the form of a patient complaint (subjective finding) or a test finding (objective finding).				
3. ✦	Look in the Index of the ICD-10-CM coding manual to find the Main Term.				
4. ✦	Look up the preliminary code(s) in the Tabular List. Confirm that the written description matches the chart notes. If in doubt, check with the physician.				
5. ✦	Read and apply the conventions in the Tabular List. Assign any additional characters required.				
6. ✦	Assign the code for each diagnosis, beginning with the appropriate first-listed diagnosis.				

Name: _____

Date: _____

Document: Enter the appropriate information in the chart below.

Grading

Points Earned	_____		
Points Possible	_____	39	39
Percent Grade (Points Earned/Points Possible)	_____		
PASS:	_____	❑ YES ❑ NO ❑ N/A	❑ YES ❑ NO ❑ N/A

Instructor Sign-Off

Instructor: _____   **Date:** _____

Procedure 17-1:

Coding for a Procedure

Objective: Assign CPT codes based on documentation.

Equipment and Supplies:
- CPT coding manual
- Superbill/encounter form
- Patient's chart

Affective Behaviors: Affective behaviors provide a professional approach to a skill that enhances the patient encounter. These behaviors may also display sensitivity to a patient's rights and enhance communication. Pay close attention to these skills, which will be in **bold, *italicized*** font.

Notes to the Student

_____

_____

_____

_____

_____

_____

Skills Assessment Requirements

Read and familiarize yourself with the procedure; complete the minimum practice requirements (MPRs). Document each MPR using proper charting technique. Complete each procedure within a reasonable amount of time, with a minimum of 85% accuracy.

Name: _____

Date: _____

POINT VALUE ✦ = 3–6 points ✶ = 7–9 points		PRACTICE TRIAL	GRADED TRIAL # 1	GRADED TRIAL # 2	NOTES
1. ✦	On the superbill, locate the procedure code the physician has circled.				
2. ✦	Identify the primary and secondary services or procedures performed, as stated in the medical record.				
3. ✦	Locate the Main Term in the Index.				
4. ✦	Review the modifying terms and instructional notes associated with the Main Term.				
5. ✶	Identify the preliminary code(s) associated with the most appropriate modifying term(s).				
6. ✦	Locate the preliminary code(s) in the Tabular List.				
7. ✦	Interpret the conventions used in the Tabular List.				
8. ✶	Select the code with the highest level of specificity.				
9. ✶	Review the code for appropriate bundling, add-on codes, and quantity.				
10. ✶	Determine if modifiers are required.				
11. ✶	Verify the final code against the documentation.				
12. ✶	Assign the code.				

Name: _____

Date: _____

Document: Enter the appropriate information in the chart below.

Grading

Points Earned	_____		
Points Possible	_____	90	90
Percent Grade (Points Earned/Points Possible)	_____		
PASS:	_____	❑ YES ❑ NO ❑ N/A	❑ YES ❑ NO ❑ N/A

Instructor Sign-Off

Instructor: _____ **Date:** _____

Name: _____

Date: _____

Procedure 18-1:

Using a Computerized Billing System

Objective: Accurately post patient accounting transactions (charges, payments, adjustments) using a computerized practice management system (PMS).

Equipment and Supplies: Computer with a PMS; source document for the transaction, such as the encounter form for charges; the check, cash, or credit card for payments; information supporting the need for an adjustment

Affective Behaviors: Affective behaviors provide a professional approach to a skill that enhances the patient encounter. These behaviors may also display sensitivity to a patient's rights and enhance communication. Pay close attention to these skills, which will be in **_bold, italicized_** font.

Notes to the Student

_____

_____

_____

_____

_____

_____

Skills Assessment Requirements

Read and familiarize yourself with the procedure; complete the minimum practice requirements (MPRs). Document each MPR using proper charting technique. Complete each procedure within a reasonable amount of time, with a minimum of 85% accuracy.

Name: _____

Date: _____

POINT VALUE ✦ = 3–6 points ✳ = 7–9 points		PRACTICE TRIAL	GRADED TRIAL # 1	GRADED TRIAL # 2	NOTES
1. ✦	Log in with your username and password previously created.				
2. ✦	Review the rules associated with the PMS for entering transactions.				
3. ✳	Access the appropriate patient account. Double-check the patient name and birth date to verify that you have the correct patient.				
	Accounts can easily be confused among patients with the same or similar names and when multiple family members are served.				
	Verify that you have the correct account for the transaction to be entered.				
4. ✳	The PMS tracks the date, time, and identity of the person making the entry, based on the login information provided. If this is not the case, add your name, date, and time in the description field of each entry made.				
5. ✳	Complete the transaction according to the steps that follow for the type of transaction.				
	To post charges:				
1. ✳	Access the menu item for entering new charges.				
2. ✳	Enter the date of service and the CPT procedure code(s) marked on the encounter form.				

Name: _____

Date: _____

POINT VALUE ✦ = 3–6 points ✳ = 7–9 points		PRACTICE TRIAL	GRADED TRIAL # 1	GRADED TRIAL # 2	NOTES
3. ✳	The PMS normally fills in the service description and dollar amount based on the CPT code. Verify that these are accurate and match what you expect.				
4. ✳	Enter or verify the ICD-10-CM diagnosis code. When a patient has a new diagnosis, enter the ICD-10-CM code. When a patient is seen repeatedly for the same condition, the diagnosis code may carry over from one encounter to the next. The PMS normally fills in the diagnosis description. Verify that the description matches the encounter form.				
5. ✳	Repeat the process for additional procedures.				
6. ✳	Review all the data entered to be sure it is correct.				
	To post payments:				
1. ✳	Access the menu item for entering new payments.				
2. ✳	Enter the date of the payment and the purpose of the payment. Examples are patient copayment, patient coinsurance, payment on account, and insurance payment.				
3. ✳	Enter the dollar amount. Some systems require you to enter a decimal point and some systems automatically enter the decimal point and assume that the last two digits you enter should be placed to the right of the decimal point. If the system enters the decimal point for you, you must enter the final two zeroes for whole dollar amounts, such as "1000" for $10.00.				

POINT VALUE ✦ = 3–6 points ✶ = 7–9 points		PRACTICE TRIAL	GRADED TRIAL # 1	GRADED TRIAL # 2	NOTES
4. ✶	Select the form of payment (check, cash, credit card) from the menu. Enter the check number in the designated spot.				
5. ✶	Repeat the process for additional payments on the same account.				
6. ✶	Review all the data entered to be sure it is correct.				
7. ✶	Save the data, if required.				
8. ✶	If the patient is making payment in person, print a receipt, following the steps required by the PMS.				
	To post adjustments:				
1. ✶	Access the menu item for entering adjustments.				
2. ✶	Enter the date of the adjustments and the purpose of the adjustments.				
3. ✶	Enter the dollar amount, being careful to indicate if it is a positive or negative adjustment.				
4. ✶	Add any necessary comments, notes, or descriptive information to document the reason for the adjustment. You may be able to do this in the description field of the adjustment entry, or you may be able to enter a free-form account note.				
5. ✦	Compare the computer screen to the source document to verify that the entry was entered correctly.				

Name: _____

Date: _____

POINT VALUE ✦ = 3–6 points ✶ = 7–9 points		PRACTICE TRIAL	GRADED TRIAL # 1	GRADED TRIAL # 2	NOTES
	After the transaction has been entered:				
1. ✦	Save the data, if required, and exit the patient's account.				
2. ✦	Write or stamp the date posted and your name or initials on the source document, according to office procedures.				
3. ✦	File the source document in the appropriate location, according to office procedures.				
4. ✦	Log off the system when you are done posting for all patients.				

Document: Enter the appropriate information in the chart below.

Grading

Points Earned	_____		
Points Possible	_____	225	225
Percent Grade (Points Earned/Points Possible)	_____		
PASS:	_____	❏ YES ❏ NO ❏ N/A	❏ YES ❏ NO ❏ N/A

Instructor Sign-Off

Instructor: _____ **Date:** _____

Procedure 18-2:

Correcting Account Posting Errors

Objective: Identify and correct a charge or payment posted to the incorrect patient account using a practice management system (PMS).

Equipment and Supplies: A description of the error identified; computer with PMS software; source document (check, encounter form, or similar) supporting the transaction affected.

Affective Behaviors: Affective behaviors provide a professional approach to a skill that enhances the patient encounter. These behaviors may also display sensitivity to a patient's rights and enhance communication. Pay close attention to these skills, which will be in **bold, *italicized*** font.

Notes to the Student

_____

_____

_____

_____

_____

_____

Skills Assessment Requirements

Read and familiarize yourself with the procedure; complete the minimum practice requirements (MPRs). Document each MPR using proper charting technique. Complete each procedure within a reasonable amount of time, with a minimum of 85% accuracy.

POINT VALUE ✦ = 3–6 points ✳ = 7–9 points		PRACTICE TRIAL	GRADED TRIAL # 1	GRADED TRIAL # 2	NOTES
1. ✦	Errors in patient accounts may be identified by a patient who reports that his or her account contains a charge or payment that is not his or hers, or that a charge or payment that should appear is missing. Errors may also be identified when posting payments that do not match up to the charges on the account.				
2. ✦	Turn on the computer. Log in to the patient accounting program with the username and password previously established.				
3. ✳	Access the account of the patient known to have an error.				
4. ✳	Identify whether the error involved a charge, payment, or adjustment.				
5. ✦	Identify the date on which the original transaction occurred or was posted.				
6. ✳	Locate the source document. For an error involving a payment, pull a copy of the patient check or insurance EOB from the paper or electronic files of past payments. For an error involving a charge, pull a copy of the encounter form from the paper or electronic files of past encounter forms.				
7. ✳	Read the details on the source document and identify the patient and account to which it should have been posted.				
8. ✳	Reverse the entry on the account posted in error. Refer to the instructions for the PMS, because functions and steps vary based on the program.				

POINT VALUE ✦ = 3–6 points ✳ = 7–9 points		PRACTICE TRIAL	GRADED TRIAL # 1	GRADED TRIAL # 2	NOTES
9. ✳	Post a correcting entry to the account that should have been posted to originally. Refer to the instructions for the PMS, because functions and steps vary based on the program.				
	For an error involving a payment, enter a negative adjustment, because you need to decrease the account balance.				
	For an error involving a charge, enter a positive adjustment, because you need to increase the account balance.				
	Add a description or account note that explains the reason for the correction.				
10. ✳	Write a note on the source document describing the correction.				
11. ✳	Double-check all entries. Refile the source document.				
12. ✳	***Place a telephone call to both patients. Briefly explain the error and apologize for any confusion. Remember not to reveal the name of the other patient whose account was involved in the error.*** Send both patients an updated account statement.				
13. ✳	If the error involves a charge, determine if the charge was billed to the insurance company. Also identify whether the claim was paid. ***Contact the insurance company that was billed in error, explain what happened, and ask how to proceed.***				

Name: _____

Date: _____

POINT VALUE ✦ = 3–6 points ✳ = 7–9 points	PRACTICE TRIAL	GRADED TRIAL # 1	GRADED TRIAL # 2	NOTES
14. ✳ If the error involves a payment that was posted to the wrong account in your system, but the visit was billed correctly to insurance, you do not need to contact the insurance company. Simply enter the necessary corrections in your patient accounting system.				
15. ✳ Log out of the patient accounting system.				

Name: _____

Date: _____

Document: Enter the appropriate information in the chart below.

Grading

Points Earned	_____		
Points Possible	_____	129	129
Percent Grade (Points Earned/Points Possible)	_____		
PASS:	_____	❑ YES ❑ NO ❑ N/A	❑ YES ❑ NO ❑ N/A

Instructor Sign-Off

Instructor: _____ **Date:** _____

Procedure 18-3:

Posting NSF Checks

Objective: Accurately post entries to a patient account that has experienced a check with non-sufficient funds (NSF).

Equipment and Supplies: Copy or image of the returned check; NSF notification from your bank that likely identifies a fee charged to your account; computer with practice management system (PMS) software

Affective Behaviors: Affective behaviors provide a professional approach to a skill that enhances the patient encounter. These behaviors may also display sensitivity to a patient's rights and enhance communication. Pay close attention to these skills, which will be in **_bold, italicized_** font.

Notes to the Student

_____

_____

_____

_____

_____

_____

Skills Assessment Requirements

Read and familiarize yourself with the procedure; complete the minimum practice requirements (MPRs). Document each MPR using proper charting technique. Complete each procedure within a reasonable amount of time, with a minimum of 85% accuracy.

Name: _____

Date: _____

POINT VALUE ✦ = 3–6 points ✶ = 7–9 points		PRACTICE TRIAL	GRADED TRIAL # 1	GRADED TRIAL # 2	NOTES
1. ✦	Log in with your username and password previously created.				
2. ✦	Access the appropriate patient account. Double-check the patient name and birth date to verify that you have the correct patient and account type.				
3. ✶	Access the appropriate menu item according to the procedures for the PMS. You may be able to reverse the payment using the payments menu, or you may need to enter it as an adjustment.				
4. ✶	Select the payment or adjustment type for an NSF check.				
5. ✦	Enter the date the check was returned and dollar amount of the original check.				
6. ✶	Enter a description such as "Check # 111 returned NSF."				
7. ✶	Access the menu for adjustments. Select an item type for "bank fees."				
8. ✶	Enter the date the check was returned and the dollar amount of the processing fee charged by your bank.				
9. ✶	Enter a description such as "Bank fee for NSF Check # 111."				
10. ✶	Review the entry to verify that the date and amount were entered correctly.				
11. ✶	Save the data, if necessary.				
12. ✶	Access the menu to create a patient statement. Print a statement.				

Name: _____

Date: _____

POINT VALUE ✦ = 3–6 points ∗ = 7–9 points		PRACTICE TRIAL	GRADED TRIAL # 1	GRADED TRIAL # 2	NOTES
13. ∗	Access the menu to create a patient letter. Select or create a letter to the patient that explains: "Your check number 999 for $00.00 was returned to our office because of lack of funds in your account. In addition, the medical office was charged a fee of $00.00 for the processing of the check. You are responsible to reimburse us for this cost, in addition to paying for the original service. A statement is enclosed that shows the current balance on your account. Please remit payment within eight days by MM/DD/YY or call the office to make payment arrangements."				
14. ∗	Make a photocopy or scanned image of the returned check for your records.				
15. ∗	Mail the letter, the patient statement, and the returned check via certified mail.				
16. ∗	Complete the steps in Procedure 18-1 **after the transaction has been entered.**				

Name: _____

Date: _____

Document: Enter the appropriate information in the chart below.

Grading

Points Earned	_____		
Points Possible	_____	135	135
Percent Grade (Points Earned/Points Possible)	_____		
PASS:	_____	❏ YES ❏ NO ❏ N/A	❏ YES ❏ NO ❏ N/A

Instructor Sign-Off

Instructor: _____   Date: _____

Procedure 18-4:

Posting Insurance Payments

Objective: Accurately post single and bulk insurance payments to patients' accounts using a practice management system (PMS).

Equipment and Supplies: Explanation of benefits (EOB); copy of check; computer with PMS

Affective Behaviors: Affective behaviors provide a professional approach to a skill that enhances the patient encounter. These behaviors may also display sensitivity to a patient's rights and enhance communication. Pay close attention to these skills, which will be in **_bold, italicized_** font.

Notes to the Student

_____

_____

_____

_____

_____

_____

Skills Assessment Requirements

Read and familiarize yourself with the procedure; complete the minimum practice requirements (MPRs). Document each MPR using proper charting technique. Complete each procedure within a reasonable amount of time, with a minimum of 85% accuracy.

Name: _____

Date: _____

POINT VALUE ✦ = 3–6 points ✶ = 7–9 points		PRACTICE TRIAL	GRADED TRIAL # 1	GRADED TRIAL # 2	NOTES
1. ✦	Log in with your username and password previously created.				
2. ✦	Access the menu item for posting payments.				
3. ✶	Enter the date the check was received, the payer, the dollar amount, and the check number in the designated fields.				
4. ✶	Select the account of the patient the payment is for. Verify that you have the correct name, the correct family member, and the correct account type for the payment to be posted.				
5. ✦	Select the date of service covered by the payment.				
6. ✶	Select the first line item for the date of service.				
7. ✶	Enter the dollar amount for the following: • Payment amount • Copayment, coinsurance, and deductible owed by patient • Non-covered items that are patient responsibility • Contractual allowance (write-off) for participating provider contracts • Disallowance that is to be billed to the patient for nonparticipating provider contracts				
8. ✶	Post additional line items in the same way.				
9. ✶	Verify that the total of line-item entries, plus any amount already paid by the patient, equals the total charge for each date of service.				

POINT VALUE ✦ = 3–6 points ✱ = 7–9 points		PRACTICE TRIAL	GRADED TRIAL # 1	GRADED TRIAL # 2	NOTES
10. ✱	If more than one date of service is included in the check, repeat the process for any additional dates of service.				
11. ✱	Verify whether the balance on the claim should be billed to the patient or to a secondary insurance policy.				
12. ✱	Review all numbers to verify that data was entered accurately. Save the data, if necessary.				
13. ✱	Repeat this process for any additional dates of service for the same patient.				
14. ✱	If the check includes payments for multiple patients, repeat this process for additional patients, until the entire amount of the check has been posted to patient accounts. Complete the steps in Procedure 18-1 **after the transaction has been entered**.				

Name: _____

Date: _____

Document: Enter the appropriate information in the chart below.

Grading

Points Earned	_____		
Points Possible	_____	129	129
Percent Grade (Points Earned/Points Possible)	_____		
PASS:	_____	❏ YES ❏ NO ❏ N/A	❏ YES ❏ NO ❏ N/A

Instructor Sign-Off

Instructor: _____   Date: _____

Procedure 18-5:

Responding to a Denied Insurance Claim

Objective: Identify the reason for a denied insurance claim, correct the error, and resubmit the claim.

Equipment and Supplies: Patient's account in the practice management system (PMS) including: patient insurance information (i.e., ID number, birth date of the insured, name and provider customer service telephone number of insurance company) and details of the procedure the doctor has performed, including CPT code, patient's diagnosis, place of service, date of service; paper and pen; copy of the explanation of benefits (EOB); any documentation of the service having been preauthorized by the office

Affective Behaviors: Affective behaviors provide a professional approach to a skill that enhances the patient encounter. These behaviors may also display sensitivity to a patient's rights and enhance communication. Pay close attention to these skills, which will be in **_bold, italicized_** font.

Notes to the Student

_____

_____

_____

_____

_____

_____

Skills Assessment Requirements

Read and familiarize yourself with the procedure; complete the minimum practice requirements (MPRs). Document each MPR using proper charting technique. Complete each procedure within a reasonable amount of time, with a minimum of 85% accuracy.

Name: _____

Date: _____

POINT VALUE ✦ = 3–6 points ✶ = 7–9 points		PRACTICE TRIAL	GRADED TRIAL # 1	GRADED TRIAL # 2	NOTES
1. ✦	Organize all materials.				
2. ✦	Call the insurance company's provider customer service phone number as listed on the patient's insurance identification card.				
3. ✶	Write down the date and time of the telephone call, the number called, and the name of the customer service representative on the phone.				
4. ✶	**Introduce yourself and your medical office to the customer service representative, and then provide the patient's identification number and date of service.**				
5. ✦	If the service was pre-authorized, give the pre-authorization number to the customer service representative.				
6. ✶	**Ask the customer service representative why the procedure was not paid as anticipated.**				
7. ✶	If there was an error in processing the service for payment, ask if any other information is needed to process the claim correctly. Also ask when the office can expect payment for the procedure.				
8. ✶	If the customer service representative says the claim was processed correctly, **request the reason for the denial.**				

POINT VALUE ✦ = 3–6 points ✶ = 7–9 points	PRACTICE TRIAL	GRADED TRIAL # 1	GRADED TRIAL # 2	NOTES
9. ✶ If the reason for the denial was lack of supporting documentation, ask if faxing the information is a solution. If the answer is yes, get the customer service representative's direct fax line and fax the needed documentation.				
10. ✶ If the reason for the denial requires an appeal to be filed, ask the customer service representative to explain the insurance company's process for appeals. Also request a written procedure for appeals.				
11. ✶ **Thank the customer service representative for the assistance. Ask if the representative can give you a direct phone number should you have any further questions**. A direct phone number is one that goes to that individual, usually with voice mail, rather than going through the call center.				
12. ✶ Write down any pertinent information, such as where to mail the appeal and what information the appeal should contain.				
13. ✶ **Call the patient with the findings and get the patient involved as needed.**				
14. ✶ Create an account note in the PMS that describes the details of the telephone call.				

Document: Enter the appropriate information in the chart below.

Grading

Points Earned	_____		
Points Possible	_____	90	90
Percent Grade (Points Earned/Points Possible)	_____		
PASS:	_____	❏ YES ❏ NO ❏ N/A	❏ YES ❏ NO ❏ N/A

Instructor Sign-Off

Instructor: _____   Date: _____

Procedure 18-6:

Preparing Patient Statements

Objective: Produce patient bills using a computerized practice management system (PMS)

Equipment and Supplies: Computer with a PMS; printer; window envelopes compatible with statement format; stamps, postage meter, or other method of applying postage

Affective Behaviors: Affective behaviors provide a professional approach to a skill that enhances the patient encounter. These behaviors may also display sensitivity to a patient's rights and enhance communication. Pay close attention to these skills, which will be in **bold, *italicized*** font.

Notes to the Student

_____

_____

_____

_____

_____

_____

Skills Assessment Requirements

Read and familiarize yourself with the procedure; complete the minimum practice requirements (MPRs). Document each MPR using proper charting technique. Complete each procedure within a reasonable amount of time, with a minimum of 85% accuracy.

POINT VALUE ✦ = 3–6 points ✳ = 7–9 points	PRACTICE TRIAL	GRADED TRIAL # 1	GRADED TRIAL # 2	NOTES
1. ✦ Fill the printer with patient statement forms, if used, or plain paper.				
2. ✦ Log in with your username and password previously created.				
3. ✦ Access the menu for creating patient statements.				
4. ✳ Select the statement format to be used.				
5. ✦ Enter the parameters for the patients to be billed, such as: • a preset definition for "cycle 1," "cycle 2," and so on • the section of the alphabet to be billed, such as "last name beginning with A" through "last name beginning with F" • the payer type, such as Medicare patients or HMO patients • the names of specific patients • patients with an account balance within a specified range, such as "accounts over $10.00" • patients with account balances over "x" days old. (This can be useful if the office policies call for printing special reminder notices, writing personal notes, or affixing a reminder sticker to such statements.)				
6. ✳ Complete any other information required by the PMS, such as a reminder message or late charge policy to be printed on the statement.				
7. ✳ Print the statements. The PMS automatically updates the patient accounts to document that a billing statement was sent.				

Name: _____

Date: _____

POINT VALUE ✦ = 3–6 points ✷ = 7–9 points		PRACTICE TRIAL	GRADED TRIAL # 1	GRADED TRIAL # 2	NOTES
8. ✷	Complete the steps in Procedure 18-1 **after the transaction has been entered.**				
9. ✦	Collect the statements from the printer and organize a work area for folding and stuffing. If special patient statement forms are used, remove the forms from the printer so that the next staff member does not unknowingly print on the forms.				
10. ✷	As you handle each statement, review it to verify that it is readable, complete, properly aligned on the paper, and undamaged. Set aside those statements that may need to be checked or reprinted.				
11. ✦	Affix any reminder stickers used by the practice. Fold each statement neatly in such a way that the address appears in the window of the envelope.				
12. ✦	Insert the statement in the envelope and check the front to verify that the entire address is visible.				
13. ✦	Seal the envelope and affix postage. Mail the statements according to office procedures.				
14. ✦	Reprint those statements that are not usable, following the preceding steps. Shred the unused statements to maintain patient privacy.				

Name: _____

Date: _____

Document: Enter the appropriate information in the chart below.

Grading

Points Earned	_____		
Points Possible	_____	99	99
Percent Grade (Points Earned/Points Possible)	_____		
PASS:	_____	❏ YES ❏ NO ❏ N/A	❏ YES ❏ NO ❏ N/A

Instructor Sign-Off

Instructor: _____   **Date:** _____

Name: _____

Date: _____

Procedure 18-7:

Processing Credit Balances and Refunds

Objective: Post the appropriate entries to a patient account that has a credit balance using a practice management system (PMS).

Equipment and Supplies: Computer with a PMS; source document that identifies the reason for the credit balance and authorizes the refund to be made; refund check, EOB, or credit card slip

Affective Behaviors: Affective behaviors provide a professional approach to a skill that enhances the patient encounter. These behaviors may also display sensitivity to a patient's rights and enhance communication. Pay close attention to these skills, which will be in **_bold, italicized_** font.

Notes to the Student

_____

_____

_____

_____

_____

_____

Skills Assessment Requirements

Read and familiarize yourself with the procedure; complete the minimum practice requirements (MPRs). Document each MPR using proper charting technique. Complete each procedure within a reasonable amount of time, with a minimum of 85% accuracy.

POINT VALUE ✦ = 3–6 points ✶ = 7–9 points	PRACTICE TRIAL	GRADED TRIAL # 1	GRADED TRIAL # 2	NOTES
1. ✦ Log in to the PMS using your previously established username and password.				
2. ✦ Access the patient's account.				
3. ✶ Locate the charge that was overpaid.				
4. ✦ Select the menu item to enter an adjustment.				
5. ✦ Enter the dollar amount to be refunded. This will be a positive adjustment (debit) that increases the account balance.				
6. ✶ Enter a description or account note to explain the reason for the adjustment. Be as detailed as possible.				
7. ✶ Verify that all entries are correct.				
8. ✶ If a check is to be sent to the insurance company or the patient, access the correspondence menu and generate a letter that explains the refund.				
9. ✶ Complete the steps in Procedure 18-1 for **after the transaction has been entered**.				
10. ✶ Mail the letter and check via certified mail.				

Name: _____

Date: _____

Document: Enter the appropriate information in the chart below.

Grading

Points Earned	_____		
Points Possible	_____	78	78
Percent Grade (Points Earned/Points Possible)	_____		
PASS:	_____	❏ YES ❏ NO ❏ N/A	❏ YES ❏ NO ❏ N/A

Instructor Sign-Off

Instructor: _____ **Date:** _____

Procedure 18-8:

Making Collection Calls

Objective: Place a call to a patient requesting payment.

Equipment and Supplies: Patient's account in the practice management system (PMS); demographic information; telephone; black ink pen

Affective Behaviors: Affective behaviors provide a professional approach to a skill that enhances the patient encounter. These behaviors may also display sensitivity to a patient's rights and enhance communication. Pay close attention to these skills, which will be in **bold, *italicized*** font.

Notes to the Student

_____

_____

_____

_____

_____

_____

Skills Assessment Requirements

Read and familiarize yourself with the procedure; complete the minimum practice requirements (MPRs). Document each MPR using proper charting technique. Complete each procedure within a reasonable amount of time, with a minimum of 85% accuracy.

Name: _____

Date: _____

POINT VALUE ✦ = 3–6 points ✳ = 7–9 points		PRACTICE TRIAL	GRADED TRIAL # 1	GRADED TRIAL # 2	NOTES
1. ✦	Based on the collection policy of the office, determine how many days overdue the bill must be before the first call is made.				
2. ✦	Access the patient's account in the PMS and review the account activity before placing the call.				
3. ✳	Find a quiet area of the office in which to work while placing collection calls.				
4. ✳	Collection calls should only be made Monday through Saturday from 8:00 a.m. to 9:00 p.m. Do not call on Sundays or holidays.				
5. ✦	Locate the patient's telephone number and place the call.				
6. ✳	**When the call is answered, confidently ask to speak with the patient.** Do not share information with anyone other than the patient or responsible party.				
7. ✳	If the patient is unavailable, you may leave a message; however, the message should simply state the caller's name, who the message is for, and the telephone number where the caller may be reached.				
8. ✳	**When speaking with the patient, politely introduce yourself and ask if this is a good time to talk. If the patient tells you it is not a good time, ask what time would be better, and make a note of that in the chart.** Call back the patient at the stated time.				

Name: _____

Date: _____

POINT VALUE ✦ = 3–6 points ✳ = 7–9 points		PRACTICE TRIAL	GRADED TRIAL # 1	GRADED TRIAL # 2	NOTES
9. ✳	**When speaking with the patient, be polite, project confidence, and state the facts and purpose of the call.** Never threaten an action you do not intend to take.				
10. ✳	**Ask the patient if there is a reason for nonpayment. If the patient is able to provide a reason, document the response.**				
11. ✳	**Ask the patient when you might expect payment and document that response as well.**				
12. ✳	**Politely thank the patient for his or her time, and repeat the terms agreed on.**				
13. ✳	Document the interaction with a note in the patient's account.				

Document: Enter the appropriate information in the chart below.

Grading

Points Earned	_____		
Points Possible	_____	108	108
Percent Grade (Points Earned/Points Possible)	_____		
PASS:	_____	❑ YES ❑ NO ❑ N/A	❑ YES ❑ NO ❑ N/A

Instructor Sign-Off

Instructor: _____   **Date:** _____

Procedure 18-9:

Writing a Collection Letter

Objective: Compose a collection letter requesting payment.

Equipment and Supplies: Patient's ledger; demographic information; computer; black ink pen

Affective Behaviors: Affective behaviors provide a professional approach to a skill that enhances the patient encounter. These behaviors may also display sensitivity to a patient's rights and enhance communication. Pay close attention to these skills, which will be in **bold, *italicized*** font.

Notes to the Student

_____

_____

_____

_____

_____

_____

Skills Assessment Requirements

Read and familiarize yourself with the procedure; complete the minimum practice requirements (MPRs). Document each MPR using proper charting technique. Complete each procedure within a reasonable amount of time, with a minimum of 85% accuracy.

Name: _____

Date: _____

POINT VALUE ✦ = 3–6 points ✳ = 7–9 points		PRACTICE TRIAL	GRADED TRIAL # 1	GRADED TRIAL # 2	NOTES
1. ✦	Based on the collection policy of the office, determine at what point the first letter is sent.				
2. ✦	Review the account activity in the patient's account in the PMS.				
3. ✳	Access the correspondence module of the PMS, or open the word processing program. Compose a rough draft of the letter, using proper formatting, grammar, and punctuation.				
4. ✳	In the first paragraph, summarize the reason for the letter and any payments the patient has made on the account.				
5. ✦	In the second paragraph, state the desired action of the patient. This may simply be to contact the office, or it may specifically state the expected payment amount and date(s) of the expected payment. Ensure that the letter is written in a polite tone without any threats for lack of compliance.				
6. ✳	In the third paragraph, or closing paragraph, thank the patient in advance for his or her prompt attention to the matter and encourage the patient to contact the office.				
7. ✳	When the rough draft is complete, read through the document again, checking for spelling, grammar, and formatting errors.				
8. ✳	Correct any errors, print, and sign the document.				

POINT VALUE ✦ = 3–6 points ✳ = 7–9 points	PRACTICE TRIAL	GRADED TRIAL # 1	GRADED TRIAL # 2	NOTES
9. ✳ Make a copy of the letter and place it in the patient's file or scan it into the computer and attach it to the patient's account.				
10. ✳ Place the letter in an addressed envelope and mail it to the patient. In the PMS, enter a note in the patient's account indicating the date the letter was mailed.				

Document: Enter the appropriate information in the chart below.

Grading

Points Earned	_____		
Points Possible	_____	81	81
Percent Grade (Points Earned/Points Possible)	_____		
PASS:	_____	❏ YES ❏ NO ❏ N/A	❏ YES ❏ NO ❏ N/A

Instructor Sign-Off

Instructor: _____   **Date:** _____

Procedure 18-10:

Posting a Payment from a Collection Agency

Objective: Accurately post payments from a collection agency in a practice management system (PMS).

Equipment and Supplies: Calculator; computer with a PMS; collection agency payment

Affective Behaviors: Affective behaviors provide a professional approach to a skill that enhances the patient encounter. These behaviors may also display sensitivity to a patient's rights and enhance communication. Pay close attention to these skills, which will be in **_bold, italicized_** font.

Notes to the Student

_____

_____

_____

_____

_____

_____

Skills Assessment Requirements

Read and familiarize yourself with the procedure; complete the minimum practice requirements (MPRs). Document each MPR using proper charting technique. Complete each procedure within a reasonable amount of time, with a minimum of 85% accuracy.

POINT VALUE ✦ = 3–6 points ✳ = 7–9 points		PRACTICE TRIAL	GRADED TRIAL # 1	GRADED TRIAL # 2	NOTES
1. ✦	Log in to the PMS using your previously established username and password.				
2. ✦	Access the patient's account or the bad debt account, depending on the method used to track accounts sent to collection.				
3. ✳	Access the menu to post a payment.				
4. ✳	Enter the date the payment was received.				
5. ✦	Choose "Collection Agency" to indicate the source of the payment.				
6. ✳	Enter the dollar amount of the check.				
7. ✳	Access the menu to post an adjustment.				
8. ✳	Post an adjustment for the amount of the collection agency fee or enter the fee as an expense in the accounting system.				
9. ✳	Post an adjustment to write off the remaining balance as bad debt.				
10. ✳	Verify that all entries are accurate.				
11. ✳	Complete the steps in Procedure 18-1 for **after the transaction has been entered.**				

Name: _____

Date: _____

Document: Enter the appropriate information in the chart below.

Grading

Points Earned	_____		
Points Possible	_____	90	90
Percent Grade (Points Earned/Points Possible)	_____		
PASS:	_____	❏ YES ❏ NO ❏ N/A	❏ YES ❏ NO ❏ N/A

Instructor Sign-Off

Instructor: _____   **Date:** _____

Procedure 19-1:

Preparing a Deposit Slip

Objective: Complete a bank deposit slip.

Equipment and Supplies: Pen; deposit slip; checks and currency to be deposited; endorsing stamp; calculator

Affective Behaviors: Affective behaviors provide a professional approach to a skill that enhances the patient encounter. These behaviors may also display sensitivity to a patient's rights and enhance communication. Pay close attention to these skills, which will be in **bold, *italicized*** font.

Notes to the Student

_____

_____

_____

_____

_____

_____

Skills Assessment Requirements

Read and familiarize yourself with the procedure; complete the minimum practice requirements (MPRs). Document each MPR using proper charting technique. Complete each procedure within a reasonable amount of time, with a minimum of 85% accuracy.

Name: _____

Date: _____

POINT VALUE ✦ = 3–6 points ✷ = 7–9 points		PRACTICE TRIAL	GRADED TRIAL # 1	GRADED TRIAL # 2	NOTES
1. ✦	Verify that each check has been endorsed. If any checks were not previously endorsed, apply the endorsing stamp to the back of the check.				
2. ✦	Complete the information on the front of the deposit slip:				
	Account name (if not preprinted)				
	Account number (if not preprinted)				
	Date of the deposit				
3. ✦	If there is cash to be deposited, enter the total amount of the cash in the designated space on the deposit slip beside the Cash indicator. In the Currency box, list the total amount of all cash paper money to be deposited. In the Coin box, list the total of all the cash coin money to be deposited. Organize the currency bills in descending order by face value, with all bills face-up. For instance, group $100 bills together face-up, then all $50 bills face-up, and so on.				
4. ✦	List each check to be deposited on a different line. If you have more checks than fit on the front, list each additional check on the reverse side of the deposit slip. List money orders last.				
5. ✦	On each numbered line, write the name of the person who wrote the check and the dollar amount of the check.				
6. ✦	List each check in a different numbered box.				

POINT VALUE ✦ = 3–6 points ✳ = 7–9 points		PRACTICE TRIAL	GRADED TRIAL # 1	GRADED TRIAL # 2	NOTES
7. ✦	Use a calculator to add all the checks entered on the reverse side of the deposit slip, and enter the total of the checks in the space at the bottom of the deposit slip that reads Total. This amount is also placed on the front of the deposit slip in the space that reads Total from Reverse Side.				
8. ✳	Use the calculator to add the total amount of the cash and the checks being deposited. List this amount in the space labeled Total and in the space labeled Net Deposit on the front of the deposit slip.				
9. ✳	Verify your totals.				
	Add up all the dollar amounts listed on the deposit slip *in reverse order* from what you did the first time. The total should be the same.				
	Then, go through the stack of checks and add up the amounts as written on each check. This total should match the one written on the deposit slip.				
	Do the same for currency and coins.				
	If there is any discrepancy, even 1 cent, check for transposition errors when writing the numbers on the deposit slip and for keying errors on the calculator. If you cannot find the error, ask someone else to review the deposit.				
10. ✦	Place the deposit slip and the cash and checks listed on the slip in an envelope for deposit to the bank.				

Document: Enter the appropriate information in the chart below.

Grading

Points Earned	_____		
Points Possible	_____	66	66
Percent Grade (Points Earned/Points Possible)	_____		
PASS:	_____	❑ YES ❑ NO ❑ N/A	❑ YES ❑ NO ❑ N/A

Instructor Sign-Off

Instructor: _____   **Date:** _____

Procedure 19-2:

Preparing Manual Checks

Objective: Correctly prepare a handwritten check.

Equipment and Supplies: Blank checks with stub or record; black ink pen; invoice, purchase order, or other supporting documentation; security envelope; postage

Affective Behaviors: Affective behaviors provide a professional approach to a skill that enhances the patient encounter. These behaviors may also display sensitivity to a patient's rights and enhance communication. Pay close attention to these skills, which will be in **_bold, italicized_** font.

Notes to the Student

_____

_____

_____

_____

_____

Skills Assessment Requirements

Read and familiarize yourself with the procedure; complete the minimum practice requirements (MPRs). Document each MPR using proper charting technique. Complete each procedure within a reasonable amount of time, with a minimum of 85% accuracy.

POINT VALUE ✦ = 3–6 points ✶ = 7–9 points		PRACTICE TRIAL	GRADED TRIAL # 1	GRADED TRIAL # 2	NOTES
1. ✦	Identify the lowest-numbered unused check.				
2. ✦	Fill in the check stub or check record before writing the check.				
3. ✦	Use a black ink pen to complete the check and stub.				
4. ✦	Write the full date in the designated place. Date the check on the day it is written. Never postdate a check. (Postdating a check means writing a future date on a check.)				
5. ✦	Write the name of the payee on the "Pay to the order of" line. Use care when spelling the name of the payee. Do not use abbreviations or titles such as MD. Leave no space either before or after the payee's name. If space remains after the name, draw a straight line from the name to the end of the space.				
6. ✶	Write the amount of the check, using numbers in the designated area. Verify that the amount agrees with the invoice.				
7. ✦	Write the dollar amount in words on the second line, usually labelled "Pay." Verify that it agrees with the numeric dollar amount.				
8. ✦	Record your account number with the vendor, invoice number, and/or purpose of the check (example: "Office Supplies") on the memo line at the bottom left of the check.				
9. ✦	Fill in all blank spaces and leave no room for anyone to add anything. Always begin writing or figures at the extreme left of the space.				

POINT VALUE ✦ = 3–6 points ✷ = 7–9 points		PRACTICE TRIAL	GRADED TRIAL # 1	GRADED TRIAL # 2	NOTES
10. ✦	It is not advisable to write checks for less than one dollar. In addition to the time spent on bookkeeping for such a small amount, many banks place a service charge for each check written. This can be costly. However, when you must write a check for less than one dollar, use care. Write out the amount with the word "only" indicating to the reader that the amount is less than one dollar. Do not cross out the word *dollars.*				
11. ✦	Prepare the check to be signed. Remove the check from the register, being careful not to tear it. Attach the invoice and any other supporting documentation behind the check with a paperclip. The individual signing checks should be the owner of the bank account or his or her authorized agent. In some offices, the office manager is authorized to sign checks for the physician.				
12. ✦	Look over the check carefully to ensure all spaces have been filled in.				
13. ✷	Subtract the amount of this check from the "Balance Brought Forward" line in the check register. Write this amount as the new balance brought forward. Check the math for accuracy.				

POINT VALUE ✦ = 3–6 points ✶ = 7–9 points		PRACTICE TRIAL	GRADED TRIAL # 1	GRADED TRIAL # 2	NOTES
14. ✦	After the check is signed, place it in an envelope with the remittance slip from the invoice. Address the envelope or, if using a window envelope, verify that the complete address is visible in the window. Seal the envelope, attach postage, and mail.				
15. ✦	File the invoice and other supporting documentation in the designated location in the office.				

Document: Enter the appropriate information in the chart below.

Grading

Points Earned	_____		
Points Possible	_____	96	96
Percent Grade (Points Earned/Points Possible)	_____		
PASS:	_____	❏ YES ❏ NO ❏ N/A	❏ YES ❏ NO ❏ N/A

Instructor Sign-Off

Instructor: _____   **Date:** _____

Procedure 19-3:

Paying Bills with Accounts Payable Software

Objective: Correctly pay bills and print checks using computerized accounting software.

Equipment and Supplies: Computer with accounts payable (AP) software; invoices; purchase orders; checks; printer; scanner; software user manual

Affective Behaviors: Affective behaviors provide a professional approach to a skill that enhances the patient encounter. These behaviors may also display sensitivity to a patient's rights and enhance communication. Pay close attention to these skills, which will be in **_bold, italicized_** font.

Notes to the Student

_____

_____

_____

_____

_____

_____

Skills Assessment Requirements

Read and familiarize yourself with the procedure; complete the minimum practice requirements (MPRs). Document each MPR using proper charting technique. Complete each procedure within a reasonable amount of time, with a minimum of 85% accuracy.

POINT VALUE ✦ = 3–6 points ✳ = 7–9 points		PRACTICE TRIAL	GRADED TRIAL # 1	GRADED TRIAL # 2	NOTES
1. ✦	Log in to the accounts payable system with your username and password previously established.				
	To enter bills:				
	Note: Some offices create electronic copies of invoices and purchase orders that require that someone scan them into the system, save the file in a specific location, and name the file according to specific rules. Other offices work directly from paper invoices and purchase orders. Some bills may be able to be paid using an online "bill pay" service offered by your bank.				
1. ✦	Organize the paper documents to be entered or access the location of the electronic images according to the instructions for your system.				
2. ✦	In the software, access the menu for entering bills or invoices. Select the task to enter a new bill.				
3. ✦	Select the name of the vendor from a preestablished list of vendors.				
	If the vendor is not in the system, select the menu item to enter a new vendor and key in the following information, according to procedures for your software: vendor name, address to which payment should be mailed, phone number, contact person, e-mail address, your account number, payment terms, and any other information requested.				

POINT VALUE ✦ = 3–6 points ✳ = 7–9 points		PRACTICE TRIAL	GRADED TRIAL # 1	GRADED TRIAL # 2	NOTES
4. ✳	Enter the following information: invoice number, dollar amount due, due date.				
5. ✦	Select the type of expense, such as shipping or office supplies. This information may be automatically completed by the system for expenses such as rent and utilities. You may need to enter an account number that identifies the type of expense.				
6. ✳	Enter the date on which you wish to be reminded to pay the bill.				
7. ✳	Verify the accuracy of all data and save, if necessary.				
8. ✳	On the source document, write "Entered by (your name) on (current date)." You may have an ink stamp that provides a format, with space to enter your name and the date.				
9. ✳	Repeat for all bills. Double-check all entries against your source documents to verify that you did not miss any invoices. File source documents in designated location. Log off the system.				
	To print checks:				
1. ✦	Load checks into the printer. Follow the procedures for your combination of printer and software regarding how to orient the checks: face-up or face-down, and top edge first or bottom edge first.				
2. ✦	Access the menu to pay invoices that were previously entered.				
3. ✦	Enter the applicable range of due dates for the invoices you wish to pay.				

POINT VALUE ✦ = 3–6 points ✱ = 7–9 points		PRACTICE TRIAL	GRADED TRIAL #1	GRADED TRIAL #2	NOTES
4. ✱	Review the screen that lists invoices to be paid and manually add or delete any, as needed.				
5. ✦	Select the menu option to print checks. Enter or confirm any other required information such as check date.				
6. ✱	Select or verify the printer and check format, if necessary. Select the menu option to begin printing.				
7. ✱	Collect the checks from the printer. Review them to verify that all documents are legible and properly aligned. Reprint any misprinted or damaged checks.				
8. ✦	Log off the system.				
9. ✦	Remove blank checks from the printer tray and put them back in their designated location. Verify that the cabinet or drawer is locked.				
10. ✦	Collate the checks with supporting documents such as purchase orders or invoices. Route to the appropriate person to sign the checks.				
	After the checks are signed:				
1. ✦	Review each check to verify that all checks have the required signature(s).				
2. ✦	Detach check stub and attach to the supporting documents. File source documents in the designated location.				
3. ✱	Place checks in window envelopes. Verify that the mailing address appears completely within the window. Apply postage and mail.				

Name: _____

Date: _____

Document: Enter the appropriate information in the chart below.

Grading

Points Earned	_____		
Points Possible	_____	159	159
	_____		
PASS:	_____	❏ YES ❏ NO ❏ N/A	❏ YES ❏ NO ❏ N/A

Instructor Sign-Off

Instructor: _____   **Date:** _____

Procedure 19-4:

Reconciling a Bank Statement

Objective: Manually reconcile a bank statement for a checking account.

Equipment and Supplies: Current and previous bank statements; cancelled checks (if returned by the bank); checkbook stubs

Affective Behaviors: Affective behaviors provide a professional approach to a skill that enhances the patient encounter. These behaviors may also display sensitivity to a patient's rights and enhance communication. Pay close attention to these skills, which will be in **_bold, italicized_** font.

Notes to the Student

_____

_____

_____

_____

_____

_____

Skills Assessment Requirements

Read and familiarize yourself with the procedure; complete the minimum practice requirements (MPRs). Document each MPR using proper charting technique. Complete each procedure within a reasonable amount of time, with a minimum of 85% accuracy.

Name: _____

Date: _____

POINT VALUE ✦ = 3–6 points ✳ = 7–9 points		PRACTICE TRIAL	GRADED TRIAL #1	GRADED TRIAL #2	NOTES
1. ✦	Compare the beginning balance of the current statement with the ending balance of the previous statement. These should be the same.				
2. ✦	Write the current ending balance in the appropriate space on the reverse side of the bank statement.				
3. ✳	Compare deposits noted on the statement against your records or receipts by making a check mark next to each correct number.				
4. ✳	List separately all outstanding deposits. These are deposits made toward the end of the month that have not been included in the current statement. Add these together and place the total on the reverse side of the statement in the space provided.				
5. ✦	Add the ending balance to the total of deposits not already included and write this amount on the Total line.				
6. ✳	Compare the value of the checks listed on the statement with the value listed in the checkbook or check stubs, and place a check mark next to each correct number.				

POINT VALUE ✦ = 3–6 points ✳ = 7–9 points		PRACTICE TRIAL	GRADED TRIAL # 1	GRADED TRIAL # 2	NOTES
7. ✳	Note all numbers missing from the sequential list of check numbers; these are checks that have not yet cleared your bank (outstanding checks). List all outstanding checks. Add the total for outstanding checks and place that figure on the line indicated on the back of the statement.				
8. ✳	Subtract the total figure for checks outstanding from the previous total on the back of the statement to determine the current balance. This amount should agree with the amount in your checkbook or stub balance.				

Name: _____

Date: _____

Document: Enter the appropriate information in the chart below.

Grading

Points Earned	_____		
Points Possible	_____	45	45
Percent Grade (Points Earned/Points Possible)	_____		
PASS:	_____	❏ YES ❏ NO ❏ N/A	❏ YES ❏ NO ❏ N/A

Instructor Sign-Off

Instructor: _____ Date: _____

Procedure 19-5:

Working with an Outside Payroll Service

Objective: Prepare the information required by an outside payroll service to process payroll.

Equipment and Supplies: Employee time records; computer or calculator; telephone or computer with Internet connection; new employee paperwork; documents regarding any changes needed to employee information, such as new address, new banking information, new pay rate, etc.; payroll journal or payroll reporting forms; contact information for the payroll service or its secure website for payroll customers

Affective Behaviors: Affective behaviors provide a professional approach to a skill that enhances the patient encounter. These behaviors may also display sensitivity to a patient's rights and enhance communication. Pay close attention to these skills, which will be in **bold, *italicized*** font.

Notes to the Student

_____

_____

_____

_____

_____

_____

_____

Skills Assessment Requirements

Read and familiarize yourself with the procedure; complete the minimum practice requirements (MPRs). Document each MPR using proper charting technique. Complete each procedure within a reasonable amount of time, with a minimum of 85% accuracy.

POINT VALUE ✦ = 3–6 points ✳ = 7–9 points		PRACTICE TRIAL	GRADED TRIAL # 1	GRADED TRIAL # 2	NOTES
	The office is responsible to transmit payroll information to the payroll service each pay period. This may be done using the Internet, telephone, or fax. The procedures for each method of transmission are different. Using the procedures for the applicable transmission method, perform the following steps.				
1. ✦	Review all employee paperwork to verify it is complete and accurate.				
2. ✦	Enter the total hours worked for each employee, indicating the number of hours to be paid at the regular pay rate and the number of hours to be paid at the overtime rate.				
3. ✳	Enter the number of hours of paid time off (PTO) for each employee. This may be divided into sick time, holidays, and vacation.				
4. ✳	Enter information regarding new employees, terminated employees, change in status, change in pay, change in withholding or deductions, etc.				
5. ✦	Verify all data entered for accuracy and omissions.				
6. ✳	Save the data if working online; transmit the data via fax; or telephone the payroll company to report the numbers verbally. Write down the confirmation number for the submission.				
7. ✳	After the payroll service processes the information, you are notified of the amount of funds needed for payroll and withholding. Transfer the designated amount of money to the appropriate bank account used for payroll.				

Document: Enter the appropriate information in the chart below.

Grading

Points Earned	_____		
Points Possible	_____	45	45
Percent Grade (Points Earned/Points Possible)	_____		
PASS:	_____	❏ YES ❏ NO ❏ N/A	❏ YES ❏ NO ❏ N/A

Instructor Sign-Off

Instructor: _____   **Date:** _____

Procedure 20-1:

Staff Meeting Procedures

Objective: Explain and present the necessary steps to preparing and running a staff meeting.

Equipment and Supplies: Agenda items received from staff; meeting agenda; means of keeping time (watch, clock, stopwatch, etc.); room for the meeting; any audio or video equipment that may be needed

Affective Behaviors: Affective behaviors provide a professional approach to a skill that enhances the patient encounter. These behaviors may also display sensitivity to a patient's rights and enhance communication. Pay close attention to these skills, which will be in **bold, *italicized*** font.

Notes to the Student

_____

_____

_____

_____

_____

_____

Skills Assessment Requirements

Read and familiarize yourself with the procedure; complete the minimum practice requirements (MPRs). Document each MPR using proper charting technique. Complete each procedure within a reasonable amount of time, with a minimum of 85% accuracy.

Name: _____

Date: _____

POINT VALUE ✦ = 3–6 points ✶ = 7–9 points		PRACTICE TRIAL	GRADED TRIAL # 1	GRADED TRIAL # 2	NOTES
1. ✦	One week before the meeting, request agenda items from the staff.				
2. ✶	Before the meeting, create a meeting agenda with all topics to be discussed. On the agenda include the date, time, and place of the meeting. Identify who will be running (facilitating) the meeting (most often, the office manager). Assign a length of time to each topic and a person who is responsible for that topic.				
3. ✦	Start the meeting on time.				
4. ✦	Begin by briefly covering the previous meeting.				
5. ✦	Try to stay on schedule as much as possible.				
6. ✦	Allow for time at the end of the meeting to have open discussion of any new business.				
7. ✦	Adjourn the meeting.				
8. ✦	After the meeting, have the minutes of the meeting typed and distributed to all involved.				

Document: Enter the appropriate information in the chart below.

Grading

Points Earned	_____		
Points Possible	_____	51	51
Percent Grade (Points Earned/Points Possible)	_____		
PASS:	_____	❑ YES ❑ NO ❑ N/A	❑ YES ❑ NO ❑ N/A

Instructor Sign-Off

Instructor: _____ **Date:** _____

Name: _____

Date: _____

Procedure 20-2:

Developing a Patient Information Booklet

Objective: Develop a booklet to inform patients about services provided by your medical office.

Supplies: Computer; design software (if including images); high-quality paper; printer (or an independent printing service)

Affective Behaviors: Affective behaviors provide a professional approach to a skill that enhances the patient encounter. These behaviors may also display sensitivity to a patient's rights and enhance communication. Pay close attention to these skills, which will be in **_bold, italicized_** font.

Notes to the Student

_____

_____

_____

_____

_____

_____

Skills Assessment Requirements

Read and familiarize yourself with the procedure; complete the minimum practice requirements (MPRs). Document each MPR using proper charting technique. Complete each procedure within a reasonable amount of time, with a minimum of 85% accuracy.

POINT VALUE ✦ = 3–6 points ✱ = 7–9 points	PRACTICE TRIAL	GRADED TRIAL # 1	GRADED TRIAL # 2	NOTES
1. ✦ Make the booklet as appealing as possible. Leave a white border around all page edges. Use large print for the elderly reader's benefit. The booklet should be small enough that it fits easily into a pocket or purse.				
2. ✦ Write the booklet with the reader in mind and at a reading level appropriate for the target audience. Avoid the use of technical medical terms. Never use medical abbreviations in patient literature.				
3. ✦ Avoid long paragraphs of explanation. Keep the sentences short and concise, and use as many bulleted points as possible.				
4. ✦ Provide a list of the regular office hours.				
5. ✦ List any special services offered by the practice or clinic, such as patient education classes or blood pressure testing programs.				
6. ✦ Explain the procedure for having a prescription refilled.				
7. ✦ Explain the procedure for processing medical insurance forms.				
8. ✦ Include a general statement about payment of fees, especially if payment is expected at the time of delivery of services. Do not discuss specific fees in patient brochures.				

POINT VALUE ✦ = 3–6 points ✳ = 7–9 points		PRACTICE TRIAL	GRADED TRIAL # 1	GRADED TRIAL # 2	NOTES
9. ✦	Provide information about the physician and the staff.				
10. ✦	State what procedure to follow in case of an emergency. For example, instruct patients to call 911 if the emergency is life threatening. Also, provide a 24-hour emergency telephone number. Ask the patient to keep this number near his or her telephone.				
11. ✦	Include a telephone number at the end of the brochure where additional information may be obtained.				
12. ✦	End the brochure by thanking the patient for taking the time to read the literature.				

Document: Enter the appropriate information in the chart below.

Grading

Points Earned	_____		
Points Possible	_____	72	72
Percent Grade (Points Earned/Points Possible)	_____		
PASS:	_____	❑ YES ❑ NO ❑ N/A	❑ YES ❑ NO ❑ N/A

Instructor Sign-Off

Instructor: _____ **Date:** _____

Procedure 34-1:

Disposal of Infectious Wastes and Substances

Objective: Student will perform the procedure without errors.

Equipment and Supplies: Infectious waste container with lid marked appropriately with universal biohazard symbol and label; red disposable plastic liners; gloves

Affective Behaviors: Affective behaviors provide a professional approach to a skill that enhances the patient encounter. These behaviors may also display sensitivity to a patient's rights and enhance communication. Pay close attention to these skills, which will be in **_bold, italicized_** font.

Notes to the Student

_____

_____

_____

_____

_____

_____

Skills Assessment Requirements

Read and familiarize yourself with the procedure; complete the minimum practice requirements (MPRs). Document each MPR using proper charting technique. Complete each procedure within a reasonable amount of time, with a minimum of 85% accuracy.

POINT VALUE ✦ = 3–6 points ✳ = 7–9 points		PRACTICE TRIAL	GRADED TRIAL # 1	GRADED TRIAL # 2	NOTES
1. ✦	Check to ensure that the infectious waste container is lined with a red disposal plastic bag.				
2. ✳	Discard *any* infectious waste into the infectious waste container.				
3. ✳	Make sure that all liquid waste is already contained in a closable device or container before putting it into the infectious waste container.				
4. ✦	Do not put contaminated glass or glass of any kind into the infectious waste bag. Instead, all glass should be placed into a puncture-proof or very highly puncture-resistant container for disposal; small glass items can be deposited into a sharps container for disposal. a. Needles and syringes should never be recapped and always placed immediately into an appropriately labeled, puncture-proof sharps container after activating the safety device mechanism on the needle or syringe.				
5. ✳	When the infectious waste container becomes full, close the red trash bag, either by tying with a securing knot, twist-tying, or otherwise securing it.				
6. ✦	Make sure that the contents of the red bag are completely contained inside the closed bag.				

POINT VALUE ✦ = 3–6 points ✳ = 7–9 points		PRACTICE TRIAL	GRADED TRIAL # 1	GRADED TRIAL # 2	NOTES
7. ✦	Make sure the red bag is not overstuffed so that it cannot be closed, and so that it does not rupture when handled or lifted, re-open, or leak. a. If necessary, double-bag the infectious waste bag if there is a small rupture or tear; or when office protocol dictates. Two people should always perform this task to ensure contamination does not occur (Figure B).				
8. ✳	Do not mix noninfectious trash in the same large bin, container, or dumpster with infectious waste or trash.				
9. ✳	Closed red bags should be transported from the point of waste generation to a dirty utility room or area and stored in a designated holding area that cannot be accessed by other than authorized staff until they are transported away from the facility. Never store trash in hallways, entrances, corridors, or other areas accessible to and used by the public.				

Name: _____

Date: _____

Document: Enter the appropriate information in the chart below.

Grading

Points Earned	_____		
Points Possible	_____	69	69
Percent Grade (Points Earned/Points Possible)	_____		
PASS:	_____	❏ YES ❏ NO ❏ N/A	❏ YES ❏ NO ❏ N/A

Instructor Sign-Off

Instructor: _____ Date: _____

Procedure 34-2:

Performing Hand Washing

Objective: Perform hand washing procedure without error.

Equipment and Supplies: Soap in liquid soap dispenser; nail cleaner (brush or orange cuticle stick); warm running water; paper towels; waste container

Affective Behaviors: Affective behaviors provide a professional approach to a skill that enhances the patient encounter. These behaviors may also display sensitivity to a patient's rights and enhance communication. Pay close attention to these skills, which will be in **bold, italicized** font.

Notes to the Student

_____

_____

_____

_____

_____

Skills Assessment Requirements

Read and familiarize yourself with the procedure; complete the minimum practice requirements (MPRs). Document each MPR using proper charting technique. Complete each procedure within a reasonable amount of time, with a minimum of 85% accuracy.

POINT VALUE ✦ = 3–6 points ✳ = 7–9 points		PRACTICE TRIAL	GRADED TRIAL # 1	GRADED TRIAL # 2	NOTES
1. ✦	Remove any jewelry (including rings, with the exception of a plain wedding band). Artificial nails must be removed to maintain infection control practices.				
2. ✳	Stand at the sink without allowing clothing to touch the sink. Turn on the faucet while holding a paper towel to prevent contamination. Or, if it is available, turn the water on with the foot or knee pedal. Adjust the running water to a moderately warm temperature.				
3. ✳	Wet hands under running water and place liquid soap (1 teaspoon, or about the size of a nickel) into the palm of hand. Work soap into a lather by moving it over the palms, sides, and backs—the entire surface—of both hands for 15 to 30 seconds. Use a circular motion and friction. Interlace the fingers and move soapy water between them.				
4. ✦	Keep the hands pointed down with hands and forearms below elbow level during the entire hand washing procedure. Water should always flow from the forearms down, never from the hands up. This also prevents contamination.				
5. ✦	Use a nail cleaner (brush or orange cuticle stick) to clean under fingernails at the start of each day and if hands are heavily soiled.				

POINT VALUE ✦ = 3–6 points ✱ = 7–9 points		PRACTICE TRIAL	GRADED TRIAL # 1	GRADED TRIAL # 2	NOTES
6. ✱	Rinse hands under running water with fingers pointed down, using care not to touch the sink or faucets.				
7. ✦	If hands are heavily soiled, reapply soap and wash them again.				
8. ✦	Rinse hands under running water.				
9. ✱	Dry hands thoroughly with a paper towel without touching the paper towel dispenser. Discard the paper towel into a trash can that can be opened with a foot pedal.				
10. ✦	Use a dry paper towel to turn the faucet off if the foot or knee pedal is not available.				
11. ✱	Apply an antibacterial hand lotion to prevent chapping of skin.				

Name: _____

Date: _____

Document: Enter the appropriate information in the chart below.

Grading

Points Earned	_____		
Points Possible	_____	81	81
Percent Grade (Points Earned/Points Possible)	_____		
PASS:	_____	❏ YES ❏ NO ❏ N/A	❏ YES ❏ NO ❏ N/A

Instructor Sign-Off

Instructor: _____ Date: _____

Name: _____

Date: _____

Procedure 34-3:

Applying and Removing Nonsterile Gloves

Objective: Apply nonsterile gloves and remove them appropriately to prevent the spread of pathogens.

Equipment and Supplies: Gloves, biohazard waste container

Affective Behaviors: Affective behaviors provide a professional approach to a skill that enhances the patient encounter. These behaviors may also display sensitivity to a patient's rights and enhance communication. Pay close attention to these skills, which will be in **_bold, italicized_** font.

Notes to the Student

_____

_____

_____

_____

_____

_____

Skills Assessment Requirements

Read and familiarize yourself with the procedure; complete the minimum practice requirements (MPRs). Document each MPR using proper charting technique. Complete each procedure within a reasonable amount of time, with a minimum of 85% accuracy.

Name: _____

Date: _____

	POINT VALUE ✦ = 3–6 points ✳ = 7–9 points		PRACTICE TRIAL	GRADED TRIAL # 1	GRADED TRIAL # 2	NOTES
1. ✦		Perform hand hygiene.				
2. ✦		Choose appropriate -size gloves for your hands. Hold a glove at the wrist opening and insert fingers, pulling the glove up to wrist.				
3. ✦		Apply the second glove in the same manner, checking for holes and other flaws. If any flaws are found, discard the gloves and obtain new gloves.				
4. ✳		To remove gloves, grasp the glove covering your nondominant hand at the palm and pull it away.				
5. ✳		Pull the glove off and hold it in the palm of the gloved dominant hand.				
6. ✦		While holding the soiled glove in your gloved hand, slide the index finger of the ungloved hand below the cuff of the remaining glove and peel it down, inverting it over the first glove. Both gloves will be in a ball and inside out.				
7. ✳		Dispose of the gloves in a biohazard container.				
8. ✦		Perform hand hygiene.				

Name: _____

Date: _____

Document: Enter the appropriate information in the chart below.

Grading

Points Earned	_____		
Points Possible	_____	63	63
Percent Grade (Points Earned/Points Possible)	_____		
PASS:	_____	❑ YES ❑ NO ❑ N/A	❑ YES ❑ NO ❑ N/A

Instructor Sign-Off

Instructor: _____   **Date:** _____

Procedure 34-4:

Performing Transmission-Based Precaution: Isolation Techniques

Objective: Provide barrier protection for caregivers to prevent the spread of infectious diseases.

Equipment and Supplies: Disposable gowns, masks, caps, nonsterile gloves, sterile gloves; sink and running water; paper towels

Affective Behaviors: Affective behaviors provide a professional approach to a skill that enhances the patient encounter. These behaviors may also display sensitivity to a patient's rights and enhance communication. Pay close attention to these skills, which will be in **bold, italicized** font.

Notes to the Student

_____

_____

_____

_____

_____

_____

Skills Assessment Requirements

Read and familiarize yourself with the procedure; complete the minimum practice requirements (MPRs). Document each MPR using proper charting technique. Complete each procedure within a reasonable amount of time, with a minimum of 85% accuracy.

POINT VALUE ✦ = 3–6 points ✳ = 7–9 points		PRACTICE TRIAL	GRADED TRIAL # 1	GRADED TRIAL # 2	NOTES
1. ✦	Review orders and agency protocols regarding isolation procedures. *Note:* Office-based medical assistants may not use transmission-based precautions often, but they should be familiar with the necessary personal protective equipment (PPE) and how to put PPE on appropriately.				
2. ✦	Assemble the necessary protective equipment that is appropriate for the level of isolation necessary based on the patient's diagnosis, signs, or symptoms.				
3. ✦	Remove lab coat and jewelry.				
4. ✦	Perform hand hygiene.				
5. ✳	Apply the appropriate disposable apparel in the following order: a. Apply the cap to cover hair and ears completely. b. Apply the gown over uniform or clothing as follows: Hold the gown in front of the body and place arms through the sleeves. Pull the sleeves on, covering the wrists. Tie the gown securely at the neck and waist. c. Apply the mask by placing the top of the mask over the bridge of the nose and pinching the metal strip to secure a snug fit on the nose, tying it if needed. Apply protective eyewear. d. Apply nonsterile gloves, pulling the cuffs of the glove up and over the cuffs of the gown, covering them completely.				

POINT VALUE ✦ = 3–6 points ✶ = 7–9 points		PRACTICE TRIAL	GRADED TRIAL # 1	GRADED TRIAL # 2	NOTES
6. ✦	Enter the isolation room and perform patient tasks as needed.				
7. ✶	Exit the isolation room and immediately remove barrier protections in the following order: a. Untie waist of the gown. b. Remove gloves. c. Wash hands. d. Untie the neck of the gown. Remove the gown by pulling it down from the shoulders. Turn the gown inside out and remove arms from the sleeves. The inside of the gown is not contaminated. e. Holding the gown away from the body with contaminated area on the inside, fold and place it in a biohazard container. *Note:* Most isolation rooms will have designated areas and appropriate receptacles near the doorway for immediate removal of protective barriers.				
8. ✶	Remove protective eyewear.				
9. ✦	Remove mask and discard in biohazard container.				
10. ✦	Perform hand hygiene for the final time.				

Document: Enter the appropriate information in the chart below.

Grading

Points Earned	_____		
Points Possible	_____	69	69
Percent Grade (Points Earned/Points Possible)	_____		
PASS:	_____	❏ YES ❏ NO ❏ N/A	❏ YES ❏ NO ❏ N/A

Instructor Sign-Off

Instructor: _____   **Date:** _____

Procedure 34-5:

Sanitizing Instruments

Objective: Learn to clean and sanitize instruments to eliminate any visible contamination.

Equipment and Supplies: Disposable gloves; rubber (utility) gloves; face shield or mask and goggles; plastic brushes (large and small), preferably disposable; disposable towels; sink; running water; container to hold all the instruments; low-sudsing (low-pH) detergent or germicidal agent; biohazard container

Note: Instruments should be rinsed under warm running water immediately after surgery to re-move blood, body fluids, and tissue. If it is not possible to clean them immediately, instruments should be submerged in water containing a low-pH detergent.

Affective Behaviors: Affective behaviors provide a professional approach to a skill that enhances the patient encounter. These behaviors may also display sensitivity to a patient's rights and enhance communication. Pay close attention to these skills, which will be in **bold, *italicized*** font.

Notes to the Student

_____

_____

_____

_____

_____

_____

Skills Assessment Requirements

Read and familiarize yourself with the procedure; complete the minimum practice requirements (MPRs). Document each MPR using proper charting technique. Complete each procedure within a reasonable amount of time, with a minimum of 85% accuracy.

POINT VALUE ✦ = 3–6 points ✳ = 7–9 points		PRACTICE TRIAL	GRADED TRIAL #1	GRADED TRIAL #2	NOTES
1. ✦	Apply both disposable and rubber gloves. a. If there is potential of splashing of infectious materials, don face shield or goggles and mask as necessary.				
2. ✦	Place a low-sudsing (low-pH) detergent or germicidal agent in a large basin with water following manufacturer's instructions.				
3. ✦	Initially rinse instruments in clear cold water in either a sink or other container. Delicate and sharp instruments should be separated from general instruments.				
4. ✳	Scrub each instrument individually with a brush and detergent under running water. Open instruments to thoroughly scrub all serrated edges, crevices, and hinge areas.				
5. ✦	Rinse instruments thoroughly under hot water.				
6. ✦	After thoroughly rinsing cleaned instruments, roll them in a towel and hand dry them.				
7. ✳	Check the condition of all instruments for defects or any remaining soil. Take appropriate action, if required.				
8. ✦	Discard disposable towels and any disposable instruments in the biohazard waste container.				
9. ✳	Remove utility gloves and disposable gloves and perform hand hygiene.				

POINT VALUE ✦ = 3–6 points ✽ = 7–9 points		PRACTICE TRIAL	GRADED TRIAL # 1	GRADED TRIAL # 2	NOTES
10. ✽	Place sanitized instruments in the appropriate area for storage or wrap instrument(s) for sterilization or place them in an ultrasonic cleaner.				
11. ✦	If necessary, perform quality assurance reporting in necessary log books regarding sanitization practices.				

Document: Enter the appropriate information in the chart below.

Grading

Points Earned	_____		
Points Possible	_____	78	78
Percent Grade (Points Earned/Points Possible)	_____		
PASS:	_____	❏ YES ❏ NO ❏ N/A	❏ YES ❏ NO ❏ N/A

Instructor Sign-Off

Instructor: _____ **Date:** _____

Name: _____

Date: _____

Procedure 34-6:

Wrapping and Labeling Instruments for Autoclaving

Objective: Wrap and label instruments properly.

Equipment and Supplies: Wrapping material; instrument(s) for autoclaving; sterilization indicator strips; autoclave tape; permanent pen; gloves

Affective Behaviors: Affective behaviors provide a professional approach to a skill that enhances the patient encounter. These behaviors may also display sensitivity to a patient's rights and enhance communication. Pay close attention to these skills, which will be in **_bold, italicized_** font.

Notes to the Student

_____

_____

_____

_____

_____

_____

Skills Assessment Requirements

Read and familiarize yourself with the procedure; complete the minimum practice requirements (MPRs). Document each MPR using proper charting technique. Complete each procedure within a reasonable amount of time, with a minimum of 85% accuracy.

POINT VALUE ✦ = 3–6 points ✷ = 7–9 points		PRACTICE TRIAL	GRADED TRIAL # 1	GRADED TRIAL # 2	NOTES
1. ✦	Wash your hands and don gloves.				
2. ✦	Place a square of wrapping material on a clean flat surface. Arrange the material so that it appears as a "diamond" shape when you look at it. Be sure the wrapping material is large enough to cover the entire article being wrapped. a. According to office policy, it might be necessary to use an additional piece of wrapping material if the material is only single layered.				
3. ✷	Place the items in the center of the wrapping material. a. If hinged items are included, be sure the instrument is in the open position. b. If sharp instruments are being autoclaved, place the tip in a piece of gauze to prevent puncture through the material.				
4. ✷	Place the sterility indicator strip in the center of the packet.				
5. ✷	Fold the bottom point of the wrapping material up and over the instruments. Fold a small portion of the point back over so that it can be used to pull back the paper when it is unwrapped.				
6. ✷	Fold the right side of the wrapping paper over until it covers the instrument(s). Fold a small portion of the point back over as in the previous step.				

POINT VALUE ✦ = 3–6 points ✴ = 7–9 points		PRACTICE TRIAL	GRADED TRIAL # 1	GRADED TRIAL # 2	NOTES
7. ✴	Fold the left side of the wrapping paper over until it covers the instrument(s). Fold a small portion of the point back over as in the previous step.				
8. ✴	Now fold the bottom of the package upward until you have reached the top point of the wrapping square.				
9. ✦	Be sure the pack is folded snugly and air pockets are not present.				
10. ✦	Secure the final point of the package with a piece of autoclave tape.				
11. ✴	Label the package with the name of the item(s) inside, your initials, and the date.				
12. ✦	If bags are used for the autoclaving procedure, place the item and an indicator strip inside the bag. (If the item has a sharp point, wrap the point in a piece of gauze.)				
13. ✴	Seal the bag. Label the bag with the name of the item(s) inside, your initials, and the date.				

Name: _____

Date: _____

Document: Enter the appropriate information in the chart below.

Grading

Points Earned	_____		
Points Possible	_____	102	102
Percent Grade (Points Earned/Points Possible)	_____		
PASS:	_____	❑ YES ❑ NO ❑ N/A	❑ YES ❑ NO ❑ N/A

Instructor Sign-Off

Instructor: _____ Date: _____

Procedure 34-7:

Sterilizing Instruments in an Autoclave

Objective: Sterilize instruments in an autoclave to prevent the spread of pathogens.

Equipment and Supplies: Autoclave; instruments sanitized and wrapped for autoclaving; distilled water; autoclave directions

Affective Behaviors: Affective behaviors provide a professional approach to a skill that enhances the patient encounter. These behaviors may also display sensitivity to a patient's rights and enhance communication. Pay close attention to these skills, which will be in **bold, _italicized_** font.

Notes to the Student

_____

_____

_____

_____

_____

_____

Skills Assessment Requirements

Read and familiarize yourself with the procedure; complete the minimum practice requirements (MPRs). Document each MPR using proper charting technique. Complete each procedure within a reasonable amount of time, with a minimum of 85% accuracy.

Name: _____

Date: _____

POINT VALUE ✦ = 3–6 points ✱ = 7–9 points		PRACTICE TRIAL	GRADED TRIAL # 1	GRADED TRIAL # 2	NOTES
1. ✦	Check the level of water in the autoclave reservoir. Add distilled water as needed to the fill line.				
2. ✱	Load the autoclave: a. Trays and packs should be loaded on their sides. b. Containers should be loaded on their sides with lids off or ajar. c. Mixed loads are loaded with hard objects on bottom racks and softer items on top racks. d. Keep large packs 2 to 4 inches apart and smaller packets 1 to 2 inches apart.				
3. ✱	Read the manufacturer's instructions and follow them exactly. Most autoclaves follow similar protocols. a. Turn the control knob to fill and observe carefully with the door open until the water reaches the chamber fill line. b. Turn the knob to autoclave position. This shuts off the water. Do not allow the water to overflow. c. Close and lock the door.				
4. ✱	When pressure reaches 15 to 17 pounds per square inch and the temperature reaches 250°F to 270°F, set the timer for the required time. Typical timing is 30 minutes for wrapped trays and packages and 15 minutes for unwrapped items. Always check the manufacturer's suggested times and facility protocol.				
5. ✦	When timing is complete, turn the control knob to vent.				

POINT VALUE ✦ = 3–6 points ✶ = 7–9 points		PRACTICE TRIAL	GRADED TRIAL # 1	GRADED TRIAL # 2	NOTES
6. ✦	When the pressure reaches zero, open the chamber door about 3/4 of an inch and allow items in the autoclave to dry completely before removing them (about 30 to 45 minutes).				
7. ✦	Turn the autoclave knob to off.				
8. ✦	Remove the wrapped items and check the autoclave tape on the outside for indicated color change. Store in a dry closed cabinet for future use. Unwrapped items must be removed using sterile transfer forceps and must be placed on a sterile field or in a sterile storage area.				
9. ✶	Perform quality assurance measures by recording the activity in the proper log book. Record date, time, and types of items autoclaved in log and initial.				

Name: _____

Date: _____

Document: Enter the appropriate information in the chart below.

Grading

Points Earned	_____		
Points Possible	_____	66	66
Percent Grade (Points Earned/Points Possible)	_____		
PASS:	_____	❏ YES ❏ NO ❏ N/A	❏ YES ❏ NO ❏ N/A

Instructor Sign-Off

Instructor: _____ Date: _____

Procedure 34-8:

Chemically Sterilizing Instruments

Objective: Chemically sterilize heat-sensitive instruments to prevent the spread of pathogens.

Supplies: Chemical disinfectant; goggles, disposable gloves, utility (rubber) gloves; sink; glass or stainless steel container with cover; sterile towels; sterile transfer forceps; sterile basin; sanitized articles

Note: Before anything can be chemically sterilized, it must be sanitized properly as described in Procedure 34-5 the earlier procedure. Always read and follow the manufacturer's directions on the original container of the chemical agent.

Affective Behaviors: Affective behaviors provide a professional approach to a skill that enhances the patient encounter. These behaviors may also display sensitivity to a patient's rights and enhance communication. Pay close attention to these skills, which will be in **_bold, italicized_** font.

Notes to the Student

_____

_____

_____

_____

_____

_____

Skills Assessment Requirements

Read and familiarize yourself with the procedure; complete the minimum practice requirements (MPRs). Document each MPR using proper charting technique. Complete each procedure within a reasonable amount of time, with a minimum of 85% accuracy.

Name: _____

Date: _____

POINT VALUE ✦ = 3–6 points ✱ = 7–9 points	PRACTICE TRIAL	GRADED TRIAL # 1	GRADED TRIAL # 2	NOTES
1. ✦ Sanitize instruments appropriately.				
2. ✱ Select the type of chemical needed to sterilize the instruments.				
3. ✱ Read the directions on the original germicidal agent label. If opening the germicide for the first time, write the date on the container and follow directions to properly prepare the chemical agent for initial use.				
4. ✦ Place the chemical agent in an appropriate container that is large enough to submerge the instrument completely.				
5. ✦ Cover the container tightly and record the time, date, and your initials.				
6. ✱ Do not open the container during the sterilization process.				
7. ✦ When sterilization timing is complete, remove the instrument from the container using sterile gloves or sterile transfer forceps.				
8. ✦ Rinse the items thoroughly with sterile water over a sterile basin. Hold the instruments over the basin for a few moments to drain excess sterile water.				
9. ✦ Dry the instruments thoroughly with a sterile towel and place onto a sterile field for use.				
10. ✦ Change the chemical agent every 7 to 14 days, or as recommended by the manufacturer.				

POINT VALUE ✦ = 3–6 points ✶ = 7–9 points		PRACTICE TRIAL	GRADED TRIAL # 1	GRADED TRIAL # 2	NOTES
11. ✦	Remove gloves and perform hand hygiene.				
12. ✶	Perform quality assurance by recording appropriate information in the appropriate log book.				

Name: _____

Date: _____

Document: Enter the appropriate information in the chart below.

Grading

Points Earned	_____		
Points Possible	_____	81	81
Percent Grade (Points Earned/Points Possible)	_____		
PASS:	_____	❏ YES ❏ NO ❏ N/A	❏ YES ❏ NO ❏ N/A

Instructor Sign-Off

Instructor: _____ **Date:** _____

Procedure 35-1:

Measuring Adult Weight and Height

Objective: Obtain height and weight measurements and perform math conversions.

Supplies: Balance scale with bar to measure height; paper towel; pen; patient's medical record

Affective Behaviors: Affective behaviors provide a professional approach to a skill that enhances the patient encounter. These behaviors may also display sensitivity to a patient's rights and enhance communication. Pay close attention to these skills, which will be in **_bold, italicized_** font.

Notes to the Student

_____

_____

_____

_____

_____

_____

Skills Assessment Requirements

Read and familiarize yourself with the procedure; complete the minimum practice requirements (MPRs). Document each MPR using proper charting technique. Complete each procedure within a reasonable amount of time, with a minimum of 85% accuracy.

POINT VALUE ✦ = 3–6 points ✳ = 7–9 points	PRACTICE TRIAL	GRADED TRIAL # 1	GRADED TRIAL # 2	NOTES
1. ✦ Perform hand hygiene.				
2. ✳ **Greet** and identify the patient.				
3. ✳ **Explain the procedure.**				
4. ✦ **Instruct the patient to remove his or her shoes and place a paper towel on the scale if the patient is in bare feet.** **a. Heavy objects such as keys should be removed, and female patients should set aside their purses.**				
5. ✳ Set all the weights to zero. The balance bar pointer should float in the center of the frame. a. If the balance bar is not centered at zero, adjustments will need to be made. Balance the scale by adjusting the small knob at one end until the balance bar pointer floats in the center of the frame. (A coin can be used to make this adjustment.)				
6. ✦ **Assist the patient onto the scale.**				
7. ✦ **Ask the patient to stand still while the measurement is being obtained.**				
8. ✳ First, move the large weight into the groove closest to the weight you estimate for the patient. (You may refer to the patient's last recorded weight in the medical record.) a. If the balance bar pointer touches the bottom of the bar, then move the large weight to the left, one notch.				

Name: _____

Date: _____

POINT VALUE ✦ = 3–6 points ✱ = 7–9 points		PRACTICE TRIAL	GRADED TRIAL # 1	GRADED TRIAL # 2	NOTES
9. ✦	Then move the small weight by tapping it gently until it reaches a point at which the pointer floats in the center of the frame.				
10. ✱	Leave the weights in place as you go on to obtain the patient's height.				
11. ✦	Ask the patient to place his or her back to the scale, stand erect, and look straight ahead. a. The patient's heels, buttocks, and back of head should be touching the scale.				
12. ✱	Raise the height bar in a collapsed position, making sure the tip is over the patient's head.				
13. ✱	Open the bar into the horizontal position and bring it down gently to touch the top of the patient's head. Leave this setting in place				
14. ✱	***Assist the patient in stepping off the scale.***				
15. ✱	Calculate the patient's weight by adding the numbers at the large and small weight groove markings. Record the weight to the nearest ¼ pound.				
16. ✦	Record this measurement on the patient's record.				
17. ✱	Read the height as marked behind the movable level of the ruled bar. a. Medical office policy will usually dictate if height is recorded in feet and inches, total inches, or total centimeters.				

Name: _____

Date: _____

POINT VALUE ✦ = 3–6 points ✶ = 7–9 points		PRACTICE TRIAL	GRADED TRIAL # 1	GRADED TRIAL # 2	NOTES
18. ✶	Record this measurement to the nearest ¼ inch on the patient's record.				
19. ✦	Return the weights to zero and the height bar to the normal position and discard the paper towel.				
20. ✦	Perform hand hygiene.				

Name: _____

Date: _____

Document: Enter the appropriate information in the chart below.

Grading

Points Earned	_____		
Points Possible	_____	153	153
Percent Grade Points Earned/Points Possible)	_____		
PASS:	_____	❏ YES ❏ NO ❏ N/A	❏ YES ❏ NO ❏ N/A

Instructor Sign-Off

Instructor: _____   **Date:** _____

Procedure 35-2:

Measuring Oral Temperature Using an Electronic Thermometer

Objective: Accurately perform all steps of the procedure and provide an accurate temperature reading.

Supplies: Electronic thermometer (rechargeable); blue (oral) probe; probe cover; waste container; pen; patient's medical record

Affective Behaviors: Affective behaviors provide a professional approach to a skill that enhances the patient encounter. These behaviors may also display sensitivity to a patient's rights and enhance communication. Pay close attention to these skills, which will be in **bold, italicized** font.

Notes to the Student

_____

_____

_____

_____

_____

_____

Skills Assessment Requirements

Read and familiarize yourself with the procedure; complete the minimum practice requirements (MPRs). Document each MPR using proper charting technique. Complete each procedure within a reasonable amount of time, with a minimum of 85% accuracy.

Name: _____

Date: _____

	POINT VALUE ✦ = 3–6 points ✷ = 7–9 points	PRACTICE TRIAL	GRADED TRIAL # 1	GRADED TRIAL # 2	NOTES
1. ✦	Perform hand hygiene.				
2. ✦	Assemble equipment, ensuring the electronic thermometer is properly charged.				
3. ✷	**Greet and identify the patient and explain the procedure.**				
4. ✦	Attach the correct probe that would be used to measure an oral temperature.				
5. ✦	Attach a disposable probe cover by inserting the thermometer probe into the disposable tip (probe cover) box and secure the disposable cover onto the probe.				
6. ✷	Insert the thermometer into the patient's mouth, under the tongue on either side of the frenulum linguae. **Instruct the patient to close his or her mouth, forming a tight seal around the thermometer.**				
7. ✷	When the temperature signal is seen or heard, remove the thermometer from the patient's mouth and read the result displayed on the LED window.				
8. ✷	Dispose of the probe cover in a waste container.				
9. ✦	Return the thermometer probe to the storage place.				
10. ✦	Return the unit to the rechargeable base.				
11. ✦	Perform hand hygiene.				
12. ✷	Document the results.				

Name: _____

Date: _____

Document: Enter the appropriate information in the chart below.

Grading

Points Earned	_____		
Points Possible	_____	87	87
Percent Grade (Points Earned/Points Possible)	_____		
PASS:	_____	❏ YES ❏ NO ❏ N/A	❏ YES ❏ NO ❏ N/A

Instructor Sign-Off

Instructor: _____   **Date:** _____

Procedure 35-3:

Measuring Rectal Temperature Using an Electronic Thermometer

Objective: Accurately perform all steps of the procedure and provide an accurate temperature reading.

Equipment and Supplies: Electronic thermometer; red (rectal) probe; disposable probe cover; disposable gloves; patient's medical record; paper and pen; tissue; water-soluble lubricant; biohazard waste container.

Affective Behaviors: Affective behaviors provide a professional approach to a skill that enhances the patient encounter. These behaviors may also display sensitivity to a patient's rights and enhance communication. Pay close attention to these skills, which will be in **bold, _italicized_** font.

Notes to the Student

_____

_____

_____

_____

_____

_____

Skills Assessment Requirements

Read and familiarize yourself with the procedure; complete the minimum practice requirements (MPRs). Document each MPR using proper charting technique. Complete each procedure within a reasonable amount of time, with a minimum of 85% accuracy.

Name: _____

Date: _____

POINT VALUE ✦ = 3–6 points ✳ = 7–9 points		PRACTICE TRIAL	GRADED TRIAL # 1	GRADED TRIAL # 2	NOTES
1. ✦	Perform hand hygiene.				
2. ✦	Don a pair of gloves.				
3. ✳	**Greet and identify the patient.**				
4. ✳	**Explain the procedure. If the patient is a child, explain the procedure to both the parent and child.**				
5. ✦	**Instruct the patient to remove appropriate clothing so that the rectal area can be accessed.** a. Excuse yourself from the room while the patient disrobes to ensure patient privacy. Provide a drape or gown, as necessary.				
6. ✦	**Assist the patient onto the exam table and help assist him or her into the Sim's position (lying on left side with top leg bent).**				
7. ✦	Because of the delicate nature of the procedure, be mindful of the patient's privacy and adjust draping as necessary to provide maximum coverage.				
8. ✦	Remove the electronic thermometer from the base and choose the correct probe for a rectal temperature.				
9. ✳	Attach a disposable probe cover on the thermometer probe.				
10. ✳	Place a small amount of lubricant on a tissue. Dip the tip of the probe in the lubricant.				

POINT VALUE ✦ = 3–6 points ✶ = 7–9 points		PRACTICE TRIAL	GRADED TRIAL # 1	GRADED TRIAL # 2	NOTES
11. ✶	With one hand, raise the upper buttock to expose the anus or anal opening. a. If unable to see the anal opening, ask the patient to bear down slightly. This will expose the opening.				
12. ✶	With the other hand, gently insert the lubricated thermometer probe ½ inch into the anal canal. a. Do not force the thermometer into the anal canal; if any resistance is felt, discontinue the procedure.				
13. ✶	Hold the thermometer still and in place until the result is signaled.				
14. ✶	Gently withdraw the thermometer and dispose of the probe cover by ejecting it into a biohazard container.				
15. ✦	Make a mental note of the temperature, which will be recorded later.				
16. ✶	Wipe the anus from front to back to remove any excess lubricant.				
17. ✶	*Assist the patient from the examination table. Instruct the patient to redress or don an examination gown. If necessary, provide assistance or excuse yourself from the room to allow patient privacy.*				
18. ✶	Remove gloves and place in a biohazard waste container.				
19. ✶	Perform hand hygiene.				

POINT VALUE ✦ = 3–6 points ✳ = 7–9 points	PRACTICE TRIAL	GRADED TRIAL # 1	GRADED TRIAL # 2	NOTES
20. ✦ Record the temperature in the patient's record using (R) to indicate a rectal temperature was obtained.				
21. ✦ Return the probe to its appropriate storage place and then return the entire thermometer unit to the rechargeable base. a. Perform appropriate sanitization of the thermometer unit either according to manufacturer's instructions or office protocol, possibly by cleaning the unit with a disinfecting wipe.				

Name: _____

Date: _____

Document: Enter the appropriate information in the chart below.

Grading

Points Earned	_____		
Points Possible	_____	159	159
Percent Grade (Points Earned/Points Possible)	_____		
PASS:	_____	❏ YES ❏ NO ❏ N/A	❏ YES ❏ NO ❏ N/A

Instructor Sign-Off

Instructor: _____ **Date:** _____

Procedure 35-4:

Measuring Axillary Temperature

Objective: Accurately perform all steps of the procedure and provide an accurate temperature reading.

Equipment and Supplies: Electronic thermometer and appropriate probe (blue oral probes are used for axillary temperatures); disposable probe cover; paper and pen; patient's medical record; tissue; biohazard waste container

Affective Behaviors: Affective behaviors provide a professional approach to a skill that enhances the patient encounter. These behaviors may also display sensitivity to a patient's rights and enhance communication. Pay close attention to these skills, which will be in **_bold, italicized_** font.

Notes to the Student

_____

_____

_____

_____

_____

_____

Skills Assessment Requirements

Read and familiarize yourself with the procedure; complete the minimum practice requirements (MPRs). Document each MPR using proper charting technique. Complete each procedure within a reasonable amount of time, with a minimum of 85% accuracy.

Name: _____

Date: _____

POINT VALUE ✦ = 3–6 points ✳ = 7–9 points		PRACTICE TRIAL	GRADED TRIAL # 1	GRADED TRIAL # 2	NOTES
1. ✦	Perform hand hygiene.				
2. ✳	**Greet and identify the patient.**				
3. ✳	**Explain the procedure. If patient is a child, then explain procedure to both the parent and child.**				
4. ✦	Remove the electronic thermometer from its charging base, select the appropriate probe, and attach a disposable probe cover.				
5. ✳	**Ask the patient to expose the axilla.** **a. If patient is an infant or child, ask parent to take child's arm out of clothing to expose axilla.**				
6. ✳	Using a tissue, pat the axilla dry of any perspiration.				
7. ✳	Place the probe with cover into the axillary space.				
8. ✦	**Ask the patient to remain still and hold the arm tightly next to the body while the temperature registers.**				
9. ✦	When the thermometer signals completion, remove the thermometer and discard the probe cover in a waste container.				
10. ✳	Record the temperature in the patient's record, making sure to note that the temperature was obtained via the axillary route (AX).				
11. ✦	Return the thermometer probe to its appropriate storage location and then return the entire unit to the rechargeable base.				
12. ✦	Perform hand hygiene.				

Document: Enter the appropriate information in the chart below.

Grading

Points Earned	_____		
Points Possible	_____	90	90
Percent Grade (Points Earned/Points Possible)	_____		
PASS:	_____	❏ YES ❏ NO ❏ N/A	❏ YES ❏ NO ❏ N/A

Instructor Sign-Off

Instructor: _____   **Date:** _____

Name: _____

Date: _____

Procedure 35-5:

Measuring Temperature Using a Tympanic Membrane (Aural) Thermometer

Objective: Accurately perform all steps of the procedure and provide an accurate temperature reading.

Equipment and Supplies: Tympanic membrane thermometer; disposable protective probe cover; paper and pen; patient's medical record; waste container

Affective Behaviors: Affective behaviors provide a professional approach to a skill that enhances the patient encounter. These behaviors may also display sensitivity to a patient's rights and enhance communication. Pay close attention to these skills, which will be in **bold, *italicized*** font.

Notes to the Student

_____

_____

_____

_____

_____

_____

Skills Assessment Requirements

Read and familiarize yourself with the procedure; complete the minimum practice requirements (MPRs). Document each MPR using proper charting technique. Complete each procedure within a reasonable amount of time, with a minimum of 85% accuracy.

POINT VALUE ✦ = 3–6 points ✳ = 7–9 points		PRACTICE TRIAL	GRADED TRIAL # 1	GRADED TRIAL # 2	NOTES
1. ✦	Perform hand hygiene.				
2. ✳	**Greet and identify the patient.**				
3. ✳	**Explain the procedure to the patient.**				
4. ✦	Remove the thermometer unit from its base. The display will read "Ready."				
5. ✦	Attach the disposable cover to the earpiece.				
6. ✳	With one hand, gently pull upward and out on the patient's outer ear if an adult or pull back and downward if an infant or child.				
7. ✦	Gently insert the plastic-covered tip of the probe into the ear canal.				
8. ✦	Press the scan button that activates the thermometer.				
9. ✦	Observe the temperature reading on the display window.				
10. ✳	Gently withdraw the thermometer from the ear canal.				
11. ✦	Eject the used probe cover into a biohazard waste container by pressing the eject button.				
12. ✳	Record the temperature in the patient's medical record, indicating a tympanic membrane temperature (T) was obtained.				
13. ✦	Return the tympanic membrane thermometer to its base.				
14. ✦	Perform hand hygiene.				

Name: _____

Date: _____

Document: Enter the appropriate information in the chart below.

Grading

Points Earned	_____		
Points Possible	_____	93	93
Percent Grade (Points Earned/Points Possible)	_____		
PASS:	_____	❑ YES ❑ NO ❑ N/A	❑ YES ❑ NO ❑ N/A

Instructor Sign-Off

Instructor: _____ Date: _____

Procedure 35-6:

Measuring Temperature Using a Heat-Sensitive Wearable Thermometer

Objective: Accurately perform all steps of the procedure and provide an accurate temperature reading.

Equipment and Supplies: Wearable heat-sensitive thermometer (chemical strip, liquid crystal); paper and pen; patient's medical record; tissue; watch with second hand; waste container

Affective Behaviors: Affective behaviors provide a professional approach to a skill that enhances the patient encounter. These behaviors may also display sensitivity to a patient's rights and enhance communication. Pay close attention to these skills, which will be in **_bold, italicized_** font.

Notes to the Student

_____

_____

_____

_____

_____

_____

Skills Assessment Requirements

Read and familiarize yourself with the procedure; complete the minimum practice requirements (MPRs). Document each MPR using proper charting technique. Complete each procedure within a reasonable amount of time, with a minimum of 85% accuracy.

Name: _____

Date: _____

POINT VALUE ✦ = 3–6 points ✱ = 7–9 points	PRACTICE TRIAL	GRADED TRIAL #1	GRADED TRIAL #2	NOTES
1. ✦ Perform hand hygiene.				
2. ✦ **Greet and identify the patient.**				
3. ✱ **Explain the procedure.**				
4. ✦ Dry the patient's forehead by patting it with a tissue.				
5. ✱ Place the thermometer strip on the forehead and begin timing for 15 seconds.				
6. ✦ After 15 seconds have passed, read the correct temperature by reading color changes.				
7. ✱ Record the temperature in the patient's chart, indicating which type of thermometer was used.				
8. ✦ Discard strip in the waste container.				
9. ✦ Perform hand hygiene.				

Document: Enter the appropriate information in the chart below.

Grading

Points Earned	_____		
Points Possible	_____	63	63
Percent Grade (Points Earned/Points Possible)	_____		
PASS:	_____	❏ YES ❏ NO ❏ N/A	❏ YES ❏ NO ❏ N/A

Instructor Sign-Off

Instructor: _____ **Date:** _____

Procedure 35-7:

Measuring Temperature Using a Temporal Artery Thermometer

Objective: Accurately measure body temperature using a temporal thermometer.

Equipment and Supplies: Paper and pen; patient's medical record; alcohol swab; temporal artery thermometer

Affective Behaviors: Affective behaviors provide a professional approach to a skill that enhances the patient encounter. These behaviors may also display sensitivity to a patient's rights and enhance communication. Pay close attention to these skills, which will be in **_bold, italicized_** font.

Notes to the Student

_____

_____

_____

_____

_____

_____

Skills Assessment Requirements

Read and familiarize yourself with the procedure; complete the minimum practice requirements (MPRs). Document each MPR using proper charting technique. Complete each procedure within a reasonable amount of time, with a minimum of 85% accuracy.

Name: _____

Date: _____

POINT VALUE ✦ = 3–6 points ✳ = 7–9 points		PRACTICE TRIAL	GRADED TRIAL # 1	GRADED TRIAL # 2	NOTES
1. ✦	Perform hand hygiene.				
2. ✦	**Greet and identify the patient.**				
3. ✳	**Explain the procedure.**				
4. ✦	**Brush aside the patient's hair, tucking it behind the ear if necessary to keep it out of the way.**				
5. ✦	Remove the cap from the probe of the thermometer and disinfect the probe by gently wiping it with an alcohol swab.				
6. ✳	**Place the probe flush on the center of the forehead and depress the red button.**				
7. ✦	**Keep the button depressed and slowly slide the probe on the midline across the forehead to the side of the head near the hairline.**				
8. ✦	**Lift the probe from the forehead and touch it on the neck just behind the earlobe.**				
9. ✦	Release the button and read the temperature.				
10. ✳	Record the results in the patient's medical record, indicating the temperature was obtained via a temporal artery measurement.				
11. ✦	Perform hand hygiene.				

Name: _____

Date: _____

Document: Enter the appropriate information in the chart below.

Grading

Points Earned	_____		
Points Possible	_____	75	75
Percent Grade (Points Earned/Points Possible)	_____		
PASS:	_____	❏ YES ❏ NO ❏ N/A	❏ YES ❏ NO ❏ N/A

Instructor Sign-Off

Instructor: _____   **Date:** _____

Procedure 35-8:

Measuring Radial Pulse

Objective: Accurately perform all steps of the procedure and provide an accurate radial pulse reading.

Equipment and Supplies: Paper and pen; patient's medical record; watch with second hand

Affective Behaviors: Affective behaviors provide a professional approach to a skill that enhances the patient encounter. These behaviors may also display sensitivity to a patient's rights and enhance communication. Pay close attention to these skills, which will be in **bold, *italicized*** font.

Notes to the Student

_____

_____

_____

_____

_____

_____

Skills Assessment Requirements

Read and familiarize yourself with the procedure; complete the minimum practice requirements (MPRs). Document each MPR using proper charting technique. Complete each procedure within a reasonable amount of time, with a minimum of 85% accuracy.

POINT VALUE ✦ = 3–6 points ✱ = 7–9 points		PRACTICE TRIAL	GRADED TRIAL # 1	GRADED TRIAL # 2	NOTES
1. ✦	Perform hand hygiene.				
2. ✱	**_Greet and identify the patient._**				
3. ✱	**_Explain the procedure._**				
4. ✦	Ask the patient if he or she has recently smoked or performed physical activity. a. Both of these factors can cause the pulse rate to increase.				
5. ✦	Ask the patient to sit down and place the arm in a comfortable, supported position. The hand should be at or below chest level with the palm facing down.				
6. ✱	Place fingertips on the radial artery on the thumb side of the wrist. a. Applying the proper amount of pressure is important; press too hard and the pulse will be interrupted and press to lightly and the pulse might not be felt at all.				
7. ✱	Check the quality of the pulse.				
8. ✦	Start counting pulse beats when the second hand on your watch is at 3, 6, 9, or 12.				
9. ✱	Count the pulse for 1 full minute to obtain an accurate and reflective measurement. a. Some medical offices may allow a count for 30 seconds, which is then multiplied by 2. When this is the case, the pulse rate will always be an even number.				
10. ✦	Immediately write the number of pulse beats per minute on a piece of paper.				

POINT VALUE ✦ = 3–6 points ✳ = 7–9 points		PRACTICE TRIAL	GRADED TRIAL # 1	GRADED TRIAL # 2	NOTES
11. ✦	Perform hand hygiene.				
12. ✳	Record the pulse beats per minute in the patient's medical record, describing any abnormalities in pulse rate.				

Name: _____

Date: _____

Document: Enter the appropriate information in the chart below.

Grading

Points Earned	_____		
Points Possible	_____	93	93
Percent Grade (Points Earned/Points Possible)	_____		
PASS:	_____	❑ YES ❑ NO ❑ N/A	❑ YES ❑ NO ❑ N/A

Instructor Sign-Off

Instructor: _____ **Date:** _____

Procedure 35-9:

Measuring Apical–Radial Pulse (Two Persons)

Objective: Accurately perform all steps of the procedure and provide an accurate apical–radial pulse reading.

Equipment and Supplies: Stethoscope; alcohol wipe/cotton balls with 70 percent isopropyl alcohol; paper and pen; patient's medical record; watch with second hand

Affective Behaviors: Affective behaviors provide a professional approach to a skill that enhances the patient encounter. These behaviors may also display sensitivity to a patient's rights and enhance communication. Pay close attention to these skills, which will be in **bold, *italicized*** font.

Notes to the Student

_____

_____

_____

_____

_____

_____

Skills Assessment Requirements

Read and familiarize yourself with the procedure; complete the minimum practice requirements (MPRs). Document each MPR using proper charting technique. Complete each procedure within a reasonable amount of time, with a minimum of 85% accuracy.

POINT VALUE ✦ = 3–6 points ✳ = 7–9 points	PRACTICE TRIAL	GRADED TRIAL # 1	GRADED TRIAL # 2	NOTES
1. ✦ Perform hand hygiene.				
2. ✳ Disinfect the stethoscope using an alcohol wipe to cleanse the earpieces and diaphragm of the scope.				
3. ✦ **Greet and identify the patient.**				
4. ✳ **Explain the procedure. If the patient is a child, explain the procedure to both the parent and child.**				
5. ✦ Uncover the left side of the patient's chest. Provide privacy with a drape, if necessary.				
6. ✳ The first person will place the earpieces of stethoscope in his or her ears, with openings of the ear tips pointing forward.				
7. ✳ Locate the apex of patient's heart by palpating to the left fifth intercostal space (between fifth and sixth ribs) at the midclavicular line. This is found just below the nipple.				
8. ✳ Warm the chest piece by holding it in the palm of the hand before placing onto patient's chest.				
9. ✦ The second person will locate the radial pulse in the thumb side of wrist, 1 inch below base of thumb.				
10. ✦ The first person places the chest piece of the stethoscope at the apex of the heart. When the heartbeat is heard, a nod is made to indicate to the second person that counting should begin. Ideally, the count should begin when the second hand is at 3, 6, 9, or 12.				

POINT VALUE ✦ = 3–6 points ✳ = 7–9 points		PRACTICE TRIAL	GRADED TRIAL # 1	GRADED TRIAL # 2	NOTES
11. ✦	Count for 1 full minute and nod to the second person that time is up and counting should cease. *Note:* Both systole and diastole (or lub/dub) that is heard in the stethoscope count as one beat.				
12. ✦	Remove the stethoscope and earpieces.				
13. ✳	Record the rate and quality of heartbeats. Include both apical and radial rates using the designation "AP" and "R." Calculate the pulse deficit by subtracting the radial pulse rate from the apical pulse rate. *Note:* A pulse deficit may indicate that the heart contractions are not strong enough to produce a palpable radial pulse.				
14. ✦	***Assist the patient with replacement of clothing, if necessary. Assist the patient from the examining table.***				
15. ✦	Wipe the earpieces and chest piece of the stethoscope with alcohol wipes or cotton balls and alcohol.				
16. ✦	Perform hand hygiene.				

Document: Enter the appropriate information in the chart below.

Grading

Points Earned	_____		
Points Possible	_____	114	114
Percent Grade (Points Earned/Points Possible)	_____		
PASS:	_____	❑ YES ❑ NO ❑ N/A	❑ YES ❑ NO ❑ N/A

Instructor Sign-Off

Instructor: _____   Date: _____

Procedure 35-10:

Measuring Respirations

Objective: Accurately perform all steps of the procedure and provide an accurate respiration measurement.

Equipment and Supplies: Patient's medical record; watch with sweeping second hand; paper and pen

Affective Behaviors: Affective behaviors provide a professional approach to a skill that enhances the patient encounter. These behaviors may also display sensitivity to a patient's rights and enhance communication. Pay close attention to these skills, which will be in **_bold, italicized_** font.

Notes to the Student

_____

_____

_____

_____

_____

_____

Skills Assessment Requirements

Read and familiarize yourself with the procedure; complete the minimum practice requirements (MPRs). Document each MPR using proper charting technique. Complete each procedure within a reasonable amount of time, with a minimum of 85% accuracy.

POINT VALUE ✦ = 3–6 points ✳ = 7–9 points		PRACTICE TRIAL	GRADED TRIAL # 1	GRADED TRIAL # 2	NOTES
1. ✦	Perform hand hygiene.				
2. ✳	**Greet and identify the patient.**				
3. ✦	**Assist the patient into a comfortable position.**				
4. ✦	Place your hand on the patient's wrist in position to take the pulse, or place your hand on the patient's chest or back.				
5. ✳	Count each breathing cycle by observing and/or feeling the rise and fall of the patient's chest or upper abdomen.				
6. ✳	Count for one full minute using a watch with a sweeping second hand. If the rate is atypical or unusual in any way, take it for another minute.				
7. ✳	Record the respiratory rate in the patient's medical record, noting any abnormality in rate, rhythm, and depth.				
8. ✦	Perform hand hygiene.				

Name: _____

Date: _____

Document: Enter the appropriate information in the chart below.

Grading

Points Earned	_____		
Points Possible	_____	60	60
Percent Grade (Points Earned/Points Possible)	_____		
PASS:	_____	❏ YES ❏ NO ❏ N/A	❏ YES ❏ NO ❏ N/A

Instructor Sign-Off

Instructor: _____ **Date:** _____

Procedure 35-11:

Measuring Blood Pressure

Objective: Obtain an accurate systolic and diastolic blood pressure reading.

Supplies: Sphygmomanometer; stethoscope; 70 percent isopropyl alcohol; alcohol sponges or cotton balls; paper and pen; patient's medical record

Affective Behaviors: Affective behaviors provide a professional approach to a skill that enhances the patient encounter. These behaviors may also display sensitivity to a patient's rights and enhance communication. Pay close attention to these skills, which will be in **bold, *italicized*** font.

Notes to the Student

_____

_____

_____

_____

_____

Skills Assessment Requirements

Read and familiarize yourself with the procedure; complete the minimum practice requirements (MPRs). Document each MPR using proper charting technique. Complete each procedure within a reasonable amount of time, with a minimum of 85% accuracy.

POINT VALUE ✦ = 3–6 points ✶ = 7–9 points		PRACTICE TRIAL	GRADED TRIAL #1	GRADED TRIAL #2	NOTES
1. ✦	Perform hand hygiene.				
2. ✦	Assemble the equipment. Thoroughly cleanse the earpieces, bell, and diaphragm pieces of the stethoscope. Use an alcohol wipe or cotton ball with 70 percent isopropyl alcohol. Allow the alcohol to dry.				
3. ✶	***Greet and identify the patient verbally, and explain the procedure.***				
4. ✦	***Assist the patient into a comfortable position. Blood pressure (BP) may be taken with the patient in a sitting or lying position.*** a. The patient's arm should be at heart level. If the patient's arm is below heart level, the BP reading will be higher than normal; if the arm is higher than heart level, the BP will be lower than normal. b. Patients should be reminded not to cross their legs or talk during the procedure.				
5. ✦	Place the sphygmomanometer on a solid surface with the gauge within 3 feet for easy viewing.				
6. ✶	Uncover the patient's arm 5 inches above the elbow. ***If the sleeve becomes constricting when rolled back, ask the patient to slip the arm out of the sleeve.*** a. Never take a BP reading through clothing. b. Sleeves that are too tight, when rolled up, will produce an inaccurate result.				

POINT VALUE ✦ = 3–6 points ✱ = 7–9 points		PRACTICE TRIAL	GRADED TRIAL # 1	GRADED TRIAL # 2	NOTES
7. ✦	Locate the brachial artery within the antecubital space by palpating with your fingertips. If the pulse is stronger in one arm than the other, use the arm with the stronger brachial artery pulse.				
8. ✦	Have the patient straighten the arm with palm up and apply the proper-size cuff of the sphygmomanometer over the brachial artery 1 to 2 inches above the antecubital space (bend in the elbow). a. Many cuffs are marked with arrows or circles to be placed over the artery. Hold the edge of the cuff in place as you wrap the remainder of the cuff tightly around the arm. If the cuff has a Velcro closure, press it into place at the end of the cuff.				
9. ✱	With the fingertips of your nondominant hand, palpate the pulse in the radial artery. Then, with your dominant hand, tighten the thumbscrew on the hand bulb and pump air into the cuff quickly and evenly. Mentally add 20–30 mmHg above the point at which the radial pulse is no longer palpable. This is the point at which the cuff will be inflated to when the actual blood pressure measurement is obtained. Then rapidly deflate the cuff and wait 60 seconds before continuing. a. The manometer should be at eye level for a more accurate reading.				

POINT VALUE ✦ = 3–6 points ✱ = 7–9 points		PRACTICE TRIAL	GRADED TRIAL # 1	GRADED TRIAL # 2	NOTES
10. ✦	Place the earpieces in your ears and the diaphragm (or bell) of the stethoscope over the area of the pulsating brachial artery. a. Hold the diaphragm in place with one hand without placing your thumb over the diaphragm. The stethoscope tubing should hang freely and not touch the patient or any object during the reading.				
11. ✦	Close the thumbscrew on the hand bulb by turning clockwise with your dominant hand. Close the thumbscrew just enough so that no air can leak out. Do not close so tightly that you will have difficulty reopening it with one hand.				
12. ✱	Slowly turn the thumbscrew counterclockwise with your dominant hand. Allow the pressure reading to fall only 2 to 3 mmHg at a time.				
13. ✦	Listen for the point at which the first clear sound is heard. Mentally note where this occurred on the manometer. This is the systolic pressure.				
14. ✱	Slowly continue to allow the cuff to deflate. The sounds will change from loud to murmur and then fade away (phases I, II, III, and IV of the Korotkoff sounds). Read the measurement on the manometer when the sound is no longer heard. This is the diastolic pressure (phase V of the Korotkoff sounds).				

POINT VALUE ✦ = 3–6 points ✷ = 7–9 points		PRACTICE TRIAL	GRADED TRIAL # 1	GRADED TRIAL # 2	NOTES
15. ✦	Quickly open the thumbscrew all the way to release the air and deflate the cuff completely.				
16. ✦	If you are unsure about the BP reading, wait at least a minute or two before attempting to take a second reading. a. Never take more than two readings in one arm, because blood stasis may have occurred, resulting in an inaccurate reading.				
17. ✷	Immediately write the BP as a fraction on paper so that it isn't forgotten before it is entered into the patient's medical record.				
18. ✦	Remove the cuff from the patient's arm.				
19. ✦	Clean the earpieces or bell of the stethoscope with an alcohol wipe.				
20. ✦	Perform hand hygiene.				
21. ✷	Chart the results in the patient's medical record.				

Name: _____

Date: _____

Document: Enter the appropriate information in the chart below.

Grading

Points Earned	_____		
Points Possible	_____	144	144
Percent Grade (Points Earned/Points Possible)	_____		
PASS:	_____	❏ YES ❏ NO ❏ N/A	❏ YES ❏ NO ❏ N/A

Instructor Sign-Off

Instructor: _____ **Date:** _____

Name: _____

Date: _____

Procedure 35-12:

Measuring Systolic Blood Pressure Using the Palpatory Method

Objective: Obtain an accurate systolic reading.

Supplies: Sphygmomanometer; paper and pen; patient's medical record

Note The American Heart Association recommends that approximate systolic BP be determined first by palpating radial pulse, then pumping up the cuff until the pulse is no longer felt. This is standard procedure in many cases.

Affective Behaviors: Affective behaviors provide a professional approach to a skill that enhances the patient encounter. These behaviors may also display sensitivity to a patient's rights and enhance communication. Pay close attention to these skills, which will be in **bold, italicized** font.

Notes to the Student

_____

_____

_____

_____

_____

_____

Skills Assessment Requirements

Read and familiarize yourself with the procedure; complete the minimum practice requirements (MPRs). Document each MPR using proper charting technique. Complete each procedure within a reasonable amount of time, with a minimum of 85% accuracy.

Name: _____

Date: _____

POINT VALUE ✦ = 3–6 points ✱ = 7–9 points		PRACTICE TRIAL	GRADED TRIAL #1	GRADED TRIAL #2	NOTES
1. ✦	Perform hand hygiene.				
2. ✱	**Greet and identify the patient, and explain the procedure.**				
3. ✦	**With the patient in a comfortable position and the hand at heart level, place the correct-size blood pressure cuff on the arm about 1–2 inches above the antecubital space.**				
4. ✦	Locate the radial pulse on the thumb side of the wrist.				
5. ✱	Inflate the blood pressure cuff until the radial pulse is unable to be palpated. Then continue to inflate about 30 mmHg above the point at which the radial artery pulse disappeared.				
6. ✱	Slowly deflate the cuff 2 to 3 mmHg per second while keeping the fingers on the pulse. The point at which the pulse is felt is the systolic blood pressure.				
7. ✦	Quickly deflate the cuff completely and remove it from the patient's arm.				
8. ✦	Perform hand hygiene.				
9. ✱	Record the systolic pressure as "palpated systolic pressure" in the patient's medical record.				

Name: _____

Date: _____

Document: Enter the appropriate information in the chart below.

Grading

Points Earned	_____		
Points Possible	_____	66	66
Percent Grade (Points Earned/Points Possible)	_____		
PASS:	_____	❏ YES ❏ NO ❏ N/A	❏ YES ❏ NO ❏ N/A

Instructor Sign-Off

Instructor: _____   **Date:** _____

Procedure 36-1:

Cleaning the Examination Room

Objective: Prepare and clean the examination room.

Supplies: Disinfectant; paper towels; disposable gloves; examination table; pillow; pillow cover; disposable gown; examination table paper

Affective Behaviors: Affective behaviors provide a professional approach to a skill that enhances the patient encounter. These behaviors may also display sensitivity to patient's rights and enhance communication. Pay close attention to these skills, which will be in **_bold, italicized_** font.

Notes to the Student

_____

_____

_____

_____

_____

_____

Skills Assessment Requirements

Read and familiarize yourself with the procedure; complete the minimum practice requirements (MPRs). Document each MPR using proper charting technique. Complete each procedure within a reasonable amount of time, with a minimum of 85% accuracy.

Name: _____

Date: _____

POINT VALUE ✦ = 3–6 points ✶ = 7–9 points		PRACTICE TRIAL	GRADED TRIAL # 1	GRADED TRIAL # 2	NOTES
1. ✦	Perform hand hygiene and don a pair of disposable gloves.				
2. ✶	Roll the soiled disposable gown into a ball and dispose of it in the appropriate waste container.				
3. ✶	Roll the soiled examination table paper into a ball and dispose of it in the appropriate waste container.				
4. ✦	Remove the soiled pillow cover and dispose of it in the appropriate waste container.				
5. ✦	Remove any other soiled items or equipment from the examination room, discarding them in the proper containers.				
6. ✦	Clean the examination table, countertops, and cabinet surfaces with disinfectant and paper towels.				
7. ✶	Dispose of the soiled paper towels in the appropriate waste container.				
8. ✦	Remove the soiled gloves and dispose of them in the appropriate waste container.				
9. ✦	Perform hand hygiene.				
10. ✦	Put clean paper on the examination table.				
11. ✦	Put a new pillow covering over the pillow.				
12. ✦	Perform a second check, making sure the examination room is clean and clutter and odor free.				

Document: Enter the appropriate information in the chart below.

Grading

Points Earned	_____		
Points Possible	_____	81	81
Percent Grade (Points Earned/Points Possible)	_____		
PASS:	_____	❏ YES ❏ NO ❏ N/A	❏ YES ❏ NO ❏ N/A

Instructor Sign-Off

Instructor: _____   **Date:** _____

Procedure 36-2:

Documenting a Chief Complaint During a Patient Interview

Objective: Accurately document the chief complaint using correct charting format and abbreviations while interviewing the patient.

Equipment and Supplies: Patient's medical record; problem list or progress notes form; black or blue pen

Note Instructor may provide a variety of patient scenarios for students to role-play for this procedure.

Affective Behaviors: Affective behaviors provide a professional approach to a skill that enhances the patient encounter. These behaviors may also display sensitivity to a patient's rights and enhance communication. Pay close attention to these skills, which will be in ***bold, italicized*** font.

Notes to the Student

_____

_____

_____

_____

_____

_____

Skills Assessment Requirements

Read and familiarize yourself with the procedure; complete the minimum practice requirements (MPRs). Document each MPR using proper charting technique. Complete each procedure within a reasonable amount of time, with a minimum of 85% accuracy.

POINT VALUE ✦ = 3–6 points ✱ = 7–9 points		PRACTICE TRIAL	GRADED TRIAL # 1	GRADED TRIAL # 2	NOTES
1. ✦	Gather supplies, including the medical record with problem list or progress notes form.				
2. ✦	Briefly review the patient's medical history form before greeting the patient.				
3. ✦	**Greet and identify the patient. Introduce yourself and escort the patient into the examination room.**				
4. ✱	**Ask open-ended questions to gather information about why the patient is being seen today. Maintain eye contact and actively listen to the patient's responses.**				
5. ✦	**Gather information about the present illness by asking questions:** a. What makes the problem better or worse? b. When did it start? c. Where does it hurt? d. Rate the pain on a pain scale of 0 to 10.				
6. ✱	Document the CC and PI correctly within the patient medical record. a. Be certain to state the chief complaint (CC) and present illness (PI) in the patient's own words when necessary.				
7. ✦	Before leaving the room, make sure that the patient is comfortable and **ask if he or she has any questions.**				
8. ✦	**Thank the patient and explain that the physician will come in shortly to perform the examination.**				

Document: Enter the appropriate information in the chart below.

Grading

Points Earned	_____		
Points Possible	_____	54	54
Percent Grade (Points Earned/Points Possible)	_____		
PASS:	_____	❏ YES ❏ NO ❏ N/A	❏ YES ❏ NO ❏ N/A

Instructor Sign-Off

Instructor: _____   **Date:** _____

Procedure 36-3:

Interviewing a New Patient to Obtain Medical History Information and Preparing for a Physical Examination

Objective: Obtain pertinent patient information for a medical history that will assist the physician in establishing cause and treatment of the present illness (PI). Include CC, past history, social history, and family history.

Equipment and Supplies: Completed medical history form and other new patient documents; clipboard; pens (black and red); gown; drape

Affective Behaviors: Affective behaviors provide a professional approach to a skill that enhances the patient encounter. These behaviors may also display sensitivity to a patient's rights and enhance communication. Pay close attention to these skills, which will be in **bold, *italicized*** font.

Notes to the Student

_____

_____

_____

_____

_____

_____

Skills Assessment Requirements

Read and familiarize yourself with the procedure; complete the minimum practice requirements (MPRs). Document each MPR using proper charting technique. Complete each procedure within a reasonable amount of time, with a minimum of 85% accuracy.

Name: _____

Date: _____

POINT VALUE ✦ = 3–6 points ✳ = 7–9 points	PRACTICE TRIAL	GRADED TRIAL # 1	GRADED TRIAL # 2	NOTES
1. ✳ **Identify the patient, greet the patient warmly, and identify yourself.**				
2. ✦ **Escort the patient to a private examination room and explain that you will be preparing the patient to be seen by the physician.**				
3. ✦ Review the medical history form with the patient. Be sure that all the sections have been appropriately filled out. a. Ask for additional information to complete any blank lines.				
4. ✦ Speak in a clear voice and avoid using medical terminology when communicating with the patient.				
5. ✳ Ask the patient why he or she is visiting the medical office today and record the chief complaint (CC) in the patient's own words, as appropriate.				
6. ✦ Gather additional information about the present illness (PI) to provide more information about the patient's CC. a. Ask the patient open-ended questions to gather more information. b. Use observation skills during the interview.				

POINT VALUE ✦ = 3–6 points ✳ = 7–9 points	PRACTICE TRIAL	GRADED TRIAL # 1	GRADED TRIAL # 2	NOTES
7. ✳ According to physician preference or office policy, gather additional information regarding the patient's social and family histories. Document this information appropriately and as stated by the patient within the patient's medical record.				
8. ✦ Inquire about the patient's allergies. Record allergy information as appropriate within the electronic health record or using red ink in a paper record. a. If the patient states he or she does not have any allergies, record NKA (no known allergies) according to the office policy and as appropriate for the method of charting.				
9. ✦ Note any other information or observations you feel are relevant to the patient's chief complaint or present illness. a. This may include illness of other family members at home or the recent loss of a loved one, for example.				
10. ✳ Record all information using correct charting guidelines according to the method of charting used in the medical office. a. Correct any errors as necessary. If using a paper medical record, draw one line through the error, and date and initial each error. Record the correct information.				

POINT VALUE ✦ = 3–6 points ✳ = 7–9 points		PRACTICE TRIAL	GRADED TRIAL # 1	GRADED TRIAL # 2	NOTES
11. ✦	**Inform the patient if a gown must be worn and which items of clothing will need to be removed. Provide the patient with a gown and drape the patient for modesty.**				
12. ✳	**Ask the patient if he or she has any questions before leaving the examination room and inform the patient that the physician will be in shortly to perform the examination.**				
13. ✳	**Thank the patient and leave the examination room, closing the door behind you to ensure privacy.**				
14. ✦	Place the medical record with completed health history form in the designated location for the physician's review and inform the physician that the patient is ready to be examined.				

Document: Enter the appropriate information in the chart below.

Grading

Points Earned	_____		
Points Possible	_____	102	102
Percent Grade (Points Earned/Points Possible)	_____		
PASS:	_____	❏ YES ❏ NO ❏ N/A	❏ YES ❏ NO ❏ N/A

Instructor Sign-Off

Instructor: _____   **Date:** _____

Procedure 36-4:

Positioning the Patient in the Supine Position

Objective: Safely assist the patient into supine position for examination of the anterior surface of the body.

Equipment and Supplies: Examination table, gown and drape

Affective Behaviors: Affective behaviors provide a professional approach to a skill that enhances the patient encounter. These behaviors may also display sensitivity to a patient's rights and enhance communication. Pay close attention to these skills, which will be in **_bold, italicized_** font.

Notes to the Student

_____

_____

_____

_____

_____

Skills Assessment Requirements

Read and familiarize yourself with the procedure; complete the minimum practice requirements (MPRs). Document each MPR using proper charting technique. Complete each procedure within a reasonable amount of time, with a minimum of 85% accuracy.

POINT VALUE ✦ = 3–6 points ✷ = 7–9 points		PRACTICE TRIAL	GRADED TRIAL # 1	GRADED TRIAL # 2	NOTES
1. ✦	Perform hand hygiene.				
2. ✷	***Greet and identify the patient.*** Explain that you will be assisting him or her into a position as required for the physical examination.				
3. ✦	Provide a gown and assist the patient if necessary. a. If the patient does not need assistance with disrobing and gowning, leave the room to maintain the patient's privacy. b. Always knock on the exam room door and ask for permission before reentering.				
4. ✦	Assist the patient onto the examination table. a. If a separate step stool is used, stabilize it with your feet as the patient steps up to prevent the stool from sliding.				
5. ✦	Ask the patient to lie back on the table and provide an arm of support near the patient's back as the patient lies down. Pull out the foot extension on the examination table.				
6. ✦	Place a pillow under the patient's head.				
7. ✦	***Cover the patient with the drape from his or her chest to ankles.***				

POINT VALUE ✦ = 3–6 points ✷ = 7–9 points		PRACTICE TRIAL	GRADED TRIAL # 1	GRADED TRIAL # 2	NOTES
8. ✦	After the examination, **assist the patient to a sitting position**. Allow and encourage the patient to remain seated to prevent dizziness from the change of position.				
9. ✦	Push the foot extension into place while supporting the patient's feet.				
10. ✦	When the patient is stable and the examination is complete, **assist the patient to a standing position and hold the patient's arm while he or she steps down off the table**. Provide assistance with redressing if necessary.				
11. ✦	After the patient has left, clean the examination room.				
12. ✦	Perform hand hygiene.				

Name: _____

Date: _____

Document: Enter the appropriate information in the chart below.

Grading

Points Earned	_____		
Points Possible	_____	75	75
Percent Grade (Points Earned/Points Possible)	_____		
PASS:	_____	❏ YES ❏ NO ❏ N/A	❏ YES ❏ NO ❏ N/A

Instructor Sign-Off

Instructor: _____ **Date:** _____

Procedure 36-5:

Positioning the Patient in the Dorsal Recumbent Position

Objective: Safely assist the patient into the dorsal recumbent position for examination of the anterior surface of the body, catheterization, or pelvic examination.

Supplies: Examination table; gown; drape

Affective Behaviors: Affective behaviors provide a professional approach to a skill that enhances the patient encounter. These behaviors may also display sensitivity to a patient's rights and enhance communication. Pay close attention to these skills, which will be in **bold, italicized** font.

Notes to the Student

_____

_____

_____

_____

_____

_____

Skills Assessment Requirements

Read and familiarize yourself with the procedure; complete the minimum practice requirements (MPRs). Document each MPR using proper charting technique. Complete each procedure within a reasonable amount of time, with a minimum of 85% accuracy.

POINT VALUE ✦ = 3–6 points ✳ = 7–9 points		PRACTICE TRIAL	GRADED TRIAL # 1	GRADED TRIAL # 2	NOTES
1. ✦	Perform hand hygiene.				
2. ✳	Greet and identify the patient. Explain that you will be assisting him or her into a position as required for the physical examination.				
3. ✦	Provide a gown and assist the patient if necessary. a. If the patient does not need assistance with disrobing and gowning, leave the room to maintain the patient's privacy. b. Always knock on the exam room door and ask for permission before reentering.				
4. ✦	Assist the patient onto the examination table. a. If a separate step stool is used, stabilize it with your feet as the patient steps up to prevent the stool from sliding.				
6. ✦	***Ask the patient to bend the knees and place the feet flat on the table.*** Push in the foot extension.				
7. ✦	***Cover the patient with the drape with the point of the drape between the patient's legs.***				
8. ✦	Place a pillow under the patient's head if needed to provide additional comfort.				
9. ✦	Position the light source and a rolling stool in place for the examiner.				

Name: _____

Date: _____

POINT VALUE ✦ = 3–6 points ✷ = 7–9 points	PRACTICE TRIAL	GRADED TRIAL # 1	GRADED TRIAL # 2	NOTES
10. ✦ **After the procedure is complete, assist the patient to a sitting position using the foot extension to support the patient's feet.**				
11. ✦ **Ask the patient to remain seated for a few moments to prevent dizziness from the change of position.**				
12. ✦ **When the patient is stable, assist the patient to a standing position and hold the patient's arm while he or she steps down off the table. Provide assistance with redressing if necessary.**				
13. ✦ After the patient has left, clean the examination room.				
14. ✦ Perform hand hygiene.				

Document: Enter the appropriate information in the chart below.

Grading

Points Earned	_____		
Points Possible	_____	87	87
Percent Grade (Points Earned/Points Possible)	_____		
PASS:	_____	❏ YES ❏ NO ❏ N/A	❏ YES ❏ NO ❏ N/A

Instructor Sign-Off

Instructor: _____   Date: _____

Procedure 36-6:

Positioning the Patient in the Lithotomy Position

Objective: Safely assist the patient into and out of the lithotomy position for a pelvic examination or catheterization.

Supplies: Examination table with stirrups, gown; drape

Affective Behaviors: Affective behaviors provide a professional approach to a skill that enhances the patient encounter. These behaviors may also display sensitivity to a patient's rights and enhance communication. Pay close attention to these skills, which will be in **_bold, italicized_** font.

Notes to the Student

_____

_____

_____

_____

_____

Skills Assessment Requirements

Read and familiarize yourself with the procedure; complete the minimum practice requirements (MPRs). Document each MPR using proper charting technique. Complete each procedure within a reasonable amount of time, with a minimum of 85% accuracy.

POINT VALUE ✦ = 3–6 points ✳ = 7–9 points		PRACTICE TRIAL	GRADED TRIAL # 1	GRADED TRIAL # 2	NOTES
1. ✦	Perform hand hygiene.				
2. ✳	**Greet and identify the patient. Explain that you will be assisting her into a position as required for the physical examination.**				
3. ✦	**Provide a gown and assist the patient if necessary.** a. If the patient does not need assistance with disrobing and gowning, leave the room to maintain the patient's privacy. b. Always knock on the exam room door and ask for permission before reentering.				
4. ✦	**Assist the patient to sit on the end of the table.**				
5. ✦	**Cover the patient's legs with a drape.**				
6. ✦	**Ask the patient to lie back on the table and provide an arm of support near the patient's back as she lies down.**				
7. ✦	Position the stirrups level with the height of the table, about 1 foot from the side of the table. Lock the stirrups in place.				
8. ✦	**Ask the patient to slide down on the table until her buttocks are on the edge of the table end.**				
9. ✦	**Assist the patient to bend the knees and place the feet in the stirrups. Position a drape for privacy with a point between the legs.**				

POINT VALUE ✦ = 3–6 points ✱ = 7–9 points		PRACTICE TRIAL	GRADED TRIAL #1	GRADED TRIAL #2	NOTES
10. ✦	Position the light source and a rolling stool for the examiner.				
11. ✦	**Place a pillow under the patient's head as needed for additional comfort.**				
12. ✦	When the examination is complete, pull out the foot extension and help the patient remove her feet from the stirrups. **Instruct the patient to lie with the feet extended out.**				
13. ✦	**Ask the patient to slide up on the table, assisting as necessary. Keep the drape in place to ensure privacy.**				
14. ✦	**Assist the patient to a sitting position and push in the foot extension.** Allow the patient to adjust to the change in position to prevent dizziness.				
15. ✦	When the patient is stable, **assist him or her to a standing position and hold the patient's arm while he or she steps down off the table. Provide assistance with redressing if necessary.**				
16. ✦	After the patient has left, clean the examination room.				
17. ✦	Perform hand hygiene.				

Name: _____

Date: _____

Document: Enter the appropriate information in the chart below.

Grading

Points Earned	_____		
Points Possible	_____	105	105
Percent Grade (Points Earned/Points Possible)	_____		
PASS:	_____	❑ YES ❑ NO ❑ N/A	❑ YES ❑ NO ❑ N/A

Instructor Sign-Off

Instructor: _____ **Date:** _____

Procedure 36-7:

Positioning the Patient in the Fowler's Position

Objective: Safely assist the patient into the Fowler's position for examination of the upper body and the head.

Equipment and Supplies: Examination table; gown; drape

Affective Behaviors: Affective behaviors provide a professional approach to a skill that enhances the patient encounter. These behaviors may also display sensitivity to a patient's rights and enhance communication. Pay close attention to these skills, which will be in **_bold, italicized_** font.

Notes to the Student

_____

_____

_____

_____

_____

_____

Skills Assessment Requirements

Read and familiarize yourself with the procedure; complete the minimum practice requirements (MPRs). Document each MPR using proper charting technique. Complete each procedure within a reasonable amount of time, with a minimum of 85% accuracy.

POINT VALUE ✦ = 3–6 points ✳ = 7–9 points		PRACTICE TRIAL	GRADED TRIAL # 1	GRADED TRIAL # 2	NOTES
1. ✦	Perform hand hygiene.				
2. ✳	**Greet and identify the patient. Explain that you will be assisting the patient into a position as required for the physical examination.**				
3. ✦	**Provide a gown and assist the patient if necessary.** a. If the patient does not need assistance with disrobing and gowning, leave the room to maintain the patient's privacy. b. Always knock on the exam room door and ask for permission before reentering.				
4. ✦	**Assist the patient up the step to sit on the end of the examination table.**				
5. ✦	**Cover the patient's legs with a drape.**				
6. ✦	Raise the head of the table to a 90-degree angle for Fowler's position and to a 45-degree angle for semi-Fowler's position.				
7. ✦	**Direct and assist the patient to slide back and lean on the raised end of the table.**				
8. ✦	Pull out the foot extension while supporting the patient's feet.				
9. ✦	**Place a pillow under the patient's knees to relieve strain on the lower back. Adjust the drape as needed.**				

POINT VALUE ✦ = 3–6 points ✱ = 7–9 points		PRACTICE TRIAL	GRADED TRIAL #1	GRADED TRIAL #2	NOTES
10. ✦	When the examination is complete, push in the foot extension. ***Ask the patient to remain seated at the end of the table to prevent dizziness.***				
11. ✦	***Ask the patient to lean forward, sitting upright, while you support the patient's back and lower the table. Inform the patient before lowering the table.***				
12. ✦	***When the patient is stable, assist the patient to a standing position and hold the patient's arm while he or she steps down off the table. Provide assistance with redressing if necessary.***				
13. ✦	After the patient as left, clean the examination room.				
14. ✦	Perform hand hygiene.				

Document: Enter the appropriate information in the chart below.

Grading

Points Earned	_____		
Points Possible	_____	87	87
Percent Grade (Points Earned/Points Possible)	_____		
PASS:	_____	❏ YES ❏ NO ❏ N/A	❏ YES ❏ NO ❏ N/A

Instructor Sign-Off

Instructor: _____ **Date:** _____

Procedure 36-8:

Positioning the Patient in the Prone Position

Objective: Safely assist the patient into the prone position for examination of the posterior of the body.

Equipment and Supplies: Examination table; gown; drape

Affective Behaviors: Affective behaviors provide a professional approach to a skill that enhances the patient encounter. These behaviors may also display sensitivity to a patient's rights and enhance communication. Pay close attention to these skills, which will be in **_bold, italicized_** font.

Notes to the Student

_____

_____

_____

_____

_____

_____

Skills Assessment Requirements

Read and familiarize yourself with the procedure; complete the minimum practice requirements (MPRs). Document each MPR using proper charting technique. Complete each procedure within a reasonable amount of time, with a minimum of 85% accuracy.

POINT VALUE ✦ = 3–6 points ✳ = 7–9 points		PRACTICE TRIAL	GRADED TRIAL #1	GRADED TRIAL #2	NOTES
1. ✦	Perform hand hygiene.				
2. ✳	**Greet and identify the patient. Explain that you will be assisting the patient into a position as required for the physical examination.**				
3. ✦	**Provide a gown and assist the patient if necessary.** a. If the patient does not need assistance with disrobing and gowning, leave the room to maintain the patient's privacy. b. Always knock on the exam room door and ask for permission before reentering.				
4. ✦	**Assist the patient up the step to sit on the end of the examination table.** a. Stabilize the step stool as needed.				
5. ✦	Cover the patient's legs with a drape.				
6. ✦	**Ask the patient to lie back on the table and provide an arm of support near the patient's back as he or she lies down.** Pull out the foot extension.				
7. ✦	Ask the patient to turn toward you onto his or her side, then onto the abdomen. Position yourself close to the middle of the side of the table to prevent the patient from falling.				

POINT VALUE ✦ = 3–6 points ✳ = 7–9 points		PRACTICE TRIAL	GRADED TRIAL # 1	GRADED TRIAL # 2	NOTES
8. ✦	Place pillows under the patient's head and feet as needed for comfort. Cover with a drape from the shoulders to the ankles.				
9. ✦	When the examination is complete, ask the patient to turn toward you, turning face up, **and then help the patient to a sitting position**. Allow the patient to remain seated to prevent dizziness.				
10. ✦	**Have the patient stay seated for a few moments to prevent dizziness from the change in position.**				
11. ✦	**When the patient is stable, assist the patient to a standing position and hold the patient's arm while he or she steps down off the table. Provide assistance with redressing if necessary.**				
12. ✦	After the patient has left, clean the examination room.				
13. ✦	Perform hand hygiene.				

Name: _____

Date: _____

Document: Enter the appropriate information in the chart below.

Grading

Points Earned	_____		
Points Possible	_____	81	81
Percent Grade (Points Earned/Points Possible)	_____		
PASS:	_____	❏ YES ❏ NO ❏ N/A	❏ YES ❏ NO ❏ N/A

Instructor Sign-Off

Instructor: _____   **Date:** _____

Procedure 36-9:

Positioning the Patient in the Sims' Position

Objective: Safely assist the patient into the Sims' position for rectal exams, rectal temperatures, enemas, and perineal and pelvic exams.

Equipment and Supplies: Examination table; gown; drape

Affective Behaviors: Affective behaviors provide a professional approach to a skill that enhances the patient encounter. These behaviors may also display sensitivity to a patient's rights and enhance communication. Pay close attention to these skills, which will be in **bold, *italicized*** font.

Notes to the Student

_____

_____

_____

_____

_____

_____

Skills Assessment Requirements

Read and familiarize yourself with the procedure; complete the minimum practice requirements (MPRs). Document each MPR using proper charting technique. Complete each procedure within a reasonable amount of time, with a minimum of 85% accuracy.

POINT VALUE ✦ = 3–6 points ✳ = 7–9 points		PRACTICE TRIAL	GRADED TRIAL # 1	GRADED TRIAL # 2	NOTES
1. ✦	Perform proper hand hygiene.				
2. ✳	**Greet and identify the patient. Explain that you will be assisting the patient into a position as required for the physical examination.**				
3. ✦	**Provide a gown and assist the patient if necessary.** a. If the patient does not need assistance with disrobing and gowning, leave the room to maintain the patient's privacy. b. Always knock on the exam room door and ask for permission before reentering.				
4. ✦	**Assist the patient up the step to sit on the end of the examination table.** a. Stabilize the step stool as needed.				
5. ✦	Cover the patient's legs with a drape.				
6. ✦	**Ask the patient to lie back on the table and provide an arm of support near the patient's back as he or she lies down.** Pull out the foot extension.				
7. ✦	**Ask the patient to turn toward you onto his or her left side with the left knee flexed slightly, placing the body weight on the chest.**				

POINT VALUE ✦ = 3–6 points ✱ = 7–9 points	PRACTICE TRIAL	GRADED TRIAL # 1	GRADED TRIAL # 2	NOTES
8. ✦ **Ask the patient to flex the right knee to a 90-degree angle. Bend the patient's right arm at the elbow with the hand toward the head. Adjust the drape to cover the patient from the shoulders to the ankles.**				
9. ✦ When the examination or procedure is complete, **ask the patient to turn toward you and onto his or her back. Ask the patient to remain seated at the end of the table for a few moments to prevent dizziness from the change in position.**				
10. ✦ **When the patient is stable, assist the patient to a standing position and hold the patient's arm while he or she steps down off the table. Provide assistance with redressing if necessary.**				
11. ✦ After the patient has left, clean the examination room.				
12. ✦ Perform hand hygiene.				

Name: _____

Date: _____

Document: Enter the appropriate information in the chart below.

Grading

Points Earned	_____		
Points Possible	_____	81	81
Percent Grade (Points Earned/Points Possible)	_____		
PASS:	_____	❏ YES ❏ NO ❏ N/A	❏ YES ❏ NO ❏ N/A

Instructor Sign-Off

Instructor: _____ Date: _____

Procedure 36-10:

Positioning the Patient in the Knee-Chest Position

Objective: Safely assist the patient into the knee–chest position for examination of the rectum, sigmoid colon, or vagina.

Equipment and Supplies: Patient gown and drape; examination table

Affective Behaviors: Affective behaviors provide a professional approach to a skill that enhances the patient encounter. These behaviors may also display sensitivity to a patient's rights and enhance communication. Pay close attention to these skills, which will be in **bold, italicized** font.

Notes to the Student

_____

_____

_____

_____

_____

_____

Skills Assessment Requirements

Read and familiarize yourself with the procedure; complete the minimum practice requirements (MPRs). Document each MPR using proper charting technique. Complete each procedure within a reasonable amount of time, with a minimum of 85% accuracy.

POINT VALUE ✦ = 3–6 points ✳ = 7–9 points		PRACTICE TRIAL	GRADED TRIAL # 1	GRADED TRIAL # 2	NOTES
1. ✦	Perform hand hygiene.				
2. ✳	**Greet and identify the patient. Explain that you will be assisting the patient into a position as required for the physical examination.**				
3. ✦	**Provide a gown and assist the patient if necessary.** a. If the patient does not need assistance with disrobing and gowning, leave the room to maintain the patient's privacy. b. Always knock on the exam room door and ask for permission before reentering.				
4. ✦	**Assist the patient up the step to sit on the end of the examination table.** a. Stabilize the step stool as needed.				
5. ✦	**Cover the legs with a drape.**				
6. ✦	**Ask the patient to lie back on the table and provide an arm of support near the patient's back as he or she lies down.** Pull out the foot extension.				
7. ✦	**Ask the patient to turn toward you onto the abdomen, providing assistance as needed.** Position yourself in the center of the side of the table to prevent the patient from falling. Adjust the drape.				

POINT VALUE ✦ = 3–6 points ✶ = 7–9 points		PRACTICE TRIAL	GRADED TRIAL # 1	GRADED TRIAL # 2	NOTES
8. ✦	**Assist the patient onto the knees, with hips bent and keeping the chest on the table.** Buttocks will be raised in the air, arms bent, head turned to the side, and hands next to the head. The patient may rest his or her weight on the elbows if it is more comfortable				
9. ✦	**Adjust the drape so the point of the drape is between the patient's legs.**				
10. ✦	When the examination is complete, **help the patient to lie flat on the abdomen. When the patient is ready, ask him or her to turn toward you and then lie on his or her back. Help the patient to sit up and remain seated for a few moments to prevent dizziness from the change of position.**				
11. ✦	**When the patient is stable, assist the patient to a standing position and hold the patient's arm while he or she steps down off the table. Provide assistance with redressing if necessary.**				
12. ✦	After the patient has left, clean the examination room.				
13. ✦	Perform hand hygiene.				

Document: Enter the appropriate information in the chart below.

Grading

Points Earned	_____		
Points Possible	_____	81	81
Percent Grade (Points Earned/Points Possible)	_____		
PASS:	_____	❏ YES ❏ NO ❏ N/A	❏ YES ❏ NO ❏ N/A

Instructor Sign-Off

Instructor: _____   **Date:** _____

Procedure 36-11:

Assisting with a Complete Physical Examination

Objective: Assist with the physical examination by preparing the necessary equipment, while observing proper sequencing and ensuring patient safety with limited direction.

Equipment and Supplies: Alcohol swabs; drape; emesis basin; examination table with clean sheet; disposable gloves; laryngeal mirror; lubricant; nasal speculum; ophthalmoscope; otoscope; pillow (with clean cover); reflex hammer; scale with height rod; Snellen chart (vision); sphygmomanometer; stethoscope; tape measure; thermometer; tissues; tongue depressors; tuning fork; urine specimen container

Note Equipment and supplies will vary, depending on the type and purpose of the examination and personal preferences of the physician.

Affective Behaviors: Affective behaviors provide a professional approach to a skill that enhances the patient encounter. These behaviors may also display sensitivity to a patient's rights and enhance communication. Pay close attention to these skills, which will be in **bold, *italicized*** font.

Notes to the Student

_____

_____

_____

_____

_____

Skills Assessment Requirements

Read and familiarize yourself with the procedure; complete the minimum practice requirements (MPRs). Document each MPR using proper charting technique. Complete each procedure within a reasonable amount of time, with a minimum of 85% accuracy.

Name: _____

Date: _____

POINT VALUE ✦ = 3–6 points ✶ = 7–9 points	PRACTICE TRIAL	GRADED TRIAL # 1	GRADED TRIAL # 2	NOTES
1. ✦ Perform hand hygiene.				
2. ✦ Assemble all equipment in the examination room.				
3. ✶ **Greet and identify the patient. Explain to the patient that the doctor will be performing a physical examination.**				
4. ✦ For comfort and efficiency during the examination, the patient should have an empty bladder. This is the time to provide the patient with a urine specimen container and appropriate instructions if a urine sample is needed for the examination. a. If a urine specimen is not required, simply offer the patient the opportunity to use the restroom. Make sure the patient knows how to find the restroom and then find his or her way back to the examination room.				
5. ✶ Obtain the patient's vital signs and measurements (temperature, pulse, respirations, blood pressure, height, and weight). a. Immediately document this information in the patient's medical record.				
6. ✦ **Provide the patient with a gown and drape and give instructions on disrobing. Inform the patient as to whether the opening of the gown should be in the front or the back. Then instruct the patient to sit on the**				

POINT VALUE ✦ = 3–6 points ✱ = 7–9 points		PRACTICE TRIAL	GRADED TRIAL # 1	GRADED TRIAL # 2	NOTES
	examination table after donning the gown. a. Excuse yourself from the room to provide patient privacy while the patient disrobes.				
7. ✱	After an adequate amount of time has passed, return to the room. **Knock on the door, identify yourself, and ask permission to enter the room. Once inside, place the drape over the patient's legs and inquire if he or she has any questions or concerns.**				
8. ✦	Inform the physician that the patient is ready to be seen. a. A female medical assistant should remain in the room if the patient is a female and the physician is a male or if the physician needs assistance. A male medical assistant may be required to remain in the room if the patient is male and the physician is female or, again, if the physician needs assistance.				
9. ✦	Assist the physician as needed by handing instruments and other supplies needed during the examination. a. Be aware of when you will need to help the patient during positional changes while ensuring that proper draping is providing for patient modesty.				
10. ✦	Use personal protective equipment (PPE), such as gloves, when appropriate.				

POINT VALUE ✦ = 3–6 points ✱ = 7–9 points		PRACTICE TRIAL	GRADED TRIAL # 1	GRADED TRIAL # 2	NOTES
11. ✦	As the physician progresses from one section of the body to the next during the ROS, reposition the drape to expose only the portion of the patient's body being examined.				
12. ✦	If collected, label all specimen slides and containers as soon as possible. Use gloves when handling specimens.				
13. ✱	When the examination is complete, assist the patient to sit up slowly, because some patients experience dizziness when they sit up suddenly. When removing legs from stirrups, take both legs down together to prevent strain on the hips and back.				
14. ✦	***Assist the patient off the examination table if necessary.*** ***a. Ask the patient if he or she requires help dressing. If help is not needed, leave the room to allow the patient to get dressed in privacy.***				
15. ✦	***Provide the patient with further instructions after he or she is done dressing.***				
16. ✦	After the patient has left, clean the examination room.				
17. ✦	Resupply the examination room, including replacing soiled linens.				
18. ✦	Complete proper documentation within the patient's medical record. CPX is commonly recognized as the abbreviation for *complete physical exam.*				

Name: _____

Date: _____

Document: Enter the appropriate information in the chart below.

Grading

Points Earned	_____		
Points Possible	_____	120	120
Percent Grade (Points Earned/Points Possible)	_____		
PASS:	_____	❏ YES ❏ NO ❏ N/A	❏ YES ❏ NO ❏ N/A

Instructor Sign-Off

Instructor: _____   **Date:** _____

Procedure 37-1:

Performing a Scratch Test

Objective: Determine specific substances that cause an allergic reaction in the patient.

Equipment and Supplies: Allergen extracts; control solution; cotton balls; alcohol; disposable sterile needles or lancets; timer; tape; ruler; cold pack or ice bag; patient's medical record; disposable gloves; biohazard waste containers, including sharps container

Affective Behaviors: Affective behaviors provide a professional approach to a skill that enhances the patient encounter. These behaviors may also display sensitivity to a patient's rights and enhance communication. Pay close attention to these skills, which will be in **_bold, italicized_** font.

Notes to the Student

_____

_____

_____

_____

_____

_____

Skills Assessment Requirements

Read and familiarize yourself with the procedure; complete the minimum practice requirements (MPRs). Document each MPR using proper charting technique. Complete each procedure within a reasonable amount of time, with a minimum of 85% accuracy.

POINT VALUE ✦ = 3–6 points ✷ = 7–9 points		PRACTICE TRIAL	GRADED TRIAL # 1	GRADED TRIAL # 2	NOTES
1. ✦	Perform hand hygiene.				
2. ✦	**Warmly greet and identify the patient**, introduce self, and explain the procedure. a. Allow the patient time to ask questions before proceeding, because the patient may have hesitation concerning the test.				
3. ✦	**Ask the patient to take a seat on the examination table. Provide support and assistance if necessary.**				
4. ✦	Apply gloves and swab the test site (either forearm or back) with alcohol and allow it to air dry.				
5. ✦	Label the skin surface with adhesive tape in rows about 1 ½ to 2 inches apart.				
6. ✷	Place a drop of allergen above or below the correct label. Be consistent.				
7. ✷	Using a separate sterile lancet or needle for each extract, make a small scratch (no more than ⅛ inch deep) on the skin below each drop.				
8. ✷	Set the timer for the specified reaction time. Time is usually 10 to 30 minutes.				
9. ✦	After the specified time period elapses, clean each site with alcohol and cotton ball. Take care not to remove labels.				
10. ✷	Examine and measure each site, and record the results in the patient's record.				

POINT VALUE ✦ = 3–6 points ✳ = 7–9 points		PRACTICE TRIAL	GRADED TRIAL # 1	GRADED TRIAL # 2	NOTES
11. ✦	Have the physician check each site and review your measurements.				
12. ✳	Apply cold packs or ice bag to relieve itching if necessary.				
13. ✦	Dispose of used material properly.				
14. ✦	**Assist the patient off the examination table and provide the patient with further instructions, as indicated by the physician.**				
15. ✦	Clean the examination room. Record any further data in the patient's record.				
16. ✦	Perform proper hand hygiene.				

Name: _____

Date: _____

Document: Enter the appropriate information in the chart below.

Grading

Points Earned	_____		
Points Possible	_____	111	111
Percent Grade (Points Earned/Points Possible)	_____		
PASS:	_____	❏ YES ❏ NO ❏ N/A	❏ YES ❏ NO ❏ N/A

Instructor Sign-Off

Instructor: _____   Date: _____

Procedure 37-2:

Taking a Wound Culture

Objective: Obtain a sample from a wound by using a swab technique without error.

Equipment and Supplies: Gloves; culture tube with sterile swab and transport media; tape for dressing; sterile water for cleansing wound; sterile 4 X 3 X 4 gauze dressing; hazardous waste container; bag for soiled dressing; prepared label for culture tube or pen for labeling tube

Affective Behaviors: Affective behaviors provide a professional approach to a skill that enhances the patient encounter. These behaviors may also display sensitivity to a patient's rights and enhance communication. Pay close attention to these skills, which will be in **_bold, italicized_** font.

Notes to the Student

_____

_____

_____

_____

_____

Skills Assessment Requirements

Read and familiarize yourself with the procedure; complete the minimum practice requirements (MPRs). Document each MPR using proper charting technique. Complete each procedure within a reasonable amount of time, with a minimum of 85% accuracy.

Name: _____

Date: _____

POINT VALUE ✦ = 3–6 points ✶ = 7–9 points		PRACTICE TRIAL	GRADED TRIAL #1	GRADED TRIAL #2	NOTES
1. ✦	**Warmly greet and identify the patient. Explain the procedure and answer any patient questions as necessary.**				
2. ✦	Assemble equipment and label the culture tube with the patient's name, date of birth, your initials, and today's date.				
3. ✶	Perform hand hygiene and don a pair of gloves.				
4. ✦	Remove the patient's wound dressing. Take note of the amount and type of exudate. Dispose of used dressing materials in a biohazard waste container.				
5. ✶	Observe the wound for redness, crusting, swelling, and odor.				
6. ✶	Remove the sterile swab from the culture tube and place it in the wound. Rotate the swab back and forth to obtain a good sample. Place the swab in the sterile culture tube. Crush the ampule of preservative that is found at the bottom of the culture tube and seal the tube.				
7. ✦	Remove gloves, perform hand hygiene, and apply sterile gloves.				
8. ✦	Clean the wound using sterile water and 4 × 3 × 4 gauze squares.				
9. ✶	Apply sterile dressing over the wound.				
10. ✦	Dispose of used gauze squares in the biohazard waste container.				

POINT VALUE ✦ = 3–6 points ✳ = 7–9 points		PRACTICE TRIAL	GRADED TRIAL #1	GRADED TRIAL #2	NOTES
11. ✳	Remove gloves and dispose of them properly in hazardous waste container.				
12. ✦	**Instruct the patient in wound care. Provide both verbal and written instructions.**				
13. ✳	Chart the procedure in the patient's medical record, taking time to make detailed notes regarding the appearance of the wound and any outstanding observations.				

Name: _____

Date: _____

Document: Enter the appropriate information in the chart below.

Grading

Points Earned	_____		
Points Possible	_____	90	90
Percent Grade (Points Earned/Points Possible)	_____		
PASS:	_____	❏ YES ❏ NO ❏ N/A	❏ YES ❏ NO ❏ N/A

Instructor Sign-Off

Instructor: _____ Date: _____

Procedure 37-3:

Assisting with a Sigmoidoscopy

Objective: Assist the physician during the sigmoidoscopic examination by positioning the patient, handling all equipment and biopsy material, and providing support for the patient throughout the procedure without error.

Equipment and Supplies: Sigmoidoscope (metal or plastic) with obturator; rectal speculum; insufflator; suction equipment; sterile specimen container with preservative; sterile biopsy forceps; cotton applicators (long); lubricating jelly; basin of warm water; patient drape; gloves; patient gown; small towel or examination table pad; tissue; biohazard waste container; patient medical record; cleaning supplies for disinfection

Affective Behaviors: Affective behaviors provide a professional approach to a skill that enhances the patient encounter. These behaviors may also display sensitivity to a patient's rights and enhance communication. Pay close attention to these skills, which will be in **bold, *italicized*** font.

Notes to the Student

_____

_____

_____

_____

_____

_____

Skills Assessment Requirements

Read and familiarize yourself with the procedure; complete the minimum practice requirements (MPRs). Document each MPR using proper charting technique. Complete each procedure within a reasonable amount of time, with a minimum of 85% accuracy.

POINT VALUE ✦ = 3–6 points ✳ = 7–9 points		PRACTICE TRIAL	GRADED TRIAL # 1	GRADED TRIAL # 2	NOTES
1. ✦	Perform hand hygiene.				
2. ✦	Prepare the equipment and supplies. a. Check all that lights and lightbulbs in equipment are properly functioning. b. Prepare a basin of warm water to receive used instruments. c. Test the suction equipment. d. Place the obturator (a rigid device inserted into the flexible tube to help guide it) within the sigmoidoscope.				
3. ✳	**Warmly greet and identify the patient and explain the steps of the procedure.**				
4. ✦	**Verify that the patient has followed the enema and diet instructions.**				
5. ✦	Verify that the patient has signed an informed consent for the procedure and biopsy of samples obtained.				
6. ✦	**Ask the patient to undress, put on a patient gown with the opening in the back, and empty the bladder.** **a. Direct the patient to the location of the restroom.** **b. Allow the patient to privately undress and don a gown. Before reentering the examination room, knock on the door and wait for permission to enter.**				

POINT VALUE ✦ = 3–6 points ✶ = 7–9 points	PRACTICE TRIAL	GRADED TRIAL # 1	GRADED TRIAL # 2	NOTES
7. ✶ **Assist the patient into the Sims', lateral, or knee–chest position or onto the proctology table. Drape the patient and place a towel or disposable examination pad under the perineal area.**				
8. ✦ Inform the physician that the patient is ready and don a pair of gloves when the physician is prepared to begin the procedure.				
9. ✶ Place lubricant on the physician's gloved fingers for a digital examination, which is initially performed.				
10. ✦ If a metal scope is being used, place it in a basin of warm water before it will be inserted into the patient. Lubricate the tip of the scope.				
11. ✦ Attach the inflation bulb (for air inflation during the procedure) and attach the light source. Turn the scope on just before the physician is ready to use it.				
12. ✶ **Remind the patient to take deep breaths and relax the abdominal muscles. Observe the patient for undue reactions.**				
13. ✶ Assist the physician by handing instruments and equipment, as they are needed, such as suction and cotton-tipped applicators. Place used equipment, including suction tubing, into the basin of water.				

POINT VALUE ✦ = 3–6 points ✳ = 7–9 points		PRACTICE TRIAL	GRADED TRIAL #1	GRADED TRIAL #2	NOTES
14. ✳	Assist with biopsy by holding open specimen containers to receive specimen while maintaining sterility of container.				
15. ✦	After the procedure is completed, clean around the patient's anal opening with tissue. Discard the tissue in a biohazard waste container.				
16. ✦	Remove gloves and perform hand hygiene.				
17. ✦	**_Assist the patient to slowly sit up._**				
18. ✦	Inform the patient that he or she may re-dress, providing assistance as needed. If assistance is not needed, exit the examination room to provide patient privacy.				
19. ✳	Label specimen container with patient's name, address, date and time of collection, source of the specimen, and ID number.				
20. ✦	Apply gloves and clean the equipment. Sterilize and sanitize equipment according to the manufacturer's recommendations and office protocol.				
21. ✦	Disinfect the examination table and clean the examination room.				
22. ✦	Remove gloves, perform hand hygiene, and document the procedure in the patient's medical record. The physician will document the results of the procedure.				

Name: _____

Date: _____

Document: Enter the appropriate information in the chart below.

Grading

Points Earned	_____		
Points Possible	_____	153	153
Percent Grade (Points Earned/Points Possible)	_____		
PASS:	_____	❏ YES ❏ NO ❏ N/A	❏ YES ❏ NO ❏ N/A

Instructor Sign-Off

Instructor: _____   **Date:** _____

Name: _____

Date: _____

Procedure 37-4:

Administering a Disposable Enema

Objective: To assist in cleansing fecal material from bowel in preparation for a diagnostic examination.

Equipment and Supplies: Examination table; disposable enema; lubricant; towel; gloves; tissues; drape; pen; patient's medical record

Affective Behaviors: Affective behaviors provide a professional approach to a skill that enhances the patient encounter. These behaviors may also display sensitivity to a patient's rights and enhance communication. Pay close attention to these skills, which will be in **bold, italicized** font.

Notes to the Student

_____

_____

_____

_____

_____

_____

Skills Assessment Requirements

Read and familiarize yourself with the procedure; complete the minimum practice requirements (MPRs). Document each MPR using proper charting technique. Complete each procedure within a reasonable amount of time, with a minimum of 85% accuracy.

POINT VALUE ✦ = 3–6 points ✳ = 7–9 points	PRACTICE TRIAL	GRADED TRIAL #1	GRADED TRIAL #2	NOTES
1. ✦ Assemble equipment. Warm the disposable enema container prior to using it to avoid causing abdominal cramping.				
2. ✳ *Warmly greet and identify the patient. Explain the procedural steps in a reassuring manner, allowing the patient to ask questions as necessary.*				
3. ✦ Perform hand hygiene.				
4. ✦ *Instruct the patient to disrobe from the waist down and cover with drape; provide assistance as necessary.* *a. If the patient doesn't need assistance undressing, exit the examination room to allow for patient privacy. Before reentering, knock on the door and wait for permission to enter.*				
5. ✦ *Assist the patient onto the examination table as needed. Ask the patient to assume the Sims' position (left side with right knee at 90-degree angle). Drape for comfort and privacy.*				
6. ✦ Apply gloves.				
7. ✦ Remove the cap from the enema container. Apply a small amount of lubricant to the tip.				
8. ✳ Separate the buttocks to expose the anus and gently insert the lubricated tip about 2 inches into the anus, with tip pointing toward patient's navel.				
9. ✳ *Instruct the patient to take deep breaths while you slowly empty the contents of the container.*				

Name: _____

Date: _____

	POINT VALUE ✦ = 3–6 points ✳ = 7–9 points	PRACTICE TRIAL	GRADED TRIAL # 1	GRADED TRIAL # 2	NOTES
10. ✦	*Ask the patient to retain the liquid as long as possible to ensure good results: 5 to 10 minutes should help the enema to work.*				
11. ✦	After withdrawing the tip, gently wipe the anal area with a tissue to remove excess lubricant.				
12. ✦	*Provide a bedpan or direct the patient to the restroom, instructing the patient not to flush the toilet until you have checked the results.*				
13. ✦	*Review instructions with the patient as necessary for the next testing procedure.*				
14. ✦	Don a new pair of gloves and clean the examination room and disinfect the examination table; discard disposable enema equipment in the biohazard waste container.				
15. ✦	Remove gloves and perform hand hygiene.				
16. ✳	Make appropriate documentation notes in the patient's medical record.				

Name: _____

Date: _____

Document: Enter the appropriate information in the chart below.

Grading

Points Earned	_____		
Points Possible	_____	105	105
Percent Grade (Points Earned/Points Possible)	_____		
PASS:	_____	❏ YES ❏ NO ❏ N/A	❏ YES ❏ NO ❏ N/A

Instructor Sign-Off

Instructor: _____ **Date:** _____

Procedure 37-5:

Instructing the Patient in Collecting a Stool Specimen

Objective: To instruct patients how to obtain an adequate stool specimen for laboratory testing.

Equipment and Supplies: Sterile specimen container with lid (for culture or ova and parasite testing); lab request form; pen; patient's medical record; label; printed instructions; tongue depressor; biohazard transport bag; bedpan or other container for the collection of stool

Affective Behaviors: Affective behaviors provide a professional approach to a skill that enhances the patient encounter. These behaviors may also display sensitivity to a patient's rights and enhance communication. Pay close attention to these skills, which will be in **bold, *italicized*** font.

Notes to the Student

Check the physician's orders for the type of test to be performed prior to collecting the specimen.

_____

_____

_____

_____

_____

Skills Assessment Requirements

Read and familiarize yourself with the procedure; complete the minimum practice requirements (MPRs). Document each MPR using proper charting technique. Complete each procedure within a reasonable amount of time, with a minimum of 85% accuracy.

Note: Check the physician's orders for the type of test to be performed before collecting the specimen.

POINT VALUE ✦ = 3–6 points ✶ = 7–9 points	PRACTICE TRIAL	GRADED TRIAL # 1	GRADED TRIAL # 2	NOTES
1. ✦ Assemble the necessary items and place them in the examination room.				
2. ✶ Label the specimen container or the occult blood slides with the patient's identifying information and fill out the laboratory request form.				
3. ✶ **Identify the patient and explain the physician orders. Give the patient a copy of the printed instructions and review them together.**				
4. ✶ **Instruct the patient on how to obtain a small amount of stool.** *Note:* For culture and ova parasites: 3–4 tablespoons are required for culture and ova, and nothing else may be placed in the container (no toilet paper, tissues, urine, or menses). To maintain sterility, patients are not to touch the inside of the cup or cover. The patient may use a sterile tongue depressor to obtain larger samples of stool from the bedpan, commode, or specipan (Figure A). Patient compliance is difficult, and it is up to you, the medical assistant, to put the patient at ease as much as possible.				

Name: _____

Date: _____

Note: Check the physician's orders for the type of test to be performed before collecting the specimen.

POINT VALUE ✦ = 3–6 points ✱ = 7–9 points	PRACTICE TRIAL	GRADED TRIAL # 1	GRADED TRIAL # 2	NOTES
5. ✱ **Instruct the patient to write the date and time of the specimen, place it in a biohazard transport bag, and bring it as soon as possible with the laboratory request form to the laboratory or office.** Storage and time of delivery directions depend on the test performed and are specified in the testing facility manual.				
6. ✱ **Have the patient or family member repeat instructions back to you to verify comprehension.**				
7. ✱ Document that instructions were given to the patient.				

Document: Enter the appropriate information in the chart below.

Grading

Points Earned	_____		
Points Possible	_____	60	60
Percent Grade (Points Earned/Points Possible)	_____		
PASS:	_____	❏ YES ❏ NO ❏ N/A	❏ YES ❏ NO ❏ N/A

Instructor Sign-Off

Instructor: _____   **Date:** _____

Procedure 37-6:

Testing for Occult Blood

Objective: To test feces for occult blood.

Equipment and Supplies: 3 occult blood slides; applicators; envelope; timer; patient's medical record; pen; gloves; color developer

Note Many test kits are available on the market. Each one has its own set of directions, color developer, slides, and control monitors. The test kit directions should be followed exactly.

Affective Behaviors: Affective behaviors provide a professional approach to a skill that enhances the patient encounter. These behaviors may also display sensitivity to a patient's rights and enhance communication. Pay close attention to these skills, which will be in ***bold, italicized*** font.

Notes to the Student

_____

_____

_____

_____

_____

_____

Skills Assessment Requirements

Read and familiarize yourself with the procedure; complete the minimum practice requirements (MPRs). Document each MPR using proper charting technique. Complete each procedure within a reasonable amount of time, with a minimum of 85% accuracy.

Name: _____

Date: _____

POINT VALUE ✦ = 3–6 points ✱ = 7–9 points		PRACTICE TRIAL	GRADED TRIAL #1	GRADED TRIAL #2	NOTES
1. ✦	Perform hand hygiene and don gloves.				
2. ✦	Place a paper towel on the area to hold the slides.				
3. ✱	Verify the patient's name and date of birth against the patient's medical record. Verify that the dates on the occult blood slides are from three different dates.				
4. ✱	Check the expiration date on the color developer.				
5. ✦	Open the window flap on the back of slide and apply 2 drops of the developer to Box A and Box B.				
6. ✱	Immediately set the timer for result interpretation according to manufacturer's instructions (usually 30–60 seconds). a. A positive result will have blue color around the edge of the specimen; a negative result will have no color change visible. Any amount of blue color indicates a positive result for occult blood.				
7. ✱	Perform quality control tests on the positive and negative controls on each card or as indicated by the manufacturer.				
8. ✦	Test the remaining slides in the same manner.				
9. ✦	Dispose of all materials in a biohazard waste container. Clean and sanitize the work area.				

POINT VALUE ✦ = 3–6 points ✶ = 7–9 points		PRACTICE TRIAL	GRADED TRIAL # 1	GRADED TRIAL # 2	NOTES
10. ✦	Remove gloves.				
11. ✦	Perform hand hygiene.				
12. ✶	Document the results in the patient's record.				

Document: Enter the appropriate information in the chart below.

Grading

Points Earned	_____		
Points Possible	_____	117	117
Percent Grade (Points Earned/Points Possible)	_____		
PASS:	_____	❏ YES ❏ NO ❏ N/A	❏ YES ❏ NO ❏ N/A

Instructor Sign-Off

Instructor: _____   **Date:** _____

Procedure 37-7:

Performing a Pupil Check on a Patient

Objective: To correctly check patients' pupils for size, dilation, constriction, accommodation, and equal reaction to light.

Equipment and Supplies: Pen light; patient's medical record; pen

Affective Behaviors: Affective behaviors provide a professional approach to a skill that enhances the patient encounter. These behaviors may also display sensitivity to a patient's rights and enhance communication. Pay close attention to these skills, which will be in **_bold, italicized_** font.

Notes to the Student

_____

_____

_____

_____

_____

_____

Skills Assessment Requirements

Read and familiarize yourself with the procedure; complete the minimum practice requirements (MPRs). Document each MPR using proper charting technique. Complete each procedure within a reasonable amount of time, with a minimum of 85% accuracy.

POINT VALUE ✦ = 3–6 points ✳ = 7–9 points	PRACTICE TRIAL	GRADED TRIAL #1	GRADED TRIAL #2	NOTES
1. ✦ **Warmly greet and identify the patient.**				
2. ✦ **Introduce yourself and observe the patient for responsiveness to your introduction.**				
3. ✳ **Explain the procedure.**				
4. ✦ **Ask the patient to look straight ahead.**				
5. ✳ Using a penlight or flashlight, approach from the side and shine light on one pupil at a time. Observe for constriction of the pupil.				
6. ✦ Shine the light on the pupil again and observe the other pupil for constriction.				
7. ✳ Hold open the eyes by gently separating the eyelids (lightly grasping near the brow bone and below the eye socket) and observe the pupils for size. They should be equal in size.				
8. ✳ Hold an object (penlight or pen) about 10 cm (4 in.) from the bridge of the patient's nose. Ask the patient to look at the top of the object and then at a different object on the wall across the room, forcing the patient to shift his or her focus. Observe for pupil response. (Pupil should constrict when looking at close object and dilate when looking across the room.)				
9. ✦ Move the pen toward the patient's nose. The pupils should converge toward the patient's nose.				

Name: _____

Date: _____

POINT VALUE ✦ = 3–6 points ✱ = 7–9 points		PRACTICE TRIAL	GRADED TRIAL # 1	GRADED TRIAL # 2	NOTES
10. ✱	Observe the pupils for shape. They should be equal or similar in shape.				
11. ✦	**Explain to the patient what other tests will be performed.**				
12. ✱	Document the results in the patient's medical record. When the pupil check is normal, the abbreviation for Pupils Equal, Round, Reactive to Light and Accommodation (PERRLA) is used. If the pupil check is not normal, document the results observed.				

Name: _____

Date: _____

Document: Enter the appropriate information in the chart below.

Grading

Points Earned	_____		
Points Possible	_____	90	90
Percent Grade (Points Earned/Points Possible)	_____		
PASS:	_____	❑ YES ❑ NO ❑ N/A	❑ YES ❑ NO ❑ N/A

Instructor Sign-Off

Instructor: _____   **Date:** _____

Procedure 37-8:

Assisting with a Neurologic Examination

Objective: Assist the physician with a neurologic screening examination.

Equipment and Supplies: Percussion hammer; safety pin; tongue depressor; Mayo tray; penlight; cotton ball; tuning fork; neurological wheel; ophthalmoscope; otoscope; hot and cold water; materials with different odors

Affective Behaviors: Affective behaviors provide a professional approach to a skill that enhances the patient encounter. These behaviors may also display sensitivity to a patient's rights and enhance communication. Pay close attention to these skills, which will be in **bold, *italicized*** font.

Notes to the Student

_____

_____

_____

_____

_____

_____

Skills Assessment Requirements

Read and familiarize yourself with the procedure; complete the minimum practice requirements (MPRs). Document each MPR using proper charting technique. Complete each procedure within a reasonable amount of time, with a minimum of 85% accuracy.

POINT VALUE ✦ = 3–6 points ✳ = 7–9 points	PRACTICE TRIAL	GRADED TRIAL # 1	GRADED TRIAL # 2	NOTES
1. ✦ Perform hand hygiene.				
2. ✦ Assemble equipment on the Mayo tray and cover the tray.				
3. ✳ ***Warmly greet and identify the patient and explain the procedure.***				
4. ✳ ***Evaluate the patient's mental status while taking a medical history, paying attention to responses, memory, coherence of thought, overall mood, and awareness. Make appropriate documentation notes within the patient's medical record.***				
5. ✳ If ordered, perform a visual acuity test.				
6. ✦ ***Assist the patient onto the examination table*** and drape as needed for comfort.				
7. ✦ The physician will test reflexes with the percussion hammer. Be prepared to hand the physician the hammer and take it back when the reflexes have been tested.				
8. ✳ Sensory abilities and skin sensations are tested using a safety pin, neurological wheel, and cotton ball and the patient's recognition of simple objects by touch (key, pen, coin). Be ready and alert to provide these items to the physician when necessary.				
9. ✦ The physician will check the cranial nerves by having the patient touch the finger to the nose, touch the heel to the shin, and move the heel down the opposite shin.				

POINT VALUE ✦ = 3–6 points ✳ = 7–9 points		PRACTICE TRIAL	GRADED TRIAL # 1	GRADED TRIAL # 2	NOTES
10. ✦	**Assist the patient off the table if the physician wants to evaluate gait or to have the patient perform the Romberg test successfully.**				
11. ✦	When the neurological exam is completed and the physician is finished, **assist the patient off the examination table and instruct him or her to re-dress. Assist and provide privacy as needed.**				
12. ✦	After the patient leaves the examination room, disinfect the items used during the exam according to office protocol. Then, clean the examination room.				
13. ✦	Perform hand hygiene.				
14. ✳	Document information in the patient's record. The physician will document the results of the neurological examination.				

Document: Enter the appropriate information in the chart below.

Grading

Points Earned	_____		
Points Possible	_____	99	99
Percent Grade (Points Earned/Points Possible)	_____		
PASS:	_____	❏ YES ❏ NO ❏ N/A	❏ YES ❏ NO ❏ N/A

Instructor Sign-Off

Instructor: _____ **Date:** _____

Procedure 38-1:

Instructing a Patient on Breast Self-Examination

Objective: *Instruct the patient how to do breast self-examination.*

Equipment and Supplies: Breast model, if available; pamphlets on breast self-examination

Affective Behaviors: Affective behaviors provide a professional approach to a skill that enhances the patient encounter. These behaviors may also display sensitivity to a patient's rights and enhance communication. Pay close attention to these skills, which will be in **bold, *italicized*** font.

Notes to the Student

_____

_____

_____

_____

_____

_____

Skills Assessment Requirements

Read and familiarize yourself with the procedure; complete the minimum practice requirements (MPRs). Document each MPR using proper charting technique. Complete each procedure within a reasonable amount of time, with a minimum of 85% accuracy.

POINT VALUE ✦ = 3–6 points ✳ = 7–9 points		PRACTICE TRIAL	GRADED TRIAL # 1	GRADED TRIAL # 2	NOTES
1. ✳	Perform hand hygiene.				
2. ✦	Assemble equipment.				
3. ✳	Identify the patient and **explain the necessity for performing the procedure correctly in three different positions each month.** *In the shower:* • Raise the right arm. Use the left hand to examine the right breast, then raise the left arm and use the right hand to examine the left breast. • Using flat fingertips, check breast tissue and underarm tissue, gently feeling for any lump or thickening. Touch every part of the breast when skin is wet; hands will move easily over the softened wet skin. *Before a mirror:* • Inspect the breasts for any irregularity in shape while arms are at the side of the body. Look for swelling, dimpling, or puckering of the skin; lumps; or changes in the nipples, such as retracting. Gently squeeze both nipples and look for discharge. • Raise the arms overhead and look for size, shape, and contour changes in each breast. • With palms resting on hips, flex chest muscles to observe for any obvious differences in breasts. *Note:* The left and right breasts on most females do not match exactly.				

POINT VALUE ✦ = 3–6 points ✳ = 7–9 points		PRACTICE TRIAL	GRADED TRIAL # 1	GRADED TRIAL # 2	NOTES
	Lying down: • To examine the right breast, place a pillow or folded towel behind the right shoulder and place the right hand behind the head. Examine the right breast with the left hand and the left breast with the right hand. • Using the hand with fingers flat, gently press the breast tissue using small circular motions starting at the outermost top of the breast in the 12:00 position and spiraling toward the nipple. An up-and-down motion can also be used, as long as all breast tissue is systematically examined. Cover all the breast tissue, feeling for lumps or any abnormal changes in breast tissue. Gently squeeze the nipple of each breast between the thumb and index finger and note lumps or discharge. • Repeat the procedure for the left breast. *With the arm resting on a firm surface:* • Use the same circular motion to examine the underarm area. (This is breast tissue, too.) Repeat the procedure for both underarm areas.				
4. ✳	Use the breast model to explain the correct application of fingertips. Instruct the patient to report any abnormalities to the physician. This self-examination is not a substitute for periodic examinations by a qualified physician.				

Name: _____

Date: _____

Document: Enter the appropriate information in the chart below.

Grading

Points Earned	_____		
Points Possible	_____	36	36
Percent Grade (Points Earned/Points Possible)	_____		
PASS:	_____	❏ YES ❏ NO ❏ N/A	❏ YES ❏ NO ❏ N/A

Instructor Sign-Off

Instructor: _____ Date: _____

Procedure 38-2:

Assisting with a Pelvic Examination and Pap Test

Objective: Set up and assist with a gynecologic examination, including collection without error of dry or liquid-based prep-method Pap smear.

Equipment and Supplies: Vaginal speculum; water-soluble lubricant; cotton-tipped applicator; patient drape; Pap smear materials: Dry Prep—cervical spatula brush, glass slides, fixative spray or liquid slide holder, identification label; Liquid-Based Prep—plastic cervical spatula, broom or brush, cytology medium transport vial, identification label; laboratory request form; cleansing tissue; gloves; container for contaminated vaginal speculum; gooseneck lamp; biohazard waste container

Affective Behaviors: Affective behaviors provide a professional approach to a skill that enhances the patient encounter. These behaviors may also display sensitivity to a patient's rights and enhance communication. Pay close attention to these skills, which will be in **_bold, italicized_** font.

Notes to the Student

The physician will chart the procedure.

_____

_____

_____

_____

_____

_____

Skills Assessment Requirements

Read and familiarize yourself with the procedure; complete the minimum practice requirements (MPRs). Document each MPR using proper charting technique. Complete each procedure within a reasonable amount of time, with a minimum of 85% accuracy.

Name: _____

Date: _____

POINT VALUE ✦ = 3–6 points ✳ = 7–9 points		PRACTICE TRIAL	GRADED TRIAL #1	GRADED TRIAL #2	NOTES
	For dry prep collection				
1. ✦	Perform hand hygiene.				
2. ✦	Assemble equipment.				
3. ✳	Label the slides and complete the laboratory form.				
4. ✳	**Identify the patient and explain the procedure.**				
5. ✳	**Direct the patient to the restroom to empty her bladder.**				
6. ✦	**Ask the patient to remover her clothing and put on the gown with the opening in front.**				
7. ✳	**Drape the patient appropriately, and assist her into the supine position for breast and abdominal examination.**				
8. ✳	When the physician is ready to collect the Pap specimen, **assist and instruct the patient to assume the dorsal lithotomy position with her buttocks at the edge of the table and her feet in the stirrups. Knees should be relaxed and rotated outward. Expose the genitalia by moving the drape away from this area while it still covers the legs.**				
9. ✦	Adjust the gooseneck lamp and place the physician's stool in the proper position at the end of examination table.				

POINT VALUE ✦ = 3–6 points ✳ = 7–9 points		PRACTICE TRIAL	GRADED TRIAL # 1	GRADED TRIAL # 2	NOTES
10. ✳	Assist the physician with the procedure: • Apply gloves. • Hand gloves and equipment to the physician as needed. Place lubricant onto the speculum as the physician holds it. • Hold the microscopic slides as the physician smears the slides. Mark the slides *C* for cervical, *V* for vaginal, and *E* for endocervical. • Spray fixative from about 6 inches away from the slide. • Place the slide into a container with the appropriate label.				
11. ✳	Hold the receptacle as the physician places the contaminated speculum into it. Set the container into the sink for later cleaning.				
12. ✳	Apply lubricant to the physician's gloved fingers in preparation for the manual examination.				
13. ✦	Properly dispose of gloves in a biohazard waste container and perform proper hygiene.				
14. ✦	Assist the patient to sit up by (a) helping her move back on the table, (b) taking her feet out of the stirrups, and (c) helping her to a sitting position.				
15. ✳	Sanitize and sterilize equipment as needed.				
16. ✳	Perform proper hand hygiene.				
17. ✳	Prepare the Pap specimen to be sent to the laboratory.				

POINT VALUE ♦ = 3–6 points ✳ = 7–9 points		PRACTICE TRIAL	GRADED TRIAL # 1	GRADED TRIAL # 2	NOTES
	For liquid-based prep collection				
18. ✳	Proceed through steps 1–9 above.				
19. ✳	Open the vial of liquid transport medium and hold it so the physician can place both the plastic spatula and either the brush or the broom containing the specimen into the vial.				
20. ✳	Rinse the broom vigorously by pushing it to the bottom of the vial 10 times.				
21. ✳	Use the spatula to scrape cells from the brush, and swirl both the spatula and brush in the vial to mix before removing.				
22. ✳	Label the vial and dispose of hazardous waste appropriately.				
23. ✳	Proceed through steps 1–17 above.				

Document: Enter the appropriate information in the chart below.

Grading

Points Earned	_____		
Points Possible	_____	189	189
Percent Grade (Points Earned/Points Possible)	_____		
PASS:	_____	❏ YES ❏ NO ❏ N/A	❏ YES ❏ NO ❏ N/A

Instructor Sign-Off

Instructor:_____ **Date:** _____

Procedure 38-3:

Instructing a Male Patient How to Perform a Testicular Self-Examination

Objective: Instruct a male patient how to perform a testicular self-examination.

Supplies: Instruction sheet; testicular examination model or illustration

Affective Behaviors: Affective behaviors provide a professional approach to a skill that enhances the patient encounter. These behaviors may also display sensitivity to a patient's rights and enhance communication. Pay close attention to these skills, which will be in **bold, italicized** font.

Notes to the Student

_____

_____

_____

_____

_____

_____

Skills Assessment Requirements

Read and familiarize yourself with the procedure; complete the minimum practice requirements (MPRs). Document each MPR using proper charting technique. Complete each procedure within a reasonable amount of time, with a minimum of 85% accuracy.

Name: _____

Date: _____

POINT VALUE ✦ = 3–6 points ✳ = 7–9 points		PRACTICE TRIAL	GRADED TRIAL # 1	GRADED TRIAL # 2	NOTES
1. ✦	**Identify the patient and introduce yourself.**				
2. ✳	**Explain to the patient that he should perform the examination in the shower or right after a warm shower, which causes the scrotal tissue to relax.**				
3. ✳	**Using the testicular model or illustration, explain that he should place his middle and index fingers underneath the scrotum and thumb on top and use a gentle motion to roll the testes between the fingers. Indicate on the model or illustration the location of the epididymis, the soft tubular cord behind the testis that stores and carries sperm. The patient should know what the epididymis feels like so he does not confuse it with a lump.**				
4. ✳	**Explain that the entire procedure should be repeated on the second testicle.**				
5. ✳	**Encourage the patient to immediately report to his physician any lumps or thickening found during an examination, because early testicular cancer cases have a high cure rate.**				
6. ✳	Document the instruction in the patient's record.				

Document: Enter the appropriate information in the chart below.

Grading

Points Earned	_____		
Points Possible	_____	51	51
Percent Grade (Points Earned/Points Possible)	_____		
PASS:	_____	❏ YES ❏ NO ❏ N/A	❏ YES ❏ NO ❏ N/A

Instructor Sign-Off

Instructor: _____   **Date:** _____

Procedure 39-1:

Testing Visual Acuity Using a Snellen Eye Chart

Objective: Screen a patient for distance acuity using a Snellen eye chart.

Equipment and Supplies: Snellen eye chart placed at a distance of 20 feet; eye shield or occluder; pointer; pen and paper; alcohol and gauze

Affective Behaviors: Affective behaviors provide a professional approach to a skill that enhances the patient encounter. These behaviors may also display sensitivity to a patient's rights and enhance communication. Pay close attention to these skills, which will be in ***bold, italicized*** font.

Notes to the Student

_____

_____

_____

_____

_____

_____

Skills Assessment Requirements

Read and familiarize yourself with the procedure; complete the minimum practice requirements (MPRs). Document each MPR using proper charting technique. Complete each procedure within a reasonable amount of time, with a minimum of 85% accuracy.

Name: _____

Date: _____

POINT VALUE ✦ = 3–6 points ✱ = 7–9 points		PRACTICE TRIAL	GRADED TRIAL # 1	GRADED TRIAL # 2	NOTES
1. ✦	Assemble equipment.				
2. ✦	Review the physician's order.				
3. ✦	Perform hand hygiene and *identify the patient*.				
4. ✱	***Explain the procedure.***				
5. ✱	***Determine the patient's ability to recognize letters.*** If the patient is unable to read letters, use an alternate chart to accommodate the patient's abilities.				
6. ✦	Place the patient 20 feet from the chart, either seated or standing, with Snellen chart at eye level.				
7. ✦	Follow office policy regarding testing with or without corrective lenses.				
8. ✦	Following office policies regarding which eye to test first, have the patient cover the other eye with a cup or occluder. The occluder should be held in such a way so as not to interfere with the normal position of a patient's glasses.				
9. ✦	***Instruct the patient to keep both eyes open even though one eye is covered.*** Have the patient read the lines with both eyes first at a distance of 20 feet.				
10. ✦	Use a pointer and point to letters or appropriate symbols in random order.				

POINT VALUE ✦ = 3–6 points ✱ = 7–9 points		PRACTICE TRIAL	GRADED TRIAL # 1	GRADED TRIAL # 2	NOTES
11. ✱	Starting with the 20/70 line, ask the patient to identify each line and proceed down the chart to the last line the patient can read without error. Observe for signs of squinting or tilting the head, which indicate difficulty identifying letters.				
12. ✱	Record the ratio numbers adjacent to the line the patient can read without error. If there is an error, note it (e.g., "Right eye 20/40—1"; or "Right eye 20/40—1 with correction," meaning glasses were worn during testing). The ISMP recommends using words instead of abbreviations for eye designations to avoid misinterpretation. Follow office protocol regarding charting.				
13. ✱	Repeat the procedure with the other eye and record result, noting any unusual symptoms such as squinting or blinking excessively.				
14. ✦	Clean the occluder with gauze and alcohol.				
15. ✦	Remove gloves. Perform hand hygiene.				
16. ✱	Document results accurately in the patient's chart.				

Name: _____

Date: _____

Document: Enter the appropriate information in the chart below.

Grading

Points Earned	_____		
Points Possible	_____	111	111
Percent Grade (Points Earned/Points Possible)	_____		
PASS:	_____	❑ YES ❑ NO ❑ N/A	❑ YES ❑ NO ❑ N/A

Instructor Sign-Off

Instructor: _____ **Date:** _____

Procedure 39-2:

Screening for Near Vision Acuity

Objective: Screen near vision acuity using the Jaeger system.

Equipment and Supplies: Jaeger near vision acuity chart; paper and pen

Affective Behaviors: Affective behaviors provide a professional approach to a skill that enhances the patient encounter. These behaviors may also display sensitivity to a patient's rights and enhance communication. Pay close attention to these skills, which will be in **_bold, italicized_** font.

Notes to the Student

_____

_____

_____

_____

_____

_____

Skills Assessment Requirements

Read and familiarize yourself with the procedure; complete the minimum practice requirements (MPRs). Document each MPR using proper charting technique. Complete each procedure within a reasonable amount of time, with a minimum of 85% accuracy.

Name: _____

Date: _____

POINT VALUE ✦ = 3–6 points ✱ = 7–9 points		PRACTICE TRIAL	GRADED TRIAL # 1	GRADED TRIAL # 2	NOTES
1. ✦	Perform hand hygiene.				
2. ✦	Review the physician's order.				
3. ✦	Assemble equipment.				
4. ✦	**Identify the patient and introduce yourself.**				
5. ✱	**Explain the procedure.**				
6. ✦	In a well-lit room, have the patient hold the Jaeger card at a distance of 14 to 16 inches.				
7. ✦	**Ask the patient** to read aloud with both eyes open the smallest paragraph or line possible without error.				
8. ✱	Document the results accurately in the patient's record, noting any unusual symptoms, such as squinting.				

Document: Enter the appropriate information in the chart below.

Grading

Points Earned	_____		
Points Possible	_____	54	54
Percent Grade (Points Earned/Points Possible)	_____		
PASS:	_____	❏ YES ❏ NO ❏ N/A	❏ YES ❏ NO ❏ N/A

Instructor Sign-Off

Instructor: _____   **Date:** _____

Procedure 39-3:

Screening for Color Vision Acuity

Objective: Screen a patient for color vision defects.

Equipment and Supplies: Ishihara screening book/cards, paper and pen

Affective Behaviors: Affective behaviors provide a professional approach to a skill that enhances the patient encounter. These behaviors may also display sensitivity to a patient's rights and enhance communication. Pay close attention to these skills, which will be in **_bold, italicized_** font.

Notes to the Student

_____

_____

_____

_____

_____

_____

Skills Assessment Requirements

Read and familiarize yourself with the procedure; complete the minimum practice requirements (MPRs). Document each MPR using proper charting technique. Complete each procedure within a reasonable amount of time, with a minimum of 85% accuracy.

Name: _____

Date: _____

		PRACTICE TRIAL	GRADED TRIAL # 1	GRADED TRIAL # 2	NOTES
POINT VALUE ✦ = 3–6 points ✶ = 7–9 points					
1. ✦	Perform hand hygiene.				
2. ✦	Review the physician's order.				
3. ✦	Assemble equipment.				
4. ✦	***Identify the patient and introduce yourself.***				
5. ✶	***Explain the procedure.***				
6. ✦	Have the patient assume a comfortable position and ask the patient to keep both eyes open.				
7. ✶	In a well-lit room at a distance of 30 inches, ***ask the patient to identify*** the number that is formed by the colored dots on each card or page within 3 seconds per page or card.				
8. ✦	***If the patient is unable to identify the numbers, have the patient trace the numbers with his or her finger.***				
9. ✶	Score each plate as it is read. If the patient is able to identify a number, then record the number seen after the plate number. If the patient is unable to identify a number on the plate, record the plate number and mark an X next to it.				
10. ✶	Note any unusual symptoms.				
11. ✶	Document the results accurately.				

Document: Enter the appropriate information in the chart below.

Grading

Points Earned	_____		
Points Possible	_____	78	78
Percent Grade (Points Earned/Points Possible)	_____		
PASS:	_____	❑ YES ❑ NO ❑ N/A	❑ YES ❑ NO ❑ N/A

Instructor Sign-Off

Instructor: _____ **Date:** _____

Procedure 39-4:

Irrigation of the Eye

Objective: Cleanse or irrigate the eye.

Equipment and Supplies: Nonsterile gloves; sterile basin; emesis basin; sterile solution; sterile irrigating syringe; sterile gauze; towel; tissues; pen and patient's chart

Affective Behaviors: Affective behaviors provide a professional approach to a skill that enhances the patient encounter. These behaviors may also display sensitivity to a patient's rights and enhance communication. Pay close attention to these skills, which will be in **_bold, italicized_** font.

Notes to the Student

_____

_____

_____

_____

_____

_____

Skills Assessment Requirements

Read and familiarize yourself with the procedure; complete the minimum practice requirements (MPRs). Document each MPR using proper charting technique. Complete each procedure within a reasonable amount of time, with a minimum of 85% accuracy.

POINT VALUE ✦ = 3–6 points ✷ = 7–9 points		PRACTICE TRIAL	GRADED TRIAL # 1	GRADED TRIAL # 2	NOTES
1. ✷	*Identify the patient and explain the procedure.*				
2. ✦	Review the physician's order.				
3. ✦	Assemble the equipment: Check the label of the irrigating solution three times to ensure it is the correct solution and concentration ordered by the physician. Check the expiration date on the label to make sure the solution has not expired. The solution should be brought to room temperature by wrapping the bottle in a dry heating pad or standing the bottle in a warm water bath.				
4. ✦	Perform hand hygiene and apply gloves.				
5. ✦	*Ask the patient which position he or she would prefer, sitting or lying down.*				
6. ✦	*Place a towel over the patient's shoulder.* If both eyes are to be irrigated, then two separate sets of equipment must be used to prevent cross-infection.				
7. ✦	Open the irrigating solution and fill the syringe.				
8. ✦	*Ask the patient to tilt the head to the affected side if seated, and hold the basin.*				
9. ✷	Open the patient's eye using the index finger and thumb of the nondominant hand.				
10. ✷	Hold a tissue on the patient's cheekbone below the lower lid and pull down and expose the conjunctiva.				

POINT VALUE ✦ = 3–6 points ✸ = 7–9 points		PRACTICE TRIAL	GRADED TRIAL #1	GRADED TRIAL #2	NOTES
11. ✸	Hold the syringe ½ inch from the eye.				
12. ✸	Gently irrigate from inner to outer canthus (corner of eye), aiming at the lower conjunctiva.				
13. ✸	Continue irrigating until the solution is used up.				
14. ✦	Dry the area around the eye with sterile gauze.				
15. ✦	Dispose of the equipment properly.				
16. ✦	Perform hand hygiene.				
17. ✦	Document information in the patient's chart in the appropriate manner.				

Name: _____

Date: _____

Document: Enter the appropriate information in the chart below.

Grading

Points Earned	_____		
Points Possible	_____	117	117
Percent Grade (Points Earned/Points Possible)	_____		
PASS:	_____	❏ YES ❏ NO ❏ N/A	❏ YES ❏ NO ❏ N/A

Instructor Sign-Off

Instructor: _____ **Date:** _____

Procedure 39-5:

Instilling Eye Medication

Objective: Instill eye medication following a physician's order.

Equipment and Supplies: Sterile medication; sterile eyedropper (if needed); tissues; sterile gauze squares; nonsterile gloves; drape or towel

Affective Behaviors: Affective behaviors provide a professional approach to a skill that enhances the patient encounter. These behaviors may also display sensitivity to a patient's rights and enhance communication. Pay close attention to these skills, which will be in **_bold, italicized_** font.

Notes to the Student

_____

_____

_____

_____

_____

_____

Skills Assessment Requirements

Read and familiarize yourself with the procedure; complete the minimum practice requirements (MPRs). Document each MPR using proper charting technique. Complete each procedure within a reasonable amount of time, with a minimum of 85% accuracy.

Name: _____

Date: _____

POINT VALUE ✦ = 3–6 points ✳ = 7–9 points	PRACTICE TRIAL	GRADED TRIAL # 1	GRADED TRIAL # 2	NOTES
1. ✦ Perform hand hygiene.				
2. ✦ Check the physician's order.				
3. ✳ **Identify the patient, introduce yourself, and explain the procedure.**				
4. ✳ Check the name of the medication, expiration date, and concentration three times.				
5. ✳ **Ask the patient if he or she has any known allergies to the medication.**				
6. ✦ Give the patient a tissue to blot cheeks.				
7. ✦ Put on gloves.				
8. ✦ Position the patient with the head tilted back and looking upward.				
9. ✳ Pull down the lower eyelid, exposing the conjunctiva.				
10. ✳ Place the dropper about ½ inch above the eyeball with the dominant hand. Insert the proper amount of drops to the center of the conjunctiva, or if ointment is used, apply as a thin strip from inner to outer canthus.				
11. ✳ Do not touch the dropper or ointment tube to the eye.				
12. ✦ **Ask the patient to gently close the eye and rotate the eyeball.**				
13. ✳ Remove excess medication from the inner canthus to the outer canthus using sterile gauze.				

Name: _____

Date: _____

POINT VALUE ✦ = 3–6 points ✳ = 7–9 points		PRACTICE TRIAL	GRADED TRIAL # 1	GRADED TRIAL # 2	NOTES
14. ✦	**Explain to the patient that his or her vision may be blurry.**				
15. ✦	Cleanse the area and dispose of unused medication.				
16. ✦	Remove gloves and perform hand hygiene.				
17. ✳	Document procedure appropriately.				

Document: Enter the appropriate information in the chart below.

Grading

Points Earned	_____		
Points Possible	_____	127	127
Percent Grade (Points Earned/Points Possible)	_____		
PASS:	_____	❏ YES ❏ NO ❏ N/A	❏ YES ❏ NO ❏ N/A

Instructor Sign-Off

Instructor: _____ **Date:** _____

Procedure 39-6:

Irrigation of the Ear

Objective: Irrigate ear following the physician's order.

Equipment and Supplies: Gloves; ear syringe; sterile basin; emesis basin; warm irrigation solution per physician's order; towels; cotton balls

Affective Behaviors: Affective behaviors provide a professional approach to a skill that enhances the patient encounter. These behaviors may also display sensitivity to a patient's rights and enhance communication. Pay close attention to these skills, which will be in **bold, *italicized*** font.

Notes to the Student

_____

_____

_____

_____

_____

_____

Skills Assessment Requirements

Read and familiarize yourself with the procedure; complete the minimum practice requirements (MPRs). Document each MPR using proper charting technique. Complete each procedure within a reasonable amount of time, with a minimum of 85% accuracy.

Name: _____

Date: _____

POINT VALUE ✦ = 3–6 points ✷ = 7–9 points		PRACTICE TRIAL	GRADED TRIAL #1	GRADED TRIAL #2	NOTES
1. ✦	Check the physician's order.				
2. ✦	Perform hand hygiene.				
3. ✦	Assemble the equipment.				
4. ✷	Check the name, concentration, and expiration date of the solution three times.				
5. ✷	***Identify the patient and explain the procedure.***				
6. ✦	Apply gloves.				
7. ✦	Have the patient sit with the affected ear tilted slightly downward.				
8. ✦	Place a towel over the patient's shoulder and ask the patient to hold the emesis basin.				
9. ✷	Clean the external ear canal with a moistened cotton ball, if necessary.				
10. ✷	Pour warmed solution into a sterile basin and fill the syringe with 50 cc of solution.				
11. ✷	For adults, pull the earlobe up and back to straighten the ear canal; for children under 3 years, pull the earlobe down and back to straighten the ear canal.				
12. ✷	Expel air from the syringe and insert the tip into the ear canal. Aim the stream of flow toward the roof of the canal.				
13. ✷	Repeat until the return from the ear canal is clear.				
14. ✦	Remove basin, dry outer ear, and remove towel.				
15. ✦	Give the patient cotton balls to wipe any external drainage.				

POINT VALUE ✦ = 3–6 points ✳ = 7–9 points		PRACTICE TRIAL	GRADED TRIAL # 1	GRADED TRIAL # 2	NOTES
16. ✳	**_Instruct the patient about home care, if needed. Ask the patient if he or she has any questions._**				
17. ✦	Dispose of waste material properly.				
18. ✦	Perform hand hygiene.				
19. ✳	Document the procedure, noting the type of drainage and any patient symptoms such as pain or dizziness.				

Name: _____

Date: _____

Document: Enter the appropriate information in the chart below.

Grading

Points Earned	_____		
Points Possible	_____	138	138
Percent Grade (Points Earned/Points Possible)	_____		
PASS:	_____	❏ YES ❏ NO ❏ N/A	❏ YES ❏ NO ❏ N/A

Instructor Sign-Off

Instructor: _____ **Date:** _____

Procedure 39-7:

Instilling Ear Medication

Objective: Instill ear medication as ordered by physician.

Equipment and Supplies: Otic drops in dropper bottle; cotton balls; disposable gloves

Affective Behaviors: Affective behaviors provide a professional approach to a skill that enhances the patient encounter. These behaviors may also display sensitivity to a patient's rights and enhance communication. Pay close attention to these skills, which will be in **_bold, italicized_** font.

Notes to the Student

_____

_____

_____

_____

_____

Skills Assessment Requirements

Read and familiarize yourself with the procedure; complete the minimum practice requirements (MPRs). Document each MPR using proper charting technique. Complete each procedure within a reasonable amount of time, with a minimum of 85% accuracy.

POINT VALUE ✦ = 3–6 points ✳ = 7–9 points		PRACTICE TRIAL	GRADED TRIAL # 1	GRADED TRIAL # 2	NOTES
1. ✦	Check the physician's order.				
2. ✦	Perform hand hygiene.				
3. ✦	Assemble the equipment.				
4. ✦	*Identify the patient.*				
5. ✳	Check the medication label three times for the name, concentration, and expiration date.				
6. ✦	If the medication is cold, warm it by rolling the bottle between the palms.				
7. ✳	*Have the patient sit or lie down with the affected ear tilted facing up.*				
8. ✳	Pull the earlobe down and back for a child, and up and back for an adult.				
9. ✳	Place the dropper in the ear canal; avoid touching the sides of the ear canal.				
10. ✳	Instill the appropriate number of drops along the sides of the ear canal.				
11. ✦	*Instruct the patient to remain in the same position for 3–5 minutes.*				
12. ✳	*Give instructions for home care if needed. Ask the patient if he or she has any questions.*				
13. ✦	Dispose of equipment and clean the area.				
14. ✦	Perform hand hygiene.				
15. ✳	Document the procedure appropriately.				

Name: _____

Date: _____

Document: Enter the appropriate information in the chart below.

Grading

Points Earned	_____		
Points Possible	_____	108	108
Percent Grade (Points Earned/Points Possible)	_____		
PASS:	_____	❏ YES ❏ NO ❏ N/A	❏ YES ❏ NO ❏ N/A

Instructor Sign-Off

Instructor: _____ **Date:** _____

Procedure 39-8:

Assisting with Audiometry

Objective: Perform audiometric test without error.

Equipment and Supplies: Audiometer with headphones; quiet room or small, enclosed cubicle; patient's record; pen

Affective Behaviors: Affective behaviors provide a professional approach to a skill that enhances the patient encounter. These behaviors may also display sensitivity to a patient's rights and enhance communication. Pay close attention to these skills, which will be in **_bold, italicized_** font.

Notes to the Student

_____

_____

_____

_____

_____

_____

Skills Assessment Requirements

Read and familiarize yourself with the procedure; complete the minimum practice requirements (MPRs). Document each MPR using proper charting technique. Complete each procedure within a reasonable amount of time, with a minimum of 85% accuracy.

POINT VALUE ✦ = 3–6 points ✳ = 7–9 points		PRACTICE TRIAL	GRADED TRIAL # 1	GRADED TRIAL # 2	NOTES
1. ✦	Check physician's orders.				
2. ✦	Perform hand hygiene.				
3. ✦	Prepare the equipment.				
4. ✳	Test the equipment and be sure that power is on.				
5. ✳	***Identify the patient and explain the procedure.***				
6. ✦	Establish the signal response the patient will give if no automatic button is available. Nodding the head or holding up a hand are common signals.				
7. ✦	***Have the patient assume a comfortable position.***				
8. ✦	Place headphones over the patient's ears.				
9. ✳	Begin with low frequency and watch the patient for indication that the sound is heard; push the button to record if the machine does not do it automatically.				
10. ✳	Gradually increase frequency until the test is completed in the first ear.				
11. ✳	Proceed to the other ear and repeat the entire procedure.				
12. ✦	Remove the headphones.				
13. ✦	Clean the equipment following the manufacturer's instructions.				
14. ✦	Perform hand hygiene.				
15. ✳	Document the procedure appropriately.				

Name: _____

Date: _____

Document: Enter the appropriate information in the chart below.

Grading

Points Earned	_____		
Points Possible	_____	108	108
Percent Grade (Points Earned/Points Possible)	_____		
PASS:	_____	❑ YES ❑ NO ❑ N/A	❑ YES ❑ NO ❑ N/A

Instructor Sign-Off

Instructor: _____   **Date:** _____

Procedure 39-9:

Instilling Nasal Medications

Objective: Instill nasal medication as ordered by the physician.

Equipment and Supplies: Physician's order; patient's record; nasal medication; sterile medicine dropper; tissues; gloves

Affective Behaviors: Affective behaviors provide a professional approach to a skill that enhances the patient encounter. These behaviors may also display sensitivity to a patient's rights and enhance communication. Pay close attention to these skills, which will be in **_bold, italicized_** font.

Notes to the Student

_____

_____

_____

_____

_____

_____

Skills Assessment Requirements

Read and familiarize yourself with the procedure; complete the minimum practice requirements (MPRs). Document each MPR using proper charting technique. Complete each procedure within a reasonable amount of time, with a minimum of 85% accuracy.

POINT VALUE ✦ = 3–6 points ✳ = 7–9 points		PRACTICE TRIAL	GRADED TRIAL # 1	GRADED TRIAL # 2	NOTES
1. ✦	Check physician's orders.				
2. ✦	Perform hand hygiene.				
3. ✦	Assemble the equipment.				
4. ✳	***Identify the patient and explain the procedure.***				
5. ✳	Position the patient with head lower than the shoulders to instill medication into the ethmoid and sphenoid sinuses. To instill medication into the maxillary and frontal sinuses, have the patient assume the same back-lying position with the head turned toward the side to be treated. Place patient in a supine position with a pillow under the neck to lower the head below the shoulders. Make the patient as comfortable as possible.				
6. ✳	Check the medication three times for correct name, dosage, and expiration date. Draw the medication into a dropper and hold it over the center of the affected nostril, taking care not to touch the dropper to the inside of the nostril.				
7. ✳	Administer the medication. Repeat in the other nostril if ordered.				
8. ✳	Tell the patient to stay in that position for 5 minutes to prevent medication from running out of the nostril.				
9. ✦	***Provide tissues for the patient to use to wipe excess from the skin.***				

POINT VALUE ✦ = 3–6 points ✳ = 7–9 points		PRACTICE TRIAL	GRADED TRIAL # 1	GRADED TRIAL # 2	NOTES
10. ✦	Discard the dropper in the biohazard waste container, recap the medication, and return it to the storage place.				
11. ✦	Clean the area and remove gloves.				
12. ✳	**Provide home instruction, if needed. Ask the patient if he or she has any questions.**				
13. ✦	Perform proper hand hygiene.				
14. ✳	Document the procedure in the patient's record.				

Document: Enter the appropriate information in the chart below.

Grading

Points Earned	_____		
Points Possible	_____	111	111
Percent Grade (Points Earned/Points Possible)	_____		
PASS:	_____	❏ YES ❏ NO ❏ N/A	❏ YES ❏ NO ❏ N/A

Instructor Sign-Off

Instructor: _____ **Date:** _____

Procedure 40-1:

Wrapping an Infant or Small Child

Objective: Wrap an infant or small child securely to restrain movement.

Equipment and Supplies: Small sheet or receiving blanket; examination table; patient's medical record; pen

Affective Behaviors: Affective behaviors provide a professional approach to a skill that enhances the patient encounter. These behaviors may also display sensitivity to a patient's rights and enhance communication. Pay close attention to these skills, which will be in **_bold, italicized_** font.

Notes to the Student

Size of sheet or blanket depends on age and size of child. Be sure to choose the appropriate size.

_____

_____

_____

_____

_____

Skills Assessment Requirements

Read and familiarize yourself with the procedure; complete the minimum practice requirements (MPRs). Document each MPR using proper charting technique. Complete each procedure within a reasonable amount of time, with a minimum of 85% accuracy.

POINT VALUE ✦ = 3–6 points ✶ = 7–9 points		PRACTICE TRIAL	GRADED TRIAL # 1	GRADED TRIAL # 2	NOTES
1. ✦	**Greet and warmly introduce yourself to both the parent and the child.**				
2. ✶	**Ask the patient's parent or guardian to verify the patient's name and date of birth.**				
3. ✦	**Speak to the infant in soft, soothing tones. Explain to the parent or guardian that you will be wrapping the infant, which is often helpful during the examination process.**				
4. ✦	Perform hand hygiene.				
5. ✦	Place a receiving blanket or small sheet on the table. Fold down the top corner. a. Fold the bottom corner up if the physician prefers the infant's feet to be free from the wrapping. Otherwise, do not fold up the bottom corner. b. If necessary, have the parent or guardian undress the infant. Provide assistance to the parent/guardian as necessary.				
6. ✶	Place the child on the blanket so the folded-down top corner is behind the neck. Ensure safety by keeping one hand on the infant's abdomen.				
7. ✦	Wrap the right corner across the torso, covering the right arm, and tuck snugly under the left arm.				

POINT VALUE ✦ = 3–6 points ✳ = 7–9 points		PRACTICE TRIAL	GRADED TRIAL #1	GRADED TRIAL #2	NOTES
8. ✦	Wrap the left corner across the torso, covering the left arm, and tuck snugly under the torso.				
9. ✳	Throughout the procedure, speak soothingly to comfort the infant and allay fears as much as possible. Many infants like being swaddled and are calmed by it.				
10. ✳	When the physician has completed the examination or other procedure, pick up and comfort the infant for a few moments. **Direct the parent/ guardian to re-dress the infant and provide assistance as necessary.**				
11. ✦	Perform hand hygiene.				

Document: Enter the appropriate information in the chart below.

Grading

Points Earned			
Points Possible	_____	78	78
Percent Grade (Points Earned/Points Possible)	_____		
PASS:	_____	❏ YES ❏ NO ❏ N/A	❏ YES ❏ NO ❏ N/A

Instructor Sign-Off

Instructor: _____   **Date:** _____

Procedure 40-2:

Measuring Pediatric Vital Signs

Objective: Perform all steps of obtaining pediatric vital signs and provide accurate readings according to the instructor's guidelines.

Equipment and Supplies: Gloves; tympanic thermometer; electronic thermometer with blue and red probes; watch with second hand; pediatric stethoscope; pediatric blood pressure cuff; patient's medical record

Affective Behaviors: Affective behaviors provide a professional approach to a skill that enhances the patient encounter. These behaviors may also display sensitivity to a patient's rights and enhance communication. Pay close attention to these skills, which will be in **_bold, italicized_** font.

Notes to the Student

_____

_____

_____

_____

_____

_____

Skills Assessment Requirements

Read and familiarize yourself with the procedure; complete the minimum practice requirements (MPRs). Document each MPR using proper charting technique. Complete each procedure within a reasonable amount of time, with a minimum of 85% accuracy.

POINT VALUE ✦ = 3–6 points ✱ = 7–9 points	PRACTICE TRIAL	GRADED TRIAL # 1	GRADED TRIAL # 2	NOTES
1. ✦ Gather the appropriate equipment.				
2. ✦ **Warmly greet and ask the parent or guardian to identify the patient, introduce yourself, and explain the procedures to the parent.**				
3. ✱ **Speak calmly and reassuringly to the child, which will help to gain trust and establish rapport with the child.**				
4. ✱ Perform hand hygiene.				
5. ✦ Explain to the parent or guardian how he or she can assist you in holding the infant patient.				
Obtaining Temperature with Tympanic Thermometer				
1. ✦ Remove the thermometer from the base and note that it reads "Ready."				
2. ✦ Attach the disposable probe cover to the earpiece.				
3. ✦ **Gently pull the patient's earlobe downward and out to straighten the ear canal.**				
4. ✦ Insert the probe into the ear canal.				
5. ✦ Press the scan button.				
6. ✦ Observe the temperature reading.				
7. ✦ Gently withdraw the thermometer and eject the probe cover into a biohazard waste container.				
8. ✱ Record the temperature reading using "T" to indicate the temperature reading was obtained via the tympanic membrane route.				
9. ✦ Return the thermometer to the charging base.				

POINT VALUE ✦ = 3–6 points ✳ = 7–9 points	PRACTICE TRIAL	GRADED TRIAL # 1	GRADED TRIAL # 2	NOTES
Obtaining Temperature Reading Using Axillary Method				
1. ✦ Remove the electronic thermometer from the charging base and attach the blue probe, which can be used for oral and axillary temperatures.				
2. ✦ Attach a disposable probe cover and make sure that the thermometer is turned on and ready to take a temperature.				
3. ✳ Place the thermometer in the infant's armpit, and hold the infant's arm across the chest, causing a tight seal in the axillary region. Hold this position until the thermometer beeps, indicating the temperature has been successfully obtained.				
4. ✳ Read the thermometer, then record the reading with "AX" to indicate that the axillary method was used.				
5. ✦ Dispose of the probe cover in a waste container and return the electronic thermometer unit to the charging base.				
Obtaining Temperature Reading Rectally by Using a Digital Thermometer with Red Probe (Rectal Use)				
1. ✦ Remove the electronic digital thermometer from the charging base and attach the red probe, used for obtaining rectal body temperatures.				
2. ✦ Perform hand hygiene and don gloves.				
3. ✦ Attach the disposable probe cover.				
4. ✦ Lubricate the tip of the thermometer to assist with insertion of the tip into the rectum.				

POINT VALUE ✦ = 3–6 points ✶ = 7–9 points		PRACTICE TRIAL	GRADED TRIAL # 1	GRADED TRIAL # 2	NOTES
5. ✶	Place the infant in the supine position and pull the feet up to expose the rectal area.				
6. ✶	Insert the thermometer ¼ inch into the rectum and hold in place with hand to prevent expelling.				
7. ✶	Hold the infant securely to restrict movement and maintain the thermometer's position until the beeping sound indicates the body temperature has been obtained. a. Make a mental note of the patient's body temperature after the thermometer beeps. You will record this number after a few additional steps have been completed.				
8. ✦	Gently remove thermometer and wipe off excessive lubricant from the infant's rectum.				
9. ✶	Dispose of the probe cover into a waste container. Remove and discard gloves. Perform hand hygiene.				
10. ✶	Record the reading in the patient's medical record using "R" to indicate the rectal method used.				
Measuring Heart Rate/Pulse by Apical Measurement					
1. ✶	Place the stethoscope on the child's chest at the midpoint between the sternum and the left nipple.				
2. ✦	Listen for the "lub-dub" of the apical pulse.				
3. ✦	Count the apical pulse for one full minute. Each lub-dub represents one complete beat.				

Name: _____

Date: _____

POINT VALUE ✦ = 3–6 points ✱ = 7–9 points		PRACTICE TRIAL	GRADED TRIAL # 1	GRADED TRIAL # 2	NOTES
4. ✱	Record the apical pulse using "AP" before the pulse measurement to indicate the apical reading was obtained.				
	Measuring Infant Respirations for One Full Minute				
1. ✦	Following the count of the apical pulse, remove the stethoscope from your ears.				
2. ✦	With the infant in the same position, place your hand gently on the child's chest.				
3. ✱	One complete respiration includes the rise and fall of the chest. Count respirations for one full minute.				
4. ✱	Record the in the patient's medical record.				
	Measuring the Infant's Blood Pressure Using a Pediatric Cuff and Stethoscope as Follows				
1. ✦	Obtain a blood pressure (BP) reading on the child if the patient is aged 5 or older, or if the physician indicates that a BP measurement should be obtained.				
2. ✦	Choose the correct-size cuff and wrap it securely around the upper arm, above the antecubital space.				
3. ✱	Feel for the brachial pulse.				
4. ✦	Place the stethoscope earpieces in your ears and place the diaphragm or bell (whichever allows you to hear the best) of the stethoscope near the brachial pulse.				
5. ✱	Tighten the valve of the pump and inflate the cuff until the pulse is no longer heard.				
6. ✱	Release the valve slowly, listening for systolic and diastolic sounds.				
7. ✱	Record the results.				

Document: Enter the appropriate information in the chart below.

Grading

Points Earned	_____		
Points Possible	_____	318	318
Percent Grade (Points Earned/Points Possible)	_____		
PASS:	_____	❏ YES ❏ NO ❏ N/A	❏ YES ❏ NO ❏ N/A

Instructor Sign-Off

Instructor: _____   **Date:** _____

Procedure 40-3:

Measuring the Weight and Length of an Infant

Objective: Safely and accurately obtain the weight and length (height) of an infant.

Equipment and Supplies: Baby scale; patient's medical record; pen; small towel or protector for scale; tape measure

Affective Behaviors: Affective behaviors provide a professional approach to a skill that enhances the patient encounter. These behaviors may also display sensitivity to a patient's rights and enhance communication. Pay close attention to these skills, which will be in **bold, *italicized*** font.

Notes to the Student

_____

_____

_____

_____

_____

_____

Skills Assessment Requirements

Read and familiarize yourself with the procedure; complete the minimum practice requirements (MPRs). Document each MPR using proper charting technique. Complete each procedure within a reasonable amount of time, with a minimum of 85% accuracy.

POINT VALUE ✦ = 3–6 points ✳ = 7–9 points		PRACTICE TRIAL	GRADED TRIAL # 1	GRADED TRIAL # 2	NOTES
	Measure Weight				
1. ✳	***Warmly greet the parent/ guardian and patient. Introduce yourself and ask the parent/ guardian to verify the patient's full name and date of birth.*** a. Have the infant remain with the parent or caregiver while you prepare the equipment and explain the procedure.				
2. ✦	Perform hand hygiene.				
3. ✦	Place a towel or paper protector on the baby scale.				
4. ✳	Balance the scale by placing all the weights to the far left side. Turn the bolt at the right edge of the scale until the balance bar pointer is at the middle of the balance bar.				
5. ✦	***Ask the parent to undress the infant, and provide assistance if necessary.*** Unless office protocol is different, remove the diaper to obtain the most accurate weight.				
6. ✳	Gently lay the infant on the scale. Always use one hand to guard the infant until the weights are adjusted.				
7. ✳	Inform the caregiver that the infant can be diapered. Keep the weights in place and remain with the infant, with a protective hand guarding, until the caregiver picks up the infant for diapering.				
8. ✳	When the infant has been removed from the scale, document the weight in the patient's medical record. Return the scale weights to the zero point, or turn off the electronic scale.				

Name: _____

Date: _____

POINT VALUE ✦ = 3–6 points ✴ = 7–9 points		PRACTICE TRIAL	GRADED TRIAL # 1	GRADED TRIAL # 2	NOTES
	Continue with Length				
9. ✴	Gently place the infant on the papered examination table. It is best, and preferred, to have two people cooperate to measure the length of an infant. The parent or caregiver can assist by holding the infant's head still.				
10. ✦	Make pencil marks on the examination table paper at the top of the child's head and at the bottom of the feet at the heels. When the child is removed, measure the area between the two marks. OR, holding the tape measure with one hand, place the tape at the top of the side of the infant's head. Stretch the infant out full length as you pull the tape measure down to the bottom of the feet. a. If you are using a table with a measure bar, place the infant's head at one end of the table with the soles of his or her feet touching the footboard so that the toes are pointing toward the ceiling.				
11. ✴	Note the infant's length in inches and fractions of an inch, and write it on the paper covering the exam table or on a scrap piece of paper so that it is not forgotten while the infant is tended to.				

Name: _____

Date: _____

Document: Enter the appropriate information in the chart below.

Grading

Points Earned	_____		
Points Possible	_____	75	75
Percent Grade (Points Earned/Points Possible)	_____		
PASS:	_____	❏ YES ❏ NO ❏ N/A	❏ YES ❏ NO ❏ N/A

Instructor Sign-Off

Instructor: _____ Date: _____

Procedure 40-4:

Measuring the Head Circumference of an Infant or Small Child

Objective: Obtain an accurate measurement of the head circumference of an infant or small child.

Equipment and Supplies: Flexible tape measure (no elasticity); patient's medical record, pen, growth chart (if an electronic medical record is not being used)

Affective Behaviors: Affective behaviors provide a professional approach to a skill that enhances the patient encounter. These behaviors may also display sensitivity to a patient's rights and enhance communication. Pay close attention to these skills, which will be in **_bold, italicized_** font.

Notes to the Student

_____

_____

_____

_____

_____

_____

Skills Assessment Requirements

Read and familiarize yourself with the procedure; complete the minimum practice requirements (MPRs). Document each MPR using proper charting technique. Complete each procedure within a reasonable amount of time, with a minimum of 85% accuracy.

Name: _____

Date: _____

POINT VALUE ✦ = 3–6 points ✳ = 7–9 points		PRACTICE TRIAL	GRADED TRIAL # 1	GRADED TRIAL # 2	NOTES
1. ✦	*Warmly greet the parent/caregiver and patient. Ask the parent/caregiver to identify the patient's full name and date of birth.*				
2. ✳	*Smile and speak gently to the infant or child to establish a positive rapport.*				
3. ✦	*Explain the procedure to the parent/caregiver and the small child.*				
4. ✦	Perform hand hygiene.				
5. ✦	Position the infant on the examination table or have the caregiver hold the infant. If measuring a small child, ask him or her to "please sit nice and tall and look straight ahead."				
6. ✳	Hold the end of tape (0 inches) on the forehead over the patient's eyebrows. Bring the tape around the head and above the ears to meet in front.				
7. ✦	Measure with accuracy to the nearest fraction of an inch or centimeter. a. If there is any doubt about the measurement, repeat the procedure.				
8. ✦	*Thank the small child for helping*, or inform the parent/caregiver of an infant that the child may now be held.				
9. ✦	Document the measurement in the patient's medical record, and (if necessary) record it on the growth chart.				
10. ✦	Perform hand hygiene.				

Document: Enter the appropriate information in the chart below.

Grading

Points Earned	_____		
Points Possible	_____	63	63
Percent Grade (Points Earned/Points Possible)	_____		
PASS:	_____	❏ YES ❏ NO ❏ N/A	❏ YES ❏ NO ❏ N/A

Instructor Sign-Off

Instructor: _____ **Date:** _____

Procedure 40-5:

Measuring the Chest Circumference of a Child

Objective: Accurately measure the circumference of a child's chest.

Equipment and Supplies: Non-elastic tape measure; examination table; patient's medical record; pen

Affective Behaviors: Affective behaviors provide a professional approach to a skill that enhances the patient encounter. These behaviors may also display sensitivity to a patient's rights and enhance communication. Pay close attention to these skills, which will be in **_bold, italicized_** font.

Notes to the Student

_____

_____

_____

_____

_____

Skills Assessment Requirements

Read and familiarize yourself with the procedure; complete the minimum practice requirements (MPRs). Document each MPR using proper charting technique. Complete each procedure within a reasonable amount of time, with a minimum of 85% accuracy.

Name: _____

Date: _____

POINT VALUE ✦ = 3–6 points ✱ = 7–9 points		PRACTICE TRIAL	GRADED TRIAL # 1	GRADED TRIAL # 2	NOTES
1. ✦	*Warmly greet the parent/ caregiver and patient. Ask the parent/caregiver to identify the patient's full name and date of birth.*				
2. ✱	*Talk to the patient soothingly to gain trust and establish a positive rapport.*				
3. ✦	Perform hand hygiene.				
4. ✦	Position the child on the examination table in a supine position. If the child is over 2 years of age, he or she may sit upright on the table for this procedure.				
5. ✱	Place the end of the tape (0) in the center of the child's chest in line with the child's nipples and slip the tape under the child's body and under the armpits. Bring it completely around to meet the other end of the tape.				
6. ✱	Take a measurement in centimeters to the nearest 0.01 of a centimeter or to the nearest ½ inch.				
7. ✦	Return the child to the parent/ caregiver's care before recording the results.				
8. ✱	Perform hand hygiene after the measurement has been documented.				

Name: _____

Date: _____

Document: Enter the appropriate information in the chart below.

Grading

Points Earned	_____		
Points Possible	_____	48	48
Percent Grade (Points Earned/Points Possible)	_____		
PASS:	_____	❏ YES ❏ NO ❏ N/A	❏ YES ❏ NO ❏ N/A

Instructor Sign-Off

Instructor: _____ **Date:** _____

Name: _____

Date: _____

Procedure 40-6:

Calculating Growth Percentiles

Objective: To plot the age, weight, and height of a patient and obtain correct percentiles.

Equipment and Supplies: Patient's record with weight and height values; pen; growth chart; ruler or straight edge

Affective Behaviors: Affective behaviors provide a professional approach to a skill that enhances the patient encounter. These behaviors may also display sensitivity to a patient's rights and enhance communication. Pay close attention to these skills, which will be in **bold, italicized** font.

Notes to the Student

_____

_____

_____

_____

_____

_____

Skills Assessment Requirements

Read and familiarize yourself with the procedure; complete the minimum practice requirements (MPRs). Document each MPR using proper charting technique. Complete each procedure within a reasonable amount of time, with a minimum of 85% accuracy.

Name: _____

Date: _____

POINT VALUE ✦ = 3–6 points ✳ = 7–9 points		PRACTICE TRIAL	GRADED TRIAL # 1	GRADED TRIAL # 2	NOTES
1. ✦	Select the proper growth chart for the patient, based on age and gender.				
2. ✳	Assume the patient is a female aged 18 months. Locate the child's age in the horizontal axis at the bottom of the chart. Draw an imaginary vertical line on the chart, using a ruler or straight edge.				
3. ✳	Assume the patient's length is 33". Draw an imaginary horizontal line on the chart that intersects with the patient's age (it should intersect at the straight edge of the ruler).				
4. ✳	Find the point at which the two imaginary lines intersect on the graph, and then place a dot there.				
5. ✳	Assume the patient's weight is 27.5 lb. Draw an imaginary horizontal line on the chart that intersects with the patient's age (it should intersect at the straight edge of the ruler).				
6. ✳	Find the point at which the two imaginary lines intersect on the graph, and then place a dot there.				
7. ✳	Follow the curved line closest to the dot upward, and then read the percentile located on the right side of the chart.				
8. ✳	If the dot you placed falls between two curved lines, interpolate or estimate the percentile that falls between the two closest percentile lines.				

Name: _____

Date: _____

Document: Enter the appropriate information in the chart below.

Grading

Points Earned	_____		
Points Possible	_____	78	78
Percent Grade (Points Earned/Points Possible)	_____		
PASS:	_____	❏ YES ❏ NO ❏ N/A	❏ YES ❏ NO ❏ N/A

Instructor Sign-Off

Instructor: _____   **Date:** _____

Name: _____

Date: _____

Procedure 40-7:

Applying a Pediatric Urine Collection Device

Objective: Properly apply a urinary collection device.

Equipment and Supplies: Pediatric urine collection bag; laboratory specimen container with label; antiseptic wipes; gloves; biohazard waste container; patient's medical record

Affective Behaviors: Affective behaviors provide a professional approach to a skill that enhances the patient encounter. These behaviors may also display sensitivity to a patient's rights and enhance communication. Pay close attention to these skills, which will be in ***bold, italicized*** font.

Notes to the Student

_____

_____

_____

_____

_____

_____

Skills Assessment Requirements

Read and familiarize yourself with the procedure; complete the minimum practice requirements (MPRs). Document each MPR using proper charting technique. Complete each procedure within a reasonable amount of time, with a minimum of 85% accuracy.

Name: _____

Date: _____

POINT VALUE ✦ = 3–6 points ✶ = 7–9 points	PRACTICE TRIAL	GRADED TRIAL # 1	GRADED TRIAL # 2	NOTES
1. ✦ Assemble all equipment and label the laboratory specimen container with the patient's name, date of birth, and today's date.				
2. ✦ ***Warmly greet and introduce yourself to the patient and the parent/caregiver. Ask the caregiver to verify the patient's full name and date of birth, and explain the procedure to the caregiver.***				
3. ✦ Perform hand hygiene and don gloves.				
4. ✦ ***Ask the parent or caregiver to place the infant on the examination table in a supine position, and then remove the diaper.***				
5. ✶ Gently cleanse the genitalia (reproductive organ) area with antiseptic wipes. Explain the importance of this delicate step to the caregiver, indicating that the lack of or improper cleansing could cause the test results to be compromised. Male: Cleanse the urinary meatus (urinary tract opening) with a circular motion, starting at the opening and progressing outward. Repeat with a clean wipe if the infant is uncircumcised, retracting the foreskin to clean the meatus. When finished cleaning, replace the foreskin to the normal position. Female: Hold the labia open with your nondominant hand, cleanse the labia from superior to inferior (front to back), wiping in one directional motion. Discard the wipe, and repeat with a new wipe.				

Name: _____

Date: _____

<table>
<tr><td rowspan="2" colspan="2">POINT VALUE
✦ = 3–6 points
✳ = 7–9 points</td><td rowspan="2">PRACTICE TRIAL</td><td rowspan="2">GRADED TRIAL # 1</td><td rowspan="2">GRADED TRIAL # 2</td><td rowspan="2">NOTES</td></tr>
<tr></tr>
<tr><td></td><td>Note: Make sure the area is dry before attempting to apply the urine collection device.</td><td></td><td></td><td></td><td></td></tr>
<tr><td>6. ✦</td><td>Unfold the collection device and remove the upper portion of paper protecting the adhesive surface. Apply to the mons pubis and press to secure. Continue removing paper and applying to perineum, securing the device and ensuring that it isn't sticking to the infant's leg.</td><td></td><td></td><td></td><td></td></tr>
<tr><td>7. ✦</td><td>Offer water or suggest that the parent try to get the infant to drink fluids to increase the likelihood he or she will produce a urine specimen.</td><td></td><td></td><td></td><td></td></tr>
<tr><td>8. ✦</td><td>When a sufficient urine sample is collected, remove the bag, wipe down the area to which the bag was attached, and re-diaper the infant. It may be advisable to have the parent/ caregiver re-diaper the infant, based on office protocol.</td><td></td><td></td><td></td><td></td></tr>
<tr><td>9. ✳</td><td>Pour the sample into a labeled laboratory specimen container and handle according to routine in your facility.</td><td></td><td></td><td></td><td></td></tr>
<tr><td>10. ✦</td><td>Dispose of all used equipment in a biohazard waste container.</td><td></td><td></td><td></td><td></td></tr>
<tr><td>11. ✦</td><td>Remove gloves and perform hand hygiene.</td><td></td><td></td><td></td><td></td></tr>
<tr><td>12. ✦</td><td>Document the procedure; specific details are encouraged.</td><td></td><td></td><td></td><td></td></tr>
</table>

Document: Enter the appropriate information in the chart below.

Grading

Points Earned	_____		
Points Possible	_____	78	78
Percent Grade (Points Earned/Points Possible)	_____		
PASS:	_____	❏ YES ❏ NO ❏ N/A	❏ YES ❏ NO ❏ N/A

Instructor Sign-Off

Instructor: _____   **Date:** _____

Procedure 41-1:

Communicating Effectively with the Elderly

Objective: Communicate effectively with a new elderly patient preparing for a physical examination.

Equipment and Supplies: Patient's medical record; pen and paper; patient history form; examination table; gown and drapes; other physical examination equipment as needed

Affective Behaviors: Affective behaviors provide a professional approach to a skill that enhances the patient encounter. These behaviors may also display sensitivity to a patient's rights and enhance communication. Pay close attention to these skills, which will be in **_bold, italicized_** font.

Notes to the Student

_____

_____

_____

_____

_____

_____

Skills Assessment Requirements

Read and familiarize yourself with the procedure; complete the minimum practice requirements (MPRs). Document each MPR using proper charting technique. Complete each procedure within a reasonable amount of time, with a minimum of 85% accuracy.

Name: _____

Date: _____

POINT VALUE ✦ = 3–6 points ✱ = 7–9 points		PRACTICE TRIAL	GRADED TRIAL # 1	GRADED TRIAL # 2	NOTES
1. ✦	When entering the reception area to call the patient back to the examination area, **have a cheerful disposition and welcoming smile on your face.**				
2. ✦	Different offices may have different policies about how to address patients, whether by their first or last name. Follow the policy of your practice.				
3. ✱	**Introduce yourself. Be sincere and polite. From this point on, when addressing the patient, use a title, such as "Mr.," "Mrs.," or "Miss." For example, "Hello, Mr. Timmons, my name is Robin. It's nice to see you this morning."**				
4. ✦	Escort the patient to the examination room. If the patient is using a walker or a cane, walk closely to the patient and offer assistance if it seems to be needed.				
5. ✱	**Build rapport with the patient by making small talk while walking in the hallway or preparing items in the examination room.** The tone of your voice must be sincere, indicating that the conversation is not forced.				
6. ✦	**Explain that you will be preparing the patient to see the doctor for a physical examination or whatever today's procedure may be. Let the patient know what will be done and if anything will be expected of him or her during the appointment.**				

POINT VALUE ✦ = 3–6 points ✳ = 7–9 points	PRACTICE TRIAL	GRADED TRIAL #1	GRADED TRIAL #2	NOTES
7. ✦ Observe the patient for cues to indicate whether your remarks have or have not been understood. a. If it appears that the patient does not comprehend, paraphrase, using other words and simple gestures.				
8. ✦ Allow enough time for the patient to process information and ask if he or she has any questions before continuing.				
9. ✦ Observe the patient's overall physical ability to comply with your requests as you progress with preparing the patient for the examination or procedure.				
10. ✦ **Offer physical assistance if it appears the patient needs it.** Allow the patient to do as much for him- or herself as possible so as not to undermine his or her independence.				
11. ✦ Ask the patient to be seated while you begin to gather information for the patient history. If you think the patient would be unsteady sitting on the examination table for an extended period of time, allow the patient to answer questions while seated in a chair in the examination room.				
12. ✳ **Speak respectfully, and convey a feeling of warmth and empathy.** If the patient's replies to questions become too lengthy, gently interrupt and bring the patient back to the subject.				

Name: _____

Date: _____

POINT VALUE ✦ = 3–6 points ✱ = 7–9 points	PRACTICE TRIAL	GRADED TRIAL # 1	GRADED TRIAL # 2	NOTES
13. ✦ If answers to some of your questions seem incorrect or inappropriate, do not correct the patient. Gently distract the patient with another topic and proceed with your examination preparations.				
14. ✦ If the patient exhibits mental confusion in regard to some of your questions, do not press the patient for immediate answers. Inform the physician and make note of questions that need clearer answers. A caregiver or family member may be able to help with these answers at a later time.				
15. ✦ Do not leave the patient unattended if he or she is physically unstable or appears confused. Remember that relaxed body language, pleasant facial expressions, and a caring touch are most important in caring for patients who are confused.				
16. ✦ Document information appropriately within the patient's medical record. Keep in mind that opinions are never to be included, only objective information, facts that you are able to observe.				

Document: Enter the appropriate information in the chart below.

Grading

Points Earned	_____		
Points Possible	_____	114	114
Percent Grade (Points Earned/Points Possible)	_____		
PASS:	_____	❏ YES ❏ NO ❏ N/A	❏ YES ❏ NO ❏ N/A

Instructor Sign-Off

Instructor: _____   **Date:** _____

Procedure 42-1:

Surgical Hand Hygiene/Surgical Scrub

Objective: Perform a surgical scrub on hands and arms using the correct technique for the appropriate length of time.

Equipment and Supplies: Nail file; germicidal dispenser soap (not bar soap); sterile scrub brush; sterile towel pack (with two to three sterile paper or cloth towels); sterile gloves (prepackaged); running water (foot pedal preferable)

Affective Behaviors: Affective behaviors provide a professional approach to a skill that enhances the patient encounter. These behaviors may also display sensitivity to a patient's rights and enhance communication. Pay close attention to these skills, which will be in **_bold, italicized_** font.

Notes to the Student

_____

_____

_____

_____

_____

_____

Skills Assessment Requirements

Read and familiarize yourself with the procedure; complete the minimum practice requirements (MPRs). Document each MPR using proper charting technique. Complete each procedure within a reasonable amount of time, with a minimum of 85% accuracy.

Name: _____

Date: _____

POINT VALUE ✦ = 3–6 points ✶ = 7–9 points		PRACTICE TRIAL	GRADED TRIAL # 1	GRADED TRIAL # 2	NOTES
1. ✦	Remove all jewelry. With a nail file, remove any gross dirt from beneath fingernails before scrubbing.				
2. ✦	Assemble equipment.				
3. ✦	Stand at the sink without allowing your body to touch it.				
4. ✦	Remove your lab coat. Roll up your sleeves above the elbows. Keep your hands and arms above waist level at all times.				
5. ✦	Regulate running water temperature to warm, not hot.				
6. ✶	Place hands under running water with hands pointed upward. Allow water to run from fingertips to elbows.				
7. ✦	Apply a circle of soap from the dispenser and lather well.				
8. ✶	Vigorously scrub your hands and wrists with a scrub brush. Wash thoroughly between fingers. Scrub under fingernails. Scrub toward the elbows for 5 minutes on each hand.				
9. ✶	Raise hands, bending at the elbow, and place them under running water to rinse off soap. Allow water to flow from fingertips to elbows.				
10. ✦	If performing a second lather and scrub is the policy in your facility, use 3 minutes for each hand.				
11. ✶	Using a sterile towel (if possible), pat hands dry moving from fingertips to wrists, and then to elbows. Hands should still be held above the elbows.				

POINT VALUE ✦ = 3–6 points ✳ = 7–9 points	PRACTICE TRIAL	GRADED TRIAL # 1	GRADED TRIAL # 2	NOTES
12. ✦ Turn off the faucet with a fresh towel if foot lever is not available.				
13. ✦ Glove immediately. Keep hands above waist and folded together until the procedure begins.				

Name: _____

Date: _____

Document: Enter the appropriate information in the chart below.

Grading

Points Earned	_____		
Points Possible	_____	87	87
Percent Grade (Points Earned/Points Possible)	_____		
PASS:	_____	❏ YES ❏ NO ❏ N/A	❏ YES ❏ NO ❏ N/A

Instructor Sign-Off

Instructor: _____ Date: _____

Procedure 42-2:

Surgical Gloving

Objective: Apply sterile gloves without a break in sterile technique.

Equipment and Supplies: Double-wrapped sterile glove pack

Affective Behaviors: Affective behaviors provide a professional approach to a skill that enhances the patient encounter. These behaviors may also display sensitivity to a patient's rights and enhance communication. Pay close attention to these skills, which will be in **_bold, italicized_** font.

Notes to the Student

This procedure follows a surgical hand scrub.

_____

_____

_____

_____

_____

_____

Skills Assessment Requirements

Read and familiarize yourself with the procedure; complete the minimum practice requirements (MPRs). Document each MPR using proper charting technique. Complete each procedure within a reasonable amount of time, with a minimum of 85% accuracy.

POINT VALUE ✦ = 3–6 points ✳ = 7–9 points		PRACTICE TRIAL	GRADED TRIAL # 1	GRADED TRIAL # 2	NOTES
1. ✦	Assemble equipment and check the tape or seal for expiration date and condition of pack.				
2. ✦	Place the pack on a flat surface at waist height with the cuffed end of the gloves toward you.				
3. ✳	Open the outside wrapper by touching only the outside of the pack. Leave the opened wrapper in place to provide a sterile work field.				
4. ✳	Open the inner wrapper without reaching over the pack or touching the inside of the wrapper. Pull inner wrapper edges to each side without touching the inside of the pack.				
5. ✳	Using the thumb and fingers of your left hand (if you are right-handed), pick up the glove on the right side of the pack by grasping the folded inside edge of the cuff. The glove can be dangled slightly off the sterile packing material for easier insertion.				
6. ✳	Pull the glove onto the right hand using only the thumb and fingers of the left hands. Do not allow fingers to touch the rest of the glove.				
7. ✦	Place the fingers of the right-gloved hand under the cuff of the left glove and pull onto the left hand and up over the left wrist.				
8. ✦	With the gloved right hand, place your fingers under the cuff of the left glove and pull up over the left wrist. The thumb should not touch the cuff.				

Name: _____

Date: _____

POINT VALUE ✦ = 3–6 points ✳ = 7–9 points		PRACTICE TRIAL	GRADED TRIAL # 1	GRADED TRIAL # 2	NOTES
9. ✦	After the gloves are in place, the fingers can be adjusted, if necessary, by using the gloved hands.				
10. ✳	Removing gloves: Remove the first glove by grasping the edge of that glove (with fingers of the other gloved hand) and pull the first glove over the hand inside out. Discard the first glove into the proper biohazard waste container. Remove the other glove by grasping the edge of the cuff with your fingers (from the ungloved hand) and pull the second glove down over the hand, inside out. Discard the gloves appropriately.				

Name: _____

Date: _____

Document: Enter the appropriate information in the chart below.

Grading

Points Earned	_____		
Points Possible	_____	75	75
Percent Grade (Points Earned/Points Possible)	_____		
PASS:	_____	❏ YES ❏ NO ❏ N/A	❏ YES ❏ NO ❏ N/A

Instructor Sign-Off

_____

Instructor: _____ Date: _____

Procedure 42-3:

Opening a Sterile Packet

Objective: Open a sterile packet (pack) and use it to set up a sterile field without a break in the sterile technique.

Equipment and Supplies: Sterile packet; Mayo stand; waste container; sterile forceps

Affective Behaviors: Affective behaviors provide a professional approach to a skill that enhances the patient encounter. These behaviors may also display sensitivity to a patient's rights and enhance communication. Pay close attention to these skills, which will be in **_bold, italicized_** font.

Notes to the Student

_____

_____

_____

_____

_____

_____

Skills Assessment Requirements

Read and familiarize yourself with the procedure; complete the minimum practice requirements (MPRs). Document each MPR using proper charting technique. Complete each procedure within a reasonable amount of time, with a minimum of 85% accuracy.

POINT VALUE ✦ = 3–6 points ✴ = 7–9 points		PRACTICE TRIAL	GRADED TRIAL # 1	GRADED TRIAL # 2	NOTES
1. ✦	Perform hand hygiene.				
2. ✦	Assemble equipment. Adjust the Mayo stand to correct height.				
3. ✦	Place packet on the Mayo stand with the folded edge on top. Position the packet on the stand so that the top flap will fold away from you.				
4. ✦	Remove the tape or fastener and check the sterilization indicator and date. Discard in a waste container.				
5. ✴	Pull the corner of the pack that is tucked under and lay this flap away from you. It will hang down over the edge of the Mayo stand.				
6. ✴	With both hands, pull the next two flaps to each side. The packet will still be covered with the last layer of the outer wrapper.				
7. ✴	Grasp the corner of the last flap, without reaching over the sterile field, and open the flap toward your body without touching it.				
8. ✦	The inside of this outer wrapper is now your sterile field. If you need to arrange items within this field, use sterile forceps. If an inner packet must be opened within an instrument setup, then someone wearing sterile gloves must open it.				

Name: _____

Date: _____

Document: Enter the appropriate information in the chart below.

Grading

Points Earned	_____		
Points Possible	_____	57	57
Percent Grade (Points Earned/Points Possible)	_____		
PASS:	_____	❏ YES ❏ NO ❏ N/A	❏ YES ❏ NO ❏ N/A

Instructor Sign-Off

Instructor: _____ **Date:** _____

Procedure 42-4:

Dropping a Sterile Item onto a Sterile Field

Objective: Place (drop) a sterile item onto a sterile field or into a gloved hand without contaminating the packet or the field.

Equipment and Supplies: Sterile pack (containing, for example, prepackaged items such as a specimen container or needle and syringe in a pull-apart packet)

Affective Behaviors: Affective behaviors provide a professional approach to a skill that enhances the patient encounter. These behaviors may also display sensitivity to a patient's rights and enhance communication. Pay close attention to these skills, which will be in **bold, italicized** font.

Notes to the Student

_____

_____

_____

_____

_____

Skills Assessment Requirements

Read and familiarize yourself with the procedure; complete the minimum practice requirements (MPRs). Document each MPR using proper charting technique. Complete each procedure within a reasonable amount of time, with a minimum of 85% accuracy.

Name: _____

Date: _____

POINT VALUE ✦ = 3–6 points ✳ = 7–9 points		PRACTICE TRIAL	GRADED TRIAL #1	GRADED TRIAL #2	NOTES
1. ✦	Assemble equipment; check expiration date and sealed condition of packet.				
2. ✦	Locate the edge on the prepackaged item and pull apart by using the thumb and forefinger of each hand. Do not let your fingers touch the inside of the packet. Rationale: The inside of the packet is sterile and the outside is considered contaminated.				
3. ✳	Pull the packet apart by securely placing the remaining three fingers of each hand against the outside of the packet on each side. The wrapper edges will be pulled back and away from the sterile item.				
4. ✳	Holding the item securely about 8 to 10 inches from the sterile field, gently drop the packet contents inside the sterile field. Instead of having you drop the item, the physician may wish to remove the item directly from the packet by grasping it firmly with his or her gloved hand.				
5. ✦	Discard the paper wrapper in a waste container.				

Name: _____

Date: _____

Document: Enter the appropriate information in the chart below.

Grading

Points Earned	_____		
Points Possible	_____	36	36
Percent Grade (Points Earned/Points Possible)	_____		
PASS:	_____	❏ YES ❏ NO ❏ N/A	❏ YES ❏ NO ❏ N/A

Instructor Sign-Off

Instructor: _____   **Date:** _____

Procedure 42-5:

Transferring Sterile Objects Using Transfer Forceps

Objective: *Move sterile objects, such as instruments and supplies, within or onto a sterile field or into a gloved hand.*

Equipment and Supplies: Sterile transfer forceps in a forceps container with a sterilant solution, such as Cidex; Mayo stand with sterile field setup; sterile 4 × 4 gauze package (opened)

Affective Behaviors: Affective behaviors provide a professional approach to a skill that enhances the patient encounter. These behaviors may also display sensitivity to a patient's rights and enhance communication. Pay close attention to these skills, which will be in **bold, *italicized*** font.

Notes to the Student

_____

_____

_____

_____

_____

_____

Skills Assessment Requirements

Read and familiarize yourself with the procedure; complete the minimum practice requirements (MPRs). Document each MPR using proper charting technique. Complete each procedure within a reasonable amount of time, with a minimum of 85% accuracy.

Name: _____

Date: _____

POINT VALUE ✦ = 3–6 points ✱ = 7–9 points		PRACTICE TRIAL	GRADED TRIAL #1	GRADED TRIAL #2	NOTES
1. ✱	Grasp forceps handles firmly without separating the tips and remove vertically from the container. Remove vertically to avoid dripping solution onto exposed contaminated portion of forceps.				
2. ✱	Holding forceps vertically with tips down, gently tap tips together to drop excess solution onto dry sterile 4 × 4 gauze or touch the sterile 4 × 4 gauze to dry the tips.				
3. ✱	Pick up the sterile item to be transferred by holding transfer forceps vertically with tips down. Do not touch the sterile field. Grasp the article to be transferred firmly at its midsection.				
4. ✦	Place sterile item within the sterile field.				
5. ✱	Place forceps back into container without touching the sides of the container.				
6. ✱	Clean and sterilize the forceps and container in the autoclave. Change the solution.				

Name: _____

Date: _____

Document: Enter the appropriate information in the chart below.

Grading

Points Earned	_____		
Points Possible	_____	48	48
Percent Grade (Points Earned/Points Possible)	_____		
PASS:	_____	❏ YES ❏ NO ❏ N/A	❏ YES ❏ NO ❏ N/A

Instructor Sign-Off

Instructor: _____   **Date:** _____

Name: _____

Date: _____

Procedure 42-6:

Transferring Sterile Solutions onto a Sterile Field

Objective: Pour sterile fluid into a sterile basin on a sterile field without spilling the solution or contaminating the field.

Equipment and Supplies: Sterile saline or other solution as ordered; sterile basin; Mayo stand or side tray; waste container

Affective Behaviors: Affective behaviors provide a professional approach to a skill that enhances the patient encounter. These behaviors may also display sensitivity to a patient's rights and enhance communication. Pay close attention to these skills, which will be in **bold, *italicized*** font.

Notes to the Student

_____

_____

_____

_____

_____

_____

Skills Assessment Requirements

Read and familiarize yourself with the procedure; complete the minimum practice requirements (MPRs). Document each MPR using proper charting technique. Complete each procedure within a reasonable amount of time, with a minimum of 85% accuracy.

POINT VALUE ✦ = 3–6 points ✳ = 7–9 points		PRACTICE TRIAL	GRADED TRIAL # 1	GRADED TRIAL # 2	NOTES
1. ✦	Perform hand hygiene.				
2. ✦	Assemble all equipment. Check expiration dates on the solution and sterile basin pack.				
3. ✦	Set up sterile basin on the Mayo tray using inside of wrapper to create a sterile field.				
4. ✳	Remove cap of the solution and place it on a clean surface with the outer edge down (inside facing up). Avoid touching the inner surface of the cap, which is considered sterile.				
5. ✳	Check the label on the bottle before pouring the solution.				
6. ✦	Pour a small amount of the liquid into a waste container for discarding. This will dislodge any bacteria that may have collected on the edge of the bottle after opening it.				
7. ✳	Pour the bottle with the label held against the palm. This protects the label from drips that can destroy the name of the solution.				
8. ✳	Hold the bottle about 6 inches above the basin and pour slowly to avoid splashing.				
9. ✦	Replace the lid immediately after using.				

Name: _____

Date: _____

Document: Enter the appropriate information in the chart below.

Grading

Points Earned	_____		
Points Possible	_____	66	66
Percent Grade (Points Earned/Points Possible)	_____		
PASS:	_____	❏ YES ❏ NO ❏ N/A	❏ YES ❏ NO ❏ N/A

Instructor Sign-Off

Instructor: _____   **Date:** _____

Procedure 42-7:

Assisting with Minor Surgery

Objective: Prepare all materials and equipment for immediate use in a surgical procedure using sterile techniques.

Equipment and Supplies: Mayo stand; side stand; transfer forceps and container; sharps container; waste container/plastic bag; biohazard waste container; anesthetic; alcohol swab; sterile specimen container, depending on type of surgery; sterile pack (2 pairs sterile gloves, towel pack, 4 × 4 sponge pack, patient drape, needle pack, and suture materials); instrument pack(s), including towel clamp pack; syringe pack; 2 sterile basin packs

Affective Behaviors: Affective behaviors provide a professional approach to a skill that enhances the patient encounter. These behaviors may also display sensitivity to a patient's rights and enhance communication. Pay close attention to these skills, which will be in **_bold, italicized_** font.

Notes to the Student

_____

_____

_____

_____

_____

_____

Skills Assessment Requirements

Read and familiarize yourself with the procedure; complete the minimum practice requirements (MPRs). Document each MPR using proper charting technique. Complete each procedure within a reasonable amount of time, with a minimum of 85% accuracy.

Name: _____

Date: _____

POINT VALUE ✦ = 3–6 points ✶ = 7–9 points		PRACTICE TRIAL	GRADED TRIAL # 1	GRADED TRIAL # 2	NOTES
1. ✦	Perform hand hygiene.				
2. ✦	Open sterile tray packs on Mayo stand and side stand. Use sterile wrapper to create a sterile field. The wrapper will hang over the edges of the tray.				
3. ✦	Use sterile transfer forceps to move instruments on tray or to place equipment from packets. Materials in peel-away packets should be flipped onto the tray.				
4. ✦	Open the sterile needle and syringe unit and drop gently onto the sterile field. Use care not to reach over the sterile field.				
5. ✦	Open the sterile drape packs and towel clamp packs.				
6. ✦	Open a set of sterile gloves for the physician.				
7. ✶	After the tray is ready with all equipment open and arranged, pull the edge of the sterile towel across the tray, using sterile transfer forceps. The sterile towel will provide a protective covering for the sterile tray until the procedure begins. The medical assistant should not leave the room once the tray is set up.				
8. ✶	When the physician has donned the sterile gloves, remove the sterile towel covering the tray of instruments.				
9. ✦	Remove the towel by standing to one side and grasping the two distal corners, then lifting the towel toward you so that you do not reach over the unprotected sterile field.				

POINT VALUE ✦ = 3–6 points ✳ = 7–9 points		PRACTICE TRIAL	GRADED TRIAL # 1	GRADED TRIAL # 2	NOTES
10. ✳	Cleanse the vial of anesthetic with a sterile alcohol swab and hold it upside down in the palm of your hand with the label facing toward the physician. Hold it steady while the physician draws up the anesthetic.				
11. ✦	Stand to one side of the patient and assist the physician as requested. Provide additional supplies as needed. If you assist by handing instruments directly to the physician, you must perform a surgical scrub and wear a sterile gown and gloves.				
12. ✦	Hold all containers for specimens, drainage, or contaminated 4 × 4s. Wear nonsterile gloves to protect yourself from contact with drainage.				
13. ✦	Collect and place all soiled instruments in a basin out of the patient's view.				
14. ✦	Place all soiled gauze sponges (4 × 4s) and dressings in a plastic bag. Do not allow wet items to remain on a sterile field.				
15. ✳	Immediately label all specimens as they are obtained. Close all specimen containers tightly.				
16. ✦	**Periodically reassure the patient by quietly asking how he or she is doing.** Do not touch the patient with soiled gloves.				

POINT VALUE ✦ = 3–6 points ✱ = 7–9 points		PRACTICE TRIAL	GRADED TRIAL # 1	GRADED TRIAL # 2	NOTES
17. ✦	When the procedure is complete, wash your hands before assisting the patient. The patient will often be moved to a recovery area so the surgical area can be cleaned. To dispose of soiled dressings, use the following steps: a. Remove gloves. b. Place one hand into the empty plastic bag. c. Using the hand covered with the plastic bag, pick up all the soiled materials. With the other hand, pull the outside of the bag over the soiled dressings. d. Dispose of the bag in a biohazard waste container. e. Perform hand hygiene and document the procedure.				
18. ✦	Allow the patient to rest and recover from the anesthetic. Periodically, check the patient's vital signs according to your office policy.				
19. ✦	***Provide clear oral and written postoperative instructions for the patient. Make sure the patient is stable before he or she leaves the office.***				
20. ✱	Send the specimen(s) to the laboratory with a requisition slip.				
21. ✱	Clean, sanitize, and sterilize the instruments. Clean and sanitize the room in preparation for the next patient.				
22. ✦	Perform hand hygiene.				

Name: _____

Date: _____

Document: Enter the appropriate information in the chart below.

Grading

Points Earned	_____		
Points Possible	_____	150	150
Percent Grade (Points Earned/Points Possible)	_____		
PASS:	_____	❏ YES ❏ NO ❏ N/A	❏ YES ❏ NO ❏ N/A

Instructor Sign-Off

Instructor: _____ **Date:** _____

Procedure 42-8:

Preparing the Patient's Skin for Surgical Procedures

Objective: Prepare the patient's skin for surgical procedure using sterile scrub and shave.

Equipment and Supplies: Antiseptic germicidal soap; sterile saline; antiseptic such as Betadine; 8 sterile applicators; Mayo tray; waste receptacle (may be included in sterile pack); biohazard waste container; plastic bag for soiled dressings; sterile pack (sterile gloves, 3 to 4 towel packs, sterile basin pack with 3 basins, patient drape, 4 × 4 gauze sponge pack with 12 to 24 sponges, shave preparation kit)

Affective Behaviors: Affective behaviors provide a professional approach to a skill that enhances the patient encounter. These behaviors may also display sensitivity to a patient's rights and enhance communication. Pay close attention to these skills, which will be in **_bold, italicized_** font.

Notes to the Student

_____

_____

_____

_____

_____

Skills Assessment Requirements

Read and familiarize yourself with the procedure; complete the minimum practice requirements (MPRs). Document each MPR using proper charting technique. Complete each procedure within a reasonable amount of time, with a minimum of 85% accuracy.

POINT VALUE ✦ = 3–6 points ✱ = 7–9 points		PRACTICE TRIAL	GRADED TRIAL #1	GRADED TRIAL #2	NOTES
1. ✦	Perform hand hygiene.				
2. ✦	Assemble equipment by placing packs on Mayo stand or side tray and opening outer wraps from all packs.				
3. ✱	**Identify the patient and explain the procedure.**				
4. ✦	**Have the patient remove appropriate clothing and put on gown. Ask the patient to void, if necessary.**				
5. ✦	Position and drape the patient to provide exposure of the operative site.				
6. ✦	Unwrap the basin pack. Pour germicidal soap solution into one basin, sterile saline into the second basin, and antiseptic into the third.				
7. ✦	Wash hands using sterile scrub, and apply sterile gloves.				
8. ✦	Drape the skin with two towels placed 3 to 5 inches above and below the surgical site.				
9. ✱	With a sterile gauze or sponge, apply soapy solution to the patient's skin. Use a circular motion starting at the site of the proposed incision and move outward. Pass over each skin area only once. Place each used sponge into a waste receptacle immediately. **Instructions for a dry shave:** Some physicians prefer the patient to receive a dry shave. To remove hair, electric clippers are preferred to razor blades because they lessen the likelihood of accidental nicks in the skin.				

POINT VALUE ✦ = 3–6 points ✴ = 7–9 points		PRACTICE TRIAL	GRADED TRIAL # 1	GRADED TRIAL # 2	NOTES
	a. Clip the hair as short as possible with scissors. b. Apply firm traction to the skin with the nondominant hand. c. Remove hair in the direction of hair growth. Never shave against the grain, as this will cause unnecessary irritation to the skin and increase the likelihood of nicks.				
10. ✴	Use a fresh sterile gauze or sponge for each cleansing wipe. Repeat this process until the area is completely washed. The last area cleansed will be the outer edges.				
11. ✴	Rinse using sterile saline on a clean gauze or sponge. Pat dry with a dry gauze only on the area that has been washed. Avoid touching any other skin area. If shaving is ordered, then proceed with the following steps: 1. Apply soap solution to the site area. Remove razor from shave preparation pack. Pull the skin taut and shave the surgical site in the same direction as the hair is growing. Rinse with a saline solution using the single-pass, circular motion as before and pat it dry. 2. Reapply soap solution to the area and repeat the preceding process according to your office policy (around 5 minutes).				

Competency Check-Offs **1059**

Name: _____

Date: _____

POINT VALUE ✦ = 3–6 points ✱ = 7–9 points		PRACTICE TRIAL	GRADED TRIAL # 1	GRADED TRIAL # 2	NOTES
	3. Pat the entire area dry with the third sterile towel. 4. Apply the antiseptic solution using two cotton applicators together in the same single-pass, circular motion. 5. Apply the antiseptic solution using two cotton applicators together in the same single-pass, circular motion. 6. Properly dispose of gloves and soiled materials in a biohazard waste container.				

Document: Enter the appropriate information in the chart below.

Grading

Points Earned	_____		
Points Possible	_____	108	108
Percent Grade (Points Earned/Points Possible)	_____		
PASS:	_____	❏ YES ❏ NO ❏ N/A	❏ YES ❏ NO ❏ N/A

Instructor Sign-Off

Instructor: _____   **Date:** _____

Name: _____

Date: _____

Procedure 42-9:

Assisting with Suturing

Objective: Assist with suture repair of an incision or laceration using sterile technique.

Equipment and Supplies: Mayo stand; side stand; anesthetic; sterile transfer forceps; sterile saline; waste container/plastic bag; biohazard waste container; sharps container; sterile gloves (2 pairs); sterile pack(s) (patient drape, towel pack with four towels, 4 × 4 gauze sponge pack); scalpel blades pack (Nos. 10 and 15); needle and syringe pack; suture and needle pack (according to physician's preference); 2 sterile basins; suture pack (scalpel handle, needle holder, thumb forceps; 2 scissors; 3 hemostats)

Affective Behaviors: Affective behaviors provide a professional approach to a skill that enhances the patient encounter. These behaviors may also display sensitivity to a patient's rights and enhance communication. Pay close attention to these skills, which will be in **bold, _italicized_** font.

Notes to the Student

_____

_____

_____

_____

_____

_____

Skills Assessment Requirements

Read and familiarize yourself with the procedure; complete the minimum practice requirements (MPRs). Document each MPR using proper charting technique. Complete each procedure within a reasonable amount of time, with a minimum of 85% accuracy.

POINT VALUE ✦ = 3–6 points ✳ = 7–9 points		PRACTICE TRIAL	GRADED TRIAL #1	GRADED TRIAL #2	NOTES
1. ✦	Use a sterile scrub and gloving procedure.				
2. ✦	Stand across from the physician.				
3. ✦	Place two sponges ready for the physician near the wound site.				
4. ✦	Assist by using additional sponges to keep the wound dry.				
5. ✳	Pass instruments, such as scissors, to the physician using a firm snap of the handle into his or her hand without letting go until the physician has a firm grasp.				
6. ✦	The blade is placed into the scalpel using a hemostat.				
7. ✳	Hand the scalpel to the physician with blade edge down to avoid cutting the physician.				
8. ✦	Continue to use sponges to keep the wound free of drainage.				
9. ✦	Pass all instruments to the physician as requested. Try to anticipate the next instruments that the physician may need, such as another hemostat or scissors for cutting a suture.				
10. ✦	Pass the toothed forceps to the physician if laceration edges need to be grasped.				
11. ✳	Mount the needle into the needle holder and pass as one unit to the physician, using care to keep the suture within the sterile field. Pass the needle holder with the needle pointing outward. Hold the suture with the other hand, and do not let go of it until the physician sees it.				

POINT VALUE ✦ = 3–6 points ✱ = 7–9 points		PRACTICE TRIAL	GRADED TRIAL # 1	GRADED TRIAL # 2	NOTES
12. ✦	Using the suture scissors, prepare to cut the suture as directed by the physician (usually ⅛ to ¼ inch from the knot).				
13. ✱	Sponge the closed wound once with a sponge and discard.				
14. ✦	Repeat this step with each suture.				
15. ✱	Apply a layer of sterile dressing over the wound, such as a sterile gauze pad. The medical assistant may use forceps if preferred. The sterile dressing should extend a minimum of 2 inches past all edges of the wound.				
16. ✦	Apply a second layer of gauze over the wound site.				
17. ✦	Add a final third layer of wound dressing, such as a SurgiPad.				
18. ✦	Secure the edges of the dressing with paper tape or similar product. Some physicians will prefer the wound to be covered with a clear, waterproof membrane such as Telfa. Paper tape is often used because it contains a less-intense adhesive, lowering the risk for adverse skin reactions.				
19. ✱	After they are used, place all soiled instruments on the sterile field if they will be used again; discard others in the instrument basin.				
20. ✦	When the procedure is complete, remove your gloves and perform hand hygiene before assisting the patient.				

Name: _____

Date: _____

POINT VALUE ✦ = 3–6 points ✳ = 7–9 points		PRACTICE TRIAL	GRADED TRIAL #1	GRADED TRIAL #2	NOTES
21. ✦	Allow the patient to rest and recover from the anesthetic. Periodically check the patient's vital signs according to your office policy.				
22. ✳	***Provide clear oral and written postoperative instructions for the patient. Make sure the patient is stable before he or she leaves the office.***				
23. ✳	Clean, sanitize, and sterilize the instruments. Clean and sanitize the room in preparation for the next patient.				
24. ✦	Perform hand hygiene.				

Name: _____

Date: _____

Document: Enter the appropriate information in the chart below.

Grading

Points Earned	_____		
Points Possible	_____	168	168
Percent Grade (Points Earned/Points Possible)	_____		
PASS:	_____	❑ YES ❑ NO ❑ N/A	❑ YES ❑ NO ❑ N/A

Instructor Sign-Off

Instructor: _____   **Date:** _____

Procedure 42-10:

Removing Sutures

Objective: Remove sutures using proper sterile technique, following the physician's order.

Equipment and Supplies: Suture removal pack (suture scissors; sterile gauze squares; thumb forceps; skin antiseptic; sterile gloves; bandages; biohazard waste container)

Affective Behaviors: Affective behaviors provide a professional approach to a skill that enhances the patient encounter. These behaviors may also display sensitivity to a patient's rights and enhance communication. Pay close attention to these skills, which will be in ***bold, italicized*** font.

Notes to the Student

_____

_____

_____

_____

_____

_____

Skills Assessment Requirements

Read and familiarize yourself with the procedure; complete the minimum practice requirements (MPRs). Document each MPR using proper charting technique. Complete each procedure within a reasonable amount of time, with a minimum of 85% accuracy.

Name: _____

Date: _____

POINT VALUE ✦ = 3–6 points ✳ = 7–9 points		PRACTICE TRIAL	GRADED TRIAL # 1	GRADED TRIAL # 2	NOTES
	Removal of Sutures				
1. ✦	Perform hand hygiene.				
2. ✦	Assemble equipment and check expiration date on pack.				
3. ✦	*Identify the patient.*				
4. ✳	*Explain the procedure to the patient, and assist him or her into a comfortable position.*				
5. ✦	Perform hand hygiene.				
6. ✦	Remove old dressing using proper technique.				
7. ✦	Perform hand hygiene.				
8. ✳	Open suture or staple removal pack using proper technique.				
9. ✦	Apply sterile gloves using proper technique.				
10. ✳	Cleanse the wound as needed.				
11. ✦	Place a gauze square next to the wound for placement of sutures or staples as they are removed.				
12. ✦	Grasp the knot of the suture with thumb forceps and lift gently.				
13. ✦	Insert the suture scissors and cut suture at skin level. Pull out the suture.				
14. ✳	Place the cut suture on the gauze.				
15. ✦	Repeat these steps until all sutures are removed.				
16. ✳	Count the sutures to make sure that all have been removed.				
	Removal of Staples				
1–10. ✦	Perform steps 1 through 10 above.				

POINT VALUE ✦ = 3–6 points ✴ = 7–9 points		PRACTICE TRIAL	GRADED TRIAL # 1	GRADED TRIAL # 2	NOTES
11. ✦	Place the lower tips of a sterile staple remover under the staple.				
12. ✴	Squeeze the handles together until they are completely closed. (Pressing the handles together causes the staple to bend in the middle and pulls the edges of the staple out of the skin.) Do not lift the staple remover when squeezing the handles.				
13. ✦	When both ends of the staple are visible, gently move the staple away from the incision site.				
14. ✦	Hold the staple remover over a disposable container, release the staple remover handles, and release the staple.				
15. ✴	Place the staple on the gauze, repeat these steps until all staples are removed, and count the number of staples to ensure all have been removed.				
	Closing Steps for Either Suture or Staple Removal				
16. ✴	Clean the wound with antiseptic and allow it to dry.				
17. ✦	Dress wound as ordered.				
18. ✦	Properly dispose of equipment and supplies.				
19. ✦	Remove gloves and perform hand hygiene.				
20. ✴	***Instruct the patient on wound care.***				
21. ✴	Document the procedure, including condition of wound, number of sutures or staples removed, and patient instructions on wound care.				

Name: _____

Date: _____

Document: Enter the appropriate information in the chart below.

Grading

Points Earned	_____		
Points Possible	_____	252	252
Percent Grade (Points Earned/Points Possible)	_____		
PASS:	_____	❏ YES ❏ NO ❏ N/A	❏ YES ❏ NO ❏ N/A

Instructor Sign-Off

Instructor: _____ Date: _____

Procedure 42-11:

Changing a Sterile Dressing

Objective: Change a wound dressing using proper sterile technique.

Equipment and Supplies: Disposable gloves; antiseptic solution; solution container; prepackaged dressing pack; thumb forceps; sterile cotton balls; sterile gloves; sterile dressing; adhesive tape; scissors, if necessary for tape; waste container/plastic bag; biohazard waste container; Mayo stand or side tray

Affective Behaviors: Affective behaviors provide a professional approach to a skill that enhances the patient encounter. These behaviors may also display sensitivity to a patient's rights and enhance communication. Pay close attention to these skills, which will be in **_bold, italicized_** font.

Notes to the Student

_____

_____

_____

_____

_____

_____

Skills Assessment Requirements

Read and familiarize yourself with the procedure; complete the minimum practice requirements (MPRs). Document each MPR using proper charting technique. Complete each procedure within a reasonable amount of time, with a minimum of 85% accuracy.

Name: _____

Date: _____

POINT VALUE ✦ = 3–6 points ✱ = 7–9 points	PRACTICE TRIAL	GRADED TRIAL # 1	GRADED TRIAL # 2	NOTES
1. ✦ Perform hand hygiene.				
2. ✦ Assemble equipment using the Mayo stand.				
3. ✦ Prepare the sterile field, using aseptic technique and prepackaged dressing packet. Employ sterile transfer forceps to place additional sterile items on the sterile field.				
4. ✱ **Explain the procedure to the patient.**				
5. ✦ **Assist the patient into a comfortable position with the area to be dressed resting on a support, such as an examination table.**				
6. ✦ Apply nonsterile gloves.				
7. ✱ Remove dressing from the wound by loosening the tape with gloved hands or forceps and pulling it from both sides toward the wound. Without passing the soiled dressing over the sterile field, place it into the soiled waste bag. Do not allow the dressing to touch the outside or edges of the bag.				
8. ✱ Inspect the wound for signs of infection and inflammation. Note any discharge by its type, amount, and odor.				
9. ✦ Discard gloves and contaminated forceps properly. Place disposable gloves and forceps in a biohazardous waste container. Reusable forceps are placed in the basin for later cleaning.				

POINT VALUE ✦ = 3–6 points ✶ = 7–9 points		PRACTICE TRIAL	GRADED TRIAL # 1	GRADED TRIAL # 2	NOTES
10. ✦	Drop the antiseptic onto several cotton balls until they are moist but not saturated.				
11. ✦	Open sterile gloves and apply properly.				
12. ✦	Cleanse the wound by using sterile forceps to hold the cotton while moving from top to bottom of the wound once. Use a new cotton ball with antiseptic for each wipe. Move from the inside of the wound to the outside edges.				
13. ✦	Pick up the sterile dressing with gloved hands and place over the wound.				
14. ✦	Discard gloves and forceps.				
15. ✦	Apply adhesive tape to hold the dressing in place. Do not apply too tightly as to restrict circulation. The strips of tape should be long enough to hold the dressing in place. Do not wrap the tape entirely around an extremity or completely cover the dressing.				
16. ✦	***Instruct the patient on dressing care, and to schedule a follow-up appointment to see the physician.***				
17. ✶	Chart the procedure, including the date, time, location, and condition of the wound and the instructions given to the patient.				

Name: _____

Date: _____

Document: Enter the appropriate information in the chart below.

Grading

Points Earned	_____		
Points Possible	_____	114	114
Percent Grade (Points Earned/Points Possible)	_____		
PASS:	_____	❏ YES ❏ NO ❏ N/A	❏ YES ❏ NO ❏ N/A

Instructor Sign-Off

Instructor: _____   **Date:** _____

Procedure 42-12:

Applying a Bandage Over a Sterile Dressing

Objective: Apply a bandage to the forearm.

Equipment and Supplies: Nonsterile gloves; bandage material prescribed by physician or office procedures; bandage scissors; tape

Affective Behaviors: Affective behaviors provide a professional approach to a skill that enhances the patient encounter. These behaviors may also display sensitivity to a patient's rights and enhance communication. Pay close attention to these skills, which will be in **bold, *italicized*** font.

Notes to the Student

_____

_____

_____

_____

_____

_____

Skills Assessment Requirements

Read and familiarize yourself with the procedure; complete the minimum practice requirements (MPRs). Document each MPR using proper charting technique. Complete each procedure within a reasonable amount of time, with a minimum of 85% accuracy.

Name: _____

Date: _____

POINT VALUE ✦ = 3–6 points ✶ = 7–9 points		PRACTICE TRIAL	GRADED TRIAL #1	GRADED TRIAL #2	NOTES
1. ✦	Identify the patient.				
2. ✦	Perform hand hygiene.				
3. ✦	Apply nonsterile gloves.				
4. ✦	***Explain the procedure to the patient.***				
5. ✦	Hold bandage against the skin with nondominant hand 1 inch below the dressing.				
6. ✦	Wrap bandage around the wrist two to three times to secure.				
7. ✶	Wrap forearm from distal (part farthest away from the body) to proximal (closest to the body) with overlapping spiral turns.				
8. ✶	Check that the bandage is not restricting blood flow.				
9. ✦	Continue wrapping to at least 1 inch above the dressing.				
10. ✦	Wrap two more times to secure the bandage, then cut.				
11. ✦	Tape the cut end to the bandage; do not tape the end to the patient's skin.				
12. ✶	Check again for any blood flow restriction.				
13. ✦	Remove gloves.				
14. ✦	Perform hand hygiene.				
15. ✦	***Explain home care to the patient.***				
16. ✶	Document the procedure accurately.				

Name: _____

Date: _____

Document: Enter the appropriate information in the chart below.

Grading

Points Earned	_____		
Points Possible	_____	108	108
Percent Grade (Points Earned/Points Possible)	_____		
PASS:	_____	❑ YES ❑ NO ❑ N/A	❑ YES ❑ NO ❑ N/A

Instructor Sign-Off

Instructor: _____ Date: _____

Procedure 43-1:

Perform Adult Rescue Breathing and One-Rescuer or Two-Rescuer CPR

Objective: Administer rescue breathing for an adult and one-rescuer CPR for an adult correctly, within the time frames designated.

Equipment and Supplies: Approved mannequin; gloves; ventilator mask; mouth guard

Affective Behaviors: Affective behaviors provide a professional approach to a skill that enhances the patient encounter. These behaviors may also display sensitivity to a patient's rights and enhance communication. Pay close attention to these skills, which will be in **_bold, italicized_** font.

Notes to the Student

_____

_____

_____

_____

_____

_____

Skills Assessment Requirements

Read and familiarize yourself with the procedure; complete the minimum practice requirements (MPRs). Document each MPR using proper charting technique. Complete each procedure within a reasonable amount of time, with a minimum of 85% accuracy.

POINT VALUE ✦ = 3–6 points ✻ = 7–9 points	PRACTICE TRIAL	GRADED TRIAL #1	GRADED TRIAL #2	NOTES
One-Rescuer Adult CPR				
1. ✻ ***Assess the patient and determine if help is needed. Shout, "Are you okay?" while gently tapping the patient's shoulders.***				
2. ✻ If you determine that the adult patient is unresponsive and not breathing or not breathing normally (agonal breathing), *activate EMS immediately* by calling 911, then get an AED if available (or shout for another office employee to call 911 and get the AED).				
3. ✻ Check a carotid pulse for no less than 5 seconds but no longer than 10 seconds. If there is definitely no pulse, begin chest compressions. Kneel at the patient's side. Place your hand in the center of the chest on the lower half of the sternum.				
4. ✻ Place your other hand on top of the first hand on the chest, interlock your fingers, and be sure to lift your fingers off the chest using only the heels of your hands to administer compressions.				
5. ✻ Kneel next to the patient and keep your shoulders directly over your hands, Compress the chest at least 2 inches and allow the chest to completely recoil after each compression. Do not lift your hands completely off the chest.				

POINT VALUE ✦ = 3–6 points ✶ = 7–9 points		PRACTICE TRIAL	GRADED TRIAL # 1	GRADED TRIAL # 2	NOTES
6. ✶	Continue to compress the chest a total of 30 times at a rate of at least 100 compressions minute.				
7. ✶	After 30 compressions are delivered, perform a head-tilt, chin-lift, or, if spine injury is suspected, a jaw-thrust maneuver to open the airway. Administer 2 breaths with each delivered over 1 second, preferably using a mouth-to-mask protective device. Continue chest compressions and ventilations.				
8. ✦	Apply the AED as soon as it becomes available. (See Procedure 43-3 regarding defibrillator use.)				
9. ✶	Repeat this sequence until a pulse has been restored or until EMS arrives.				
10. ✶	If breathing is absent, but a pulse has been restored, administer 2 rescue breaths, preferably using a mouth-to-mask device. If your breaths do not cause the chest to rise, reestablish the head-tilt, chin-lift or jaw-thrust maneuver. If you suspect choking, look in the patient's mouth and remove an object if you see one. If you see no obstruction, continue with rescue breathing. If an obstruction is present, perform the steps for an obstructed airway.				
11. ✶	Wash your hands and document the incident in the patient's chart.				

POINT VALUE ✦ = 3–6 points ✳ = 7–9 points		PRACTICE TRIAL	GRADED TRIAL #1	GRADED TRIAL #2	NOTES
	Two-Rescuer Adult CPR				
1. ✳	Follow the steps just described for one-rescuer adult CPR until a second rescuer certified in professional-level CPR can join you.				
2. ✳	Continue performing chest compressions while the second rescuer positions him- or herself by kneeling above the patient's head. After you have completed a cycle of 30 compressions, the second rescuer will administer 2 breaths, as described in the steps for one-rescuer CPR.				
3. ✳	Switch positions with the second rescuer every 5 cycles (approximately every 2 minutes), with the ventilator taking over chest compressions while the compressor takes over ventilations.				
4. ✳	Repeat this sequence until a pulse has been restored or until EMS arrives.				
5. ✳	If breathing is absent but a pulse has been restored, administer 2 rescue breaths as described in step 10 for one-rescuer CPR.				
6. ✳	Wash your hands and document the incident in the patient's chart.				

Document: Enter the appropriate information in the chart below.

Grading

Points Earned	_____		
Points Possible	_____	102	102
Percent Grade (Points Earned/Points Possible)	_____		
PASS:	_____	❑ YES ❑ NO ❑ N/A	❑ YES ❑ NO ❑ N/A

Instructor Sign-Off

Instructor: _____   **Date:** _____

Name: _____

Date: _____

Procedure 43-2:

Perform Infant Rescue Breathing

Objective: Correctly administer rescue breathing for a child and one-rescuer CPR for a child, within the designated time frame.

Equipment and Supplies: Approved mannequin; gloves; ventilator mask; mouth guard

Affective Behaviors: Affective behaviors provide a professional approach to a skill that enhances the patient encounter. These behaviors may also display sensitivity to a patient's rights and enhance communication. Pay close attention to these skills, which will be in **bold, italicized** font.

Notes to the Student

_____

_____

_____

_____

_____

Skills Assessment Requirements

Read and familiarize yourself with the procedure; complete the minimum practice requirements (MPRs). Document each MPR using proper charting technique. Complete each procedure within a reasonable amount of time, with a minimum of 85% accuracy.

Name: _____

Date: _____

POINT VALUE ✦ = 3–6 points ✳ = 7–9 points		PRACTICE TRIAL	GRADED TRIAL # 1	GRADED TRIAL # 2	NOTES
1. ✳	Assess for responsiveness and breathing. Never shake an infant.				
2. ✦	If you determine that the infant is not breathing or not breathing normally but has a pulse, perform rescue breathing. *Immediately* activate EMS by calling 911.				
3. ✳	Carefully place the patient in a supine position. If a spine injury is suspected, keep the head and neck in line with the navel.				
4. ✦	With the palm of one hand, tilt the patient's head back. With two to three fingers of the other hand, lift the lower jaw forward to open the airway.				
5. ✳	If possible, place a face mask for mouth-to-mask ventilation over the patient's mouth and nose. If two rescuers are present, one may cradle the infant in a supine position while the other administers ventilations. Administer 2 rescue breaths. If your breaths do not cause the chest to rise, reestablish the head-tilt, chin-lift or jaw-thrust maneuver. If you suspect choking, look in the patient's mouth and remove an object if you see one. If you see no obstruction, continue with rescue breathing. If an obstruction is present, perform the steps for an obstructed airway.				

POINT VALUE ✦ = 3–6 points ✱ = 7–9 points		PRACTICE TRIAL	GRADED TRIAL # 1	GRADED TRIAL # 2	NOTES
6. ✱	Once the obstruction is clear, begin rescue breathing by administering 1 breath every 3 to 5 seconds or 12 to 20 breaths every minute.				
7. ✱	Continue breaths until the infant recovers or EMS arrives.				
8. ✱	Wash hands and document the incident in the patient's chart.				

Name: _____

Date: _____

Document: Enter the appropriate information in the chart below.

Grading

Points Earned	_____		
Points Possible	_____	69	69
Percent Grade (Points Earned/Points Possible)	_____		
PASS:	_____	❑ YES ❑ NO ❑ N/A	❑ YES ❑ NO ❑ N/A

Instructor Sign-Off

Instructor: _____   Date: _____

Procedure 43-3:

Use an Automated External Defibrillator

Objective: Use an automated external defibrillator (AED) correctly within the time frame designated by the instructor.

Equipment and Supplies: AED machine; patient chart

Affective Behaviors: Affective behaviors provide a professional approach to a skill that enhances the patient encounter. These behaviors may also display sensitivity to a patient's rights and enhance communication. Pay close attention to these skills, which will be in **_bold, italicized_** font.

Notes to the Student

_____

_____

_____

_____

_____

_____

Skills Assessment Requirements

Read and familiarize yourself with the procedure; complete the minimum practice requirements (MPRs). Document each MPR using proper charting technique. Complete each procedure within a reasonable amount of time, with a minimum of 85% accuracy.

POINT VALUE ✦ = 3–6 points ✶ = 7–9 points		PRACTICE TRIAL	GRADED TRIAL # 1	GRADED TRIAL # 2	NOTES
1. ✶	Place the AED next to the patient's left ear. This position allows the rescuers clear access to the chest and airway for continued CPR while the AED is being set up. (One provider may continue one-person CPR while the other sets up the AED.)				
2. ✶	Turn the AED on and follow the voice prompts.				
3. ✶	You will be prompted to attach the electrode pads to the patient's chest, following the diagram provided for correct placement. Use adult-size electrode pads on patients 8 years of age and older. Child-size electrode pads are used for patients less than 8 years of age. (Use adult-size pads on a patient less than 8 years of age if child-size pads are not available.)				
4. ✶	Next, you will be directed to clear the patient to allow the machine to analyze the heart rhythm to determine if a shockable rhythm is present. CPR should cease while the machine is analyzing, and no one should be in contact with the patient for any reason.				
5. ✶	If a shockable rhythm is present, the AED will automatically begin a charging sequence and warn rescuers to stand back and not to touch the patient. The voice prompt will then tell you to press the SHOCK button to administer the electrical current to the patient.				

Name: _____

Date: _____

POINT VALUE ✦ = 3–6 points ✱ = 7–9 points		PRACTICE TRIAL	GRADED TRIAL # 1	GRADED TRIAL # 2	NOTES
6. ✱	If the machine indicates "No shock is advised," continue CPR beginning with chest compressions. After 2 minutes, the AED will prompt you to stand clear and will reanalyze the rhythm. Repeat step 5 if a shockable rhythm is present or continue CPR, beginning with chest compressions. Repeat this sequence until advanced medical personnel arrive or the patient regains a pulse.				

Name: _____

Date: _____

Document: Enter the appropriate information in the chart below.

Grading

Points Earned	_____		
Points Possible	_____	45	45
Percent Grade (Points Earned/Points Possible)	_____		
PASS:	_____	❑ YES ❑ NO ❑ N/A	❑ YES ❑ NO ❑ N/A

Instructor Sign-Off

Instructor: _____ Date: _____

Name: _____

Date: _____

Procedure 43-4:

Respond to an Adult with an Obstructed Airway

Objective: Administer abdominal thrusts to an adult correctly, within the time frame designated.

Equipment and Supplies: Approved mannequin; gloves; ventilation mask with one-way valve for unconscious patient

Affective Behaviors: Affective behaviors provide a professional approach to a skill that enhances the patient encounter. These behaviors may also display sensitivity to a patient's rights and enhance communication. Pay close attention to these skills, which will be in **_bold, italicized_** font.

Notes to the Student

_____

_____

_____

_____

_____

_____

Skills Assessment Requirements

Read and familiarize yourself with the procedure; complete the minimum practice requirements (MPRs). Document each MPR using proper charting technique. Complete each procedure within a reasonable amount of time, with a minimum of 85% accuracy.

Name: _____

Date: _____

POINT VALUE ✦ = 3–6 points ✳ = 7–9 points		PRACTICE TRIAL	GRADED TRIAL #1	GRADED TRIAL #2	NOTES
1. ✦	Once it has been established that the patient is choking, with no air exchange, direct someone to call 911 and shout "Are you choking?" If the answer is yes—as indicated by a head nod—tell the patient you are going to begin emergency treatment.				
2. ✳	Stand behind the patient with your feet slightly apart, placing one foot between the patient's feet and one to the outside. This stance will give you greater stability, and if the patient should pass out, you can safely guide him or her to the ground by sliding him or her down your thigh.				
3. ✳	Place the index finger of one hand at the person's navel or belt buckle to mark that spot. If the patient is an obviously pregnant woman or is obese, perform chest thrusts (see step 7).				
4. ✳	Make a fist with your other hand and place it, thumb side to patient, above your other hand.				
5. ✳	Place your marking hand over your curled fist and begin to give quick inward and upward thrusts.				
6. ✳	There is no set number of thrusts to give to an adult who remains conscious. Continue to give thrusts until the object is removed or the patient becomes unconscious.				

POINT VALUE ✦ = 3–6 points ✳ = 7–9 points		PRACTICE TRIAL	GRADED TRIAL # 1	GRADED TRIAL # 2	NOTES
7. ✦	If the patient is an obviously pregnant woman or is obese, help her to lie on the ground in a supine position and perform chest thrusts.				
8. ✳	If the patient becomes unconscious, gently lower him or her to the ground.				
9. ✳	Activate EMS and put on gloves.				
10. ✳	Immediately begin CPR with 30 chest compressions followed by 2 rescue breaths. Before administering the rescue breaths, open the airway with the head-tilt, chin-lift maneuver (review Figure 43-5). Look for a foreign body in the patient's mouth and remove it if it is visible. Blind finger sweeps are no longer recommended and should not be performed.				
11. ✳	Continue with cycles of 30 compressions and 2 rescue breaths until the foreign body is expelled or advanced medical personal arrive to relieve you. Check for the foreign object each time the airway is opened to deliver the rescue breaths.				
12. ✦	Perform hand hygiene and document the event in the patient's chart.				

Name: _____

Date: _____

Document: Enter the appropriate information in the chart below.

Grading

Points Earned	_____		
Points Possible	_____	99	99
Percent Grade (Points Earned/Points Possible)	_____		
PASS:	_____	❑ YES ❑ NO ❑ N/A	❑ YES ❑ NO ❑ N/A

Instructor Sign-Off

Instructor: _____ Date: _____

Procedure 43-5:

Administering Oxygen

Objective: Administer oxygen therapy to an adult correctly within the time frame designated by the instructor.

Equipment and Supplies: Portable oxygen tank; pressure regulator; oxygen flow meter; sterile, prepackaged, disposable nasal cannula with tubing; gloves; oximeter; patient chart

Affective Behaviors: Affective behaviors provide a professional approach to a skill that enhances the patient encounter. These behaviors may also display sensitivity to a patient's rights and enhance communication. Pay close attention to these skills, which will be in **bold, italicized** font.

Notes to the Student
_____

_____

_____

_____

_____

_____

Skills Assessment Requirements

Read and familiarize yourself with the procedure; complete the minimum practice requirements (MPRs). Document each MPR using proper charting technique. Complete each procedure within a reasonable amount of time, with a minimum of 85% accuracy.

Name: _____

Date: _____

POINT VALUE ✦ = 3–6 points ✳ = 7–9 points		PRACTICE TRIAL	GRADED TRIAL # 1	GRADED TRIAL # 2	NOTES
1. ✦	Gather all needed equipment.				
2. ✦	Perform hand hygiene.				
3. ✳	**Identify the patient, and confirm the physician's order for oxygen therapy.**				
4. ✳	Check the pressure reading on the oxygen tank to ensure it has enough oxygen in it.				
5. ✦	Start the flow of oxygen by opening the cylinder.				
6. ✦	Attach the cannula tubing to the flow meter. Adjust the oxygen flow to the physician's order.				
7. ✦	Hold the cannula tips over the inside of your wrist, without touching the skin, to determine if the oxygen is flowing.				
8. ✦	Apply gloves if necessary. You may prefer to wear gloves with patients who demonstrate a chronic cough, have a nasal drip, or exhibit other characteristics of potential exposure.				
9. ✦	Place the tips of the nasal cannula into the patient's nostrils. Wrap the tubing behind the patient's ears.				
10. ✳	**Instruct the patient to breathe normally through the mouth and nose.**				

Name: _____

Date: _____

POINT VALUE ✦ = 3–6 points ✳ = 7–9 points		PRACTICE TRIAL	GRADED TRIAL # 1	GRADED TRIAL # 2	NOTES
11. ✳	Check the patient's oxygen level with an oximeter. Place the probe over the index finger and record the reading. If necessary, have the patient take a short walk to verify that the oxygen flow rate is sufficient for activity.				
12. ✳	Perform hand hygiene and document the procedure in the patient's chart.				

Name: _____

Date: _____

Document: Enter the appropriate information in the chart below.

Grading

Points Earned	_____		
Points Possible	_____	78	78
Percent Grade (Points Earned/Points Possible)	_____		
PASS:	_____	❏ YES ❏ NO ❏ N/A	❏ YES ❏ NO ❏ N/A

Instructor Sign-Off

Instructor: _____   Date: _____

Name: _____

Date: _____

Procedure 43-6:

Demonstrate the Application of a Pressure Bandage

Objective: Correctly demonstrate the application of a pressure dressing.

Equipment and Supplies: Dressing supplies or makeshift materials; gloves and other available PPE

Affective Behaviors: Affective behaviors provide a professional approach to a skill that enhances the patient encounter. These behaviors may also display sensitivity to a patient's rights and enhance communication. Pay close attention to these skills, which will be in **_bold, italicized_** font.

Notes to the Student

_____

_____

_____

_____

_____

_____

Skills Assessment Requirements

Read and familiarize yourself with the procedure; complete the minimum practice requirements (MPRs). Document each MPR using proper charting technique. Complete each procedure within a reasonable amount of time, with a minimum of 85% accuracy.

Name: _____

Date: _____

POINT VALUE ✦ = 3–6 points ✷ = 7–9 points		PRACTICE TRIAL	GRADED TRIAL # 1	GRADED TRIAL # 2	NOTES
1. ✦	Escort the patient immediately to an examination room.				
2. ✦	Perform hand hygiene.				
3. ✦	Put on disposable gloves.				
4. ✷	Under the physician's supervision, apply direct pressure with a dressing placed on the open wound. If possible, elevate the affected part.				
5. ✦	After assessment, the physician will decide if EMS should be contacted.				
6. ✦	Apply additional dressings as needed. Do not remove the original dressing.				
7. ✷	Apply pressure to pressure points as necessary and with the physician's supervision.				
8. ✷	If bleeding is controlled, anchor the dressing to maintain pressure.				
9. ✦	If the physician orders, prepare the patient for transport to an emergency care facility.				
10. ✦	Dispose of waste in a biohazard waste container.				
11. ✦	Remove and discard gloves.				
12. ✷	Perform hand hygiene and document the procedure in the patient's chart.				

Name: _____

Date: _____

Document: Enter the appropriate information in the chart below.

Grading

Points Earned	_____		
Points Possible	_____	84	84
Percent Grade (Points Earned/Points Possible)	_____		
PASS:	_____	❏ YES ❏ NO ❏ N/A	❏ YES ❏ NO ❏ N/A

Instructor Sign-Off

Instructor: _____ **Date:** _____

Procedure 43-7:

Demonstrate the Application of Triangular, Figure-Eight, and Tubular Bandages

Objective: Correctly apply triangular, figure-eight, and tubular bandages.

Equipment and Supplies: Elastic bandage; roller bandage; Kling bandage; tubular gauze and applicator; triangular bandage; tape; scissors

Affective Behaviors: Affective behaviors provide a professional approach to a skill that enhances the patient encounter. These behaviors may also display sensitivity to a patient's rights and enhance communication. Pay close attention to these skills, which will be in **_bold, italicized_** font.

Notes to the Student

_____

_____

_____

_____

_____

_____

Skills Assessment Requirements

Read and familiarize yourself with the procedure; complete the minimum practice requirements (MPRs). Document each MPR using proper charting technique. Complete each procedure within a reasonable amount of time, with a minimum of 85% accuracy.

Name: _____

Date: _____

POINT VALUE ✦ = 3–6 points ✷ = 7–9 points		PRACTICE TRIAL	GRADED TRIAL # 1	GRADED TRIAL # 2	NOTES
1. ✦	Escort the patient immediately to an examination room. You may need to assist the patient, depending on the severity, location, and type of injury.				
2. ✷	***Explain the procedure to the patient.***				
3. ✦	Perform hand hygiene.				
4. ✦	Gather necessary supplies.				
5. ✷	Apply the bandage as follows.				
	Triangular Bandage				
	Keep the injured arm as immobile as possible.				
	Carefully slide the triangular bandage under the area to be held. The two shorter sides of the triangle should be pointing toward the elbow, and the remaining longer edge should be parallel to the opposite body side.				
	Bring the lowest side of the triangle up and over the arm.				
	Tie the ends of the bandage behind and slightly to the side of the neck. Tuck the peak of the bandage in toward the elbow point of the bandage.				
	The triangular bandage may also be wrapped around the head as a turban to anchor dressings onto the head.				
	Figure-Eight Bandage				
	Place the thumb of one hand on one end of the bandage.				
	Anchor the bandage with your other hand, and then complete one circle around the extremity or body.				

POINT VALUE ✦ = 3–6 points ✳ = 7–9 points	PRACTICE TRIAL	GRADED TRIAL # 1	GRADED TRIAL # 2	NOTES
	Continue to alternate wrapping above and below the body joint or dressing and circling behind the joint or dressing area until the injured area is covered adequately. If applying a bandage to a foot, ensure that toes are exposed to evaluate circulation.			
	Tubular Bandage			
	Choose an applicator that is larger than the extremity to be bandaged.			
	Cut an approximate amount of tubular gauze bandage and slide the gathered bandage onto the applicator.			
	Slide the applicator over the extremity.			
	Hold the bandage against the proximal end of the extremity and pull the applicator approximately 1 inch past the distal end.			
	Twist the bandage gauze one complete turn.			
	Next, slide the applicator toward the proximal end of the injury.			
	Hold the proximal end of the tubular bandage gauze in place, and pull the applicator toward the distal end.			
	After pulling past the distal end, complete one twist.			
	Slide back and forth, and twist the distal end of the dressing until the injured area is adequately covered.			

Name: _____

Date: _____

POINT VALUE ✦ = 3–6 points ✱ = 7–9 points		PRACTICE TRIAL	GRADED TRIAL # 1	GRADED TRIAL # 2	NOTES
	Cut excess dressing but remember to anchor the bandage at the proximal end.				
6. ✱	**Instruct the patient to watch for signs of circulation impairment.**				
7. ✦	Perform hand hygiene.				
8. ✱	Document the procedure and patient teaching.				

Document: Enter the appropriate information in the chart below.

Grading

Points Earned	_____		
Points Possible	_____	57	57
Percent Grade (Points Earned/Points Possible)	_____		
PASS:	_____	❏ YES ❏ NO ❏ N/A	❏ YES ❏ NO ❏ N/A

Instructor Sign-Off

Instructor: _____   **Date:** _____

Name: _____

Date: _____

Procedure 43-8:

Respond to a Patient Who Has Fainted

Objective: Correctly care for a patient who has fainted, within the time limit set by the instructor.

Equipment and Supplies: Blanket; foot stool or box

Affective Behaviors: Affective behaviors provide a professional approach to a skill that enhances the patient encounter. These behaviors may also display sensitivity to a patient's rights and enhance communication. Pay close attention to these skills, which will be in **_bold, italicized_** font.

Notes to the Student

_____

_____

_____

_____

_____

_____

Skills Assessment Requirements

Read and familiarize yourself with the procedure; complete the minimum practice requirements (MPRs). Document each MPR using proper charting technique. Complete each procedure within a reasonable amount of time, with a minimum of 85% accuracy.

POINT VALUE ✦ = 3–6 points ✳ = 7–9 points		PRACTICE TRIAL	GRADED TRIAL # 1	GRADED TRIAL # 2	NOTES
1. ✦	If the patient communicates a faint feeling, help the patient sit, bend forward, and place the head on the knees. If the patient collapses with no warning, do not move the patient. The patient may have sustained a neck or back injury.				
2. ✦	Immediately notify the physician.				
3. ✦	Loosen any tight clothing, and cover the patient with a blanket for warmth.				
4. ✦	If the physician directs, use the foot stool to support the patient's legs in a raised position.				
5. ✦	If the physician directs, call for EMS.				
6. ✳	Once the emergency passes, obtain a full set of vital signs and document all activities in the patient's medical record.				

Name: _____

Date: _____

Document: Enter the appropriate information in the chart below.

Grading

Points Earned	_____		
Points Possible	_____	39	39
Percent Grade (Points Earned/Points Possible)	_____		
PASS:	_____	❑ YES ❑ NO ❑ N/A	❑ YES ❑ NO ❑ N/A

Instructor Sign-Off

Instructor: _____   **Date:** _____

Name: _____

Date: _____

Procedure 43-9:

Document an Incident

Objective: Correctly document an incident that occurred in the medical office.

Equipment and Supplies: Paper; pen; incident report template

Affective Behaviors: Affective behaviors provide a professional approach to a skill that enhances the patient encounter. These behaviors may also display sensitivity to a patient's rights and enhance communication. Pay close attention to these skills, which will be in ***bold, italicized*** font.

Notes to the Student

_____

_____

_____

_____

_____

_____

Skills Assessment Requirements

Read and familiarize yourself with the procedure; complete the minimum practice requirements (MPRs). Document each MPR using proper charting technique. Complete each procedure within a reasonable amount of time, with a minimum of 85% accuracy.

Name: _____

Date: _____

POINT VALUE ✦ = 3–6 points ✳ = 7–9 points		PRACTICE TRIAL	GRADED TRIAL # 1	GRADED TRIAL # 2	NOTES
1. ✳	Complete an incident report, reporting the care that you rendered for the patient who fainted in the office in Procedure 43-8.				
2. ✦	Store the incident report separate from the patient chart.				

Name: _____

Date: _____

Document: Enter the appropriate information in the chart below.

Grading

Points Earned	_____		
Points Possible	_____	157	157
Percent Grade (Points Earned/Points Possible)	_____		
PASS:	_____	❑ YES ❑ NO ❑ N/A	❑ YES ❑ NO ❑ N/A

Instructor Sign-Off

Instructor: _____   **Date:** _____

Procedure 43-10:

Demonstrate the Application of a Splint

Objective: To correctly apply a splint with minimal movement to the affected extremity and without impairment to circulation or neurological status.

Equipment and Supplies: Makeshift or sterile dressing supplies; stiff or solid materials to immobilize the extremity; bandages or strips of material to secure splint materials

Affective Behaviors: Affective behaviors provide a professional approach to a skill that enhances the patient encounter. These behaviors may also display sensitivity to a patient's rights and enhance communication. Pay close attention to these skills, which will be in **_bold, italicized_** font.

Notes to the Student

_____

_____

_____

_____

_____

_____

Skills Assessment Requirements

Read and familiarize yourself with the procedure; complete the minimum practice requirements (MPRs). Document each MPR using proper charting technique. Complete each procedure within a reasonable amount of time, with a minimum of 85% accuracy.

Name: _____

Date: _____

POINT VALUE ✦ = 3–6 points ✳ = 7–9 points	PRACTICE TRIAL	GRADED TRIAL # 1	GRADED TRIAL # 2	NOTES
1. ✦ **Identify the patient and introduce yourself.**				
2. ✦ Obtain vital signs.				
3. ✦ Ask the patient, if conscious, to speak his or her name.				
4. ✳ **Ask about medication allergies and any prescription or over-the-counter medications the patient may be taking. Also inquire about the patient's medical history.**				
5. ✳ Assess the area of suspected fracture for bruising, bleeding, and open areas or protruding bones.				
6. ✦ Moving the limb as little as possible, and with gentle traction on the distal side, place the splint with padding under the limb or alongside the limb. You may have to ask an other clinical staff member for help to ensure the least amount of discomfort for the least amount of time.				
7. ✦ Place sterile dressings or clean makeshift dressings gently over open areas.				
8. ✳ Secure the splint by wrapping bandages or strips of material around the splint and the limb. The ties must be above and below the joints on both sides of the suspected fracture.				
9. ✦ Add additional ties as necessary along the length of the splint.				

Name: _____

Date: _____

POINT VALUE ✦ = 3–6 points ✴ = 7–9 points		PRACTICE TRIAL	GRADED TRIAL # 1	GRADED TRIAL # 2	NOTES
10. ✴	If possible, leave an exposed area, such as toes or fingers, so that circulation can be monitored.				
11. ✴	The splint should be snug enough to immobilize the limb but not tight.				

Document: Enter the appropriate information in the chart below.

Grading

Points Earned	_____		
Points Possible	_____	81	81
Percent Grade (Points Earned/Points Possible)	_____		
PASS:	_____	❏ YES ❏ NO ❏ N/A	❏ YES ❏ NO ❏ N/A

Instructor Sign-Off

Instructor: _____   **Date:** _____

Procedure 43-11:

Create a Medical Emergency Plan

Objective: To create a medical emergency plan.

Equipment and Supplies: Pen; paper; emergency kit composed of water, canned food, can opener, snacks, personal hygiene products, first aid kit, trash bag, gloves, battery-powered radio, flashlight, extra batteries, whistle, tools, protective masks, diapers, powdered milk, formula, baby wipes, crash cart

Affective Behaviors: Affective behaviors provide a professional approach to a skill that enhances the patient encounter. These behaviors may also display sensitivity to a patient's rights and enhance communication. Pay close attention to these skills, which will be in **bold, italicized** font.

Notes to the Student

_____

_____

_____

_____

_____

_____

Skills Assessment Requirements

Read and familiarize yourself with the procedure; complete the minimum practice requirements (MPRs). Document each MPR using proper charting technique. Complete each procedure within a reasonable amount of time, with a minimum of 85% accuracy.

POINT VALUE ✦ = 3–6 points ✶ = 7–9 points		PRACTICE TRIAL	GRADED TRIAL # 1	GRADED TRIAL # 2	NOTES
1. ✦	Develop an emergency kit using the above listed supplies and any others you desire, explaining what each supply item might be used for in an emergency.				
2. ✦	Document a policy that would cover the actions needed in each of the following situations that might occur in the medical office: a. Choking b. Lack of pulse c. Shortness of breath d. Shock e. Bleeding f. Epistaxis g. Superficial burn h. Hyperthermia i. Seizures j. Fainting				
3. ✦	Determine the best location to store your medical emergency policy and kit.				
4. ✶	Develop a memorandum to the physician stating that you have developed the Medical Emergency Plan.				

Name: _____

Date: _____

Document: Enter the appropriate information in the chart below.

Grading

Points Earned	_____		
Points Possible	_____	27	27
Percent Grade (Points Earned/Points Possible)	_____		
PASS:	_____	❏ YES ❏ NO ❏ N/A	❏ YES ❏ NO ❏ N/A

Instructor Sign-Off

Instructor: _____ Date: _____

Procedure 43-12:

Develop an Environmental Exposure Safety Plan

Objective: To develop an environmental exposure plan that can be used in all hazards.

Equipment and Supplies: Pen; paper; computer; copy machine; various emergency supplies—waterproof containers, flashlights, batteries, bottles of water, nonperishable food, duct tape, plastic sheeting, masks, bandages, alcohol wipes, blankets, gloves, tweezers, scissors, self-powered radio, assorted medications; map of a hypothetical medical office; hypothetical staff chart

Affective Behaviors: Affective behaviors provide a professional approach to a skill that enhances the patient encounter. These behaviors may also display sensitivity to a patient's rights and enhance communication. Pay close attention to these skills, which will be in ***bold, italicized*** font.

Notes to the Student

_____

_____

_____

_____

_____

_____

Skills Assessment Requirements

Read and familiarize yourself with the procedure; complete the minimum practice requirements (MPRs). Document each MPR using proper charting technique. Complete each procedure within a reasonable amount of time, with a minimum of 85% accuracy.

POINT VALUE ✦ = 3–6 points ✴ = 7–9 points	PRACTICE TRIAL	GRADED TRIAL # 1	GRADED TRIAL # 2	NOTES
1. ✦ Create an emergency kit that can be used by your office in the event of an environmental emergency. Supplies may include flashlights, batteries, bottles of water, nonperishable food, manual can opener, bandages, alcohol wipes, blankets, vinyl or latex gloves, tweezers, scissors, self-powered radio, and medications (ibuprofen, acetaminophen, antihistamines, antibiotic ointment, tetanus vaccines, etc.).				
2. ✦ Enclose the kit in a waterproof container.				
3. ✦ Place the kit in a safe area, such as a medicine closet or storage closet.				
4. ✴ Create evacuation plans for every room in the sample medical office that has been given to you.				
5. ✴ Create a delineation chart that outlines responsibilities of office staff members in the event of an environmental emergency.				
6. ✴ Create a list of safety zones that can be used in the event of an emergency (e.g., a safety zone in the event of a tornado, an outdoor safety zone in the event of a fire, a safety zone in the event of a flood).				
7. ✴ Document development of policy for physician.				

Name: _____

Date: _____

Document: Enter the appropriate information in the chart below.

Grading

Points Earned	_____		
Points Possible	_____	54	54
Percent Grade (Points Earned/Points Possible)	_____		
PASS:	_____	❏ YES ❏ NO ❏ N/A	❏ YES ❏ NO ❏ N/A

Instructor Sign-Off

Instructor: _____   **Date:** _____

Procedure 44-1:

Completing a Laboratory Requisition and Preparing a Specimen for Transport to an Outside Laboratory

Objective: Accurately complete a laboratory requisition form for testing as ordered by the physician, obtain the required specimen(s), and prepare specimen(s) for transport to an outside laboratory.

Equipment and Supplies: Physician's order for laboratory tests; patient's record; pen; laboratory requisition form; gloves; specimen container; laboratory logbook; biohazard waste container

Affective Behaviors: Affective behaviors provide a professional approach to a skill that enhances the patient encounter. These behaviors may also display sensitivity to a patient's rights and enhance communication. Pay close attention to these skills, which will be in **bold, *italicized*** font.

Notes to the Student

_____

_____

_____

_____

_____

_____

Skills Assessment Requirements

Read and familiarize yourself with the procedure; complete the minimum practice requirements (MPRs). Document each MPR using proper charting technique. Complete each procedure within a reasonable amount of time, with a minimum of 85% accuracy.

POINT VALUE ✦ = 3–6 points ✱ = 7–9 points		PRACTICE TRIAL	GRADED TRIAL # 1	GRADED TRIAL # 2	NOTES
1. ✦	Check the patient's record for orders for specific lab tests.				
2. ✦	Verify which lab will be doing the testing and locate the lab's required requisition form.				
3. ✦	Complete the patient demographic section.				
4. ✦	Complete the section requiring the physician's name, address, phone number, and account number.				
5. ✦	Complete the patient's insurance and billing information.				
6. ✱	Mark each box to indicate each test ordered by the physician. If a test is ordered that is not listed on the requisition, write in the name of the test on the lines provided.				
7. ✱	Indicate the type and source of the specimen to be tested.				
8. ✱	Enter the patient's diagnosis on the requisition as needed. If no diagnosis has been made, then code the patient's symptoms.				
9. ✱	Complete the patient authorization to release and assign the benefits as needed.				
10. ✦	Assemble the equipment and supplies needed to obtain the specimen.				
11. ✦	Perform hand hygiene and apply gloves.				

Name: _____

Date: _____

POINT VALUE ✦ = 3–6 points ✳ = 7–9 points		PRACTICE TRIAL	GRADED TRIAL # 1	GRADED TRIAL # 2	NOTES
12. ✳	Obtain the specimen required after explaining the procedure to the patient.				
13. ✳	Label the specimen with the patient's name, date, physician's name, time of collection, and other information required by the facility.				
14. ✳	Initial the laboratory requisition and complete the date and time the specimen was obtained.				
15. ✳	Process the specimens, and if they are not to be sent out until later in the day, store them according to laboratory policies and procedures manual requirements.				
16. ✳	Attach the laboratory requisition securely to the specimen before sending.				
17. ✦	Remove gloves; dispose of them in the biohazard waste container. Perform hand hygiene.				
18. ✦	Document the information in the patient's record.				
19. ✳	Record the specimen in the laboratory logbook, indicating date, time of collection, type and source of the specimen, tests ordered, where samples were sent, and the date they were sent.				

Document: Enter the appropriate information in the chart below.

Grading

Points Earned	_____		
Points Possible	_____	141	141
Percent Grade (Points Earned/Points Possible)	_____		
PASS:	_____	❏ YES ❏ NO ❏ N/A	❏ YES ❏ NO ❏ N/A

Instructor Sign-Off

Instructor: _____ **Date:** _____

Procedure 44-2:

Monitoring and Following Up on Laboratory Test Results

Objective: Review incoming laboratory results and follow up with patient per physician's orders.

Equipment and Supplies: Patient's record; laboratory test results; pen; log of patient's laboratory results

Affective Behaviors: Affective behaviors provide a professional approach to a skill that enhances the patient encounter. These behaviors may also display sensitivity to a patient's rights and enhance communication. Pay close attention to these skills, which will be in **bold, _italicized_** font.

Notes to the Student

_____

_____

_____

_____

_____

_____

Skills Assessment Requirements

Read and familiarize yourself with the procedure; complete the minimum practice requirements (MPRs). Document each MPR using proper charting technique. Complete each procedure within a reasonable amount of time, with a minimum of 85% accuracy.

POINT VALUE ✦ = 3–6 points ✶ = 7–9 points		PRACTICE TRIAL	GRADED TRIAL # 1	GRADED TRIAL # 2	NOTES
	Note: Follow the facility policy on contacting patients when results are abnormal. Results are not to be released to the patient unless authorized by the physician.				
1. ✶	Review incoming lab results and compare with the reference values provided by the analyzing laboratory. Many laboratories highlight or indicate abnormal results on the lab result sheets with H or L.				
2. ✦	Highlight any abnormal results per facility policy.				
3. ✶	Obtain the patient's medical record, attach the new laboratory results, and submit the chart to the physician for review. Accuracy when documenting results is critical.				
4. ✦	Follow the physician's orders regarding scheduling, appointments, or repeat testing.				
5. ✦	Document the patient's record accordingly.				

Name: _____

Date: _____

Document: Enter the appropriate information in the chart below.

Grading

Points Earned	_____		
Points Possible	_____	39	39
Percent Grade (Points Earned/Points Possible)	_____		
PASS:	_____	❏ YES ❏ NO ❏ N/A	❏ YES ❏ NO ❏ N/A

Instructor Sign-Off

Instructor: _____   **Date:** _____

Procedure 44-3:

Evaluating a Contour TS Glucometer Using Control Solutions

Objective: Determine the effectiveness of a glucometer through quality control testing.

Equipment and Supplies: Bayer Contour TS glucometer, testing strips, and control solutions; wax paper; pen; lab coat; quality control log

Affective Behaviors: Affective behaviors provide a professional approach to a skill that enhances the patient encounter. These behaviors may also display sensitivity to a patient's rights and enhance communication. Pay close attention to these skills, which will be in *bold, italicized* font.

Notes to the Student

_____

_____

_____

_____

_____

Skills Assessment Requirements

Read and familiarize yourself with the procedure; complete the minimum practice requirements (MPRs). Document each MPR using proper charting technique. Complete each procedure within a reasonable amount of time, with a minimum of 85% accuracy.

POINT VALUE ✦ = 3–6 points ✳ = 7–9 points		PRACTICE TRIAL	GRADED TRIAL # 1	GRADED TRIAL # 2	NOTES
1. ✦	Assemble the equipment and supplies. Check the expiration and discard dates for the control solutions and test strips. Make sure the test strip is dry, clean, and intact.				
2. ✳	Hold the test strip with the gray end facing up and insert into the orange port at the front of the meter.				
3. ✦	The machine will automatically turn on. Once the test strip and the drop of blood appear on the screen, wait for the blood drop to flash.				
4. ✦	Before opening, gently rock the control bottle to mix the solution evenly.				
5. ✳	Squeeze a small drop of the control solution onto a piece of wax paper and recap the solution. Do not apply the solution directly onto the test strip.				
6. ✳	Immediately touch the tip of the test strip to the drop of control solution. Hold it in place until the machine beeps.				
7. ✳	Compare the test result with the control range printed on the bottom of the test strip bottle label. If the result falls outside the specified range, consult the manufacturer's instructions for the error codes and symbols chart. Compare the code or symbol that appears on the screen. Repeat the test, if necessary.				

Name: _____

Date: _____

		PRACTICE TRIAL	GRADED TRIAL #1	GRADED TRIAL #2	NOTES
8. ✳	Record the results in the quality control log.				
9. ✳	Remove the test strip and dispose.				
10. ✳	Repeat the above steps with a different control solution, as required.				

Document: Enter the appropriate information in the chart below.

Grading

Points Earned	_____		
Points Possible	_____	81	81
Percent Grade (Points Earned/Points Possible)	_____		
PASS:	_____	❏ YES ❏ NO ❏ N/A	❏ YES ❏ NO ❏ N/A

Instructor Sign-Off

Instructor: _____ **Date:** _____

Procedure 44-4:

Using and Cleaning the Microscope

Objective: Observe a slide under 10×, 40×, and oil immersion properly, and clean and store microscope correctly.

Equipment and Supplies: Binocular compound microscope; specimen slide; lens paper; lens cleaner; dust cover for microscope

Affective Behaviors: Affective behaviors provide a professional approach to a skill that enhances the patient encounter. These behaviors may also display sensitivity to a patient's rights and enhance communication. Pay close attention to these skills, which will be in **bold, *italicized*** font.

Notes to the Student

_____

_____

_____

_____

_____

_____

Skills Assessment Requirements

Read and familiarize yourself with the procedure; complete the minimum practice requirements (MPRs). Document each MPR using proper charting technique. Complete each procedure within a reasonable amount of time, with a minimum of 85% accuracy.

POINT VALUE		PRACTICE TRIAL	GRADED TRIAL # 1	GRADED TRIAL # 2	NOTES
✦ = 3–6 points ✴ = 7–9 points					
1. ✦	Always carry the microscope with one hand on the arm and one hand under the base.				
2. ✦	Make sure the stage is in the down position before starting.				
3. ✦	Clean objectives with lens paper starting with 10× and ending with oil immersion.				
4. ✴	Turn on the light and rotate the nosepiece until the 10× objective is directly over the slide. Place the prepared slide on the stage.				
5. ✦	Use the coarse adjustment knob to raise the stage until the objective is close to the slide on the stage.				
6. ✴	Look through the eyepiece and adjust the coarse focus knob until the microscope field is seen (a round circle of bright light).				
7. ✴	Use the fine adjustment knob for a clearer image.				
8. ✴	Open the diaphragm and, if necessary, adjust the rheostat to focus.				
9. ✴	Raise or lower the condenser to alter light refraction. The condenser is usually lowered when using 10× power.				
10. ✴	Observe the slide.				
11. ✴	Change the objective to 40× and readjust as needed. Move the objective and place a drop of oil on the slide before completing the turn to oil immersion lens.				

Name: _____

Date: _____

Document: Enter the appropriate information in the chart below.

Grading

Points Earned	_____		
Points Possible	_____	84	84
Percent Grade (Points Earned/Points Possible)	_____		
PASS:	_____	❏ YES ❏ NO ❏ N/A	❏ YES ❏ NO ❏ N/A

Instructor Sign-Off

Instructor: _____   Date: _____

Name: _____

Date: _____

Procedure 45-1:

Obtaining a Throat Culture

Objective: Collect a throat or nasopharyngeal culture without contaminating the specimen.

Equipment and Supplies: Culturette system; laboratory requisition; tongue depressor; gloves; biohazard waste container

Affective Behaviors: Affective behaviors provide a professional approach to a skill that enhances the patient encounter. These behaviors may also display sensitivity to a patient's rights and enhance communication. Pay close attention to these skills, which will be in *bold, italicized* font.

Notes to the Student

Follow Standard Precautions and safety guidelines when working with body fluid samples. Use care to avoid splashing or spilling body fluids. Wipe up all spills using guidelines established by OSHA.

_____

_____

_____

_____

_____

_____

Skills Assessment Requirements

Read and familiarize yourself with the procedure; complete the minimum practice requirements (MPRs). Document each MPR using proper charting technique. Complete each procedure within a reasonable amount of time, with a minimum of 85% accuracy.

Name: _____

Date: _____

POINT VALUE ✦ = 3–6 points ✶ = 7–9 points		PRACTICE TRIAL	GRADED TRIAL # 1	GRADED TRIAL # 2	NOTES
1. ✦	Assemble equipment and Culturette system.				
2. ✶	**Identify the patient and explain the procedure.**				
3. ✦	Perform hand hygiene and apply gloves.				
4. ✶	**Position the patient facing a light source and have the patient open his or her mouth as wide as possible.** The gag reflex may be diminished if the patient says "Aaaah."				
5. ✦	Remove the sterile swab from the culturette.				
6. ✶	Depress the tongue, insert the swab, and roll it firmly across the back of the patient's throat or nasopharyngeal area where infected. Be careful not to contaminate the swab on the teeth, lips, tongue, or inside of the cheeks. Avoid touching the uvula to prevent gagging.				
7. ✶	Insert the swab into a plastic vial. Crush the internal vial of transport medium, making sure that the swab is saturated.				
8. ✶	Place the transport medium in labeled mailing or transporting envelope and staple shut if necessary. If being evaluated in the POL, immediately inoculate the culture plate, and apply a bacitracin disk according to office procedure.				

Name: _____

Date: _____

POINT VALUE ✦ = 3–6 points ✱ = 7–9 points		PRACTICE TRIAL	GRADED TRIAL # 1	GRADED TRIAL # 2	NOTES
9. ✦	Remove and dispose of gloves.				
10. ✦	Perform hand hygiene.				
11. ✱	Document the procedure in the patient's record.				

Name: _____

Date: _____

Document: Enter the appropriate information in the chart below.

Grading

Points Earned	_____		
Points Possible	_____	87	87
Percent Grade (Points Earned/Points Possible)	_____		
PASS:	_____	❏ YES ❏ NO ❏ N/A	❏ YES ❏ NO ❏ N/A

Instructor Sign-Off

Instructor: _____   **Date:** _____

Procedure 45-2:

Obtaining a Sputum Specimen for Culture

Objective: Collect a sputum specimen without contaminating the specimen.

Equipment and Supplies: Sterile labeled sputum container with lid; lab requisition form; gloves; biohazard waste container

Affective Behaviors: Affective behaviors provide a professional approach to a skill that enhances the patient encounter. These behaviors may also display sensitivity to a patient's rights and enhance communication. Pay close attention to these skills, which will be in **bold, *italicized*** font.

Notes to the Student

Follow Standard Precautions and safety guidelines when working with body fluid samples. Use care to avoid splashing or spilling body fluids. Wipe up all spills using the guidelines established by OSHA.

_____

_____

_____

_____

_____

_____

Skills Assessment Requirements

Read and familiarize yourself with the procedure; complete the minimum practice requirements (MPRs). Document each MPR using proper charting technique. Complete each procedure within a reasonable amount of time, with a minimum of 85% accuracy.

POINT VALUE ✦ = 3–6 points ✳ = 7–9 points		PRACTICE TRIAL	GRADED TRIAL # 1	GRADED TRIAL # 2	NOTES
1. ✦	**_Identify the patient._**				
2. ✳	**_Explain the procedure and give written instructions that the patient can take home, if necessary. Explain that the patient should breathe in or out deeply 2 to 4 times and perform a few low, deep coughs to raise sputum._** This avoids getting only saliva. The first morning specimen, collected before eating or drinking, usually provides **_the best sample._** a. Cough deeply and expel fluid into center of container and close lid immediately. b. Make sure no other fluids, such as tears, nasal mucus, or saliva, find their way into the cup. c. Fit the lid securely, then write the time and date the specimen was obtained. d. Bring the specimen into the physician's office as soon as possible, or place it in a refrigerator for no longer than 2 hours.				
3. ✦	Perform hand hygiene and apply gloves.				
4. ✳	Label the transport envelope with information, staple it shut, and transport sample immediately.				
5. ✦	Remove and dispose of gloves and perform hand hygiene.				
6. ✳	Document the procedure in the patient's record.				

Name: _____

Date: _____

Document: Enter the appropriate information in the chart below.

Grading

Points Earned	_____		
Points Possible	_____	45	45
Percent Grade (Points Earned/Points Possible)	_____		
PASS:	_____	❏ YES ❏ NO ❏ N/A	❏ YES ❏ NO ❏ N/A

Instructor Sign-Off

Instructor: _____   **Date:** _____

Procedure 45-3:

Obtaining a Stool Specimen for Ova and Parasites

Objective: Instruct a patient to collect a stool sample for ova and parasites using the correct infection control and procedure. Both fresh and preserved specimens are required.

Equipment and Supplies: Stool collection kit with container for fresh specimen and vials for preserved specimen (formalin and polyvinyl alcohol); bedpan or container for collection of stool; tongue depressors; sterile applicator sticks; mailing container; labels; laboratory request form; gloves; biohazard waste container

Affective Behaviors: Affective behaviors provide a professional approach to a skill that enhances the patient encounter. These behaviors may also display sensitivity to a patient's rights and enhance communication. Pay close attention to these skills, which will be in **_bold, italicized_** font.

Notes to the Student

Follow Standard Precautions and safety guidelines when working with body fluid samples. Use care to avoid splashing or spilling body fluids. Wipe up all spills using guidelines established by OSHA.

_____

_____

_____

_____

_____

_____

Skills Assessment Requirements

Read and familiarize yourself with the procedure; complete the minimum practice requirements (MPRs). Document each MPR using proper charting technique. Complete each procedure within a reasonable amount of time, with a minimum of 85% accuracy.

POINT VALUE ✦ = 3–6 points ✳ = 7–9 points		PRACTICE TRIAL	GRADED TRIAL # 1	GRADED TRIAL # 2	NOTES
1. ✦	Perform hand hygiene.				
2. ✦	Check orders and assemble equipment and supplies.				
3. ✳	*Identify the patient and explain the procedure, giving written instructions as well. Do not overuse medical terminology, which might cause the patient to misunderstand your instructions. Remind the patient not to urinate or put toilet tissue into container.*				
4. ✳	*Instruct the patient to defecate in a container or bedpan, if available.* If the patient is collecting the specimen at home, give the patient written instructions including diagrams.				
5. ✦	When the patient returns with the specimen, apply gloves.				
6. ✳	Using a tongue depressor, take a small amount of stool from different parts of the specimen and place in each vial, using a new depressor or sterile wooden applicator stick for each vial. Make sure that no other contaminants are included (toilet paper, toilet water, or urine).				
7. ✳	Fill out the lab request form and wrap it around the container, securing it with a rubber band.				
8. ✳	Place the specimen container in a proper mailing container.				
9. ✦	Deliver or mail the specimen container to the outside laboratory facility.				

Name: _____

Date: _____

Document: Enter the appropriate information in the chart below.

Grading

Points Earned	_____		
Points Possible	_____	69	69
Percent Grade (Points Earned/Points Possible)	_____		
PASS:	_____	❏ YES ❏ NO ❏ N/A	❏ YES ❏ NO ❏ N/A

Instructor Sign-Off

Instructor: _____   **Date:** _____

Procedure 45-4:

Obtaining a Stool Specimen for Examination for Pinworms

Objective: Collect a rectal swab using cellulose tape for pinworm examination.

Equipment and Supplies: Glass slide; clear tape (not transparent or double-sided); tongue depressor; gauze; microscope; small square of paper; lab requisition form

Affective Behaviors: Affective behaviors provide a professional approach to a skill that enhances the patient encounter. These behaviors may also display sensitivity to a patient's rights and enhance communication. Pay close attention to these skills, which will be in **bold, italicized** font.

Notes to the Student

_____

_____

_____

_____

_____

_____

Skills Assessment Requirements

Read and familiarize yourself with the procedure; complete the minimum practice requirements (MPRs). Document each MPR using proper charting technique. Complete each procedure within a reasonable amount of time, with a minimum of 85% accuracy.

Name: _____

Date: _____

POINT VALUE ✦ = 3–6 points ✳ = 7–9 points		PRACTICE TRIAL	GRADED TRIAL # 1	GRADED TRIAL # 2	NOTES
1. ✦	Gather equipment and supplies.				
2. ✳	Label one end of the microscope slide with the patient's name and date. Prepare slide by attaching the sticky side of a piece of cellulose tape to the slide surface. Put the microscope slide on top of a tongue depressor and loop the tape back over the end of the tongue depressor to expose the sticky side of the tape.				
3. ✦	Perform hand hygiene and apply gloves.				
4. ✳	Prepare the patient on examination table or parent's lap with the anal area exposed.				
5. ✳	Press the tape to the area around both sides of the anus, using the tongue depressor to help press on the tape.				
6. ✳	Remove the tape from the patient's skin and fold it back over the slide, sticky side against the slide.				
7. ✦	Smooth the tape against the slide with gauze.				
8. ✦	The physician will examine the slide for presence of pinworms or ova.				
9. ✦	Dispose of all waste; perform hand hygiene.				
10. ✳	Fill out the lab requisition form and document the procedure appropriately.				

Document: Enter the appropriate information in the chart below.

Grading

Points Earned	_____		
Points Possible	_____	75	75
Percent Grade (Points Earned/Points Possible)	_____		
PASS:	_____	❏ YES ❏ NO ❏ N/A	❏ YES ❏ NO ❏ N/A

Instructor Sign-Off

Instructor: _____   Date: _____

Procedure 45-5:

Preparing a Smear

Objective: Prepare a smear for microscopic examination without error.

Equipment and Supplies: Frosted slides; specimen from Culturette applicator or inoculating loop; Bunsen burner; inoculating loop (or swab); microscope; oil immersion; gloves; biohazard waste container.

Affective Behaviors: Affective behaviors provide a professional approach to a skill that enhances the patient encounter. These behaviors may also display sensitivity to a patient's rights and enhance communication. Pay close attention to these skills, which will be in *bold, italicized* font.

Notes to the Student

Follow Standard Precautions and safety guidelines when working with body fluid samples. Use care to avoid splashing or spilling body fluids. Wipe up all spills using guidelines established by OSHA.

_____

_____

_____

_____

_____

_____

Skills Assessment Requirements

Read and familiarize yourself with the procedure; complete the minimum practice requirements (MPRs). Document each MPR using proper charting technique. Complete each procedure within a reasonable amount of time, with a minimum of 85% accuracy.

POINT VALUE ✦ = 3–6 points ✶ = 7–9 points		PRACTICE TRIAL	GRADED TRIAL # 1	GRADED TRIAL # 2	NOTES
1. ✦	Perform hand hygiene and apply gloves.				
2. ✦	Assemble equipment.				
3. ✶	Label a clean slide with patient's name, date, and type of specimen.				
4. ✶	Collect a specimen sample. To transfer a swabbed specimen to a slide, roll the swab over the entire slide. To transfer a specimen from a culture medium, use a sterile needle or loop to pick up the material from one type of colony, place it in a drop of sterile saline on the slide, and spread it gently over two-thirds of the slide.				
5. ✦	Allow the slide to air dry for 20 to 30 minutes.				
6. ✶	Hold the slide with thumb forceps and pass the slide over the Bunsen burner flame. This heat fixes the specimen to the slide in the process known as smear fixation. Let the slide cool. If open flame is unavailable, flood the dry smear with methanol and let it dry to fix the slide.				
7. ✦	The slide is then ready to be stained.				

Name: _____

Date: _____

Document: Enter the appropriate information in the chart below.

Grading

Points Earned	_____		
Points Possible	_____	51	51
Percent Grade (Points Earned/Points Possible)	_____		
PASS:	_____	❏ YES ❏ NO ❏ N/A	❏ YES ❏ NO ❏ N/A

Instructor Sign-Off

Instructor: _____   **Date:** _____

Name: _____

Date: _____

Procedure 45-6:

Prepare a Wet Mount Slide

Objective: Prepare a wet mount slide.

Equipment and Supplies: Clean, dry slide, frosted; cover slip; saline; specimen from a Culturette applicator or swab; paper/pen; microscope; gloves

Affective Behaviors: Affective behaviors provide a professional approach to a skill that enhances the patient encounter. These behaviors may also display sensitivity to a patient's rights and enhance communication. Pay close attention to these skills, which will be in **bold, _italicized_** font.

Notes to the Student

Follow Standard Precautions and safety guidelines when working with body fluid samples. Use care to avoid splashing or spilling body fluids. Wipe up all spills using guidelines established by OSHA.

_____

_____

_____

_____

_____

Skills Assessment Requirements

Read and familiarize yourself with the procedure; complete the minimum practice requirements (MPRs). Document each MPR using proper charting technique. Complete each procedure within a reasonable amount of time, with a minimum of 85% accuracy.

POINT VALUE ✦ = 3–6 points ✱ = 7–9 points		PRACTICE TRIAL	GRADED TRIAL # 1	GRADED TRIAL # 2	NOTES
1. ✦	Perform hand hygiene and apply gloves.				
2. ✱	Label dry slide with the patient's name and date.				
3. ✱	Inoculate the dry slide by rolling a swab containing the specimen across the surface.				
4. ✱	Place a drop of saline solution on top of the specimen.				
5. ✱	Place the cover slip on top of the smeared slide. Note: The following steps would be performed by a physician or laboratory specialist.				
6. ✱	Observe the wet mount slide immediately under the microscope.				
7. ✦	Special stains may be used to enhance characteristics.				
8. ✦	Note what is observed, remove the slide, and dispose of it properly.				
9. ✦	Remove gloves and perform hand hygiene.				
10. ✱	Chart the findings on the patient's record.				

Name: _____

Date: _____

Document: Enter the appropriate information in the chart below.

Grading

Points Earned	_____		
Points Possible	_____	78	78
Percent Grade (Points Earned/Points Possible)	_____		
PASS:	_____	❏ YES ❏ NO ❏ N/A	❏ YES ❏ NO ❏ N/A

Instructor Sign-Off

Instructor: _____   Date: _____

Procedure 45-7:

Perform a Gram Stain

Objective: Prepare a slide for a Gram stain to differentiate a gram-positive organism from a gram-negative organism.

Equipment and Supplies: Gram-stain kit with decolorizer; culture specimen; slides; Bunsen burner or methanol; staining rack; water wash bottle; water; immersion oil; stopwatch; gloves; slide stand; paper towels; biohazard waste container

Affective Behaviors: Affective behaviors provide a professional approach to a skill that enhances the patient encounter. These behaviors may also display sensitivity to a patient's rights and enhance communication. Pay close attention to these skills, which will be in **_bold, italicized_** font.

Notes to the Student

Follow Standard Precautions and safety guidelines when working with body fluid samples. Use care to avoid splashing or spilling body fluids. Wipe up all spills using guidelines established by OSHA.

_____

_____

_____

_____

_____

Skills Assessment Requirements

Read and familiarize yourself with the procedure; complete the minimum practice requirements (MPRs). Document each MPR using proper charting technique. Complete each procedure within a reasonable amount of time, with a minimum of 85% accuracy.

POINT VALUE ✦ = 3–6 points ✳ = 7–9 points		PRACTICE TRIAL	GRADED TRIAL # 1	GRADED TRIAL # 2	NOTES
1. ✦	Perform hand hygiene and apply gloves.				
2. ✦	Assemble equipment.				
3. ✳	Make a smear, label it, air dry the smear, and use heat or methanol to fix.				
4. ✦	Place slide on staining rack, smear side up.				
5. ✳	Pour crystal violet solution all over the slide; let it stand for 1 minute.				
6. ✳	Tilt the slide to drain the excess crystal violet stain and rinse with water.				
7. ✳	Pour Gram's iodine stain all over the slide; let it stand for 1 minute.				
8. ✳	Tilt the slide to drain excess iodine and rinse with water.				
9. ✳	Gently pour decolorizer with alcohol-acetone all over the slide for 15 seconds or until the color blue stops running.				
10. ✳	Rinse with water.				
11. ✳	Pour safranine stain all over the slide; let it stand for 30 seconds.				
12. ✳	Tilt the slide to drain the excess safranine and rinse with water. Wipe the back of the slide.				

POINT VALUE ✦ = 3–6 points ✶ = 7–9 points		PRACTICE TRIAL	GRADED TRIAL # 1	GRADED TRIAL # 2	NOTES
13. ✶	Stand the slide on end on a paper towel or in a slide drying rack, and air dry. *Note:* Examination of a Gram-stained slide is beyond the scope of practice of the medical assistant. It should be performed by a physician or laboratory specialist.				
14. ✶	Examine under the microscope, using oil immersion lens and oil.				

Document: Enter the appropriate information in the chart below.

Grading

Points Earned	_____		
Points Possible	_____	117	117
Percent Grade (Points Earned/Points Possible)	_____		
PASS:	_____	❏ YES ❏ NO ❏ N/A	❏ YES ❏ NO ❏ N/A

Instructor Sign-Off

_____

Instructor: _____   **Date:** _____

Procedure 45-8:

Perform Rapid Group A Strep Testing

Objective: Test a throat swab specimen for Group A Strep.

Equipment and Supplies: Labeled throat swab specimen; BD Check Group A Strep Kit; personal protective equipment; timer; biohazard waste container

Affective Behaviors: Affective behaviors provide a professional approach to a skill that enhances the patient encounter. These behaviors may also display sensitivity to a patient's rights and enhance communication. Pay close attention to these skills, which will be in **_bold, italicized_** font.

Notes to the Student

Follow Standard Precautions and safety guidelines when working with body fluid samples. Use care to avoid splashing or spilling body fluids. Wipe up all spills using the guidelines.

_____

_____

_____

_____

_____

Skills Assessment Requirements

Read and familiarize yourself with the procedure; complete the minimum practice requirements (MPRs). Document each MPR using proper charting technique. Complete each procedure within a reasonable amount of time, with a minimum of 85% accuracy.

POINT VALUE ✦ = 3–6 points ✱ = 7–9 points		PRACTICE TRIAL	GRADED TRIAL # 1	GRADED TRIAL # 2	NOTES
1. ✦	Wash your hands and gather supplies.				
2. ✦	Verify that the name on the throat swab container and lab requisition form matches.				
3. ✦	Perform hand hygiene and apply gloves.				
4.	Remove the test strip from the sealed foil pouch and begin testing immediately.				
5. ✱	Add 4 full drops of Reagent A bottle (red) to the extraction test tube. Add 4 full drops of Reagent B bottle (clear) to the extraction test tube. Tap the bottom of the tube to mix; the solution should turn yellow.				
6. ✱	Insert the specimen swab into the test tube solution and rotate it 10 times. Leave it in place for 1 minute, then slowly remove while squeezing the swab along the side of the container so that most of the liquid remains. Discard the swab.				
7. ✱	Insert the test strip into the solution with the arrows pointing down; leave in place. Start the timer.				
8. ✱	Read results in 5 minutes. A pink or red line should be noted in the control area; if not present, the test is invalid and must be repeated. If a second line appears (any shade of pink or red), the test is positive for Strep. The more concentrated the sample is, the darker the second line will be.				

POINT VALUE ✦ = 3–6 points ✱ = 7–9 points		PRACTICE TRIAL	GRADED TRIAL # 1	GRADED TRIAL # 2	NOTES
9. ✦	Remove and dispose of gloves and perform hand hygiene.				
10. ✱	Document the procedure in the patient's record.				

Name: _____

Date: _____

Document: Enter the appropriate information in the chart below.

Grading

Points Earned	_____		
Points Possible	_____	78	78
Percent Grade (Points Earned/Points Possible)	_____		
PASS:	_____	❑ YES ❑ NO ❑ N/A	❑ YES ❑ NO ❑ N/A

Instructor Sign-Off

Instructor: _____ **Date:** _____

Procedure 46-1:

Collecting a 24-Hour Urine Specimen

Objective: Instruct a patient how to properly collect a 24-hour urine specimen.

Equipment and Supplies: 24-hour urine containers (2 may be necessary for some patients); toilet insert for collection; funnel for pouring; label; chemical hazard label as needed; preservatives as required by specific test; graduated cylinder; 10-mL pipette; gloves; written instruction sheet for specific test; requisition slip; patient's record; pen

Affective Behaviors: Affective behaviors provide a professional approach to a skill that enhances the patient encounter. These behaviors may also display sensitivity to a patient's rights and enhance communication. Pay close attention to these skills, which will be in **_bold, italicized_** font.

Notes to the Student

_____

_____

_____

_____

_____

Skills Assessment Requirements

Read and familiarize yourself with the procedure; complete the minimum practice requirements (MPRs). Document each MPR using proper charting technique. Complete each procedure within a reasonable amount of time, with a minimum of 85% accuracy.

POINT VALUE ✦ = 3–6 points ✳ = 7–9 points		PRACTICE TRIAL	GRADED TRIAL # 1	GRADED TRIAL # 2	NOTES
1. ✦	Check the patient's record for orders for specific test.				
2. ✦	Assemble equipment and supplies needed.				
3. ✦	Consult the laboratory directory for special instructions regarding dietary restrictions and preservative for test ordered.				
4. ✦	Perform hand hygiene.				
5. ✳	Label the container with patient's name and dates and times to start and stop collection of specimen.				
6. ✦	If required, add the exact amount of preservative using a pipette. If preservative is caustic, add a chemical hazard label.				

Name: _____

Date: _____

POINT VALUE ✦ = 3–6 points ✳ = 7–9 points		PRACTICE TRIAL	GRADED TRIAL # 1	GRADED TRIAL # 2	NOTES
7. ✳	**Identify the patient and explain thoroughly the directions for collection as follows:** • Upon waking, urinate into the toilet and flush. • Note the exact time and date as the beginning of the 24-hour collection and write it on the container. • Collect all voided urine after the start time for the next 24-hour period ending exactly 24 hours after the start time on the following day. At exactly the same time that was noted on the first day (written on the container), empty the bladder and add it to the collection. • Note the times and dates on the label. • **Instruct the patient not to urinate directly into the container or place anything other than urine in the container. Ask the patient to use a toilet or urinal insert for collection of the specimen, and then to pour the urine into the 24-hour container. Explain that the specimen may need refrigeration, depending on the test.** The patient is to return the container(s) as soon as possible after ending the collection to ensure accurate results.				
8. ✳	Provide a written copy of instructions to the patient along with the prepared container(s).				

POINT VALUE ✦ = 3–6 points ✶ = 7–9 points		PRACTICE TRIAL	GRADED TRIAL # 1	GRADED TRIAL # 2	NOTES
9. ✦	Record the supplies and instructions given to the patient and the name of the test requested.				
10. ✶	Verify the collection dates and times with the patient when the specimen is returned to the facility.				
11. ✶	Check to see if any other additives are to be included before sending the specimen to the testing laboratory.				
12. ✦	Before accepting the container from the patient, apply gloves.				
13. ✶	Mix the urine sample by swirling carefully. Measure the volume of urine collected exactly by pouring into a large graduated cylinder that holds 1 liter. Record the total volume of urine collected and the preservative added.				
14. ✶	Pour a portion of the urine into an appropriate container for delivery to a testing facility. Dispose of the remainder of the urine according to laboratory directions.				
15. ✶	Record the date, time, volume of urine, and where the specimen was sent.				
16. ✦	Clean the cylinder as appropriate. Dispose of the container in a biohazard waste container.				
17. ✦	Clean the area.				
18. ✦	Remove gloves and perform hand hygiene.				

Document: Enter the appropriate information in the chart below.

Grading

Points Earned	_____		
Points Possible	_____	132	132
Percent Grade (Points Earned/Points Possible)	_____		
PASS:	_____	❏ YES ❏ NO ❏ N/A	❏ YES ❏ NO ❏ N/A

Instructor Sign-Off

Instructor: _____   **Date:** _____

Procedure 46-2:

Collecting a Clean-Catch Midstream Urine Specimen

Objective: Instruct both male and female patients to correctly obtain a contaminant-free, clean-catch midstream urine specimen.

Equipment and Supplies: Sterile midstream urine container; antiseptic towelettes; written patient instructions

Affective Behaviors: Affective behaviors provide a professional approach to a skill that enhances the patient encounter. These behaviors may also display sensitivity to a patient's rights and enhance communication. Pay close attention to these skills, which will be in **bold, *italicized*** font.

Notes to the Student

_____

_____

_____

_____

_____

_____

Skills Assessment Requirements

Read and familiarize yourself with the procedure; complete the minimum practice requirements (MPRs). Document each MPR using proper charting technique. Complete each procedure within a reasonable amount of time, with a minimum of 85% accuracy.

POINT VALUE ✦ = 3–6 points ✳ = 7–9 points		PRACTICE TRIAL	GRADED TRIAL # 1	GRADED TRIAL # 2	NOTES
1. ✦	Perform hand hygiene.				
2. ✦	Assemble equipment. Always label the specimen container before use.				
3. ✳	**Identify and greet the patient. Explain the procedure to a male patient as follows:** • Perform hand hygiene. • Expose the penis. Pull foreskin back if uncircumcised (and hold back until specimen has been collected). • Cleanse each side of the urethral opening from top to bottom using a separate antiseptic wipe, wiping in one direction only. Cleanse across the top of the urethral opening with a third antiseptic, wiping in one direction only. Be certain to avoid having any body part touch the specimen container. • Void a small amount of urine into the toilet and then void into the container, taking care not to touch the insides of the container. Remove the container. • Continue voiding the remainder of urine into the toilet. • Recap the container immediately, taking care not to contaminate the inside of the lid. • Deliver the specimen as instructed.				

POINT VALUE ✦ = 3–6 points ✱ = 7–9 points		PRACTICE TRIAL	GRADED TRIAL # 1	GRADED TRIAL # 2	NOTES
	Explain the procedure to a female patient as follows: • Perform hand hygiene and remove underwear. • Expose the urinary meatus by pulling apart the labia and holding the area open with the nondominant hand. • If menstruation is apparent, insert a clean tampon and pull the string to the side. • Use the dominant hand to cleanse around one side of the urinary meatus from front to back with one antiseptic wipe. Use second wipe to cleanse the other side in the same manner. Using a third wipe, cleanse across the opening of the meatus itself. Continue holding the labia apart until the procedure is complete. • Begin voiding into the toilet. Place the container into position and void into the container without touching the inside. • Remove the container and continue voiding into toilet. • Wipe in the usual manner and cover the container with lid, avoiding contaminating the inside of the lid. • Deliver the specimen as instructed.				
4. ✦	Perform hand hygiene.				
5. ✱	Document the patient's chart appropriately.				

Name: _____

Date: _____

Document: Enter the appropriate information in the chart below.

Grading

Points Earned	_____		
Points Possible	_____	36	36
Percent Grade (Points Earned/Points Possible)	_____		
PASS:	_____	❑ YES ❑ NO ❑ N/A	❑ YES ❑ NO ❑ N/A

Instructor Sign-Off

Instructor: _____ Date: _____

Procedure 46-3:

Assisting with Straight Catheter Insertion and Collecting a Sterile Urine Specimen

Objective: Assist with catheterization and urine collection.

Equipment and Supplies: Catheter kit with sterile drapes, gloves, swabs, cleansing solution, lubricant, specimen container, and catheter (size and type as ordered). Precautionary: extra sterile gloves and an extra catheter, in case of the need for replacement.

Affective Behaviors: Affective behaviors provide a professional approach to a skill that enhances the patient encounter. These behaviors may also display sensitivity to a patient's rights and enhance communication. Pay close attention to these skills, which will be in **bold, italicized** font.

Notes to the Student

_____

_____

_____

_____

_____

_____

Skills Assessment Requirements

Read and familiarize yourself with the procedure; complete the minimum practice requirements (MPRs). Document each MPR using proper charting technique. Complete each procedure within a reasonable amount of time, with a minimum of 85% accuracy.

POINT VALUE ✦ = 3–6 points ✱ = 7–9 points	PRACTICE TRIAL	GRADED TRIAL # 1	GRADED TRIAL # 2	NOTES
1. ✦ Check the patient's record for orders for specific test.				
2. ✦ Assemble equipment and supplies needed.				
3. ✦ Consult the laboratory directory for special instructions regarding dietary restrictions and preservative for test ordered.				
4. ✦ Perform hand hygiene.				
5. ✱ **Identify the patient; explain the procedure and the reason for performing it. Explain that most people experience mild burning and pressure, with the sensation of urinating, during the insertion.**				
6. ✱ **Ask if there are any latex, betadine, or iodine allergies.** Notify the nurse or physician if there are patient allergies and collect alternative supplies.				
7. ✦ Visually inspect the product packaging for deterioration or perforations and verify expiration dates. If any damage, the package is not well sealed, or the expiration date has passed, do not use the package.				
8. ✱ **Assist the male patient into a dorsal recumbent position or the female patient into the lithotomy position.** Use draping to ensure privacy and diminish embarrassment.				
9. ✦ Perform hand hygiene.				

POINT VALUE ✦ = 3–6 points ✳ = 7–9 points		PRACTICE TRIAL	GRADED TRIAL # 1	GRADED TRIAL # 2	NOTES
10. ✳	If visibly soiled, don nonsterile gloves and gently wash the patient's genital area with body cleanser. Discard gloves and wash hands.				
11. ✳	Using aseptic technique, open the kit, peeling the lid away from (not toward) your body. Place the underpad beneath the patient, plastic side down. Place the fenestrated drape around the patient's genitalia.				
12. ✳	Apply sterile gloves and observe strict sterile technique for the remainder of the procedure.				
13. ✳	Dispense lubricating gel into a portion of the tray and open cleansing swab packages (or pour solution over cotton balls, if provided). Remove the plastic sleeve from the catheter and arrange on the sterile field.				
14. ✳	The health care practitioner will don sterile gloves and use the nondominant hand to hold back the labia (for females) or foreskin (for males). The dominant hand will first cleanse the meatus, using a different swab for each stroke: one down one side, another down the other side, and a third. The practitioner will then dip the tip of the catheter into the lubricating gel and carefully insert it into the urethra, advancing slowly.				

Name: _____

Date: _____

POINT VALUE ✦ = 3–6 points ✳ = 7–9 points		PRACTICE TRIAL	GRADED TRIAL # 1	GRADED TRIAL # 2	NOTES
15. ✳	The medical assistant should be prepared to collect the urine from the other end of the catheter by holding a sterile cup beneath it. When the cup is ¾ full, the catheter end should be placed in the tray to drain. Immediately seal the urine container. The practitioner will remove the catheter and discard.				
16. ✦	Remove supplies and assist the patient with privacy measures.				
17. ✦	Label the collection container for delivery to a testing facility. Measure and dispose of the remainder of the urine according to laboratory directions.				
18. ✳	Record the date, time, color, clarity, odor, and volume of urine expressed, and where the specimen was sent. The procedure itself should be charted by the person who inserted the catheter.				
19. ✦	Clean the area.				
20. ✦	Remove gloves and perform hand hygiene.				

Name: _____

Date: _____

Document: Enter the appropriate information in the chart below.

Grading

Points Earned	_____		
Points Possible	_____	147	147
Percent Grade (Points Earned/Points Possible)	_____		
PASS:	_____	❏ YES ❏ NO ❏ N/A	❏ YES ❏ NO ❏ N/A

Instructor Sign-Off

Instructor: _____   Date: _____

Competency Check-Offs **1195**

Name: _____

Date: _____

Procedure 46-4:

Evaluating the Physical Characteristics of Urine

Objective: Evaluate the physical characteristics of urine, and properly record the results.

Equipment and Supplies: Urine specimen; centrifuge tube; laboratory slip; personal protective equipment as needed

Affective Behaviors: Affective behaviors provide a professional approach to a skill that enhances the patient encounter. These behaviors may also display sensitivity to a patient's rights and enhance communication. Pay close attention to these skills, which will be in **bold, italicized** font.

Notes to the Student

_____

_____

_____

_____

_____

_____

Skills Assessment Requirements

Read and familiarize yourself with the procedure; complete the minimum practice requirements (MPRs). Document each MPR using proper charting technique. Complete each procedure within a reasonable amount of time, with a minimum of 85% accuracy.

POINT VALUE ✦ = 3–6 points ✶ = 7–9 points		PRACTICE TRIAL	GRADED TRIAL #1	GRADED TRIAL #2	NOTES
1. ✦	Perform hand hygiene and apply gloves.				
2. ✶	Label the centrifuge tube with the patient's name.				
3. ✶	Mix the urine by carefully swirling, avoiding spills.				
4. ✶	Assess the color of the specimen and record observations, using appropriate terms: straw, yellow, dark yellow, amber (other colors if noted).				
5. ✶	Assess and record the clarity using appropriate terms: clear, slightly cloudy, cloudy, and turbid. Transparency can also be evaluated by holding the container over some text and reading through an inch of urine.				
6. ✦	Clean the area.				
7. ✦	Remove gloves and perform hand hygiene unless proceeding with complete urinalysis.				
8. ✶	Document the results.				

Name: _____

Date: _____

Document: Enter the appropriate information in the chart below.

Grading

Points Earned	_____		
Points Possible	_____	63	63
Percent Grade (Points Earned/Points Possible)	_____		
PASS:	_____	❏ YES ❏ NO ❏ N/A	❏ YES ❏ NO ❏ N/A

Instructor Sign-Off

Instructor: _____   **Date:** _____

Procedure 46-5:

Measuring the Specific Gravity of Urine with a Refractometer

Objective: Measure the specific gravity of urine with a refractometer and without error.

Equipment and Supplies: Antiseptic cleaner; biohazard waste container; blood and body fluid protection—lab coat, protective eyewear, nonsterile gloves; distilled water; medicine dropper/pipette; paper, pen/pencil; paper towels; refractometer; urine specimen

Affective Behaviors: Affective behaviors provide a professional approach to a skill that enhances the patient encounter. These behaviors may also display sensitivity to a patient's rights and enhance communication. Pay close attention to these skills, which will be in ***bold, italicized*** font.

Notes to the Student

_____

_____

_____

_____

_____

_____

Skills Assessment Requirements

Read and familiarize yourself with the procedure; complete the minimum practice requirements (MPRs). Document each MPR using proper charting technique. Complete each procedure within a reasonable amount of time, with a minimum of 85% accuracy.

POINT VALUE ✦ = 3–6 points ✱ = 7–9 points		PRACTICE TRIAL	GRADED TRIAL #1	GRADED TRIAL #2	NOTES
1. ✦	Perform hand hygiene.				
2. ✦	Apply gloves and protective clothing.				
3. ✦	Assemble equipment and materials.				
4. ✱	Before using the refractometer, perform a quality control check by using a sample of distilled water first. The value with distilled water should be 1.000. a. Clean the prism and refractometer cover with distilled water. Wipe dry. b. Close the cover. Using the medicine dropper or pipette, place a drop of distilled water on the notched area of the cover. If the refractometer does not have an attached cover, place the water directly onto the prism, and then place a cover plate on top of the prism. c. Tilt the refractometer to allow light to enter. Read the specific gravity by noting the division line between the light and dark area. This reading should be 1.000. If it is not, retest with fresh distilled water.				
5. ✱	To test the urine sample, swirl the urine specimen gently to avoid splashing. Using the medicine dropper, remove a small sample and place 1 to 2 drops onto the notched area of the cover.				
6. ✦	Follow the instructions in step 4c to read the specific gravity.				

POINT VALUE ✦ = 3–6 points ✱ = 7–9 points		PRACTICE TRIAL	GRADED TRIAL # 1	GRADED TRIAL # 2	NOTES
7. ✦	Record the reading on a piece of paper.				
8. ✱	Discard the urine appropriately.				
9. ✱	Remove gloves and protective clothing, and dispose of them properly.				
10. ✦	Perform hand hygiene.				
11. ✱	Document findings in the patient record.				
12. ✦	Clean the work area and equipment.				

Document: Enter the appropriate information in the chart below.

Grading

Points Earned	_____		
Points Possible	_____	87	87
Percent Grade (Points Earned/Points Possible)	_____		
PASS:	_____	❏ YES ❏ NO ❏ N/A	❏ YES ❏ NO ❏ N/A

Instructor Sign-Off

Instructor: _____   Date: _____

Procedure 46-6:

Testing the Chemical Characteristics of Urine with Reagent Strips

Objective: Perform chemical testing on urine using chemical reagent strips.

Equipment and Supplies: Urine specimen; reagent test strips; timer; paper towel; laboratory slip; pen/pencil; personal protective equipment as needed

Affective Behaviors: Affective behaviors provide a professional approach to a skill that enhances the patient encounter. These behaviors may also display sensitivity to a patient's rights and enhance communication. Pay close attention to these skills, which will be in **bold, *italicized*** font.

Notes to the Student

_____

_____

_____

_____

_____

_____

Skills Assessment Requirements

Read and familiarize yourself with the procedure; complete the minimum practice requirements (MPRs). Document each MPR using proper charting technique. Complete each procedure within a reasonable amount of time, with a minimum of 85% accuracy.

Name: _____

Date: _____

POINT VALUE ✦ = 3–6 points ✱ = 7–9 points		PRACTICE TRIAL	GRADED TRIAL # 1	GRADED TRIAL # 2	NOTES
1. ✦	Perform hand hygiene and don personal protective gear.				
2. ✦	Check the specimen for patient identity, date, and time of collection.				
3. ✦	Check the expiration date on the chemical reagent strips.				
4. ✦	Bring the specimen to room temperature and swirl gently to mix.				
5. ✱	Dip the chemical reagent strip in the urine, making sure all pads on the strip are moistened.				
6. ✱	Read each pad by comparing it to the chart on the side of the bottle, appropriately timing each test. (Do not touch the test strip against the side of the bottle, because contamination will result.) Ignore color changes until prescribed time has elapsed.				
7. ✱	Record the results on the patient's laboratory slip.				
8. ✦	Clean the work area, remove gloves, and perform hand hygiene.				

Name: _____

Date: _____

Document: Enter the appropriate information in the chart below.

Grading

Points Earned	_____		
Points Possible	_____	57	57
Percent Grade (Points Earned/Points Possible)	_____		
PASS:	_____	❏ YES ❏ NO ❏ N/A	❏ YES ❏ NO ❏ N/A

Instructor Sign-Off

Instructor: _____   **Date:** _____

Procedure 46-7:

Testing for Glucose in Urine Using the Tablet Method

Objective: Perform procedure to test for sugar in the urine without error.

Equipment and Supplies: Antiseptic cleaner; biohazard waste container; body and body fluid protection—lab coat, goggles, nonsterile gloves; clean glass test tube; Clinitest tablets; distilled water; medicine dropper/pipette; urine specimen

Affective Behaviors: Affective behaviors provide a professional approach to a skill that enhances the patient encounter. These behaviors may also display sensitivity to a patient's rights and enhance communication. Pay close attention to these skills, which will be in **bold, *italicized*** font.

Notes to the Student

_____

_____

_____

_____

_____

_____

Skills Assessment Requirements

Read and familiarize yourself with the procedure; complete the minimum practice requirements (MPRs). Document each MPR using proper charting technique. Complete each procedure within a reasonable amount of time, with a minimum of 85% accuracy.

POINT VALUE ✦ = 3–6 points ✳ = 7–9 points		PRACTICE TRIAL	GRADED TRIAL # 1	GRADED TRIAL # 2	NOTES
1. ✦	Perform hand hygiene.				
2. ✦	Apply gloves and protective clothing.				
3. ✦	Assemble equipment and materials.				
4. ✳	Using the medicine dropper or a pipette, place 5 drops of the urine specimen into a clean test tube.				
5. ✳	Add 10 drops of water. Mix drops together, using the pipette and being careful not to splash the urine.				
6. ✳	Drop one Clinitest tablet into the urine and water solution. Observe the solution (do not shake) as it reacts in the test tube. Do not touch the bottom of the tube during this chemical process, because it becomes very hot.				
7. ✳	At 15 seconds after the reaction (boiling) stops, gently shake the tube to mix the contents.				
8. ✳	Immediately match the color of the liquid against the color chart on the side of the Clinitest container.				
9. ✦	Discard the urine according to Occupational Safety and Health Administration (OSHA) guidelines.				

POINT VALUE ✦ = 3–6 points ✶ = 7–9 points		PRACTICE TRIAL	GRADED TRIAL #1	GRADED TRIAL #2	NOTES
10. ✦	Remove gloves and protective clothing, and dispose of them properly.				
11. ✦	Perform hand hygiene.				
12. ✶	Document findings in patient record.				
13. ✦	Clean work area and equipment according to OSHA guidelines.				

Name: _____

Date: _____

Document: Enter the appropriate information in the chart below.

Grading

Points Earned	_____		
Points Possible	_____	96	96
Percent Grade (Points Earned/Points Possible)	_____		
PASS:	_____	❏ YES ❏ NO ❏ N/A	❏ YES ❏ NO ❏ N/A

Instructor Sign-Off

Instructor: _____ Date: _____

Name: _____

Date: _____

Procedure 46-8:

Preparing a Urine Specimen for Microscopic Examination (for Classroom Evaluation Only)

Objective: Perform microscopic examination of urine sediment for casts and cells.

Equipment and Supplies: Biohazard waste container; body and body fluid protection—lab coat, goggles, nonsterile gloves; capillary pipette; centrifuge; centrifuge tube; microscope; microscope slide; paper, pen/pencil; Sedi-stain (optional); urine specimen
Note: Medical assistants are not expected to perform a microscopic examination. They may be requested by the physician to prepare the specimen to step 11.

Affective Behaviors: Affective behaviors provide a professional approach to a skill that enhances the patient encounter. These behaviors may also display sensitivity to a patient's rights and enhance communication. Pay close attention to these skills, which will be in **bold, *italicized*** font.

Notes to the Student

_____

_____

_____

_____

_____

_____

Skills Assessment Requirements

Read and familiarize yourself with the procedure; complete the minimum practice requirements (MPRs). Document each MPR using proper charting technique. Complete each procedure within a reasonable amount of time, with a minimum of 85% accuracy.

POINT VALUE ✦ = 3–6 points ✳ = 7–9 points		PRACTICE TRIAL	GRADED TRIAL # 1	GRADED TRIAL # 2	NOTES
1. ✦	Perform hand hygiene.				
2. ✦	Apply gloves and protective clothing.				
3. ✦	Assemble equipment and materials.				
4. ✳	Mix the specimen gently to stir up the sediment that has settled to the bottom.				
5. ✳	Place 10 mL of urine into the centrifuge tube. Place cap on tube. Place the tube in the centrifuge and balance this with another tube of 10 mL of water on the opposite side of the machine.				
6. ✳	Set centrifuge timer for 5 minutes.				
7. ✳	After the centrifuge has stopped, remove the tube and pour off the supernatant fluid (the clear liquid left on the top of the specimen after centrifuging), leaving only the sediment. Alternate Method: Some medical assistants prefer using stain (such as Sedi-stain) to help identify sediment more easily. Place 1 drop of the commercially prepared stain in the test tube.				
8. ✳	Mix the sediment by holding the top of the tube and tapping the bottom with a finger, mixing well to ensure a correct reading.				
9. ✳	Use a capillary pipette to transfer 1 drop of sediment to a clean slide.				
10. ✳	Cover the drop of sediment with a coverslip.				

POINT VALUE ✦ = 3–6 points ✷ = 7–9 points		PRACTICE TRIAL	GRADED TRIAL # 1	GRADED TRIAL # 2	NOTES
11. ✷	Place the slide on the microscope stage.				
12. ✷	Focus under low power and reduced light for casts and epithelial cells.				
13. ✷	Carefully examine for anything abnormal, paying close attention to the edges, which are where casts are seen if present.				
14. ✷	Examine 10 to 15 fields using low power. Count the number of casts or other abnormalities seen in each field. If there is nothing in one field, then record 0 (zero). Average the count from the 10 to 15 fields for the final result.				
15. ✷	Using high-power magnification and adjusting for more light, review the 10 to 15 fields. Identify casts if present. Count RBCs, WBCs, round cells, transitional cells, and squamous epithelial cells. Average the count from the 10 to 15 fields for each formed element seen, and record appropriately.				
16. ✷	Observe for crystals and identify. Observe for bacteria, sperm, yeast, and parasites. Report them as few, moderate, or many.				
17. ✦	Discard the urine according to OSHA guidelines.				
18. ✦	Remove gloves and protective clothing, and dispose of them properly.				
19. ✦	Perform hand hygiene.				
20. ✷	Document findings in patient record.				
21. ✦	Clean work area and equipment according to OSHA guidelines.				

Document: Enter the appropriate information in the chart below. _____

Grading

Points Earned	_____		
Points Possible	_____	171	171
Percent Grade (Points Earned/Points Possible)	_____		
PASS:	_____	❏ YES ❏ NO ❏ N/A	❏ YES ❏ NO ❏ N/A

Instructor Sign-Off

Instructor: _____ **Date:** _____

Procedure 46-9:

Performing a Urine Pregnancy Test Using the Enzyme Immunoassay Method

Objective: Perform a urine pregnancy test for hCG using an EIA test and interpret results correctly.

Equipment and Supplies: Patient's first a.m. urine specimen; EIA test kit for hCG; timer; gloves; laboratory report

Affective Behaviors: Affective behaviors provide a professional approach to a skill that enhances the patient encounter. These behaviors may also display sensitivity to a patient's rights and enhance communication. Pay close attention to these skills, which will be in **_bold, italicized_** font.

Notes to the Student

_____

_____

_____

_____

_____

_____

Skills Assessment Requirements

Read and familiarize yourself with the procedure; complete the minimum practice requirements (MPRs). Document each MPR using proper charting technique. Complete each procedure within a reasonable amount of time, with a minimum of 85% accuracy.

POINT VALUE ✦ = 3–6 points ✳ = 7–9 points		PRACTICE TRIAL	GRADED TRIAL # 1	GRADED TRIAL # 2	NOTES
1. ✦	Perform hand hygiene and apply gloves.				
2. ✦	Gather supplies and equipment.				
3. ✦	Allow the testing materials and specimen to come to room temperature.				
4. ✳	Label the test with patient name or ID number.				
5. ✳	Label one area positive and one negative for controls.				
6. ✳	Place the patient's urine on test chamber following manufacturer's directions.				
7. ✳	Place positive and negative controls in correct areas.				
8. ✳	Time the test according to the manufacturer's directions.				
9. ✳	Interpret results correctly.				
10. ✳	Record results on patient's laboratory slip.				
11. ✳	Record positive and negative controls in quality control logbook according to office policy.				
12. ✦	Dispose of equipment and perform hand hygiene.				

Document: Enter the appropriate information in the chart below.

Grading

Points Earned	_____		
Points Possible	_____	96	96
Percent Grade (Points Earned/Points Possible)	_____		
PASS:	_____	❏ YES ❏ NO ❏ N/A	❏ YES ❏ NO ❏ N/A

Instructor Sign-Off

Instructor: _____   **Date:** _____

Procedure 46-10:

Performing a Chain of Custody Urine Collection for Drug Analysis

Objective: Prepare for and instruct the patient to properly collect a urine sample for drug analysis, following a chain of custody procedure.

Equipment and Supplies: Urine collection cup with a built-in thermometer; gloves; bluing; paper tape; laboratory report

Affective Behaviors: Affective behaviors provide a professional approach to a skill that enhances the patient encounter. These behaviors may also display sensitivity to a patient's rights and enhance communication. Pay close attention to these skills, which will be in **bold, *italicized*** font.

Notes to the Student

To avoid distraction that could compromise security, the medical assistant should conduct a collection for only one patient at a time.

_____

_____

_____

_____

_____

_____

Skills Assessment Requirements

Read and familiarize yourself with the procedure; complete the minimum practice requirements (MPRs). Document each MPR using proper charting technique. Complete each procedure within a reasonable amount of time, with a minimum of 85% accuracy.

POINT VALUE ✦ = 3–6 points ✶ = 7–9 points		PRACTICE TRIAL	GRADED TRIAL # 1	GRADED TRIAL # 2	NOTES
	Step 1: Prepare the Bathroom Facility (used when the medical assistant is not required to be present during urination):				
1. ✦	Gather supplies and equipment.				
2. ✦	Secure any water sources by turning off the water inlet or taping handles to prevent opening faucets.				
3. ✦	Add bluing to the toilet and tank.				
4. ✦	Remove soap, disinfectants, and any cleaning agents; inspect the site to ensure that no foreign or unauthorized substances are present.				
5. ✦	Ensure that undetected access is not possible.				
6. ✦	Secure areas and items that may be suitable for concealing contaminants, such as under-sink areas, trash receptacles, ledges, and paper towel dispenser.				
	Step 2: Prepare the Patient				
1. ✦	Photocopy patient's ID and sign it.				
2. ✶	***Explain the procedure to the patient. Have the consent form and questionnaire signed.***				
3. ✦	***Instruct the patient to leave coats and bags in a secure area.***				

POINT VALUE ✦ = 3–6 points ✶ = 7–9 points		PRACTICE TRIAL	GRADED TRIAL # 1	GRADED TRIAL # 2	NOTES
4. ✦	**Provide the patient with a container that is labeled with the patient's name and date.**				
5. ✶	**Ask the patient to use the bathroom and void into a container. Tell the patient to fill the container only two-thirds of the way to avoid spillage.**				
6. ✶	**Explain where you want the patient to leave the container of urine. Place a paper towel in the designated area to avoid contamination of the work area.**				
Step 3: Process the Specimen					
1. ✶	Immediately after the patient opens the door, inspect the room for irregularities.				
2. ✦	Wearing nonsterile gloves, take the specimen. The urine sample should remain within view until sealed for delivery or tested on-site. Do not allow anyone else to handle or process it. The patient should sign to verify that the sample is his or hers.				
3. ✶	Record the temperature of the urine.				
4. ✶	Analyze the urine immediately if using a CLIA-waived test. Follow manufacturer's directions exactly. Carefully and accurately record results.				

POINT VALUE ✦ = 3–6 points ✳ = 7–9 points		PRACTICE TRIAL	GRADED TRIAL # 1	GRADED TRIAL # 2	NOTES
5. ✳	If the specimen is being sent to an outside facility, immediately record the temperature, then apply the tamper-evident seal and secure the specimen for transport according to the facility's policy.				
6. ✦	Dispose of equipment and perform hand hygiene.				
7. ✦	Prevent unauthorized personnel from entering any part of the site in which urine specimens are collected or stored.				

Name: _____

Date: _____

Document: Enter the appropriate information in the chart below.

Grading

Points Earned	_____		
Points Possible	_____	141	141
Percent Grade (Points Earned/Points Possible)	_____		
PASS:	_____	❑ YES ❑ NO ❑ N/A	❑ YES ❑ NO ❑ N/A

Instructor Sign-Off

Instructor: _____ **Date:** _____

Procedure 47-1:

Perform a Capillary Puncture (Manual)

Objective: Perform a capillary stick using a lancet or spring-loaded lancet following correct aseptic technique and obtaining an adequate sample.

Equipment and Supplies: Biohazard sharps container; gloves; alcohol sponge; 2 × 2 gauze square, or cotton balls; lancet or spring-loaded lancet; capillary tubes; sealing clay; ammonia ampules; bandage; lab coat

Affective Behaviors: Affective behaviors provide a professional approach to a skill that enhances the patient encounter. These behaviors may also display sensitivity to a patient's rights and enhance communication. Pay close attention to these skills, which will be in **bold, italicized** font.

Notes to the Student

Lancets come in a variety of sizes and needle gauges for specific purposes. The majority of capillary punctures performed on adults, requiring only a few drops of blood, can be performed with needle gauges 21G, 25G, or 28G. Pediatrics and microcollections will require specific lancets and blades.

Follow Standard Precautions and safety guidelines. Use care to avoid splashing or spilling blood. Wipe up all spills using guidelines established by OSHA.

_____

_____

_____

_____

_____

Skills Assessment Requirements

Read and familiarize yourself with the procedure; complete the minimum practice requirements (MPRs). Document each MPR using proper charting technique. Complete each procedure within a reasonable amount of time, with a minimum of 85% accuracy.

POINT VALUE ✦ = 3–6 points ✳ = 7–9 points		PRACTICE TRIAL	GRADED TRIAL # 1	GRADED TRIAL # 2	NOTES
1. ✳	Perform hand hygiene.				
2. ✦	Assemble equipment.				
3. ✳	**Identify the patient and explain the procedure. Have the patient either sit or lie down.**				
4. ✦	Apply gloves.				
5. ✳	Select either the ring or great finger on the nondominant hand for an adult. Select a heel for a newborn. Briskly rub the finger or heel between your palms, to warm it up. Wipe the site with alcohol. Let the alcohol evaporate.				
6. ✳	Remove plastic protective tip to expose the lancet.				
7. ✳	**Grasp patient's hand (or infant's heel) and gently squeeze 1 inch below the chosen puncture site.**				
8. ✳	Puncture the site using a quick, jabbing motion to obtain a full round drop of blood. Do not puncture the direct center. Immediately discard the lancet in a sharps container. (A spring-loaded lancet may also be used.)				
9. ✳	Wipe away the first drop of blood with a gauze square or cotton ball.				

POINT VALUE ✦ = 3–6 points ✳ = 7–9 points		PRACTICE TRIAL	GRADED TRIAL # 1	GRADED TRIAL # 2	NOTES
10. ✳	Obtain the sample using a microhematocrit capillary tube. The finger or foot may be gently massaged or lowered below the level of the heart, to increase blood flow. Seal one end of the capillary tube in a clay sealer.				
11. ✳	Apply clean gauze over the site and ask the patient to apply firm, continuous pressure until the bleeding stops.				
12. ✦	Assess the patient and the site. Apply a bandage, if needed, but never on an infant (choking hazard). Ask the patient if he or she is dizzy or light-headed.				
13. ✦	Remove gloves and perform hand hygiene.				
14. ✳	Record the procedure on the patient's medical record.				

Document: Enter the appropriate information in the chart below.

Grading

Points Earned	_____		
Points Possible	_____	111	111
Percent Grade (Points Earned/Points Possible)	_____		
PASS:	_____	❏ YES ❏ NO ❏ N/A	❏ YES ❏ NO ❏ N/A

Instructor Sign-Off

Instructor: _____ **Date:** _____

Procedure 47-2:

Obtaining Venous Blood with a Sterile Syringe and Needle

Objective: Perform a venipuncture using the syringe and needle method.

Equipment and Supplies: Sterile 22-gauge needle and 10- to 20-mL syringe; appropriate vacuum specimen tubes for tests ordered; tourniquet; gloves; alcohol wipe; 2 × 2 gauze square; adhesive bandage; patient's record; pen; lab coat; biohazard sharps container

Affective Behaviors: Affective behaviors provide a professional approach to a skill that enhances the patient encounter. These behaviors may also display sensitivity to a patient's rights and enhance communication. Pay close attention to these skills, which will be in **bold, *italicized*** font.

Notes to the Student

_____

_____

_____

_____

_____

_____

Skills Assessment Requirements

Read and familiarize yourself with the procedure; complete the minimum practice requirements (MPRs). Document each MPR using proper charting technique. Complete each procedure within a reasonable amount of time, with a minimum of 85% accuracy.

POINT VALUE ✦ = 3–6 points ✳ = 7–9 points		PRACTICE TRIAL	GRADED TRIAL # 1	GRADED TRIAL # 2	NOTES
1. ✦	Prepare necessary equipment and work area on an aseptic field. Check expiration dates.				
2. ✦	Perform hand hygiene and apply gloves.				
3. ✦	Securely attach the sterile needle to the syringe, if required. Pump the plunger several times, to ensure that it moves freely. Depress the plunger completely, to expel the air from within.				
4. ✳	**Identify the patient and explain the procedure, making sure he or she understands the procedure.**				
5. ✳	**Confirm that the patient has followed any pretest preparation requirements. Verify allergies, the last time the patient ate, and if there is a history of complications (syncope, hematoma, etc.). Ensure that the patient does not have anything in his or her mouth, such as candy or gum, to prevent choking in the case of syncope.**				
6. ✳	Apply a tourniquet 3 to 4 inches above the antecubital space. Palpate the area to locate the vein of choice.				
7. ✳	Remove the tourniquet if the vein of choice is not located immediately and the specimen(s) cannot be collected within 60 seconds.				

POINT VALUE ✦ = 3–6 points ✳ = 7–9 points		PRACTICE TRIAL	GRADED TRIAL # 1	GRADED TRIAL # 2	NOTES
8. ✳	Clean the venipuncture site with an alcohol wipe and allow to air dry. Leave the opened alcohol wipe on the aseptic field within reach.				
9. ✦	Reapply the tourniquet, if necessary.				
10. ✦	**Have the patient make a gentle fist and hold it shut until told to release it. Instruct the patient not to pump vigorously.**				
11. ✳	Verify that there is no air in the syringe and remove the needle guard.				
12. ✳	From beneath the puncture site, pull the skin down so that it is taut. With the bevel facing up, insert the needle into the vein.				
13. ✳	Slowly pull back the syringe plunger until the proper amount of blood has been obtained. Do not force it to fill quickly.				
14. ✳	Instruct the patient to open his or her fist.				
15. ✳	Release the tourniquet and withdraw the needle quickly. Immediately cover with gauze. **Instruct the patient to keep firm pressure on the site and raise the arm to prevent hematomas from occurring.**				

POINT VALUE ✦ = 3–6 points ✳ = 7–9 points		PRACTICE TRIAL	GRADED TRIAL #1	GRADED TRIAL #2	NOTES
16. ✳	(A) If using a transfer device, engage the safety mechanism over the needle; safely remove the needle from the syringe and place it in the sharps container. Apply the blood transfer device to the end of the syringe. (B) If no transfer device is available, place the vacuum-sealed tube in a tube rack so that it is standing upright. Do not hold the tube or the rack. Gently pierce the tube stopper with the needle. For either (A) or (B), allow the vacuum to pull blood into the tube until filled to the desired level. Do not push on the plunger to speed the process. Be sure to use the appropriate collection tube for the ordered tests, following the correct order of the draw.				
17. ✦	Discard the syringe in a sharps container, always inserting the needle end first to avoid injury.				
18. ✳	Gently invert the tubes, as required by the manufacturer; do not shake them. Immediately label the specimen with the patient's name, date and time of collection, test's name, and the name of the person collecting the specimen.				
19. ✦	Follow correct procedures for decontaminating the work area and equipment according to OSHA guidelines.				

POINT VALUE ✦ = 3–6 points ✳ = 7–9 points	PRACTICE TRIAL	GRADED TRIAL # 1	GRADED TRIAL # 2	NOTES
20. ✦ Remove gloves and dispose in appropriate container. Perform hand hygiene. Dispose of all used needles and other equipment in a biohazard waste container.				
21. ✦ **Thank the patient and observe for any signs or symptoms of inappropriate response to the procedure.**				
22. ✳ Document the procedure in the patient's chart.				
23. ✦ If the specimen is to be transported to an outside laboratory, prepare it for transport in the proper container, with all the appropriate information according to OSHA guidelines.				

Document: Enter the appropriate information in the chart below. _____

Grading

Points Earned	_____		
Points Possible	_____	177	177
Percent Grade (Points Earned/Points Possible)	_____		
PASS:	_____	❏ YES ❏ NO ❏ N/A	❏ YES ❏ NO ❏ N/A

Instructor Sign-Off

Instructor: _____   **Date:** _____

Procedure 47-3:

Performing Venipuncture Using the Vacutainer Method

Objective: Perform venipuncture by correctly assembling, locating, and entering vein and withdrawing blood sample.

Equipment and Supplies: Biohazard sharps container; Vacutainer tubes; multisample needle; two or three 2-inch gauze squares; alcohol pads; examination gloves; Vacutainer sleeve; tourniquet; bandage; ink pen; lab coat; patient record

Note: Follow Standard Precautions and safety guidelines when working with blood samples. Use care to avoid splashing or spilling blood. Wipe up all spills using guidelines established by OSHA.

Affective Behaviors: Affective behaviors provide a professional approach to a skill that enhances the patient encounter. These behaviors may also display sensitivity to a patient's rights and enhance communication. Pay close attention to these skills, which will be in **bold, italicized** font.

Notes to the Student

_____

_____

_____

_____

_____

_____

Skills Assessment Requirements

Read and familiarize yourself with the procedure; complete the minimum practice requirements (MPRs). Document each MPR using proper charting technique. Complete each procedure within a reasonable amount of time, with a minimum of 85% accuracy.

Name: _____

Date: _____

POINT VALUE ✦ = 3–6 points ✱ = 7–9 points		PRACTICE TRIAL	GRADED TRIAL # 1	GRADED TRIAL # 2	NOTES
1. ✦	Perform hand hygiene.				
2. ✦	Assemble equipment.				
3. ✱	**Identify the patient and explain the procedure. Have the patient either sit or lie down.**				
4. ✱	Apply gloves.				
5. ✱	Screw the Vacutainer needle into the plastic sleeve. Insert the tube into the other end of the sleeve. The top of the colored stopper should reach the thin guideline on the sleeve. Do not press the tube. If the tube exceeds the line, discard the tube; it may not have a vacuum.				
6. ✱	Apply the tourniquet about 2 inches above the antecubital space. Place the middle of the tourniquet on the posterior (elbow) side of the arm. Crisscross the ends. While holding one end stable, tuck in the other end. This creates a tie that can be quickly released with one hand. In addition, the tourniquet should apply enough tension to engorge the vein with blood.				
7. ✱	The arm should be in an extended position with the palm facing up. Palpate the vein with your fingertips. If a vein cannot be felt in one arm, try the other. Release the tourniquet.				

POINT VALUE ✦ = 3–6 points ✳ = 7–9 points		PRACTICE TRIAL	GRADED TRIAL # 1	GRADED TRIAL # 2	NOTES
8. ✳	Wipe the site with an alcohol pad in a circular pattern, beginning at the insertion site. Let the alcohol evaporate. Cleanse your gloved finger with alcohol in case you need to re-palpate after the site is cleansed. Reapply the tourniquet.				
9. ✳	Anchor the vein by placing the thumb of the nondominant hand 2 inches below the insertion site and pulling the skin toward the hand.				
10. ✳	While holding onto the tube's sleeve with your dominant hand, insert the needle smoothly and rapidly at a 15- to 20-degree angle with the bevel up. The needle only needs to be inserted just past the bevel. If inserted too far, it will puncture both vein walls. Also keep the needle in line with the vein. The dominant hand is now considered "fixed," meaning you may not remove it from the tube sleeve until the procedure is over. All other movements must be done with the nondominant hand.				
11. ✳	While the dominant hand is stabilizing the sleeve, use the nondominant hand to push the tube into the sleeve. Use your thumb to push the tube and hold the sleeve with the index and middle fingers on the flange.				

POINT VALUE ✦ = 3–6 points ✱ = 7–9 points		PRACTICE TRIAL	GRADED TRIAL # 1	GRADED TRIAL # 2	NOTES
12. ✱	Allow the tube to fill. The vacuum will automatically fill the tube to the manufacturer's recommended level for the specific tube used. You should familiarize yourself with the adequate fill level of the individual tubes. Blood collection tubes may contain a weak vacuum caused by processing errors, and you will need to redraw those specimens.				
13. ✱	Remove the tube very carefully without moving the needle and apply a second tube if needed. Gently invert the tube 5 to 6 times after removing it from the sleeve to allow the blood to mix with the additive. Only use the tubes needed for the tests ordered. Fill these tubes following the correct order of the draw.				
14. ✱	Release the tourniquet once the last tube has been inserted into the adaptor. Fill the last tube, remove it, swiftly remove the needle, and cover the site with a clean gauze pad. Be careful not to push on the needle when covering the puncture site, because that may cause the needle to scratch the patient's arm. Gently invert the collection tube.				
15. ✱	Immediately have the patient apply firm, continuous pressure using a gauze square.				
16. ✦	Properly dispose of needle in biohazard container.				

POINT VALUE ✦ = 3–6 points ✳ = 7–9 points		PRACTICE TRIAL	GRADED TRIAL # 1	GRADED TRIAL # 2	NOTES
17. ✳	Assess the patient. Check the venipuncture site for bleeding, and then apply a bandage. **Ask if the patient is dizzy or light-headed.**				
18. ✳	Label the tubes with the patient's name, date, time, ID number, specimen type, tests to be done, and the phlebotomist's initials. Fill out the laboratory requisition sheet.				
19. ✦	Remove gloves. Perform hand hygiene.				
20. ✳	Record the procedure on the patient's medical record.				

Name: _____

Date: _____

Document: Enter the appropriate information in the chart below.

Grading

Points Earned	_____		
Points Possible	_____	165	165
Percent Grade (Points Earned/Points Possible)	_____		
PASS:	_____	❏ YES ❏ NO ❏ N/A	❏ YES ❏ NO ❏ N/A

Instructor Sign-Off

Instructor: _____   Date: _____

Procedure 48-1:

Determining Hemoglobin Using the Hemoglobinometer

Objective: Perform a blood test to determine hemoglobin levels using the hemoglobinometer.

Equipment and Supplies: Hemoglobinometer; glass slide chamber; hemolysis applicator (plastic or wooden); sterile manual or spring-loaded lancet; cotton balls; dry gauze square; alcohol sponges; gloves; patient's record; lab coat; biohazard sharps container

Note: Follow Standard Precautions and safety guidelines when working with blood samples. Use care to avoid splashing or spilling blood. Wipe up all spills using guidelines established by OSHA.

Affective Behaviors: Affective behaviors provide a professional approach to a skill that enhances the patient encounter. These behaviors may also display sensitivity to a patient's rights and enhance communication. Pay close attention to these skills, which will be in **bold, *italicized*** font.

Notes to the Student

_____

_____

_____

_____

_____

_____

Skills Assessment Requirements

Read and familiarize yourself with the procedure; complete the minimum practice requirements (MPRs). Document each MPR using proper charting technique. Complete each procedure within a reasonable amount of time, with a minimum of 85% accuracy.

Name: _____

Date: _____

POINT VALUE ✦ = 3–6 points ✱ = 7–9 points		PRACTICE TRIAL	GRADED TRIAL #1	GRADED TRIAL #2	NOTES
1. ✦	Perform hand hygiene and apply gloves.				
2. ✦	Gather the necessary equipment and supplies.				
3. ✦	Clean the puncture site with an alcohol sponge.				
4. ✦	Using a manual or spring-loaded lancet, obtain capillary blood.				
5. ✦	Pull the glass chamber out of the hemoglobinometer, and position the lower part of the slide so that it is slightly offset.				
6. ✦	Place a large drop of capillary blood onto the slide.				
7. ✱	***Wipe the patient's puncture site with a cotton ball and provide the patient with a dry gauze square to apply mild pressure to the puncture.*** This should stop further bleeding.				
8. ✱	Mix blood with the hemolysis applicator until the blood becomes clear.				
9. ✦	Push the glass chamber into the clip and place it into the slot on the left side of the hemoglobinometer.				
10. ✱	Hold the hemoglobinometer in your left hand at eye level while using your left thumb to turn on the light by depressing the bottom button. Look into the instrument to see a split green field.				

Name: _____

Date: _____

POINT VALUE ✦ = 3–6 points ✶ = 7–9 points		PRACTICE TRIAL	GRADED TRIAL # 1	GRADED TRIAL # 2	NOTES
11. ✦	Slide the button on the right side of the meter with your right thumb and index finger while looking into the meter until a matching green field occurs. Leave the sliding scale on the calibrated line where the solid green field appeared.				
12. ✶	Read the hemoglobin value at the top of the scale. The results are read as grams of hemoglobin per 100 mL of blood (g/dL).				
13. ✦	Wash the chamber and reusable hemolysis applicator with a detergent solution, rinse, dry, and return to the instrument for the next test.				
14. ✦	Remove gloves and perform hand hygiene. Discard gloves and nonreusable supplies in appropriate containers.				
15. ✶	Record the results in the patient's record.				

Document: Enter the appropriate information in the chart below.

Grading

Points Earned	_____		
Points Possible	_____	105	105
Percent Grade (Points Earned/Points Possible)	_____		
PASS:	_____	❏ YES ❏ NO ❏ N/A	❏ YES ❏ NO ❏ N/A

Instructor Sign-Off

Instructor: _____ **Date:** _____

Procedure 48-2:

Performing a Microhematocrit

Objective: Perform a microhematocrit on a capillary blood sample using proper aseptic technique.

Equipment and Supplies: Biohazard sharps container; gloves; capillary tubes; sealing clay; microhematocrit centrifuge; whole blood; hematocrit card or other reader

Note: Follow Standard Precautions and safety guidelines when working with blood samples. Use care to avoid splashing or spilling blood. Wipe up all spills using guidelines established by OSHA.

Affective Behaviors: Affective behaviors provide a professional approach to a skill that enhances the patient encounter. These behaviors may also display sensitivity to a patient's rights and enhance communication. Pay close attention to these skills, which will be in **bold, italicized** font.

Notes to the Student

_____

_____

_____

_____

_____

_____

Skills Assessment Requirements

Read and familiarize yourself with the procedure; complete the minimum practice requirements (MPRs). Document each MPR using proper charting technique. Complete each procedure within a reasonable amount of time, with a minimum of 85% accuracy.

Name: _____

Date: _____

POINT VALUE ✦ = 3–6 points ✱ = 7–9 points	PRACTICE TRIAL	GRADED TRIAL # 1	GRADED TRIAL # 2	NOTES
1. ✦ Perform hand hygiene and apply gloves.				
2. ✦ Assemble equipment.				
3. ✱ Fill two capillary tubes three-quarters full. The blood specimen can be obtained from a vacuum tube of anticoagulated blood using a plain capillary tube or directly from a finger-stick site using a heparinized capillary tube. Seal one end in the sealing clay.				
4. ✱ Place capillary tubes in the centrifuge with the sealed ends against the rubber gasket. If more than one patient's blood is being tested, mark down the number of the slot the patient's tube is in. Spin for 3 to 5 minutes at 10,000 rpm. (Always check the manufacturer's recommendations for proper time and speed.) After centrifuging, the sample will be separated into three layers: • The top layer is the plasma. • The middle layer, or the buffy coat, is made up of WBCs and platelets. • The bottom layer is packed RBCs.				
5. ✱ Remove the tubes immediately after centrifuge stops. If the tubes are not removed immediately, blood may begin to mix together.				

POINT VALUE ✦ = 3–6 points ✳ = 7–9 points		PRACTICE TRIAL	GRADED TRIAL # 1	GRADED TRIAL # 2	NOTES
6. ✳	Determine the results. Use the Hct card by placing the sealing clay just below the zero line on both tubes. Then, on both tubes, match the top of the plasma with the 100 line. Read results on both tubes directly below the buffy coat. Then add those results together and divide by 2.				
7. ✦	Discard the tubes into the sharps container.				
8. ✦	Remove gloves and perform hand hygiene.				
9. ✳	Record the value as a percentage on the patient's medical record.				

Name: _____

Date: _____

Document: Enter the appropriate information in the chart below.

Grading

Points Earned	_____		
Points Possible	_____	69	69
Percent Grade (Points Earned/Points Possible)	_____		
PASS:	_____	❏ YES ❏ NO ❏ N/A	❏ YES ❏ NO ❏ N/A

Instructor Sign-Off

Instructor: _____   Date: _____

Procedure 48-3:

Perform an Erythrocyte Sedimentation Rate Test Using the Wintrobe Tube Method

Objective: Perform an ESR using the Wintrobe tube method and aseptic technique.

Equipment and Supplies: Gloves; whole blood (EDTA); Wintrobe tube; Wintrobe rack; ink pen; patient's record; lab coat; biohazard sharps container

Note: Follow Standard Precautions and safety guidelines when working with blood samples. Use care to avoid splashing or spilling blood. Wipe up all spills using guidelines established by OSHA.

Affective Behaviors: Affective behaviors provide a professional approach to a skill that enhances the patient encounter. These behaviors may also display sensitivity to a patient's rights and enhance communication. Pay close attention to these skills, which will be in **bold, *italicized*** font.

Notes to the Student

_____

_____

_____

_____

_____

_____

Skills Assessment Requirements

Read and familiarize yourself with the procedure; complete the minimum practice requirements (MPRs). Document each MPR using proper charting technique. Complete each procedure within a reasonable amount of time, with a minimum of 85% accuracy.

Name: _____

Date: _____

POINT VALUE ✦ = 3–6 points ✱ = 7–9 points		PRACTICE TRIAL	GRADED TRIAL # 1	GRADED TRIAL # 2	NOTES
1. ✦	Perform hand hygiene and apply gloves.				
2. ✦	Assemble equipment.				
3. ✱	Obtain a whole-blood sample using a purple-top tube. Mix well. EDTA is the anticoagulant of choice.				
4. ✱	Slowly fill Wintrobe tube with blood. Avoid air bubbles.				
5. ✱	Adjust the meniscus of the specimen to the zero line at the top of the tube.				
6. ✦	Maintain the tube in an upright vertical position for 1 hour.				
7. ✱	After 1 hour, record the number of RBCs that settle. Read the ESR on the same side of the tube as the zero line at the top.				
8. ✦	Remove gloves and perform hand hygiene.				
9. ✱	Record the procedure on the patient's medical record.				

Name: _____

Date: _____

Document: Enter the appropriate information in the chart below.

Grading

Points Earned	_____		
Points Possible	_____	69	69
Percent Grade (Points Earned/Points Possible)	_____		
PASS:	_____	❑ YES ❑ NO ❑ N/A	❑ YES ❑ NO ❑ N/A

Instructor Sign-Off

Instructor: _____   **Date:** _____

Procedure 48-4:

Preparing Slides

Objective: Prepare a slide for a differential WBC count using correct aseptic procedure, for educational purposes.

Equipment and Supplies: Clean, glass slides; whole blood (EDTA); gloves; biohazard container; eye dropper; Wright's stain; lab coat; ink pen; patient record

Note: Follow Standard Precautions and safety guidelines when working with blood samples. Use care to avoid splashing or spilling blood. Wipe up all spills using guidelines established by OSHA.

Affective Behaviors: Affective behaviors provide a professional approach to a skill that enhances the patient encounter. These behaviors may also display sensitivity to a patient's rights and enhance communication. Pay close attention to these skills, which will be in **bold, *italicized*** font.

Notes to the Student

_____

_____

_____

_____

_____

_____

Skills Assessment Requirements

Read and familiarize yourself with the procedure; complete the minimum practice requirements (MPRs). Document each MPR using proper charting technique. Complete each procedure within a reasonable amount of time, with a minimum of 85% accuracy.

Name: _____

Date: _____

POINT VALUE ✦ = 3–6 points ✳ = 7–9 points		PRACTICE TRIAL	GRADED TRIAL # 1	GRADED TRIAL # 2	NOTES
1. ✦	Perform hand hygiene and apply gloves.				
2. ✦	Assemble equipment.				
3. ✳	Obtain a whole-blood sample using EDTA as the anticoagulant of choice. Blood must be mixed thoroughly before use.				
4. ✳	Using a dropper, place 1 drop of room-temperature blood on the end of a clean glass slide.				
5. ✳	Using the short side of another clean glass slide, back the slide to the drop of blood. Allow the blood to spread across the short side of the slide. Holding the spreader slide at a 30-degree angle, spread the blood across the length of the slide. Use gentle, continuous pressure and a smooth gliding motion to create a smear. Notice that the smear has a thick side that gradually changes to a thin side. The thin side has a feathered edge, and the blood covers one-half to three-quarters the length of the slide.				
6. ✦	Allow the slide to air dry on a rack.				
7. ✳	Label the patient's name and the date on the frosted edge of the slide.				
8. ✳	Stain slide using Wright's staining method. Flood slide with stain for exactly 45 seconds or amount of time indicated by manufacturer.				

Name: _____

Date: _____

POINT VALUE ✦ = 3–6 points ✶ = 7–9 points	PRACTICE TRIAL	GRADED TRIAL # 1	GRADED TRIAL # 2	NOTES
9. ✶ Rinse with distilled water. Rinse until water is clear.				
10. ✦ Allow slide to air dry before examining under the microscope.				

Document: Enter the appropriate information in the chart below.

Grading

Points Earned	_____		
Points Possible	_____		
Percent Grade (Points Earned/Points Possible)	_____	78	78
PASS:	_____	❏ YES ❏ NO ❏ N/A	❏ YES ❏ NO ❏ N/A

Instructor Sign-Off

Instructor: _____ Date: _____

Name: _____

Date: _____

Procedure 48-5:

Perform a Glycosylated Hemoglobin A1C Test Using a Bayer DCA Vantage Analyzer

Objective: Perform a glycosylated hemoglobin A1C test on a capillary blood sample using proper aseptic technique.

Equipment and Supplies: DCA Vantage Analyzer; DCA Vantage Reagent Kit with capillary holder, reagent cartridge, calibration code; alcohol pad; 2 × 2 sterile gauze; lancet; biohazard sharps container; gloves; pen; patient record

Note: Follow Standard Precautions and safety guidelines when working with blood samples. Use care to avoid splashing or spilling blood. Wipe up all spills using guidelines established by OSHA.

Affective Behaviors: Affective behaviors provide a professional approach to a skill that enhances the patient encounter. These behaviors may also display sensitivity to a patient's rights and enhance communication. Pay close attention to these skills, which will be in ***bold, italicized*** font.

Notes to the Student

_____

_____

_____

_____

_____

_____

Skills Assessment Requirements

Read and familiarize yourself with the procedure; complete the minimum practice requirements (MPRs). Document each MPR using proper charting technique. Complete each procedure within a reasonable amount of time, with a minimum of 85% accuracy.

POINT VALUE ✦ = 3–6 points ✳ = 7–9 points		PRACTICE TRIAL	GRADED TRIAL # 1	GRADED TRIAL # 2	NOTES
1. ✦	Verify physician orders and check for allergies. Perform hand hygiene and apply gloves.				
2. ✦	Inspect and assemble equipment and supplies. If a seal is loose or the containers are damaged, discard and replace.				
3. ✳	Cleanse skin with alcohol and allow to air dry. Perform capillary puncture and wipe the first drop of blood. (You may alternatively use venipuncture blood from a tube with EDTA, heparin, citrate, or fluoride/oxylate after inverting the sample several times to properly mix it.) Dispose of sharps properly.				
4. ✳	Touch the tip of the capillary tube into blood until filled. Wipe the sides of the tube with gauze to remove excess. Inspect the sample for bubbles; if present, discard and begin again. Once a sample is properly collected, analysis must be performed within 5 minutes.				
5. ✳	With the flat side toward the cartridge, gently insert the capillary tube into the cartridge until it snaps into place. Use caution not to contaminate or touch the optical window on the bottom corner of the cartridge. Do not remove the foil.				

POINT VALUE ✦ = 3–6 points ✶ = 7–9 points		PRACTICE TRIAL	GRADED TRIAL # 1	GRADED TRIAL # 2	NOTES
6. ✶	Hold the reagent cartridge so that the barcode faces to the right. Using the track on the left side of the analyzer, scan the cartridge by inserting it into the track above the blue dot and sliding it down quickly. If no beep is heard, try again.				
7. ✶	Open the compartment door on the front of the machine. Hold the cartridge with the barcode facing right and insert until a snap is heard or felt. It will fit only when held in the right direction.				
8. ✶	Using a smooth, continuous motion, pull the foil tab completely out of the cartridge and close the door. Within 5 seconds, a beep should sound.				
9. ✶	Read the results, when ready.				
10. ✶	Open the cartridge door. Push/hold the button on the right side of the cartridge while pushing the cartridge tab to the right and gently pull the cartridge out. Discard in a sharps container.				
11. ✦	Remove gloves and perform hand hygiene.				
12. ✶	Record the value as a percentage on the patient's medical record.				

Name: _____

Date: _____

Document: Enter the appropriate information in the chart below.

Grading

Points Earned	_____		
Points Possible	_____	99	99
Percent Grade (Points Earned/Points Possible)	_____		
PASS:	_____	❑ YES ❑ NO ❑ N/A	❑ YES ❑ NO ❑ N/A

Instructor Sign-Off

Instructor: _____   **Date:** _____

Procedure 48-6:

Perform a PKU Test

Objective: Collect blood specimen for PKU testing.

Equipment and Supplies: Sterile lancet; alcohol sponge; gloves; sterile dry gauze; special filter paper card, typically supplied by the state health department

Affective Behaviors: Affective behaviors provide a professional approach to a skill that enhances the patient encounter. These behaviors may also display sensitivity to a patient's rights and enhance communication. Pay close attention to these skills, which will be in **bold, italicized** font.

Notes to the Student

_____

_____

_____

_____

_____

_____

Skills Assessment Requirements

Read and familiarize yourself with the procedure; complete the minimum practice requirements (MPRs). Document each MPR using proper charting technique. Complete each procedure within a reasonable amount of time, with a minimum of 85% accuracy.

Name: _____

Date: _____

POINT VALUE ✦ = 3–6 points ✳ = 7–9 points		PRACTICE TRIAL	GRADED TRIAL # 1	GRADED TRIAL # 2	NOTES
1. ✦	Perform hand hygiene and apply gloves.				
2. ✦	***Cleanse the infant's heel with an alcohol sponge.***				
3. ✳	Puncture the lateral portion of the infant's heel with a sterile disposable lancet.				
4. ✳	Wipe away the first drop of blood with dry sterile gauze.				
5. ✳	Allow a large blood droplet to form.				
6. ✳	Touch the blood droplet to the center of the circle on one side of the special filter paper card.				
7. ✳	Ensure the blood has completely soaked through the paper card by looking at the reverse side.				
8. ✳	Fill all required five circles on the paper card.				
9. ✳	***Do not squeeze the heel excessively to avoid collecting tissue fluid mixed with blood.***				
10. ✦	Set the card in an appropriate area to air dry for 2 hours at room temperature.				
11. ✦	When completely dry, place in the state-provided envelope and mail within 48 hours.				

Name: _____

Date: _____

Document: Enter the appropriate information in the chart below.

Grading

Points Earned	_____		
Points Possible	_____	87	87
Percent Grade (Points Earned/Points Possible)	_____		
PASS:	_____	❑ YES ❑ NO ❑ N/A	❑ YES ❑ NO ❑ N/A

Instructor Sign-Off

Instructor: _____ Date: _____

Procedure 48-7:

Perform a Mono Test

Objective: Perform a mono test.

Equipment and Supplies: Biohazard waste container; disposable lancet; gloves; capillary tube; test tube; mono test diluent; mono test stick(s); blood specimen

Affective Behaviors: Affective behaviors provide a professional approach to a skill that enhances the patient encounter. These behaviors may also display sensitivity to a patient's rights and enhance communication. Pay close attention to these skills, which will be in **_bold, italicized_** font.

Notes to the Student

_____

_____

_____

_____

_____

_____

Skills Assessment Requirements

Read and familiarize yourself with the procedure; complete the minimum practice requirements (MPRs). Document each MPR using proper charting technique. Complete each procedure within a reasonable amount of time, with a minimum of 85% accuracy.

POINT VALUE ✦ = 3–6 points ✲ = 7–9 points	PRACTICE TRIAL	GRADED TRIAL # 1	GRADED TRIAL # 2	NOTES
1. ✦ Perform hand hygiene.				
2. ✦ Apply gloves.				
3. ✦ Assemble equipment and supplies.				
4. ✲ Perform a capillary puncture.				
5. ✲ Fill a capillary tube end to end, dispensing all the blood into the test tube.				
6. ✲ Slowly add 1 drop of diluent to the bottom of the test tube.				
7. ✲ Mix.				
8. ✲ Remove the test stick(s) from the container. Recap the container immediately.				
9. ✲ Place the absorbent end of the test stick into the treated sample. Leave the test stick in the test tube.				
10. ✲ Read results at 5 minutes. Positive results may be read as soon as the red control line appears.				
11. ✦ Discard used test tubes, lancet, and test sticks in the biohazard waste container.				
12. ✲ Remove gloves and dispose of them correctly. Perform hand hygiene.				
13. ✲ Document findings in the patient record: Positive: A blue test line and a red control line indicate a positive result. Negative: A red control line but no blue test line indicates a negative result.				
14. ✲ Clean the work area and equipment according to OSHA guidelines.				

Name: _____

Date: _____

Document: Enter the appropriate information in the chart below.

Grading

Points Earned	_____		
Points Possible	_____	114	114
Percent Grade (Points Earned/Points Possible)	_____		
PASS:	_____	❏ YES ❏ NO ❏ N/A	❏ YES ❏ NO ❏ N/A

Instructor Sign-Off

Instructor: _____ **Date:** _____

Procedure 49-1:

General X-Ray Examination

Objective: Assist with a radiologic procedure under the supervision of a physician or radiologic technologist.

Equipment and Supplies: Order for X-ray examination; dosimeter badge; appropriate X-ray equipment—X-ray film, holder, and machine; processing equipment; drape; lead patient shield

Affective Behaviors: Affective behaviors provide a professional approach to a skill that enhances the patient encounter. These behaviors may also display sensitivity to a patient's rights and enhance communication. Pay close attention to these skills, which will be in **bold, italicized** font.

Notes to the Student

_____

_____

_____

_____

_____

_____

Skills Assessment Requirements

Read and familiarize yourself with the procedure; complete the minimum practice requirements (MPRs). Document each MPR using proper charting technique. Complete each procedure within a reasonable amount of time, with a minimum of 85% accuracy.

POINT VALUE ✦ = 3–6 points ✳ = 7–9 points		PRACTICE TRIAL	GRADED TRIAL #1	GRADED TRIAL #2	NOTES
1. ✦	Check X-ray examination order.				
2. ✦	Check necessary X-ray equipment as needed.				
3. ✦	Identify the patient.				
4. ✳	Determine patient compliance with procedure preparation instructions.				
5. ✳	*Explain the procedure to the patient.*				
6. ✦	*Instruct the patient to remove all clothing as appropriate for the procedure.*				
7. ✦	*Ask the patient to remove all jewelry and metals as needed for the procedure.*				
8. ✦	The following steps will most likely be performed by a radiologic technologist.				
9. ✳	Position and drape the patient correctly.				
10. ✳	Align the X-ray tube and cassette at the correct distance and set the controls.				
11. ✳	*Ask the patient to hold his or her breath as necessary.*				
12. ✳	Leave the room and stand behind the lead shield to take the X-ray(s).				
13. ✦	*Ask the patient to take a comfortable position while all X-rays are processed and reviewed.*				
14. ✦	*Instruct the patient to dress if the X-rays are satisfactory.*				
15. ✦	Label the X-rays and place them in an envelope, according to office procedures.				
16. ✳	Document appropriately.				

Name: _____

Date: _____

Document: Enter the appropriate information in the chart below.

Grading

Points Earned	_____		
Points Possible	_____	117	117
Percent Grade (Points Earned/Points Possible)	_____		
PASS:	_____	❏ YES ❏ NO ❏ N/A	❏ YES ❏ NO ❏ N/A

Instructor Sign-Off

Instructor: _____   Date: _____

Name: _____

Date: _____

Procedure 50-1:

Recording a 12-Lead Electrocardiograph

Objective: Perform an accurate ECG without assistance.

Equipment and Supplies: ECG machine lead wires and patient cables, and power cord; ECG paper; electrode sensors; alcohol wipes; screwdriver, for adjustments, if needed; patient gown, if needed; razor if needed

Affective Behaviors: Affective behaviors provide a professional approach to a skill that enhances the patient encounter. These behaviors may also display sensitivity to a patient's rights and enhance communication. Pay close attention to these skills, which will be in **_bold, italicized_** font.

Notes to the Student

_____

_____

_____

_____

_____

_____

Skills Assessment Requirements

Read and familiarize yourself with the procedure; complete the minimum practice requirements (MPRs). Document each MPR using proper charting technique. Complete each procedure within a reasonable amount of time, with a minimum of 85% accuracy.

POINT VALUE ✦ = 3–6 points ✳ = 7–9 points	PRACTICE TRIAL	GRADED TRIAL #1	GRADED TRIAL #2	NOTES
1. ✦ Assemble necessary supplies and perform hand hygiene.				
2. ✦ **_Greet and identify the patient, having the patient verify his or her full name and date of birth._**				
3. ✳ **_Introduce yourself and explain the procedure to the patient._**				
4. ✳ Begin technical preparation of the ECG machine by attaching the power cord and plugging in the machine to a grounded outlet.				
5. ✦ Turn on the machine, allowing it time to warm up. Following office policy and manufacturer instructions, ensure that the machine is properly calibrated. a. Enter necessary patient data into the ECG machine.				
6. ✦ Prepare the patient for the procedure. a. Offer female patients gowns to be worn with the opening down the front. Instruct female patients to remove the bra. b. Instruct male patients to remove the shirt so that the chest can be exposed. c. Both male and female patients should be instructed to remove shoes and socks or stockings. d. Instruct patients to roll up their pant legs to expose their lower legs. e. Instruct patients to remove any metal jewelry, because it can interfere with the electrical current of the EKG.				

POINT VALUE ✦ = 3–6 points ✳ = 7–9 points		**PRACTICE TRIAL**	**GRADED TRIAL # 1**	**GRADED TRIAL # 2**	**NOTES**
7. ✦	Position the patient in a supine position, flat on the examination table. Provide pillows for comfort, if necessary.				
8. ✳	Prepare the patient's skin for electrodes by wiping the areas with alcohol swabs. Shave excessively hairy areas using a razor, if necessary.				
9. ✳	Attach the electrodes to the appropriate anatomical landmarks.				
10. ✳	Connect all lead wires to the electrodes, making sure the wires remain untangled.				
11. ✳	Instruct the patient to relax, breathe normally, and refrain from speaking during the procedure.				
12. ✦	For automatic machines, depress AUTO-RUN; for manual machines, select the leads in sequence and depress the correct button to run each individual lead. Use problem-solving skills if you encounter artifacts and repeat the recording if necessary so that the final tracing is clean and clear of artifacts.				
13. ✦	Remove the lead wires from the electrodes and carefully put away the patient cable box with attached lead wires.				
14. ✦	Carefully remove the electrodes from the patient's skin and wipe away any excess adhesive residue.				
15. ✦	Perform hand hygiene.				

POINT VALUE ✦ = 3–6 points ✳ = 7–9 points	PRACTICE TRIAL	GRADED TRIAL # 1	GRADED TRIAL # 2	NOTES
16. ✦ **Inform the patient that he or she may get dressed.** Leave the room for privacy, taking the EKG machine and test with you.				
17. ✦ In a quiet area, mount the EKG, if necessary, and transfer necessary patient information.				
18. ✦ Chart the procedure in the patient's medical record.				
19. ✦ Give the ECG to the physician for interpretation.				
20. ✳ Clean the machine and accessories according to manufacturer's instructions.				

Name: _____

Date: _____

Document: Enter the appropriate information in the chart below.

Grading

Points Earned	_____		
Points Possible	_____	135	135
Percent Grade (Points Earned/Points Possible)	_____		
PASS:	_____	❏ YES ❏ NO ❏ N/A	❏ YES ❏ NO ❏ N/A

Instructor Sign-Off

Instructor: _____ **Date:** _____

Procedure 50-2:

Applying a Holter Monitor

Objective: Apply a Holter monitor, instruct the patient.

Equipment and Supplies: Holter monitor with sensors; patient cable; patient activity diary; fresh batteries or charging device; blank recording tape or digital flash card or microchip; adhesive tape; razor; alcohol

Affective Behaviors: Affective behaviors provide a professional approach to a skill that enhances the patient encounter. These behaviors may also display sensitivity to a patient's rights and enhance communication. Pay close attention to these skills, which will be in **_bold, italicized_** font.

Notes to the Student

_____

_____

_____

_____

_____

_____

Skills Assessment Requirements

Read and familiarize yourself with the procedure; complete the minimum practice requirements (MPRs). Document each MPR using proper charting technique. Complete each procedure within a reasonable amount of time, with a minimum of 85% accuracy.

Name: _____

Date: _____

POINT VALUE ✦ = 3–6 points ✶ = 7–9 points		PRACTICE TRIAL	GRADED TRIAL #1	GRADED TRIAL #2	NOTES
1. ✦	Assemble all necessary supplies.				
2. ✶	Install new batteries; depending on the model, make sure the digital storage unit (flashcard or microchip) has the maximum amount of memory. For older models, insert a new blank cassette tape.				
3. ✦	Verify that the machine is operational.				
4. ✶	***Introduce yourself and then identify, interview, and instruct the patient according to office protocol. Explain the importance of accurately recording in the diary as well as depressing the event button at the correct times.***				
5. ✦	Have the patient remove clothing to the waist (female patients may wear a gown open down the front) and sit on an examination table.				
6. ✦	Perform hand hygiene.				
7. ✦	Prepare the electrode sites by shaving small patches of chest hair where the electrodes will be placed (if necessary). Using alcohol pads, wipe the skin to remove any residue that could interfere with electrode placement. Allow the skin to air dry.				
8. ✦	Using a dry washcloth or other abrasive material, rub the skin where the electrodes will be placed. This will help the electrodes stick to the skin more effectively.				

POINT VALUE ✦ = 3–6 points ✳ = 7–9 points		PRACTICE TRIAL	GRADED TRIAL #1	GRADED TRIAL #2	NOTES
9. ✦	Attach the electrodes according to the manufacturer's instructions. The sensors will be placed in these locations: third intercostal space 2 or 3 inches to the right of the sternum, third intercostal space 2 or 3 inches to the left of the sternum, fifth intercostal space at the left sternum margin, sixth intercostal space at the right anterior axillary line, and sixth intercostal space at the left anterior axillary line.				
10. ✦	Attach the wires so that they point toward the feet, and then connect the patient cable.				
11. ✦	Secure each sensor with adhesive tape.				
12. ✦	**Assist the patient with replacing his or her shirt.** Extend the cable between the buttons or under the hem.				
13. ✦	Place the recorder in the carrying case, and either attach to the patient's belt or place the neck strap around the patient's neck. Check that there is no tension on the wires.				
14. ✳	Plug the cable into the recorder.				
15. ✳	Record the starting time in the diary.				
16. ✳	Ensure that the patient understands what to do by having him or her repeat the instructions for pressing the event button as well as what to record in the diary.				
17. ✳	Confirm the time for the patient to return to the clinic for removal of the Holter monitor.				
18. ✳	Chart the procedure in the patient's record. Sign or initial your work.				

Name: _____

Date: _____

Document: Enter the appropriate information in the chart below.

Grading

Points Earned	_____		
Points Possible	_____	123	123
Percent Grade (Points Earned/Points Possible)	_____		
PASS:	_____	❏ YES ❏ NO ❏ N/A	❏ YES ❏ NO ❏ N/A

Instructor Sign-Off

Instructor: _____ Date: _____

Procedure 51-1:

Performing a Spirometry Test to Measure Forced Vital Capacity

Objective: Perform a forced vital capacity test.

Equipment and Supplies: Functioning spirometry machine; nose clip; disposable patient mouthpiece; spirometric tubing; disinfectant; biohazard waste container; paper and pencil; scale for height and weight; sphygmomanometer, stethoscope and blood pressure cuff; patient medical record

Affective Behaviors: Affective behaviors provide a professional approach to a skill that enhances the patient encounter. These behaviors may also display sensitivity to a patient's rights and enhance communication. Pay close attention to these skills, which will be in **_bold, italicized_** font.

Notes to the Student

_____

_____

_____

_____

_____

_____

Skills Assessment Requirements

Read and familiarize yourself with the procedure; complete the minimum practice requirements (MPRs). Document each MPR using proper charting technique. Complete each procedure within a reasonable amount of time, with a minimum of 85% accuracy.

POINT VALUE ✦ = 3–6 points ✶ = 7–9 points		PRACTICE TRIAL	GRADED TRIAL # 1	GRADED TRIAL # 2	NOTES
1. ✦	Perform hand hygiene.				
2. ✦	Assemble all equipment, attaching the tubing and mouthpiece to the spirometer as necessary.				
3. ✶	Calibrate spirometer as necessary, according to manufacturer's instructions. Turn on the machine and ensure that the spirometer is properly functioning.				
4. ✦	***Warmly greet and identify the patient.***				
5. ✦✶	***Question the patient about having prepared for the test.*** a. Make sure the patient has not eaten a large meal and has not smoked within the past 4 to 6 hours. b. Also, the patient should not have used any bronchodilator medications within 6 hours of the test.				
6. ✦	***Inquire about general health at present and notify the physician if the patient has a fever, active allergies, a cough, or cold or flu symptoms.***				
7. ✦✶	***Explain and demonstrate the procedure to the patient. Instruct the patient that he or she will need to complete three of these maneuvers.***				
8. ✦	Obtain the patient's height and weight and measure and record all vital signs.				

POINT VALUE ✦ = 3–6 points ✳ = 7–9 points	PRACTICE TRIAL	GRADED TRIAL # 1	GRADED TRIAL # 2	NOTES
9. ✳ **Explain the proper positioning and, if necessary, assist with loosening any tight clothing that could cause constriction.** a. Ideally, the patient should be seated with feet flat on the floor. The patient's head and chin should be slightly elevated during the procedure.				
10. ✳ Enter all appropriate patient data into the spirometry machine. This will likely include the patient's name, date of birth, height, weight, and blood pressure. Medications may also be entered on some spirometer models.				
11. ✦ **For the second time, review the procedure with the patient. Be sure that the patient knows to breathe forcibly several times into the spirometer.**				
12. ✦ **Have the patient place the mouthpiece in his or her mouth and seal his or her lips around the mouthpiece.**				
13. ✦ Apply nose clips.				
14. ✳ **Have the patient inhale deeply.**				
15. ✦ Push the start button at the same time as you give the following instruction to the patient.				
16. ✳ **Encourage the patient to exhale and blast breath out as hard, fast, and long as possible.**				

POINT VALUE ✦ = 3–6 points ✱ = 7–9 points		PRACTICE TRIAL	GRADED TRIAL # 1	GRADED TRIAL # 2	NOTES
17. ✱	***Make recommendations to improve the outcome of the next maneuvers, if necessary.***				
18. ✦	Obtain the second set of maneuvers.				
19. ✦	***Again, make recommendations for improvement and obtain the third set of maneuvers.***				
20. ✦	Continue until you have three acceptable outcomes. You may facilitate up to eight attempts, if needed, to obtain three good trials. Some computerized machines will automatically select the best attempt and print the results.				
21. ✦	***Remove the nose clip and ask the patient to remain in the examination room until the physician reviews the results.***				
22. ✦	Give the physician the trial information.				
23. ✱	Record performance of the test and the results (if instructed to do so by the physician) in the patient's medical record.				
24. ✦	Clean the tubing and dispose of the mouthpieces using Standard Precautions and following the manufacturer's directions.				
25. ✦	Properly shut down the computerized spirometry machine according to manufacturer's directions and place the machine in its proper storage location.				
26. ✦	Clean the examination room in preparation for the next patient.				

Name: _____

Date: _____

Document: Enter the appropriate information in the chart below.

Grading

Points Earned	_____		
Points Possible	_____	186	186
Percent Grade (Points Earned/Points Possible)	_____		
PASS:	_____	❏ YES ❏ NO ❏ N/A	❏ YES ❏ NO ❏ N/A

Instructor Sign-Off

Instructor: _____   Date: _____

Procedure 51-2:

Instructing Patients According to Their Needs:
Teaching Peak Flow Measurement

Objective: Instruct the patient to correctly monitor peak flow and to record results.

Equipment and Supplies: Peak flow meter; documentation diary/chart; diagram of lungs and breathing processes; pen; patient's medical record

Affective Behaviors: Affective behaviors provide a professional approach to a skill that enhances the patient encounter. These behaviors may also display sensitivity to a patient's rights and enhance communication. Pay close attention to these skills, which will be in *bold, italicized* font.

Notes to the Student

_____

_____

_____

_____

_____

_____

Skills Assessment Requirements

Read and familiarize yourself with the procedure; complete the minimum practice requirements (MPRs). Document each MPR using proper charting technique. Complete each procedure within a reasonable amount of time, with a minimum of 85% accuracy.

POINT VALUE ✦ = 3–6 points ✳ = 7–9 points		PRACTICE TRIAL	GRADED TRIAL # 1	GRADED TRIAL # 2	NOTES
1. ✦	Perform proper hand hygiene.				
2. ✦	Assemble peak flow meter with disposable mouthpiece or individual peak flow meter for patient use at home.				
3. ✳	**Warmly greet and identify the patient and explain the procedure. Include an explanation of breathing processes and importance to overall health**. A diagram of the lungs can be beneficial. Demonstrate how the mouthpiece fits onto the meter and explain what the numbers on the side mean. The peak flow meter should always be set on zero to start. a. The numbers on the side of the meter measure the amount of liters exhaled per second or per minute, depending on the calibration of the given meter.				
4. ✦✳	**Explain that results are best obtained if the patient is standing with the mouthpiece in his or her mouth and with a tight seal formed by the lips.**				
5. ✳	**Instruct the patient to stand, take as deep a breath as possible, place the mouthpiece in the mouth without biting down on it, and exhale as completely and forcibly as possible.**				

POINT VALUE ✦ = 3–6 points ✳ = 7–9 points		PRACTICE TRIAL	GRADED TRIAL # 1	GRADED TRIAL # 2	NOTES
6. ✦	The exhalation will move the marker up the side and scale on the meter. ***Instruct the patient to note the number at which the sliding gauge stopped and to record the results.*** This reading is the peak expiratory flow rate (PEFR). Reset the gauge to zero.				
7. ✦	Repeat steps 5 and 6 two more times so that there are three acceptable results.				
8. ✦	Inform the physician of the patient's results.				
9. ✳	***Instruct the patient to follow the physician's orders about when and how often to perform peak flow measurement. Instruct him or her to record the "best" result, of three attempts, in the diary.***				
10. ✦	Demonstrate how to properly care for the peak flow meter, including how to disinfect and care for the meter according to manufacturer's instructions.				
11. ✳	Verify that the patient understands how to obtain peak flow measurements, how to document and record results in the diary, and how to properly care for and maintain the peak flow meter. Allow time for the patient to ask questions.				
12. ✳	Document that patient instruction was provided.				
13. ✦	Perform hand hygiene.				

Name: _____

Date: _____

Document: Enter the appropriate information in the chart below.

Grading

Points Earned	_____		
Points Possible	_____	93	93
Percent Grade (Points Earned/Points Possible)	_____		
PASS:	_____	❏ YES ❏ NO ❏ N/A	❏ YES ❏ NO ❏ N/A

Instructor Sign-Off

Instructor: _____   **Date:** _____

Procedure 51-3:

Measuring Oxygen Saturation

Objective: Attach and measure the oxygen saturation of patient.

Equipment and Supplies: Pulse oximeter, nail polish remover, alcohol wipes, patient's medical record

Affective Behaviors: Affective behaviors provide a professional approach to a skill that enhances the patient encounter. These behaviors may also display sensitivity to a patient's rights and enhance communication. Pay close attention to these skills, which will be in **bold, italicized** font.

Notes to the Student

_____

_____

_____

_____

_____

_____

Skills Assessment Requirements

Read and familiarize yourself with the procedure; complete the minimum practice requirements (MPRs). Document each MPR using proper charting technique. Complete each procedure within a reasonable amount of time, with a minimum of 85% accuracy.

POINT VALUE ✦ = 3–6 points ✳ = 7–9 points		PRACTICE TRIAL	GRADED TRIAL # 1	GRADED TRIAL # 2	NOTES
1. ✦	Perform hand hygiene.				
2. ✦	Assemble equipment based on the type of sensor that will be used.				
3. ✳	**_Warmly greet and identify the patient and explain the procedure._** When oxygen saturation is performed routinely in a medical office, it is often performed as a part of the patient's vital sign measurements.				
4. ✳	Choose the correct site to apply the sensor for the patient. If circulation is poor in the patient's hands or feet, select an alternative location such as the patient's earlobe or bridge of the nose. In the medical office, the most common site for pulse oximetry reading is the fingertip. The rest of the procedure will be based on the assumption that this site will be used.				
5. ✦	Remove nail polish as needed.				
6. ✦	Wipe the selected finger with an alcohol wipe and allow it to air dry.				
7. ✦	Turn on the oximeter device and verify it is functioning properly.				
8. ✦	When prompted, attach the device to the patient's finger and wait for the beep.				
9. ✳	Record the oxygen saturation level in the patient's medical record as SpO_2 and a percentage.				

POINT VALUE ✦ = 3–6 points ✳ = 7–9 points		PRACTICE TRIAL	GRADED TRIAL # 1	GRADED TRIAL # 2	NOTES
10. ✦	If the oxygen saturation level is abnormal, notify the physician of the results.				
11. ✦	Perform hand hygiene and return the oximeter to its storage location.				

Name: _____

Date: _____

Document: Enter the appropriate information in the chart below.

Grading

Points Earned	_____		
Points Possible	_____	75	75
Percent Grade (Points Earned/Points Possible)	_____		
PASS:	_____	❑ YES ❑ NO ❑ N/A	❑ YES ❑ NO ❑ N/A

Instructor Sign-Off

Instructor: _____ Date: _____

Name: _____

Date: _____

Procedure 51-4:

Administer a Nebulizer Treatment

Objective: To assist the physician through patient care by administering a nebulizer treatment to a patient.

Equipment and Supplies: Medication as ordered by the physician; diluent (either sterile saline or water); nebulizer machine; disposable tubing with medication cup or dispenser; disposable mask or mouthpiece; biohazard waste container; patient's medical record

Affective Behaviors: Affective behaviors provide a professional approach to a skill that enhances the patient encounter. These behaviors may also display sensitivity to a patient's rights and enhance communication. Pay close attention to these skills, which will be in **bold, italicized** font.

Notes to the Student

_____

_____

_____

_____

_____

_____

_____

Skills Assessment Requirements

Read and familiarize yourself with the procedure; complete the minimum practice requirements (MPRs). Document each MPR using proper charting technique. Complete each procedure within a reasonable amount of time, with a minimum of 85% accuracy.

Name: _____

Date: _____

POINT VALUE ✦ = 3–6 points ✶ = 7–9 points		PRACTICE TRIAL	GRADED TRIAL # 1	GRADED TRIAL # 2	NOTES
1. ✦	Gather all necessary equipment, including the nebulizer machine, disposable mask or mouthpiece, connecting disposable tubing, and medicine cap/dispenser. Plug the machine into an outlet in the examination room.				
2. ✦	**Warmly greet and identify the patient.**				
3. ✶	Explain the procedure and the treatment that will be administered.				
4. ✶	Verify the order for medication as written by the physician. The medication should be checked and reviewed three times before administering the medication.				
5. ✦	Perform hand hygiene.				
6. ✶	Correctly measure the dosage of medication and diluent and place this mixture in the medication dispenser cup. Secure the lid on the medication cup.				
7. ✦	Ensure that the patient is either sitting upright on the examination table or positioned in the semi-Fowler's position.				
8. ✶	Connect the disposable tubing to both the nebulizer machine and the medication cup.				
9. ✦	Turn on the nebulizer machine and wait for the aerosol mist to form. It will either fill the mask or come out of the opposite end of the mouthpiece.				

POINT VALUE ✦ = 3–6 points ✳ = 7–9 points	PRACTICE TRIAL	GRADED TRIAL # 1	GRADED TRIAL # 2	NOTES
10. ✳ Instruct the patient in the following manner: a. If a mouthpiece is used, instruct the patient to gently bite the mouthpiece and purse the lips around the mouthpiece. b. If a mask is used, assist the patient in comfortably securing the mask in the proper position.				
11. ✳ Ask the patient to take deep and slow breaths and frequently hold these breaths for 3 to 5 seconds at a time, allowing the medication to disperse deep into the lungs. a. The treatment will continue until the aerosol mist no longer forms.				
12. ✦ Turn off the machine when the treatment is completed.				
13. ✳ **Encourage the patient to produce deep breaths and coughs in order to facilitate removing loosened secretions.** a. If sputum is produced after the treatment, take note of amount and characteristics such as color and viscosity.				
14. ✦ Detach and dispose of the tubing and mouthpiece in the biohazard waste container.				
15. ✦ Perform hand hygiene.				
16. ✳ Provide patient education, both written and verbal, if the patient is to continue nebulizing treatments at home.				
17. ✳ Document the administration of the nebulizing treatment and the completion of patient education.				

Name: _____

Date: _____

Document: Enter the appropriate information in the chart below.

Grading

Points Earned	_____		
Points Possible	_____	123	123
Percent Grade (Points Earned/Points Possible)	_____		
PASS:	_____	❏ YES ❏ NO ❏ N/A	❏ YES ❏ NO ❏ N/A

Instructor Sign-Off

Instructor: _____ **Date:** _____

Name: _____

Date: _____

Procedure 52-1:

Assisting with Assessing Gait, Using a Gait Belt

Objective: Assist patient with ambulation to assess gait.

Equipment and Supplies: Gait belt

Affective Behaviors: Affective behaviors provide a professional approach to a skill that enhances the patient encounter. These behaviors may also display sensitivity to a patient's rights and enhance communication. Pay close attention to these skills, which will be in **bold, italicized** font.

Notes to the Student

_____

_____

_____

_____

_____

_____

Skills Assessment Requirements

Read and familiarize yourself with the procedure; complete the minimum practice requirements (MPRs). Document each MPR using proper charting technique. Complete each procedure within a reasonable amount of time, with a minimum of 85% accuracy.

Name: _____

Date: _____

POINT VALUE ✦ = 3–6 points ✱ = 7–9 points		PRACTICE TRIAL	GRADED TRIAL #1	GRADED TRIAL #2	NOTES
1. ✦	Perform hand hygiene.				
2. ✦	Assemble the equipment.				
3. ✱	*Identify and explain the procedure to the patient.*				
4. ✦	Place the belt around the patient's waist, but over clothing, with the buckle at the front. Do not place over women's breasts.				
5. ✦	Thread the belt through the teeth of the buckle, putting the belt through the other two openings to lock it. Make sure it is snug, with just enough room for a couple of fingers to insert under it.				
6. ✦	Ambulate patient, holding gently onto the gait belt for safety, so the physician can assess gait.				
7. ✦	Perform hand hygiene and return the equipment.				
8. ✦	Document the procedure in the patient's record.				

Name: _____

Date: _____

Document: Enter the appropriate information in the chart below.

Grading

Points Earned	_____		
Points Possible	_____	51	51
Percent Grade (Points Earned/Points Possible)	_____		
PASS:	_____	❏ YES ❏ NO ❏ N/A	❏ YES ❏ NO ❏ N/A

Instructor Sign-Off

Instructor: _____   Date: _____

Procedure 52-2:

Assisting with Assessing Ability to Use Stairs

Objective: Assist patient with stair assessment, using a gait belt and step stool.

Equipment and Supplies: Step stool; gait belt

Affective Behaviors: Affective behaviors provide a professional approach to a skill that enhances the patient encounter. These behaviors may also display sensitivity to a patient's rights and enhance communication. Pay close attention to these skills, which will be in **bold, *italicized*** font.

Notes to the Student

_____

_____

_____

_____

_____

_____

Skills Assessment Requirements

Read and familiarize yourself with the procedure; complete the minimum practice requirements (MPRs). Document each MPR using proper charting technique. Complete each procedure within a reasonable amount of time, with a minimum of 85% accuracy.

POINT VALUE ✦ = 3–6 points ✳ = 7–9 points		PRACTICE TRIAL	GRADED TRIAL # 1	GRADED TRIAL # 2	NOTES
1. ✦	Perform hand hygiene.				
2. ✦	Assemble the equipment.				
3. ✳	*Identify and explain the procedure to the patient.*				
4. ✦	Place the belt around the patient's waist, but over clothing, with the buckle at the front. Do not place over women's breasts.				
5. ✳	Thread the belt through the teeth of the buckle, putting the belt through the other two openings to lock it. Make sure it is snug, with just enough room for a couple of fingers to insert under it.				
6. ✦	*Assist patient to step onto stool while facing the stool, gently holding onto the gait belt for safety.*				
7. ✦	*Ask the patient to step off the stool, while gently holding onto the gait belt for safety.*				
8. ✦	Perform hand hygiene and return the equipment.				
9. ✦	Document the procedure in the patient's record.				

Name: _____

Date: _____

Document: Enter the appropriate information in the chart below.

Grading

Points Earned	_____		
Points Possible	_____	48	48
Percent Grade (Points Earned/Points Possible)	_____		
PASS:	_____	❑ YES ❑ NO ❑ N/A	❑ YES ❑ NO ❑ N/A

Instructor Sign-Off

Instructor: _____   Date: _____

Procedure 52-3:

Application of a Hot Compress

Objective: Perform application of a hot compress and document the procedure.

Equipment and Supplies: Soaking solution (or water) as ordered by physician; basin; bath thermometer; absorbent cloths such as washcloths or gauze squares; waterproof cover such as plastic wrap

Affective Behaviors: Affective behaviors provide a professional approach to a skill that enhances the patient encounter. These behaviors may also display sensitivity to a patient's rights and enhance communication. Pay close attention to these skills, which will be in **bold, italicized** font.

Notes to the Student

_____

_____

_____

_____

_____

_____

Skills Assessment Requirements

Read and familiarize yourself with the procedure; complete the minimum practice requirements (MPRs). Document each MPR using proper charting technique. Complete each procedure within a reasonable amount of time, with a minimum of 85% accuracy.

POINT VALUE ✦ = 3–6 points ✳ = 7–9 points		PRACTICE TRIAL	GRADED TRIAL # 1	GRADED TRIAL # 2	NOTES
1. ✦	Perform proper hand hygiene.				
2. ✦	Assemble all equipment and materials. Use sterile equipment and Standard Precautions if open wound is present.				
3. ✳	**Identify the patient and explain the procedure.**				
4. ✦	Fill the basin half full of warm water or medicated solution prepared according to the physician's directions.				
5. ✦	Request that the patient remove any clothing; compresses must be on bare skin. **Assist the patient, if necessary**.				
6. ✳	Check the temperature of the solution with a bath thermometer. The temperature range for an adult is between 105° and 110°F (41° and 44°C).				
7. ✳	**Position the patient comfortably and in a well-supported position.**				
8. ✦	Place the cloths in the basin of hot water solution. Wring out one cloth until it is wet but not dripping.				
9. ✦	Gradually place the compress on the patient's body part; **ask the patient how the temperature feels.**				
10. ✳	Frequently test the temperature of the solution. Replace the water with warm water as the solution cools.				

POINT VALUE ✦ = 3–6 points ✳ = 7–9 points		PRACTICE TRIAL	GRADED TRIAL # 1	GRADED TRIAL # 2	NOTES
11. ✳	Time the procedure according to the physician's order, usually 15–30 minutes. Check the patient periodically for signs of increased redness, swelling, or pain.				
12. ✦	Gently dry the affected body part.				
13. ✦	**Instruct the patient on any further care, such as continued warm compresses at home.**				
14. ✦	Place towels in the laundry. If an open wound is present, then handle the linens according to Standard Precautions.				
15.	Clean all the equipment.				
16. ✦	Perform hand hygiene.				
17. ✳	Document the procedure in the patient's record.				

Name: _____

Date: _____

Document: Enter the appropriate information in the chart below.

Grading

Points Earned	_____		
Points Possible	_____	120	120
Percent Grade (Points Earned/Points Possible)	_____		
PASS:	_____	❏ YES ❏ NO ❏ N/A	❏ YES ❏ NO ❏ N/A

Instructor Sign-Off

Instructor: _____ **Date:** _____

Procedure 52-4:

Application of a Hot Soak

Objective: Perform hot soak application and document the procedure without error.

Equipment and Supplies: Soaking solution or water; basin or tub; bath thermometer; towels

Affective Behaviors: Affective behaviors provide a professional approach to a skill that enhances the patient encounter. These behaviors may also display sensitivity to a patient's rights and enhance communication. Pay close attention to these skills, which will be in **_bold, italicized_** font.

Notes to the Student

_____

_____

_____

_____

_____

_____

Skills Assessment Requirements

Read and familiarize yourself with the procedure; complete the minimum practice requirements (MPRs). Document each MPR using proper charting technique. Complete each procedure within a reasonable amount of time, with a minimum of 85% accuracy.

Name: _____

Date: _____

POINT VALUE ✦ = 3–6 points ✱ = 7–9 points		PRACTICE TRIAL	GRADED TRIAL # 1	GRADED TRIAL # 2	NOTES
1. ✦	Perform proper hand hygiene.				
2. ✦	Assemble all equipment and materials.				
3. ✱	***Identify and explain the procedure to the patient.***				
4. ✦	Fill the basin or tub half full of water or medicated solution prepared according to directions of the physician.				
5. ✦	***Request the patient to remove any obstructing clothing because soaks are applied to the bare skin. Assist the patient if necessary.***				
6. ✱	Check the temperature of the solution with a bath thermometer. The temperature range for an adult is between 105° and 110°F (41° and 44°C).				
7. ✦	***Position the patient in a comfortable, well-supported position.***				
8. ✦	***Pad the side of the basin or tub with a towel to prevent the patient's body from rubbing on the edge.***				
9. ✦	Gradually place the patient's body part in the solution. ***Ask the patient to tell you how the temperature feels.***				

POINT VALUE ✦ = 3–6 points ✳ = 7–9 points	PRACTICE TRIAL	GRADED TRIAL # 1	GRADED TRIAL # 2	NOTES
10. ✳ Frequently test the temperature of the solution. Using a pitcher, remove part of the liquid every 5 minutes and replace it with hot water. Pour the hot water at the edge of the basin or tub, and protect the patient by placing your hand between the patient's body part and the hot water as it is poured. Swirl the water while pouring to mix the hot and cool fluids together.				
11. ✳ Time the procedure according to the physician's order, usually 15–30 minutes. **Check the patient periodically for signs of increased redness, swelling, or pain.**				
12. ✦ Gently dry the affected body part.				
13. ✦ Instruct the patient on any aftercare, such as performing warm soaks at home.				
14. ✦ Place towels in the laundry. If an open wound is present, then handle linens according to Standard Precautions.				
15. ✦ Clean all equipment.				
16. ✦ Perform hand hygiene and return equipment.				
17. ✳ Document the procedure in the patient's record.				

Document: Enter the appropriate information in the chart below.

Grading

Points Earned	_____		
Points Possible	_____	117	117
Percent Grade (Points Earned/Points Possible)	_____		
PASS:	_____	❏ YES ❏ NO ❏ N/A	❏ YES ❏ NO ❏ N/A

Instructor Sign-Off

Instructor: _____ **Date:** _____

Procedure 52-5:

Application of a Heating Pad

Objective: Perform a heating pad application and document the procedure.

Equipment and Supplies: Heating pad with protective covering or pillowcase

Affective Behaviors: Affective behaviors provide a professional approach to a skill that enhances the patient encounter. These behaviors may also display sensitivity to a patient's rights and enhance communication. Pay close attention to these skills, which will be in **_bold, italicized_** font.

Notes to the Student

Perform a preliminary check of the heating pad without bending it to determine that the wires are in good condition.

_____

_____

_____

_____

_____

Skills Assessment Requirements

Read and familiarize yourself with the procedure; complete the minimum practice requirements (MPRs). Document each MPR using proper charting technique. Complete each procedure within a reasonable amount of time, with a minimum of 85% accuracy.

Name: _____

Date: _____

POINT VALUE ✦ = 3–6 points ✳ = 7–9 points		PRACTICE TRIAL	GRADED TRIAL # 1	GRADED TRIAL # 2	NOTES
1. ✦	Perform hand hygiene.				
2. ✦	Assemble and test the equipment.				
3. ✳	***Identify and instruct the patient concerning the procedure. The patient should be cautioned against using pins, bending the heating elements within the pad, or lying on the heating pad.***				
4. ✦	Place the heating pad in a protective covering or pillow case.				
5. ✦	Connect the heating pad cord to an electrical plug. Set the temperature at the setting ordered by the physician (low or medium).				
6. ✦	Place the heating pad over the patient's affected area. ***Ask the patient to tell you how it feels. Adjust the temperature as necessary.***				
7. ✦	***Instruct the patient regarding the proper temperature setting. Tell him or her not to change the setting.***				
8. ✳	Leave the heating pad in place for the amount of time ordered by the physician (15 to 20 minutes). ***Check the patient periodically for any signs of redness, swelling, or pain.***				
9. ✦	Remove the heating pad when the procedure is complete. ***Instruct the patient on any after-care procedures, such as heat treatments at home.***				

POINT VALUE ✦ = 3–6 points ✶ = 7–9 points		PRACTICE TRIAL	GRADED TRIAL # 1	GRADED TRIAL # 2	NOTES
10. ✦	Place the protective covering in the laundry.				
11. ✦	Perform hand hygiene and return all used equipment.				
12. ✶	Document the procedure in the patient's record.				

Name: _____

Date: _____

Document: Enter the appropriate information in the chart below.

Grading

Points Earned	_____		
Points Possible	_____	81	81
Percent Grade (Points Earned/Points Possible)	_____		
PASS:	_____	❏ YES ❏ NO ❏ N/A	❏ YES ❏ NO ❏ N/A

Instructor Sign-Off

Instructor: _____   **Date:** _____

Name: _____

Date: _____

Procedure 52-6:

Application of a Cold Compress

Objective: Perform a cold compress application and document the procedure.

Equipment and Supplies: Water; absorbent cloths or gauze squares; waterproof cover or plastic wrap; basin; ice

Affective Behaviors: Affective behaviors provide a professional approach to a skill that enhances the patient encounter. These behaviors may also display sensitivity to a patient's rights and enhance communication. Pay close attention to these skills, which will be in **_bold, italicized_** font.

Notes to the Student

_____

_____

_____

_____

_____

_____

Skills Assessment Requirements

Read and familiarize yourself with the procedure; complete the minimum practice requirements (MPRs). Document each MPR using proper charting technique. Complete each procedure within a reasonable amount of time, with a minimum of 85% accuracy.

POINT VALUE ✦ = 3–6 points ✳ = 7–9 points		PRACTICE TRIAL	GRADED TRIAL # 1	GRADED TRIAL # 2	NOTES
1. ✦	Perform hand hygiene.				
2. ✦	Assemble all equipment. If an open wound is present, use sterile equipment and Standard Precautions.				
3. ✳	***Identify and instruct the patient concerning the procedure.***				
4. ✦	Fill the basin half full of cold water. Add ice cubes and compresses.				
5. ✳	Wring out the compress until wet but not dripping. Wrap the compress in a plastic or waterproof covering to prevent further dripping. Gently place the compress on the patient's affected body part.				
6. ✦	Check the compress every 3–5 minutes and replace it with another cold compress when it is no longer cool. Add more ice as the water warms.				
7. ✦	Leave the compress in place for the time specified by the physician (usually 15–20 minutes).				
8. ✦	Gently dry the affected body part.				
9. ✦	Place the linens in the proper container. Clean all the equipment.				
10. ✦	Perform hand hygiene and return all equipment.				
11. ✳	Document the procedure in the patient's record.				

Document: Enter the appropriate information in the chart below.

Grading

Points Earned	_____		
Points Possible	_____	75	75
Percent Grade (Points Earned/Points Possible)	_____		
PASS:	_____	❏ YES ❏ NO ❏ N/A	❏ YES ❏ NO ❏ N/A

Instructor Sign-Off

Instructor: _____ **Date:** _____

Procedure 52-7:

Application of an Ice Bag

Objective: Perform application of an ice bag and document the procedure without error.

Equipment and Supplies: Ice bag with protective cover; ice chips or crushed ice

Affective Behaviors: Affective behaviors provide a professional approach to a skill that enhances the patient encounter. These behaviors may also display sensitivity to a patient's rights and enhance communication. Pay close attention to these skills, which will be in **bold, *italicized*** font.

Notes to the Student

_____

_____

_____

_____

_____

_____

Skills Assessment Requirements

Read and familiarize yourself with the procedure; complete the minimum practice requirements (MPRs). Document each MPR using proper charting technique. Complete each procedure within a reasonable amount of time, with a minimum of 85% accuracy.

POINT VALUE ✦ = 3–6 points ✲ = 7–9 points		PRACTICE TRIAL	GRADED TRIAL # 1	GRADED TRIAL # 2	NOTES
1. ✦	Perform hand hygiene.				
2. ✦	Assemble and test equipment.				
3. ✲	**_Identify and instruct the patient concerning the procedure._**				
4. ✦	Fill the ice bag one-half to two-thirds full of ice. Expel air by squeezing the empty portion of the ice bag. Replace the cap.				
5. ✦	Dry the bag, and place it in a protective cover or small hand towel.				
6. ✦	Place the ice bag over the patient's affected body part. **_Ask the patient how the ice bag feels._**				
7. ✦	Refill the bag with ice, as needed.				
8. ✲	Leave the bag in place for the time specified by the physician's order (15–20 minutes).				
9. ✦	Clean the equipment. Allow the bag to air dry.				
10. ✦	Perform hand hygiene.				
11. ✲	Document the procedure in the patient's record.				

Name: _____

Date: _____

Document: Enter the appropriate information in the chart below.

Grading

Points Earned	_____		
Points Possible	_____	75	75
Percent Grade (Points Earned/Points Possible)	_____		
PASS:	_____	❑ YES ❑ NO ❑ N/A	❑ YES ❑ NO ❑ N/A

Instructor Sign-Off

Instructor: _____   **Date:** _____

Procedure 52-8:

Application of a Cold Chemical Pack

Objective: Perform a cold chemical pack application and document the procedure without error.

Equipment and Supplies: Cold chemical pack; soft cloth

Affective Behaviors: Affective behaviors provide a professional approach to a skill that enhances the patient encounter. These behaviors may also display sensitivity to a patient's rights and enhance communication. Pay close attention to these skills, which will be in **bold, _italicized_** font.

Notes to the Student

_____

_____

_____

_____

_____

_____

Skills Assessment Requirements

Read and familiarize yourself with the procedure; complete the minimum practice requirements (MPRs). Document each MPR using proper charting technique. Complete each procedure within a reasonable amount of time, with a minimum of 85% accuracy.

POINT VALUE ✦ = 3–6 points ✳ = 7–9 points		PRACTICE TRIAL	GRADED TRIAL # 1	GRADED TRIAL # 2	NOTES
1. ✦	Perform hand hygiene.				
2. ✦	Assemble the equipment.				
3. ✳	*Identify and instruct the patient concerning the procedure.*				
4. ✳	Shake the bag to allow crystals to fall to the bottom. Squeeze the pack until the inner bag ruptures. Shake the bag to mix contents. The bag should become cold immediately and remain cold for about 30 minutes.				
5. ✦	Place the bag inside a soft cloth.				
6. ✦	Place the cloth-protected bag over the patient's affected body part.				
7. ✦	Check the patient every 3 to 5 minutes.				
8. ✦	Leave the cold pack in place for the time specified by the physician (usually 15–20 minutes).				
9. ✦	Discard the ice pack in a proper waste container after use.				
10. ✦	Perform hand hygiene.				
11. ✳	Document the procedure in the patient's record.				

Name: _____

Date: _____

Document: Enter the appropriate information in the chart below.

Grading

Points Earned	_____		
Points Possible	_____	75	75
Percent Grade (Points Earned/Points Possible)	_____		
PASS:	_____	❏ YES ❏ NO ❏ N/A	❏ YES ❏ NO ❏ N/A

Instructor Sign-Off

Instructor: _____   **Date:** _____

Procedure 52-9:

Instructing a Patient to Use Crutches Correctly

Objective: Instruct a patient on the correct use of crutches.

Equipment and Supplies: Crutches; gait belt

Affective Behaviors: Affective behaviors provide a professional approach to a skill that enhances the patient encounter. These behaviors may also display sensitivity to a patient's rights and enhance communication. Pay close attention to these skills, which will be in **bold, *italicized*** font.

Notes to the Student

_____

_____

_____

_____

_____

_____

Skills Assessment Requirements

Read and familiarize yourself with the procedure; complete the minimum practice requirements (MPRs). Document each MPR using proper charting technique. Complete each procedure within a reasonable amount of time, with a minimum of 85% accuracy.

POINT VALUE ✦ = 3–6 points ✶ = 7–9 points		PRACTICE TRIAL	GRADED TRIAL # 1	GRADED TRIAL # 2	NOTES
1. ✦	Assemble all equipment requested by the physician's order.				
2. ✦	Check the crutches to determine that they are in good working order.				
3. ✦	Perform hand hygiene.				
4. ✶	**Identify the patient and explain the procedure.**				
5. ✶	**Check to see if the patient is wearing sturdy, nonskid shoes.**				
6. ✦	Demonstrate the correct position.				
7. ✦	**Attach the gait belt requested by the physician.**				
8. ✦	**Have the patient stand against the wall or near a chair for support.**				
9. ✶	Adjust the crutch length to the appropriate height. The distance between the top of the crutch and axilla should be equivalent to three finger widths.				
10. ✦	**Instruct the patient to keep his or her head up, stand straight with abdomen in, and keep feet straight with a slight (5-degree) bend at the knee joint. Remind the patient to look ahead and not down while walking with crutches.** This will prevent the patient from bending forward.				

Name: _____

Date: _____

POINT VALUE ✦ = 3–6 points ✶ = 7–9 points	PRACTICE TRIAL	GRADED TRIAL # 1	GRADED TRIAL # 2	NOTES
11. ✶ **Explain to the patient that the weight should be supported by the hands, not the underarms.** The patient should practice standing to maintain balance and place weight on the palms of the hands, not on the axillae, at the hand bars. **Instruct the patient not to rest body weight on the axillary bars for more than 1 or 2 minutes to prevent injury to the brachial plexus.**				
12. ✦ **Instruct the patient to assume basic crutch stance, or tripod, to provide a firm base of support.** Feet are slightly apart, and the tips of the crutches are 4 to 6 inches in front of and 4 to 6 inches to the side of the toes. An imaginary line drawn from the two crutch points to an area behind the center of the feet will form a triangle (tripod).				
13. ✦ **Instruct the patient to take small steps and swing through when first learning to use crutches.** The crutches should only move about 12 inches forward with each step to prevent the crutches from slipping. Have the patient move slowly at first.				
14. ✦ **Have the patient practice his or her gait.**				

POINT VALUE ✦ = 3–6 points ✶ = 7–9 points		PRACTICE TRIAL	GRADED TRIAL # 1	GRADED TRIAL # 2	NOTES
15. ✶	Remind the patient to report any numbness or tingling in the arms. The crutch shoulders and hand bars can be padded for extra comfort with either sponge rubber or a soft cloth. The patient should then remeasure and adjust the crutches for the correct length.				
16. ✦	Crutches should always be moved forward and to the side so the feet can swing through.				
17. ✦	**Remind the patient to periodically check the nuts and wing bolts to maintain tightness and to check the rubber tips frequently for cracks.**				
18. ✦	**Make corrections on the patient's use of crutches as needed.**				
19. ✶	Chart appropriately.				

Document: Enter the appropriate information in the chart below.

Grading

Points Earned	_____		
Points Possible	_____	132	132
Percent Grade (Points Earned/Points Possible)	_____		
PASS:	_____	❏ YES ❏ NO ❏ N/A	❏ YES ❏ NO ❏ N/A

Instructor Sign-Off

Instructor: _____   **Date:** _____

Name: _____

Date: _____

Procedure 52-10:

Instructing a Patient to Use a Cane

Objective: Instruct a patient on the correct use of a cane.

Equipment and Supplies: Cane suited to the patient's needs; gait belt

Affective Behaviors: Affective behaviors provide a professional approach to a skill that enhances the patient encounter. These behaviors may also display sensitivity to a patient's rights and enhance communication. Pay close attention to these skills, which will be in **bold, italicized** font.

Notes to the Student

_____

_____

_____

_____

_____

_____

_____

Skills Assessment Requirements

Read and familiarize yourself with the procedure; complete the minimum practice requirements (MPRs). Document each MPR using proper charting technique. Complete each procedure within a reasonable amount of time, with a minimum of 85% accuracy.

Name: _____

Date: _____

POINT VALUE ✦ = 3–6 points ✶ = 7–9 points		PRACTICE TRIAL	GRADED TRIAL # 1	GRADED TRIAL # 2	NOTES
1. ✦	Assemble the equipment according to the physician's order.				
2. ✦	Check the cane height and condition of the cane tip.				
3. ✦	***Identify the patient.***				
4. ✶	Perform hand hygiene and ***explain the procedure.***				
5. ✶	Be sure that the patient is wearing sturdy, nonskid shoes.				
6. ✦	Demonstrate the correct position.				
7. ✦	Demonstrate the gait.				
8. ✦	***Instruct the patient to hold the cane (or single crutch) on the opposite side of the injury or affected limb.*** As the affected leg moves forward, the cane (or crutch) on the opposite side will move forward to provide support.				
9. ✶	Place the cane (or single crutch) 6 inches in front of and slightly to one side of the unaffected side. Make sure the cane tip is firmly on the floor and the weight is supported on the strong leg and the cane. The patient's elbow should be slightly flexed during weight bearing.				
10. ✦	Have the patient look straight ahead, not down at his or her feet.				

POINT VALUE ✦ = 3–6 points ✳ = 7–9 points		PRACTICE TRIAL	GRADED TRIAL # 1	GRADED TRIAL # 2	NOTES
11. ✦	Have the patient move the cane (or single crutch) forward 6 to 12 inches and bring the affected leg forward until it is even with the cane. The weight should be placed on the strong foot and leg.				
12. ✳	**Instruct the patient to move the strong leg forward past the cane and weaker leg.** As the unaffected foot moves forward, the weight is shifted to the weak or affected foot and the cane. Thus the cane will provide support for weight bearing on the weaker leg.				
13. ✦	Have the patient repeat the walking pattern. Evaluate his or her balance and endurance.				
14. ✳	Document the procedure correctly.				

Document: Enter the appropriate information in the chart below.

Grading

Points Earned	_____		
Points Possible	_____	96	96
Percent Grade (Points Earned/Points Possible)	_____		
PASS:	_____	❏ YES ❏ NO ❏ N/A	❏ YES ❏ NO ❏ N/A

Instructor Sign-Off

Instructor: _____   Date: _____

Procedure 52-11:

Teaching a Patient to Correctly Use a Walker

Objective: Teach a patient to correctly use a walker.

Equipment and Supplies: Walker suited to patient's needs; gait belt

Affective Behaviors: Affective behaviors provide a professional approach to a skill that enhances the patient encounter. These behaviors may also display sensitivity to a patient's rights and enhance communication. Pay close attention to these skills, which will be in **bold, *italicized*** font.

Notes to the Student

_____

_____

_____

_____

_____

Skills Assessment Requirements

Read and familiarize yourself with the procedure; complete the minimum practice requirements (MPRs). Document each MPR using proper charting technique. Complete each procedure within a reasonable amount of time, with a minimum of 85% accuracy.

Name: _____

Date: _____

POINT VALUE ✦ = 3–6 points ✳ = 7–9 points		PRACTICE TRIAL	GRADED TRIAL #1	GRADED TRIAL #2	NOTES
1. ✦	Assemble the equipment according to the physician's order.				
2. ✦	Check the condition of the walker.				
3. ✦	Perform hand hygiene.				
4. ✳	*Identify the patient and explain the procedure.*				
5. ✳	Check to see if the patient is wearing sturdy, nonskid shoes.				
6. ✦	Demonstrate the correct stance and gait with the walker.				
7. ✦	*Assist the patient into the walker.*				
8. ✳	*Evaluate the walker for proper height and fit.*				
9. ✳	*Instruct the patient to distribute his or her weight evenly between the walker and both legs.*				
10. ✦	Have the patient move the walker 6–8 inches ahead, with all four legs of the walker hitting the floor at the same time.				
11. ✦	*Instruct the patient to bring the weaker foot into the walker.*				
12. ✦	*Instruct the patient to bring the stronger foot forward, even with the weaker foot.*				
13. ✦	Have the patient continue walking with the walker while you evaluate the patient's balance and endurance.				
14. ✳	Document properly.				

Document: Enter the appropriate information in the chart below.

Grading

Points Earned	_____		
Points Possible	_____	99	99
Percent Grade (Points Earned/Points Possible)	_____		
PASS:	_____	❏ YES ❏ NO ❏ N/A	❏ YES ❏ NO ❏ N/A

Instructor Sign-Off

Instructor: _____   **Date:** _____

Procedure 52-12:

Wheelchair Transfer to a Chair or Examination Table

Objective: Move the patient from a wheelchair to a chair or examination table without error.

Equipment and Supplies: Chair or examination table; gait belt, if needed; step stool, if needed

Affective Behaviors: Affective behaviors provide a professional approach to a skill that enhances the patient encounter. These behaviors may also display sensitivity to a patient's rights and enhance communication. Pay close attention to these skills, which will be in **_bold, italicized_** font.

Notes to the Student

_____

_____

_____

_____

_____

_____

Skills Assessment Requirements

Read and familiarize yourself with the procedure; complete the minimum practice requirements (MPRs). Document each MPR using proper charting technique. Complete each procedure within a reasonable amount of time, with a minimum of 85% accuracy.

POINT VALUE ✦ = 3–6 points ✶ = 7–9 points		PRACTICE TRIAL	GRADED TRIAL # 1	GRADED TRIAL # 2	NOTES
1. ✦	Perform hand hygiene.				
2. ✶	***Identify the patient and introduce yourself.***				
3. ✶	***Explain what you are going to do before you start. Discuss what the patient can do to assist you.***				
4. ✦	Place the wheelchair at a 45-degree angle to the chair or exam table.				
5. ✦	Put the wheelchair brakes in the lock position on both sides. The patient's legs should be moved off the pedals by supporting the ankle and lower leg. Gently place the patient's feet on the floor and have the patient shift forward in the chair, if possible. Move the foot pedals up and out of the way so the patient has a clear path to move forward.				
6. ✶	Make sure the examination table or chair is stable before attempting the transfer.				
7. ✦	Position yourself near the patient's nonparalyzed side so you can provide support and the patient can use his or her stronger limb. You will move the patient toward the stronger side. Do not refer to the patient's "good" or "bad" side.				
8. ✶	Place one of your feet forward to establish a firm base of support for your body. Move down toward the patient while keeping your back straight.				

POINT VALUE ✦ = 3–6 points ✶ = 7–9 points	PRACTICE TRIAL	GRADED TRIAL # 1	GRADED TRIAL # 2	NOTES
9. ✦ Have the patient place his or her hands on the arm supports of the wheelchair. ***Then, ask the patient to lean forward and push up as you assist the patient to a standing position, on the count of three.***				
10. ✦ Position yourself so that the patient's paralyzed leg is between your knees. Support the paralyzed leg with your knees, if necessary, so the leg will not slip as the patient stands.				
11. ✦ Place your hands under the patient's armpits and help the patient to stand. Use the muscles in your legs to push your body upward. Do not bend over and use your back muscles.				
12. ✦ Allow the patient to stand for a few moments before attempting to move into the chair or onto the examination table.				
13. ✶ ***Assist the patient to pivot (turn) toward the nonparalyzed side*** by pivoting your own body as you hold the patient under his or her armpits. Do not twist your body. Turn it as a unit.				
14. ✶ Gently lower the patient into the chair by bending your knees and keeping your back straight.				

POINT VALUE ✦ = 3–6 points ✷ = 7–9 points		PRACTICE TRIAL	GRADED TRIAL # 1	GRADED TRIAL # 2	NOTES
15. ✦	If the patient must move up onto an examination table and can assist you, then support the weak side as the patient places his or her stronger leg onto the step stool. Pivot the patient around so he or she can then sit on the edge of the table. Encourage the patient to move back on the table to eliminate the danger of falling.				
16. ✦	If the patient is unable to assist you, then ask for another assistant to hold one side of the patient as you support the other side. Count aloud "one," "two," "three," and then lift the patient together. Do not attempt to lift—by yourself—a patient who is unable to help you.				
17. ✦	When assisting the patient into a supine position, support the paralyzed leg gently onto the table.				
18. ✦	Never leave a physically challenged (disabled) patient unattended.				

Name: _____

Date: _____

Document: Enter the appropriate information in the chart below.

Grading

Points Earned	_____		
Points Possible	_____	126	126
Percent Grade (Points Earned/Points Possible)	_____		
PASS:	_____	❏ YES ❏ NO ❏ N/A	❏ YES ❏ NO ❏ N/A

Instructor Sign-Off

Instructor: _____   **Date:** _____

Procedure 55-1:

Administering Oral Medications

Objective: Administer oral medication.

Equipment and Supplies: Medication order signed by physician; oral medication; calibrated paper cup or receptacle for medication; water in glass; patient instruction sheet; biohazard waste container; pen

Affective Behaviors: Affective behaviors provide a professional approach to a skill that enhances the patient encounter. These behaviors may also display sensitivity to a patient's rights and enhance communication. Pay close attention to these skills, which will be in **bold, italicized** font.

Notes to the Student

_____

_____

_____

_____

_____

_____

Skills Assessment Requirements

Read and familiarize yourself with the procedure; complete the minimum practice requirements (MPRs). Document each MPR using proper charting technique. Complete each procedure within a reasonable amount of time, with a minimum of 85% accuracy.

POINT VALUE ✦ = 3–6 points ✳ = 7–9 points		**PRACTICE TRIAL**	**GRADED TRIAL # 1**	**GRADED TRIAL # 2**	**NOTES**
1. ✦	Assemble equipment.				
2. ✦	Perform hand hygiene.				
3. ✳	Select the correct medication using the "three befores" technique. If you are not familiar with the medication, look it up in a reference book, read the package insert, and/or consult the physician.				
4. ✳	Always double-check the label to make sure the strength is correct.				
5. ✳	Correctly calculate the dosage in writing. Double-check your calculations with someone else.				
6. ✦	Place a medicine cup or container on a flat surface.				
7. ✦	Gently shake the medication if it is in liquid form.				
8. ✳	Hold the bottle so that the label is in the palm of your hand to prevent damaging the label with liquid medication.				
9. ✳	Recheck the label.				
10. ✳	Remove the cap from the medicine container and place it upside down on a clean surface.				

POINT VALUE ✦ = 3–6 points ✳ = 7–9 points	PRACTICE TRIAL	GRADED TRIAL # 1	GRADED TRIAL # 2	NOTES
11. ✳ **Liquid Medication:** Hold the calibrated medicine cup at eye level and pour the medication into the cup, stopping at the correct dosage line. Pour the medication away from the label side of the bottle. If too much medication is poured into the calibrated cup, do not return it to the bottle. Discard it into a sink. **Table or Capsule Medication:** Shake out the correct number of tablets or pills into the bottle cap. Then, place the tablets or pills in the medicine cup. If you accidentally pour out an extra tablet, do not return it to the medication bottle; discard it.				
12. ✦ Check the medication again to make sure the dosage is the same as the medication order.				
13. ✦ Replace the cap on the medication bottle and return the bottle to the storage shelf.				
14. ✳ Take the prepared medication and a glass of water to the patient.				
15. ✳ *Warmly greet and identify the patient both by stating his or her name and by examining any printed identification such as a wrist name band or medical record. Introduce yourself to the patient and ask the patient if he or she has any allergies.*				

POINT VALUE ✦ = 3–6 points ✶ = 7–9 points		PRACTICE TRIAL	GRADED TRIAL # 1	GRADED TRIAL # 2	NOTES
16. ✶	Tell the patient the name of the medication and dosage that you are administering per the physician's order. **Ask the patient if he or she has any questions prior to taking the medication.**				
17. ✶	**Provide the patient with written follow-up instructions if further medication is to be taken.**				
18. ✶	Document the medication administration, on the correct patient's record, noting in the patient's record the time, medication name, dosage route, and your name. After giving medication to the patient, it is best to have the patient wait in the office for 30 minutes.				

Name: _____

Date: _____

Document: Enter the appropriate information in the chart below.

Grading

Points Earned	_____		
Points Possible	_____	147	147
Percent Grade (Points Earned/Points Possible)	_____		
PASS:	_____	❏ YES ❏ NO ❏ N/A	❏ YES ❏ NO ❏ N/A

Instructor Sign-Off

Instructor: _____ Date: _____

Procedure 55-2:

Administering Sublingual or Buccal Medication

Objective: Administer a medication to a patient under the tongue or between the cheek and gum.

Equipment and Supplies: Medication order signed by physician on the patient's medical record; oral medication; paper cup or receptacle for medication; patient instruction sheet; biohazard waste container; pen

Affective Behaviors: Affective behaviors provide a professional approach to a skill that enhances the patient encounter. These behaviors may also display sensitivity to a patient's rights and enhance communication. Pay close attention to these skills, which will be in **_bold, italicized_** font.

Notes to the Student

_____

_____

_____

_____

_____

Skills Assessment Requirements

Read and familiarize yourself with the procedure; complete the minimum practice requirements (MPRs). Document each MPR using proper charting technique. Complete each procedure within a reasonable amount of time, with a minimum of 85% accuracy.

POINT VALUE ✦ = 3–6 points ✳ = 7–9 points		PRACTICE TRIAL	GRADED TRIAL # 1	GRADED TRIAL # 2	NOTES
1. ✦	Assemble equipment.				
2. ✦	Perform hand hygiene.				
3. ✳	Select the correct medication using the "three befores" technique. If you are not familiar with the medication, look it up in a reference book, read the package insert, and/or consult the physician.				
4. ✳	Always double-check the label to make sure the strength is correct.				
5. ✳	Correctly calculate the dosage in writing. Double-check your calculations with someone else.				
6. ✦	Place a medicine cup/container on a flat surface.				
7. ✳	Shake the tablet ordered into the bottle cap and then into a medication container.				
8. ✳	Check the dosage again against the medication order.				
9. ✦	Replace the cap on the medication bottle, and return the bottle to the storage shelf after reading the label *again*.				
10. ✳	***Introduce yourself and warmly greet and identify the patient, both by stating his or her name and by examining any printed identification such as a wrist name band or medical record. Ask the patient if he or she has any allergies.***				

POINT VALUE ✦ = 3–6 points ✶ = 7–9 points	PRACTICE TRIAL	GRADED TRIAL # 1	GRADED TRIAL # 2	NOTES
11. ✶ **Tell the patient the name of the medication and dosage you are administering per the physician's order. Ask the patient if he or she has any questions prior to taking the medication.**				
12. ✶ **Sublingual Medication:** Have the patient place the tablet under the tongue. **Instruct the patient not to swallow until the tablet has dissolved.** **Buccal Medication:** Have the patient place the tablet between the cheek and gum. **Instruct the patient not to swallow until the tablet is dissolved.**				
13. ✦ **Tell the patient not to take fluids until the tablet is dissolved.**				
14. ✶ **Remain with the patient until the medication has dissolved.**				
15. ✶ **Provide the patient with written follow-up instructions if further medication is to be taken.**				
16. ✶ Chart the medication administration on the correct patient's record, noting the time, medication name, dosage route, and your name. After giving medication to the patient, it is best to have the patient wait in the office for 30 minutes.				

Document: Enter the appropriate information in the chart below.

Grading

Points Earned	_____		
Points Possible	_____	120	120
Percent Grade (Points Earned/Points Possible)	_____		
PASS:	_____	❏ YES ❏ NO ❏ N/A	❏ YES ❏ NO ❏ N/A

Instructor Sign-Off

Instructor: _____ **Date:** _____

Procedure 55-3:

Administering a Rectal or Vaginal Suppository

Objective: Insert a suppository as ordered by the physician.

Equipment and Supplies: Medication order signed by physician; lubricant; water; biohazard waste container; patient instructions; vaginal suppository or cream; sanitary napkin; rectal suppository; nonsterile gloves; 4 × 4 gauze square; pen

Affective Behaviors: Affective behaviors provide a professional approach to a skill that enhances the patient encounter. These behaviors may also display sensitivity to a patient's rights and enhance communication. Pay close attention to these skills, which will be in **bold, *italicized*** font.

Notes to the Student

_____

_____

_____

_____

_____

_____

Skills Assessment Requirements

Read and familiarize yourself with the procedure; complete the minimum practice requirements (MPRs). Document each MPR using proper charting technique. Complete each procedure within a reasonable amount of time, with a minimum of 85% accuracy.

Name: _____

Date: _____

POINT VALUE ✦ = 3–6 points ✶ = 7–9 points		PRACTICE TRIAL	GRADED TRIAL # 1	GRADED TRIAL # 2	NOTES
1. ✦	Assemble equipment.				
2. ✦	Perform hand hygiene.				
3. ✦	Select the medication using the "three befores." If you are not familiar with the medication, look it up in a reference book, read the package insert, and/or consult the physician.				
4. ✶	Always double-check the suppository label to validate that the strength is correct, because medications are manufactured with different strengths.				
5. ✶	Correctly calculate the dosage in writing. Double-check your calculations with someone else.				
6. ✶	Check the dosage again against the medication order.				
7. ✦	Replace the cap on the medication bottle and return the bottle to the storage shelf or refrigerator after reading the label again.				
8. ✶	***Warmly greet and identify the patient both by stating his or her name and by examining any printed identification such as a wrist name band or medical record. Introduce yourself to the patient and ask the patient if he or she has any allergies.***				

POINT VALUE ✦ = 3–6 points ✳ = 7–9 points	PRACTICE TRIAL	GRADED TRIAL # 1	GRADED TRIAL # 2	NOTES
9. ✦ Give the patient a gown or sheet. Have the patient remove all clothing from the waist down. Assist the patient, as necessary, **and provide reassurance if the patient seems uncomfortable with the administration of a suppository**.				
10. ✦ Tell the patient the name of the medication and dosage that you are administering, per the physician's order. **Ask the patient if he or she has any questions prior to receiving the medication.**				
11. ✳ a. *Rectal suppository:* Have the patient lie on the left side, if possible, with top leg bent. Drape a sheet over the patient. Apply nonsterile gloves. Open the suppository wrapper and place the suppository on a gauze square. Moisten the suppository with a small amount of lubricant or water. With one hand, separate the buttocks. Pick up the suppository with the other hand. **Ask the patient to breathe slowly as you insert the suppository from 1 to 1 ½ inches through the rectal sphincter.** Hold the buttocks together and instruct the patient not to bear down or push out the suppository. Wipe the anal area with the gauze and discard gauze into a biohazard waste container. Have the patient remain in the side position for about 20 minutes until the suppository melts.				

POINT VALUE ✦ = 3–6 points ✶ = 7–9 points		PRACTICE TRIAL	GRADED TRIAL # 1	GRADED TRIAL # 2	NOTES
	b. *Vaginal suppository:* Have the patient lie supine (face up) with legs apart and place a clean pad between the patient's legs for placement of supplies. Drape the patient for privacy. Apply nonsterile disposable gloves. Peel open the suppository container and drop the suppository on the clean pad. If an applicator is provided, drop it on the clean pad. With one gloved hand, separate the labia minora and hold the folds apart. Using the other hand, insert the suppository one finger length into the vagina. If an applicator is used, place the suppository into the applicator and insert it in a downward direction. ***Instruct the patient to remain in the supine,*** legs-apart position for at least 10 minutes for the suppository to dissolve. Place the applicator into the glove wrapper. Remove one glove by pulling inside out from the cuff. With the remaining gloved hand, roll the contaminated wrapper and contents. Hold these waste items as you remove the remaining glove over them. Dispose of all materials in a biohazard waste container. ***Offer the patient a sanitary napkin.***				

POINT VALUE ✦ = 3–6 points ✳ = 7–9 points	PRACTICE TRIAL	GRADED TRIAL # 1	GRADED TRIAL # 2	NOTES
12. ✳ **Remain with the patient until the medication has dissolved.**				
13. ✳ **Provide the patient with written follow-up instructions if further medication is to be taken.**				
14. ✳ Chart the medication administration in the patient's record, noting time, medication name, dosage, injection site, route, and your name.				

Name: _____

Date: _____

Document: Enter the appropriate information in the chart below.

Grading

Points Earned	_____		
Points Possible	_____	108	108
Percent Grade (Points Earned/Points Possible)	_____		
PASS:	_____	❑ YES ❑ NO ❑ N/A	❑ YES ❑ NO ❑ N/A

Instructor Sign-Off

Instructor: _____ **Date:** _____

Procedure 55-4:

Withdrawing Medication from Single-Dose or Multiple-Dose Vials

Objective: Withdraw medication from single-dose and multiple-dose vials.

Equipment and Supplies: Disposable gloves; biohazard waste container; biohazard sharps container; soap; needle; syringe; alcohol sponge; medication vial; pen

Affective Behaviors: Affective behaviors provide a professional approach to a skill that enhances the patient encounter. These behaviors may also display sensitivity to a patient's rights and enhance communication. Pay close attention to these skills, which will be in **bold, italicized** font.

Notes to the Student

_____

_____

_____

_____

_____

_____

Skills Assessment Requirements

Read and familiarize yourself with the procedure; complete the minimum practice requirements (MPRs). Document each MPR using proper charting technique. Complete each procedure within a reasonable amount of time, with a minimum of 85% accuracy.

POINT VALUE ✦ = 3–6 points ✻ = 7–9 points		**PRACTICE TRIAL**	**GRADED TRIAL # 1**	**GRADED TRIAL # 2**	**NOTES**
1. ✦	Check the medication using the "three befores" technique before beginning. Compare the medication vial (bottle) against the physician's order.				
2. ✻	Select the correct syringe and needle based on the type of medication and the location of the injection site.				
3. ✦	Perform hand hygiene and apply gloves.				
4. ✦	Roll the medication vial between your hands to mix any medication that has settled at the bottom.				
5. ✻	Wipe the rubber stopper with an alcohol sponge, firmly and using a circular motion. Then set the vial on a clean surface while you prepare the syringe.				
6. ✦	Remove the protective cap from the needle on the syringe. Be sure to maintain the sterility of the inner surface of the protective cap, since it will be needed to cover the needle again after you have filled the syringe.				
7. ✻	Withdraw the syringe plunger, and allow air to enter the syringe barrel equal to the amount of medication to be withdrawn. Because the vials are vacuum sealed, this will allow for easier withdrawal of fluid.				

POINT VALUE ✦ = 3–6 points ✳ = 7–9 points		PRACTICE TRIAL	GRADED TRIAL # 1	GRADED TRIAL # 2	NOTES
8. ✳	Turning the vial upside down at eye level, and using care not to touch the rubber stopper, insert the needle into the rubber stopper and inject the air into the vial. Be extremely cautious concerning contamination as you enter the multiple-dose bottle.				
9. ✳	Keeping the vial upside down at eye level with the needle still inserted into the rubber stopper, slowly withdraw the correct amount of medication.				
10. ✳	While the needle is still in the vial, check to make sure that the dosage is accurate. Any air bubbles in the syringe will give you an inaccurate dose, because they take up the space needed for medication. To remove air bubbles, flick your fingers against the side of the syringe until the air bubbles go back into the tip of the syringe.				
11. ✦	Remove the needle from the vial.				
12. ✳	If you have accidentally withdrawn too much fluid, discard the excess fluid by shooting it into a sink or waste receptacle. Never return medications to the vial or bottle from which they came.				

POINT VALUE ✦ = 3–6 points ✳ = 7–9 points		PRACTICE TRIAL	GRADED TRIAL # 1	GRADED TRIAL # 2	NOTES
13. ✳	Check the medication vial after you have withdrawn the dosage to make sure you are correct. This is the last step of the "three befores" for checking medications. Also, check to see if the multiple-dose vial should be refrigerated after opening.				
14. ✦	Remove gloves and perform hand hygiene.				
15. ✳	Document the medication and procedure in the patient's record.				

Name: _____

Date: _____

Document: Enter the appropriate information in the chart below.

Grading

Points Earned	_____		
Points Possible	_____	117	117
Percent Grade (Points Earned/Points Possible)	_____		
PASS:	_____	❏ YES ❏ NO ❏ N/A	❏ YES ❏ NO ❏ N/A

Instructor Sign-Off

Instructor: _____   **Date:** _____

Name: _____

Date: _____

Procedure 55-5:

Withdrawing Medication from an Ampule

Objective: Open and withdraw medication from an ampule.

Equipment and Supplies: Ampule containing medication; soap; alcohol sponge; needle; syringe; disposable gloves; biohazard waste container; pen

Affective Behaviors: Affective behaviors provide a professional approach to a skill that enhances the patient encounter. These behaviors may also display sensitivity to a patient's rights and enhance communication. Pay close attention to these skills, which will be in *bold, italicized* font.

Notes to the Student

_____

_____

_____

_____

_____

_____

Skills Assessment Requirements

Read and familiarize yourself with the procedure; complete the minimum practice requirements (MPRs). Document each MPR using proper charting technique. Complete each procedure within a reasonable amount of time, with a minimum of 85% accuracy.

POINT VALUE ✦ = 3–6 points ✳ = 7–9 points		PRACTICE TRIAL	GRADED TRIAL # 1	GRADED TRIAL # 2	NOTES
1. ✦	Check the medication against the physician's medication order, following the "three befores" technique.				
2. ✦	Do not open the ampule until you are ready to withdraw the fluid.				
3. ✦	Perform hand hygiene and apply gloves.				
4. ✳	Snap your thumb and middle finger gently against the tip of the ampule to move all the medication away from the neck and into the bottom of the ampule.				
5. ✦	Clean the neck of the ampule using an alcohol swab.				
6. ✳	Use gauze between the ampule and your thumb when breaking the ampule. Using one hand to hold the bottom of the vial, snap the top off with the other hand using a gauze square to prevent a cut when the glass neck breaks.				
7. ✦	If the top of the ampule does not snap off easily, you may have to use a file to create a cut or "score" the ampule at the neck. Once scored, the glass ampule should break easily.				
8. ✳	Insert a filter needle (attached to a syringe) into the ampule and withdraw the fluid without touching the sides of the ampule.				

Name: _____

Date: _____

POINT VALUE ✦ = 3–6 points ✶ = 7–9 points		PRACTICE TRIAL	GRADED TRIAL #1	GRADED TRIAL #2	NOTES
9. ✶	Withdraw all the medication from the ampule. It may be necessary to tip the ampule slightly to withdraw all of the fluid.				
10. ✦	Discard the broken ampule into a biohazard waste container.				
11. ✶	Remove the filter needle from the syringe and discard it into the sharps container. Place the correct-size needle necessary for medication administration.				
12. ✦	Remove and discard gloves and perform hand hygiene.				

Name: _____

Date: _____

Document: Enter the appropriate information in the chart below.

Grading

Points Earned	_____		
Points Possible	_____	87	87
Percent Grade (Points Earned/Points Possible)	_____		
PASS:	_____	❏ YES ❏ NO ❏ N/A	❏ YES ❏ NO ❏ N/A

Instructor Sign-Off

Instructor: _____ **Date:** _____

Name: _____

Date: _____

Procedure 55-6:

Administering a Z-Track Injection

Objective: Administer a Z-track injection using proper technique.

Equipment and Supplies: Alcohol sponges; biohazard sharps container; biohazard waste container; disposable gloves; medication order signed by the physician; pen; sterile needle and syringe; medication vial

Affective Behaviors: Affective behaviors provide a professional approach to a skill that enhances the patient encounter. These behaviors may also display sensitivity to a patient's rights and enhance communication. Pay close attention to these skills, which will be in **_bold, italicized_** font.

Notes to the Student

_____

_____

_____

_____

_____

_____

Skills Assessment Requirements

Read and familiarize yourself with the procedure; complete the minimum practice requirements (MPRs). Document each MPR using proper charting technique. Complete each procedure within a reasonable amount of time, with a minimum of 85% accuracy.

POINT VALUE ✦ = 3–6 points ✱ = 7–9 points		PRACTICE TRIAL	GRADED TRIAL #1	GRADED TRIAL #2	NOTES
1–15. ✦	Follow steps 1–15 of Procedure 55-7 for intramuscular injection.				
16. ✦	After withdrawing the medication from the vial, change to a fresh needle. This will prevent any irritating medication that may be within the needle from coming into contact with the patient's tissue until the needle is placed into the muscle layer.				
17. ✱	When ready to administer the medication, pull the skin of the buttocks to one side and hold it in place with your nondominant hand. *Note:* You may wish to use a dry gauze sponge if the skin is slippery.				
18. ✱	With your dominant hand and using a dartlike grip on the syringe, insert the needle up to the hub quickly into the gluteus medius muscle. Do not move the needle once it is in place.				
19. ✱	While still maintaining a firm hold on the taut skin with your nondominant hand, pull back on the plunger of the syringe to check for blood return. To do this, simply move your fingers up the syringe, while keeping the needle steady within the patient's buttocks, until your thumb and index finger reach the top of the plunger. If blood appears in the hub of the syringe, use the correct technique to withdraw the syringe, discard it, and begin with step 1 again.				

POINT VALUE ✦ = 3–6 points ✳ = 7–9 points		PRACTICE TRIAL	GRADED TRIAL # 1	GRADED TRIAL # 2	NOTES
20. ✳	If there is no blood return, very slowly inject the medication into the muscle.				
21. ✳	Wait several seconds after injecting the medication before you withdraw the needle. Cover the area with the alcohol sponge, and withdraw the needle at the same angle of insertion. Wait at least 10 seconds before releasing the skin being held by the nondominant hand.				
22. ✳	Do not massage the area. Observe the patient for at least 15 minutes for any adverse reaction. *You may advise the patient to walk around to assist in the medication's absorption process.*				
23. ✦	Correctly dispose of all materials.				
24. ✦	Remove and discard gloves, and perform proper hand hygiene.				
25. ✦	Chart the medication administration in the patient's record, noting the time, medication name, dosage, route, injection site, and your name.				

Name: _____

Date: _____

Document: Enter the appropriate information in the chart below.

Grading

Points Earned	_____		
Points Possible	_____	168	168
Percent Grade (Points Earned/Points Possible)	_____		
PASS:	_____	❑ YES ❑ NO ❑ N/A	❑ YES ❑ NO ❑ N/A

Instructor Sign-Off

Instructor: _____ **Date:** _____

Procedure 55-7:

Administering Parenteral, Subcutaneous, or Intramuscular Injections

Objective: Administer subcutaneous (SubQ) and intramuscular (IM) injections.

Equipment and Supplies: Medication order signed by physician; vial of medication; disposable gloves; alcohol sponges; biohazard sharps container; biohazard waste container

Subcutaneous injection: 25-gauge, 5/8-inch needle for small arm; 23-gauge, 1-inch needle for average arm; disposable 3-mL syringe

Intramuscular injection: 22-gauge, 11/2-inch needle; disposable 3-mL syringe; pen

Affective Behaviors: Affective behaviors provide a professional approach to a skill that enhances the patient encounter. These behaviors may also display sensitivity to a patient's rights and enhance communication. Pay close attention to these skills, which will be in **bold, *italicized*** font.

Notes to the Student

_____

_____

_____

_____

_____

_____

Skills Assessment Requirements

Read and familiarize yourself with the procedure; complete the minimum practice requirements (MPRs). Document each MPR using proper charting technique. Complete each procedure within a reasonable amount of time, with a minimum of 85% accuracy.

Name: _____

Date: _____

		PRACTICE TRIAL	GRADED TRIAL #1	GRADED TRIAL #2	NOTES
POINT VALUE ✦ = 3–6 points ✳ = 7–9 points					
1. ✦	Perform hand hygiene.				
2. ✦	Apply gloves and follow standard blood and body fluid precautions.				
3. ✦	Select the correct medication using the "three befores."				
4. ✦	Gently roll the medication between your hands to mix any medication that may have settled. Refrigerated medication can be rolled between your hands to warm it slightly.				
5. ✳	Prepare the syringe using the correct technique. Carefully carry the covered needle and syringe to the patient.				
6. ✳	***Warmly greet and identify the patient both by stating his or her name and examining any printed identification such as a wrist name band or medical record. Introduce yourself to the patient and ask the patient if he or she has any allergies.***				
7. ✦	***Tell the patient the name of the medication and dosage. Ask the patient if he or she has any questions prior to receiving the medication.***				
8. ✦	Position the patient depending on the site you are using.				
9. ✳	Using a circular motion, cleanse the patient's skin with an alcohol sponge. Wipe the skin with a sweeping motion from the center of the area outward.				

POINT VALUE ✦ = 3–6 points ✳ = 7–9 points		PRACTICE TRIAL	GRADED TRIAL #1	GRADED TRIAL #2	NOTES
10. ✳	Once again check the medication dosage against the patient's order to determine if this is the correct time to administer the dose (one of the "ten rights").				
11. ✦	Remove the protective cover from the needle, taking care not to touch the needle. *Note:* If you accidentally touch the needle, excuse yourself to the patient. Then, return to the preparation area and change the needle on the syringe. If you are using a self-contained syringe and needle unit that does not come apart, discard the entire syringe with the medication and start the process over again.				
12. ✦	When you are prepared to administer the injection, place a new alcohol sponge or cotton ball between two fingers of your nondominant hand so that you can easily grasp it when you are finished with the injection.				
13. ✳	Firmly grasp the syringe in your dominant hand, like a pencil is held.				
14. ✳	a. To administer a subcutaneous injection: With your nondominant hand, grasp the skin at the injection site and form a small mass of tissue. b. To administer an intramuscular injection: With your nondominant hand, stretch the skin tightly where you will insert the needle.				

Name: _____

Date: _____

POINT VALUE ✦ = 3–6 points ✶ = 7–9 points		PRACTICE TRIAL	GRADED TRIAL # 1	GRADED TRIAL # 2	NOTES
15. ✶	Grasp the syringe in a dart-like fashion and insert the entire needle quickly with one swift movement.				
16. ✶	a. For a subcutaneous injection: Insert into the subcutaneous tissue at a 45-degree angle b. For an intramuscular injection: Insert directly into the muscle at a 90-degree angle.				
17. ✶	Do not move the needle once you have inserted it. If the needle is pushed in farther, contaminants are carried into the skin from the exposed needle.				
18. ✶	Aspirate to determine if you have entered a blood vessel. To do this, pull back slightly on the plunger with the hand holding the syringe while holding the needle steady in the muscle. If blood appears in the hub area of the syringe, it means that you are in a blood vessel. You will then have to withdraw the needle using correct technique and discard the syringe containing the blood and medication. Begin the procedure again with step 1 and fresh supplies.				

POINT VALUE ✦ = 3–6 points ✴ = 7–9 points		PRACTICE TRIAL	GRADED TRIAL # 1	GRADED TRIAL # 2	NOTES
19. ✴	If you do not see a return of blood in the syringe when you aspirate, slowly inject the medication without moving the needle. Do not move the needle until you have completed injecting all of the medication. (See Figures B and C for illustrations of intramuscular injections.) *Note:* Insert and withdraw the needle quickly to minimize pain but administer the medication slowly.				
20. ✴	Taking the alcohol sponge (or cotton ball) from between the last two fingers of your nondominant hand, place it over the area containing the needle. Withdraw the needle at the same angle you used for insertion, using care not to stick yourself with the needle.				
21. ✴	With one hand, place the sponge firmly over the injection site. With the other hand, discard the needle in a biohazard sharps container.				
22. ✴	***You may gently massage the injection site to assist absorption and ease the patient's pain.***				
23. ✴	***Make sure the patient is safe before leaving him or her unattended. Observe the patient for any adverse effect of the medication for at least 15 minutes.***				
24. ✦	Correctly dispose of all materials.				

Name: _____

Date: _____

POINT VALUE ✦ = 3–6 points ✱ = 7–9 points	PRACTICE TRIAL	GRADED TRIAL # 1	GRADED TRIAL # 2	NOTES
25. ✦ Remove gloves and discard them into a biohazard waste bag. Perform hand hygiene.				
26. ✱ Chart the medication administration on the patient's record, noting the time, medication name, dosage, injection site, route, lot number on the immunizations, and your name.				

Document: Enter the appropriate information in the chart below.

Grading

Points Earned	_____		
Points Possible	_____	204	204
Percent Grade (Points Earned/Points Possible)	_____		
PASS:	_____	❏ YES ❏ NO ❏ N/A	❏ YES ❏ NO ❏ N/A

Instructor Sign-Off

Instructor: _____   **Date:** _____

Procedure 55-8:

Administering an Intradermal Injection

Objective: Administer an intradermal injection.

Equipment and Supplies: Disposable gloves; hazardous waste container; alcohol sponges; sterile needle; sterile syringe; vial of medication; medication order signed by physician; pen

Affective Behaviors: Affective behaviors provide a professional approach to a skill that enhances the patient encounter. These behaviors may also display sensitivity to a patient's rights and enhance communication. Pay close attention to these skills, which will be in **bold, *italicized*** font.

Notes to the Student

_____

_____

_____

_____

_____

_____

Skills Assessment Requirements

Read and familiarize yourself with the procedure; complete the minimum practice requirements (MPRs). Document each MPR using proper charting technique. Complete each procedure within a reasonable amount of time, with a minimum of 85% accuracy.

Name: _____

Date: _____

POINT VALUE ✦ = 3–6 points ✳ = 7–9 points		PRACTICE TRIAL	GRADED TRIAL # 1	GRADED TRIAL # 2	NOTES
	I. Preparation				
1. ✦	Perform hand hygiene.				
2. ✦	Apply gloves, and follow standard blood and body fluid precautions.				
3. ✳	Select the correct medication using the "three befores." Always double-check the label to make sure the strength is correct, because medications are manufactured with different strengths (e.g., 1:10, 1:100, or 1:1,000 dilutions).				
4. ✦	Gently roll the medication between your hands to mix any medication that may have settled. Refrigerated medication can be rolled between your hands to warm it slightly.				
5. ✳	Prepare the syringe using the correct technique. Carefully carry the covered needle and syringe to the patient.				
6. ✳	***Warmly greet and identify the patient both by stating his or her name and by examining any printed identification, such as a wrist name band or medical record. Introduce yourself to the patient and ask the patient if he or she has any allergies.***				

POINT VALUE ✦ = 3–6 points ✶ = 7–9 points		PRACTICE TRIAL	GRADED TRIAL # 1	GRADED TRIAL # 2	NOTES
7. ✦	***Tell the patient the name of the medication and dosage ordered by the physician. Explain the process of the PPD skin test. Ask the patient if he or she has any questions prior to receiving the medication.***				
8. ✶	Select the proper site (center of forearm, upper chest, or upper back) for an intradermal skin injection.				
9. ✶	Using a circular motion, clean the patient's skin with an alcohol sponge. Wipe the skin with a sweeping motion from the center of the area outward. This prevents recontamination of the injection site by the alcohol sponge.				
10. ✦	Allow time for the antiseptic on the sponge to dry to reduce the possibility of it reacting with the medication.				
11. ✶	Check the medication Dosage against the patient's order to determine if this is the correct time to administer the dose (one of the "ten rights").				
12. ✦	Remove the protective covering from the needle, using care not to touch the needle.				
II. Injection					
13. ✶	Hold the syringe between the first two fingers and thumb of your dominant hand with the palm down and the bevel of the needle up.				

Name: _____

Date: _____

POINT VALUE ◆ = 3–6 points ✳ = 7–9 points		PRACTICE TRIAL	GRADED TRIAL # 1	GRADED TRIAL # 2	NOTES
14. ✳	Hold the skin taut with the fingers of your nondominant hand. If you are using the center of the forearm, place the nondominant hand under the patient's arm and pull the skin taut. This will allow the needle to slip into the skin more easily.				
15. ✳	Using a 15-degree angle, insert the needle through the skin to about one-eighth of an inch. The bevel of the needle will be facing upward and covered with skin. The needle will still show through the skin. Do not aspirate.				
16. ✳	Slowly inject the medication beneath the surface of the skin. A small elevation of skin, or wheal, will occur where you have injected the medication.				
17. ✳	Quickly withdraw the needle. With the other hand, discard the needle into the biohazard sharps container.				
	III. Patient Follow-Up				
18. ✳	Do not massage the area or place a bandage or tape on it, because this may irritate the site and lead to a false reading.				

POINT VALUE ✦ = 3–6 points ✶ = 7–9 points		PRACTICE TRIAL	GRADED TRIAL # 1	GRADED TRIAL # 2	NOTES
19. ✶	Make sure the patient is safe before leaving him or her unattended. Observe the patient for any untoward effect, such as an allergic reaction to the medication, for at least 20 to 30 minutes. Tell the patient not to rub the area. Instruct the patient to return to the office within 48 to 72 hours for the reading of the skin test. Make certain that the patient understands the directions and does not have any questions.				
20. ✦	Correctly dispose of all materials.				
21. ✦	Remove and discard gloves, and perform hand hygiene.				
22. ✶	Chart the medication administration on the patient's record, noting the time, medication name, dosage, injection site, route, appearance of the intradermal site after injection, and your name.				

Name: _____

Date: _____

Document: Enter the appropriate information in the chart below.

Grading

Points Earned	_____		
Points Possible	_____	174	174
Percent Grade (Points Earned/Points Possible)	_____		
PASS:	_____	❑ YES ❑ NO ❑ N/A	❑ YES ❑ NO ❑ N/A

Instructor Sign-Off

Instructor:_____ **Date:** _____

Procedure 55-9:

Preparing an Intravenous Tray

Objective: Prepare an intravenous (IV) tray.

Equipment and Supplies: Absorbent disposable sheet; alcohol prep pads; Betadine swabs; disposable tourniquet; IV setup: IV tubing with attached filter; IV catheter; bag of IV fluid labeled with type and patient's name, date, time; paper tape; syringe; port cap; disposable gloves; gauze (2 × 2 or 4 × 4); IV setup tray; IV pole with pump

Affective Behaviors: Affective behaviors provide a professional approach to a skill that enhances the patient encounter. These behaviors may also display sensitivity to a patient's rights and enhance communication. Pay close attention to these skills, which will be in **_bold, italicized_** font.

Notes to the Student

_____

_____

_____

_____

_____

_____

Skills Assessment Requirements

Read and familiarize yourself with the procedure; complete the minimum practice requirements (MPRs). Document each MPR using proper charting technique. Complete each procedure within a reasonable amount of time, with a minimum of 85% accuracy.

POINT VALUE ✦ = 3–6 points ✳ = 7–9 points		PRACTICE TRIAL	GRADED TRIAL # 1	GRADED TRIAL # 2	NOTES
1. ✦	Perform hand hygiene.				
2. ✦	Apply gloves.				
3. ✳	Prepare IV fluid administration set: a. Inspect the fluid bag to make sure it contains desired fluid, that the fluid is clear, and that the bag is free from any leaks and has not expired. b. Select the correct administration set (either mini or macro drip) and uncoil the tubing, being careful that the ends of the tubing do not become contaminated. c. Close the flow regulator to the fluid bag. d. Remove the protective covering from the port of the fluid bag and the protective covering from the spike of the administration set. e. Insert the spike of the administration set into the port of the fluid bag with a quick twisting motion, being careful not to puncture yourself. f. While holding the fluid bag higher than the drip chamber of the administration set, squeeze the drip chamber once or twice to start the flow of the fluid. Fill the chamber to the marker line. If the chamber is overfilled, quickly lower the bag below the level of the drip chamber and squeeze some of the fluid back into the fluid bag.				

POINT VALUE ✦ = 3–6 points ✳ = 7–9 points		PRACTICE TRIAL	GRADED TRIAL # 1	GRADED TRIAL # 2	NOTES
	g. Open the flow regulator and allow the fluid to flush all the air from the tubing. A trash can or the wrapper the fluid came in can be used for the overflow of fluid. h. Turn off the flow and place the sterile cap back on the end of the administration set (if you had to remove it). Then place this end nearby so it can be easily reached by the person ready to connect it to the IV catheter in the patient's arm.				
4. ✦	Place an absorbent disposable sheet on the tray.				
5. ✦	Assemble equipment and supplies on the tray in order of use.				
6. ✳	If using an IV pole or pump, hang the IV solution (bag) on the pole; do not set it up or calculate drops in the pump; this will be done by the person starting the IV.				
7. ✦	Notify the appropriate personnel (RN, LVN, physician) that the IV tray setup is ready for administration.				
8. ✦	Remove and dispose of gloves. Perform hand hygiene.				
9. ✳	Document the procedure.				
10. ✦	Clean the work area and equipment according to OSHA guidelines.				

Document: Enter the appropriate information in the chart below.

Grading

Points Earned	_____		
Points Possible	_____	69	69
Percent Grade (Points Earned/Points Possible)	_____		
PASS:	_____	❏ YES ❏ NO ❏ N/A	❏ YES ❏ NO ❏ N/A

Instructor Sign-Off

Instructor: _____   **Date:** _____

Name: _____

Date: _____

Procedure 55-10:

Reconstituting a Powdered Medication for Administration

Objective: Reconstitute a powdered medication.

Equipment and Supplies: Alcohol swab; disposable gloves; medication label; medication order signed by physician; pen; sterile needle; biohazard sharps container; vial of medication

Affective Behaviors: Affective behaviors provide a professional approach to a skill that enhances the patient encounter. These behaviors may also display sensitivity to a patient's rights and enhance communication. Pay close attention to these skills, which will be in ***bold, italicized*** font.

Notes to the Student

_____

_____

_____

_____

_____

_____

Skills Assessment Requirements

Read and familiarize yourself with the procedure; complete the minimum practice requirements (MPRs). Document each MPR using proper charting technique. Complete each procedure within a reasonable amount of time, with a minimum of 85% accuracy.

Name: _____

Date: _____

POINT VALUE ✦ = 3–6 points ✳ = 7–9 points		PRACTICE TRIAL	GRADED TRIAL # 1	GRADED TRIAL # 2	NOTES
1. ✦	Gather supplies, perform hand hygiene, and apply gloves.				
2. ✳	Select the correct medication and diluent, perform the "three befores" technique, verify the dosage against the physician's order, and calculate dosage (if necessary).				
3. ✦	Remove the top from the powder medication and the top from the diluent, and then wipe the tops of both vials with separate alcohol swabs.				
4. ✳	Insert a sterile needle through the rubber stopper on the vial of diluent.				
5. ✳	Withdraw the appropriate amount of diluent and add it to the powder medication.				
6. ✦	Remove the needle from the medication vial and discard it in the sharps container.				
7. ✳	To ensure that the medication is mixed well, roll the vial between the palms of your hands.				
8. ✳	Label the mixed vial with the strength of the prepared medication, time, date, your initials, and the expiration date.				

Document: Enter the appropriate information in the chart below. _____

Grading

Points Earned	_____		
Points Possible	_____	63	63
Percent Grade (Points Earned/Points Possible)	_____		
PASS:	_____	❏ YES ❏ NO ❏ N/A	❏ YES ❏ NO ❏ N/A

Instructor Sign-Off

Instructor: _____   **Date:** _____

Procedure 56-1:

Creating a Community Resource Brochure

Objective: Create a brochure that educates patients about available community resources.

Equipment and Supplies: Computer; computer software program that allows the creation of a brochure; printer; pen; phone book; Internet access; newspaper

Affective Behaviors: Affective behaviors provide a professional approach to a skill that enhances the patient encounter. These behaviors may also display sensitivity to a patient's rights and enhance communication. Pay close attention to these skills, which will be in **_bold, italicized_** font.

Notes to the Student

_____

_____

_____

_____

_____

_____

Skills Assessment Requirements

Read and familiarize yourself with the procedure; complete the minimum practice requirements (MPRs). Document each MPR using proper charting technique. Complete each procedure within a reasonable amount of time, with a minimum of 85% accuracy.

Name: _____

Date: _____

POINT VALUE ✦ = 3–6 points ✱ = 7–9 points		PRACTICE TRIAL	GRADED TRIAL # 1	GRADED TRIAL # 2	NOTES
1. ✦	Choose a specific topic for which you will create a community resource brochure. Your topic might focus on disease prevention or health promotion, such as smoking cessation or weight loss.				
2. ✦	Using the Internet, local telephone books, and even the local newspaper, identify community resources that are available to help patients regarding your topic.				
3. ✱	Create an attractive brochure for distribution to patients that includes the name, location, phone number, and services offered by the selected resources.				
4. ✦	Check your brochure for spelling and grammar errors before printing.				
5. ✦	Print one copy and do another spelling and grammar check on the printed document.				
6.	After the brochure has been edited for errors and is polished, obtain approval from the physician to print and then distribute the brochures to patients as necessary or to display them in the office reception area.				
7.	Turn your brochure in to your instructor.				

Document: Enter the appropriate information in the chart below.

Grading

Points Earned	_____		
Points Possible	_____	45	45
Percent Grade (Points Earned/Points Possible)	_____		
PASS:	_____	❏ YES ❏ NO ❏ N/A	❏ YES ❏ NO ❏ N/A

Instructor Sign-Off

Instructor: _____   **Date:** _____

Procedure 56-2:

Creating a Public Relations Brochure

Objective: Promote the office by creating a brochure for distribution to current and potential patients.

Equipment and Supplies: Computer; printer; office information; pen

Affective Behaviors: Affective behaviors provide a professional approach to a skill that enhances the patient encounter. These behaviors may also display sensitivity to a patient's rights and enhance communication. Pay close attention to these skills, which will be in *bold, italicized* font.

Notes to the Student

_____

_____

_____

_____

_____

_____

_____

Skills Assessment Requirements

Read and familiarize yourself with the procedure; complete the minimum practice requirements (MPRs). Document each MPR using proper charting technique. Complete each procedure within a reasonable amount of time, with a minimum of 85% accuracy.

Name: _____

Date: _____

POINT VALUE ✦ = 3–6 points ✳ = 7–9 points		PRACTICE TRIAL	GRADED TRIAL # 1	GRADED TRIAL # 2	NOTES
1. ✳	Gather the necessary data and create a brochure to advertise your office. Be sure to include the following: • Office name (e.g., Pearson Physicians Group) • Type of practice (e.g., family medicine) • Office hours • Office address • Names and information about physicians • Insurance plans accepted • Payment expectations (e.g., copayments are expected before visit begins; all methods of payment are acceptable except cash) • Emergency management procedures (after hours, contact the answering service at xxx-xxx-xxxx) • Prescription refill procedures (allow 24 hours for a prescription to be refilled, some medications will not be refilled and require an office appointment, etc.) • Local hospital affiliations and privileges				
2. ✦	Check your brochure for spelling and grammatical errors before printing.				
3. ✦	Print one copy, and perform another spelling and grammar check on the printed document.				
4. ✦	After the brochure has been polished, obtain approval from the office manager or physician to print and then distribute the brochures to patients.				

Document: Enter the appropriate information in the chart below.

Grading

Points Earned	_____		
Points Possible	_____	27	27
Percent Grade (Points Earned/Points Possible)	_____		
PASS:	_____	❏ YES ❏ NO ❏ N/A	❏ YES ❏ NO ❏ N/A

Instructor Sign-Off

Instructor: _____ **Date:** _____

Procedure 56-3:

Instructing Patients According to Their Needs for Health Maintenance and Promotion

Objective: Instruct a hearing-impaired individual to prepare for outpatient surgery by creating a packet of information for postoperative care.

Equipment and Supplies: Computer; printer; pen; stapler

Affective Behaviors: Affective behaviors provide a professional approach to a skill that enhances the patient encounter. These behaviors may also display sensitivity to a patient's rights and enhance communication. Pay close attention to these skills, which will be in **bold, *italicized*** font.

Notes to the Student

_____

_____

_____

_____

_____

_____

Skills Assessment Requirements

Read and familiarize yourself with the procedure; complete the minimum practice requirements (MPRs). Document each MPR using proper charting technique. Complete each procedure within a reasonable amount of time, with a minimum of 85% accuracy.

POINT VALUE ✦ = 3–6 points ✱ = 7–9 points		PRACTICE TRIAL	GRADED TRIAL #1	GRADED TRIAL #2	NOTES
1. ✦	Using a computer with word processing software, create a postoperative instruction packet for a hearing-impaired patient, include the following information: • When to resume activities such as walking, driving, or exercising • Incision wound care and dressing changes • Postoperative diet • Medications • Follow-up care				
2. ✱	Double-check the information for accuracy, spelling, and grammatical errors.				
3. ✦	Print a copy for the patient and save one copy in the patient's health record. Save a digital file for electronic health records or place a printed copy in a paper health record. a. Have the physician review and approve the packet before giving it to the patient.				
4. ✱	*Face the patient so your lips can be read easily.*				
5. ✱	*Greet and identify the patient. Introduce yourself if you haven't worked with the patient yet.*				
6. ✱	*Discuss the contents of the postoperative instructions with the patient.* a. During discussion, always face the patient. b. Do not read the information from the packet in a hurried manner; take frequent breaks, and make eye contact with the patient to ensure understanding.				

POINT VALUE ✦ = 3–6 points ✳ = 7–9 points		PRACTICE TRIAL	GRADED TRIAL #1	GRADED TRIAL #2	NOTES
7. ✳	**_Obtain feedback from the patient to show understanding._** Have a notepad and pen available so that the patient can write down questions and answers.				
8. ✦	Give a copy of the information to the patient.				
9. ✳	If paper health records are used by the facility, have the patient sign one copy of the packet and file it in the health record. If electronic health records are used, scan a copy of the signed brochure into the health record and save it to the appropriate location within the record.				
10. ✦	Document that patient education was completed and that the patient received and demonstrated understanding of the information.				

Name: _____

Date: _____

Document: Enter the appropriate information in the chart below. _____

Grading

Points Earned	_____		
Points Possible	_____	78	78
Percent Grade (Points Earned/Points Possible)	_____		
PASS:	_____	❏ YES ❏ NO ❏ N/A	❏ YES ❏ NO ❏ N/A

Instructor Sign-Off

Instructor: _____ Date: _____

Procedure 57-1:

Calculating Adult Body Mass Index

Objective: Accurately calculate adult body mass following the steps in the procedure.

Equipment and Supplies: Patient's record; paper and pen; scale or height and weight; BMI formula or nomogram or chart for BMI

Affective Behaviors: Affective behaviors provide a professional approach to a skill that enhances the patient encounter. These behaviors may also display sensitivity to a patient's rights and enhance communication. Pay close attention to these skills, which will be in **bold, *italicized*** font.

Notes to the Student

_____

_____

_____

_____

_____

_____

Skills Assessment Requirements

Read and familiarize yourself with the procedure; complete the minimum practice requirements (MPRs). Document each MPR using proper charting technique. Complete each procedure within a reasonable amount of time, with a minimum of 85% accuracy.

Name: _____

Date: _____

POINT VALUE ✦ = 3–6 points ✶ = 7–9 points		PRACTICE TRIAL	GRADED TRIAL #1	GRADED TRIAL #2	NOTES
1. ✦	Perform hand hygiene.				
2. ✦	*Greet and identify the patient; introduce yourself if you have not already done so.*				
3. ✦	If the recent height and weight measurements are not available, obtain the patient's height and weight.				
4. ✶	Insert the patient's height and weight into the formula, using pounds and inches or kilograms and meters according to facility policy.				
5. ✦	Record results in the patient's record.				
6. ✦	Submit record to your instructor.				

Name: _____

Date: _____

Document: Enter the appropriate information in the chart below.

Grading

Points Earned	_____		
Points Possible	_____	39	39
Percent Grade (Points Earned/Points Possible)	_____		
PASS:	_____	❑ YES ❑ NO ❑ N/A	❑ YES ❑ NO ❑ N/A

Instructor Sign-Off

Instructor: _____ **Date:** _____

Procedure 57-2:

Instruct a Patient According to Dietary Needs

Objective: Provide patient instruction regarding a BRAT diet to treat diarrhea.

Equipment and Supplies: Patient's health record; printed handout of BRAT diet; pen

Affective Behaviors: Affective behaviors provide a professional approach to a skill that enhances the patient encounter. These behaviors may also display sensitivity to a patient's rights and enhance communication. Pay close attention to these skills, which will be in **bold, italicized** font.

Notes to the Student

_____

_____

_____

_____

_____

_____

Skills Assessment Requirements

Read and familiarize yourself with the procedure; complete the minimum practice requirements (MPRs). Document each MPR using proper charting technique. Complete each procedure within a reasonable amount of time, with a minimum of 85% accuracy.

POINT VALUE ✦ = 3–6 points ✱ = 7–9 points		PRACTICE TRIAL	GRADED TRIAL # 1	GRADED TRIAL # 2	NOTES
1. ✦	**Warmly greet and identify the patient. Introduce yourself if you have not already done so.** a. If the patient is a child, direct the education toward the caregiver but do not exclude the patient during instruction.				
2. ✦	**Confirm that the patient is experiencing gastrointestinal (GI) upset, such as diarrhea or vomiting.**				
3. ✱	**Explain that the physician has recommended that the patient follow a BRAT diet.** During the explanation, review that the foods in this diet include bananas, rice, applesauce, and toast. Explain that the toast should be eaten plain or with a very small amount of butter or margarine. Jellies, honey, jam, and peanut butter are not allowed on the BRAT diet.				
4. ✱	Review the allowed beverages with the patient. The physician may likely encourage the patient to increase fluid consumption to prevent dehydration.				
5. ✦	Provide the patient or caregiver with a printed handout that includes information about the BRAT diet and allowed beverages.				

POINT VALUE ✦ = 3–6 points ✳ = 7–9 points		PRACTICE TRIAL	GRADED TRIAL # 1	GRADED TRIAL # 2	NOTES
6. ✦	**Inform the patient or caregiver to contact the office if the patient does not show signs of improvement within 48–72 hours.** Always ask the physician to clarify if you are not sure.				
7. ✦	**Ask the patient/caregiver if he or she has any questions and, if so, answer them to the best of your ability.**				
8. ✦	Have the patient/caregiver sign the handout indicating receipt of a copy.				
9. ✦	Place a copy of the signed handout in the patient's health record, or if electronic health records (EHRs) are used, scan the document into the patient's EHR.				
10. ✦	Perform hand hygiene.				
11. ✳	Document the teaching in the patient's health record.				
12. ✦	Turn your completed work in to your instructor.				

Name: _____

Date: _____

Document: Enter the appropriate information in the chart below.

Grading

Points Earned	_____		
Points Possible	_____	120	120
Percent Grade (Points Earned/Points Possible)	_____		
PASS:	_____	❏ YES ❏ NO ❏ N/A	❏ YES ❏ NO ❏ N/A

Instructor Sign-Off

Instructor: _____   Date: _____

Procedure 58-1:

Role-Playing a Situation in Which a Patient Is from Another Culture

Objective: Learn how to communicate with patients from another culture.

Equipment and Supplies: Pen or pencil; paper

Affective Behaviors: Affective behaviors provide a professional approach to a skill that enhances the patient encounter. These behaviors may also display sensitivity to a patient's rights and enhance communication. Pay close attention to these skills, which will be in **bold, *italicized*** font.

Notes to the Student

_____

_____

_____

_____

_____

_____

Skills Assessment Requirements

Read and familiarize yourself with the procedure; complete the minimum practice requirements (MPRs). Document each MPR using proper charting technique. Complete each procedure within a reasonable amount of time, with a minimum of 85% accuracy.

Name: _____

Date: _____

POINT VALUE ✦ = 3–6 points ✶ = 7–9 points		PRACTICE TRIAL	GRADED TRIAL # 1	GRADED TRIAL # 2	NOTES
1. ✦	Choose a classmate.				
2. ✦	Select a quiet part of the classroom to conduct the procedure.				
3. ✦	Determine who will be the medical assistant and who will be the patient.				
4. ✦	Have the "patient" act as if he or she speaks very little English.				
5. ✦	*Be calm, respectful, and considerate.*				
6. ✶	*Use simple and common words.*				
7. ✶	*Avoid using medical terms.*				
8. ✶	*Never use slang.*				
9. ✶	*Be attentive to eye contact, facial expressions, and use of hand gestures.*				
10. ✦	*Make the patient as comfortable as possible.*				
11. ✦	Document the interaction in the patient's chart.				

Name: _____

Date: _____

Document: Enter the appropriate information in the chart below.

Grading

Points Earned	_____		
Points Possible	_____	72	72
Percent Grade (Points Earned/Points Possible)	_____		
PASS:	_____	❑ YES ❑ NO ❑ N/A	❑ YES ❑ NO ❑ N/A

Instructor Sign-Off

Instructor: _____   **Date:** _____

Procedure 58-2:

Role-Playing a Situation in Which a Patient Is Frightened, Angry, or Anxious

Objective: Learn how to deal with a patient who is frightened, angry, or depressed.

Equipment and Supplies: Pen; medical record

Affective Behaviors: Affective behaviors provide a professional approach to a skill that enhances the patient encounter. These behaviors may also display sensitivity to a patient's rights and enhance communication. Pay close attention to these skills, which will be in **bold, *italicized*** font.

Notes to the Student

_____

_____

_____

_____

_____

_____

Skills Assessment Requirements

Read and familiarize yourself with the procedure; complete the minimum practice requirements (MPRs). Document each MPR using proper charting technique. Complete each procedure within a reasonable amount of time, with a minimum of 85% accuracy.

Name: _____

Date: _____

POINT VALUE ✦ = 3–6 points ✲ = 7–9 points		PRACTICE TRIAL	GRADED TRIAL #1	GRADED TRIAL #2	NOTES
1. ✦	Choose a classmate.				
2. ✦	Select a quiet part of the classroom to conduct the procedure.				
3. ✦	Determine who will be the medical assistant and who will be the patient.				
4. ✦	Have the student who is pretending to be the patient express the emotion of fear, anger, or depression.				
5. ✦	*Once you recognize one of these emotions, remain calm.*				
6. ✲	*If the patient is not displaying destructive behavior, continue to allow the patient to express his or her feelings without being interrupted.*				
7. ✦	*Let the patient know that you understand.*				
8. ✲	*Inquire about the issue so that you can attempt to resolve the issue.*				
9. ✦	During the conversation, *express empathy; let the patient see that you are concerned about his or her issue.*				
10. ✦	Notify the physician of the conversation.				
11. ✲	Document the conversation in the patient's record.				

Name: _____

Date: _____

Document: Enter the appropriate information in the chart below.

Grading

Points Earned	_____		
Points Possible	_____	75	75
Percent Grade (Points Earned/Points Possible)	_____		
PASS:	_____	❏ YES ❏ NO ❏ N/A	❏ YES ❏ NO ❏ N/A

Instructor Sign-Off

Instructor: _____   Date: _____

Procedure 58-3:

Develop a Patient Teaching Handout About Stress

Objective: Develop an appropriate teaching tool about stress.

Equipment and Supplies: Computer; word processor; printer; pen; paper

Affective Behaviors: Affective behaviors provide a professional approach to a skill that enhances the patient encounter. These behaviors may also display sensitivity to a patient's rights and enhance communication. Pay close attention to these skills, which will be in **bold, *italicized*** font.

Notes to the Student

_____

_____

_____

_____

_____

_____

_____

Skills Assessment Requirements

Read and familiarize yourself with the procedure; complete the minimum practice requirements (MPRs). Document each MPR using proper charting technique. Complete each procedure within a reasonable amount of time, with a minimum of 85% accuracy.

Name: _____

Date: _____

POINT VALUE ✦ = 3–6 points ✱ = 7–9 points		PRACTICE TRIAL	GRADED TRIAL # 1	GRADED TRIAL # 2	NOTES
1. ✱	Decide what information should be included on the patient teaching handout.				
2. ✦	Develop an outline of the information you plan to include on the patient teaching handout.				
3. ✦	Using a word processing program to develop a patient teaching handout.				
4. ✱	Make sure your patient teaching includes at a minimum the definition of stress, causes of stress, and ways to cope with stress.				
5. ✱	Proofread the patient teaching handout on the computer screen.				
6. ✦	Make any necessary corrections to the patient teaching handout.				
7. ✦	Print your patient teaching handout.				
8. ✱	Proofread the hard copy of your patient teaching handout.				
9. ✦	Make any necessary corrections to the patient teaching handout.				
10. ✦	Turn in the patient teaching handout to your instructor.				

Name: _____

Date: _____

Document: Enter the appropriate information in the chart below.

Grading

Points Earned	_____		
Points Possible	_____	69	69
Percent Grade (Points Earned/Points Possible)	_____		
PASS:	_____	❏ YES ❏ NO ❏ N/A	❏ YES ❏ NO ❏ N/A

Instructor Sign-Off

Instructor: _____   **Date:** _____

Procedure 60-1:

Conducting a Job Search

Objective: Conduct a job search.

Equipment and Supplies: Computer; Internet access; newspaper; medical assisting publication; printer; pen; paper; dictionary; thesaurus; telephone book; job search organizer or folder; calendar; contact log

Affective Behaviors: Affective behaviors provide a professional approach to a skill that enhances the patient encounter. These behaviors may also display sensitivity to a patient's rights and enhance communication. Pay close attention to these skills, which will be in **bold, italicized** font.

Notes to the Student

In your journal, document how you felt about the job search.

_____

_____

_____

_____

_____

_____

Skills Assessment Requirements

Read and familiarize yourself with the procedure; complete the minimum practice requirements (MPRs). Document each MPR using proper charting technique. Complete each procedure within a reasonable amount of time, with a minimum of 85% accuracy.

Name: _____

Date: _____

POINT VALUE ✦ = 3–6 points ✳ = 7–9 points		PRACTICE TRIAL	GRADED TRIAL # 1	GRADED TRIAL # 2	NOTES
1. ✦	Determine two sources you will use to conduct a job search.				
2. ✳	Determine a plan for your job search.				
3. ✳	Prepare a list of information sources for identifying job opportunities.				
4. ✳	Update your résumé.				
5. ✳	Rehearse interviewing with a close family member or friend.				
6. ✳	Plan your professional attire for the interview process.				
7. ✦	Perform a self-assessment.				
8. ✦	Develop a job search organizer or folder.				
9. ✦	Develop a contact log.				
10. ✦	Use a calendar to determine what times are available for job searching and interviewing.				
11. ✦	Select two sources you will use to conduct your job searches.				
12. ✦	Conduct your job searches.				

Name: _____

Date: _____

Document: Enter the appropriate information in the chart below.

Grading

Points Earned	_____		
Points Possible	_____	87	87
Percent Grade (Points Earned/Points Possible)	_____		
PASS:	_____	❏ YES ❏ NO ❏ N/A	❏ YES ❏ NO ❏ N/A

Instructor Sign-Off

Instructor: _____   **Date:** _____

Procedure 60-2:

Preparing Your Résumé and References

Objective: Prepare a résumé and references.

Equipment and Supplies: Computer; printer; pen; paper; dictionary; thesaurus; telephone book; current and past employment information; current and past educational information

Affective Behaviors: Affective behaviors provide a professional approach to a skill that enhances the patient encounter. These behaviors may also display sensitivity to a patient's rights and enhance communication. Pay close attention to these skills, which will be in **_bold, italicized_** font.

Notes to the Student

_____

_____

_____

_____

_____

_____

Skills Assessment Requirements

Read and familiarize yourself with the procedure; complete the minimum practice requirements (MPRs). Document each MPR using proper charting technique. Complete each procedure within a reasonable amount of time, with a minimum of 85% accuracy.

Name: _____

Date: _____

POINT VALUE ✦ = 3–6 points ✳ = 7–9 points	PRACTICE TRIAL	GRADED TRIAL # 1	GRADED TRIAL # 2	NOTES
1. ✦ Gather equipment and supplies.				
2. ✦ Prepare your résumé.				
3. ✦ Using a word processing program, complete the standard parts of a résumé: heading; objective; education; employment; professional organizations and memberships; credentials; and references.				
4. ✦ Proofread your résumé.				
5. ✦ Have a close family member or friend proofread your résumé.				
6. ✦ Make any corrections to errors found on the résumé.				
7. ✦ Using good-quality white or off-white 8½ × 11 paper, print your résumé.				
8. ✦ On a separate piece of paper, list at least three references with their titles, addresses, and phone numbers.				
9. ✳ Proofread your references.				
10. ✦ Have a close family member or friend proofread your references.				
11. ✦ Make any corrections to errors found on your references.				
12. ✦ Using good-quality white or off-white 8½ × 11 paper, print your references.				
13. ✦ Save your résumé and list of references on a disk, USB drive, computer hard drive, or other storage device.				

POINT VALUE ✦ = 3–6 points ✶ = 7–9 points		PRACTICE TRIAL	GRADED TRIAL # 1	GRADED TRIAL # 2	NOTES
14. ✦	Update your résumé whenever changes occur.				
15. ✦	Turn in your résumé and references to your instructor.				

Document: Enter the appropriate information in the chart below.

Grading

Points Earned	_____		
Points Possible	_____	93	93
Percent Grade (Points Earned/Points Possible)	_____		
PASS:	_____	❑ YES ❑ NO ❑ N/A	❑ YES ❑ NO ❑ N/A

Instructor Sign-Off

Instructor: _____   **Date:** _____

Procedure 60-3:

Preparing a Cover Letter

Objective: Prepare a cover letter.

Equipment and Supplies: Computer; printer; pen; paper; dictionary; thesaurus; telephone book

Affective Behaviors: Affective behaviors provide a professional approach to a skill that enhances the patient encounter. These behaviors may also display sensitivity to a patient's rights and enhance communication. Pay close attention to these skills, which will be in *bold, italicized* font.

Notes to the Student

_____

_____

_____

_____

_____

_____

Skills Assessment Requirements

Read and familiarize yourself with the procedure; complete the minimum practice requirements (MPRs). Document each MPR using proper charting technique. Complete each procedure within a reasonable amount of time, with a minimum of 85% accuracy.

Name: _____

Date: _____

POINT VALUE ✦ = 3–6 points ✷ = 7–9 points		PRACTICE TRIAL	GRADED TRIAL # 1	GRADED TRIAL # 2	NOTES
1. ✦	Gather equipment and supplies.				
2. ✦	Prepare a cover letter using a word processing program.				
3. ✷	Proofread your cover letter.				
4. ✷	Have a close family member or friend proofread your cover letter.				
5. ✷	Make any corrections to errors found on the cover letter.				
6. ✦	Using good-quality white or off-white 8 ½ × 11 paper, print your cover letter.				
7. ✦	Turn your cover letter in to your instructor.				

Document: Enter the appropriate information in the chart below.

Grading

Points Earned	_____		
Points Possible	_____	54	54
Percent Grade (Points Earned/Points Possible)	_____		
PASS:	_____	❏ YES ❏ NO ❏ N/A	❏ YES ❏ NO ❏ N/A

Instructor Sign-Off

Instructor: _____ **Date:** _____

Procedure 60-4:

Role-Playing an Interview

Objective: Successfully role-play a job interview.

Equipment and Supplies: Pen and paper

Affective Behaviors: Affective behaviors provide a professional approach to a skill that enhances the patient encounter. These behaviors may also display sensitivity to a patient's rights and enhance communication. Pay close attention to these skills, which will be in **_bold, italicized_** font.

Notes to the Student

_____

_____

_____

_____

_____

_____

Skills Assessment Requirements

Read and familiarize yourself with the procedure; complete the minimum practice requirements (MPRs). Document each MPR using proper charting technique. Complete each procedure within a reasonable amount of time, with a minimum of 85% accuracy.

Name: _____

Date: _____

POINT VALUE ✦ = 3–6 points ✳ = 7–9 points		PRACTICE TRIAL	GRADED TRIAL #1	GRADED TRIAL #2	NOTES
1. ✦	Determine five questions that may be asked during a job interview.				
2. ✦	Choose a classmate.				
3. ✦	Select a quiet part of the classroom to conduct the interview.				
4. ✦	Determine who will be the interviewer and who will be the interviewee.				
5. ✦	The interviewer will begin the interview process by giving the interviewee a general idea about the medical office and the employees who work there.				
6. ✦	The interviewer will ask the interviewee the five questions he or she selected in step 1.				
7. ✦	The interviewer will gather information about the interviewee's past work experience.				
8. ✦	The interviewer will gather information about the interviewee's educational experience.				
9. ✦	The interviewee will answer the interviewer's questions.				
10. ✦	The interviewee will ask the interviewer questions about the medical office and the position.				
11. ✦	The interviewer will answer the interviewee's questions.				
12. ✦	Repeat the process, with students reversing roles. (Each student should play the part of the interviewer and the interviewee once.)				

POINT VALUE ✦ = 3–6 points ✳ = 7–9 points		PRACTICE TRIAL	GRADED TRIAL # 1	GRADED TRIAL # 2	NOTES
13. ✦	Now discuss the 10 most common mistakes made in an interview. Did either student make any of these mistakes?				
14. ✦	Each student will assess his or her own interviewing skills.				
15. ✦	Each student will discuss the appropriate attire to wear to a job interview.				
16. ✦	Each student will discuss the successful interviewing guidelines derived from the textbook.				

Document: Enter the appropriate information in the chart below.

Grading

Points Earned	———		
Points Possible	———	96	96
Percent Grade (Points Earned/Points Possible)	———		
PASS:	———	❏ YES ❏ NO ❏ N/A	❏ YES ❏ NO ❏ N/A

Instructor Sign-Off

Instructor: _____   Date: _____

Procedure 60-5:

Preparing a Follow-Up Thank-You Letter

Objective: Prepare an interview follow-up thank-you letter.

Equipment and Supplies: Computer; printer; pen; paper; dictionary; thesaurus; telephone book

Affective Behaviors: Affective behaviors provide a professional approach to a skill that enhances the patient encounter. These behaviors may also display sensitivity to a patient's rights and enhance communication. Pay close attention to these skills, which will be in **bold, *italicized*** font.

Notes to the Student

_____

_____

_____

_____

_____

_____

Skills Assessment Requirements

Read and familiarize yourself with the procedure; complete the minimum practice requirements (MPRs). Document each MPR using proper charting technique. Complete each procedure within a reasonable amount of time, with a minimum of 85% accuracy.

POINT VALUE ✦ = 3–6 points ✳ = 7–9 points		PRACTICE TRIAL	GRADED TRIAL # 1	GRADED TRIAL # 2	NOTES
1. ✦	Prepare a follow-up thank-you letter.				
2. ✦	Proofread your follow-up thank-you letter.				
3. ✦	Have a close family member or friend proofread your follow-up thank-you letter.				
4. ✦	Make any corrections to errors found on the follow-up thank-you letter.				
5. ✦	Using good-quality white or off-white 8½ × 11 paper, print your follow-up thank-you letter.				
6. ✦	Turn in your follow-up thank-you letter to your instructor.				

Name: _____

Date: _____

Document: Enter the appropriate information in the chart below.

Grading

Points Earned	————		
Points Possible	————	36	36
Percent Grade (Points Earned/Points Possible)	————		
PASS:	————	❏ YES ❏ NO ❏ N/A	❏ YES ❏ NO ❏ N/A

Instructor Sign-Off

Instructor: _____ Date: _____